IARC MONOGRAPHS
ON THE
EVALUATION OF THE
CARCINOGENIC RISK
OF CHEMICALS TO HUMANS

Some Halogenated Hydrocarbons

VOLUME 20

This publication represents the views and expert opinions
of an IARC Working Group on the
Evaluation of the Carcinogenic Risk of Chemicals to Humans
which met in Lyon,
6-13 June 1978

October 1979

INTERNATIONAL AGENCY FOR RESEARCH ON CANCER

IARC MONOGRAPHS

In 1971, the International Agency for Research on
Cancer (IARC) initiated a programme on the evaluation
of the carcinogenic risk of chemicals to humans involving
the production of critically evaluated monographs on
individual chemicals.

The objective of the programme is to elaborate and
publish in the form of monographs critical reviews of
data on carcinogenicity for groups of chemicals to which
humans are known to be exposed, to evaluate these data
in terms of human risk with the help of international
working groups of experts in chemical carcinogenesis and
related fields, and to indicate where additional research
efforts are needed.

International Agency for Research on Cancer 1979

ISBN 92 832 1220 7

PRINTED IN SWITZERLAND

CONTENTS

IARC WORKING GROUP ON THE EVALUATION OF THE CARCINOGENIC

RISK OF CHEMICALS TO HUMANS:

SOME HALOGENATED HYDROCARBONS

Lyon, 6-13 June 1978

Members

O. Axelson, Department of Occupational Medicine, University Hospital, S-581 85 Linköping, Sweden

J.R.P. Cabral[1], MRC Toxicology Unit, Medical Research Council Laboratories, Woodmansterne Road, Carshalton, Surrey SM5 4EF, UK

I. Chernozemsky, Chief, Laboratory of Carcinogenesis, Institute of Oncology, Medical Academy, Sofia 1156, Bulgaria

C. Cueto, Jr, Chief, Toxicology Branch, Carcinogenesis Testing Program, Division of Cancer Cause and Prevention, National Cancer Institute, Bethesda, Maryland 20014, USA

S.S. Epstein, Professor of Occupational and Environmental Medicine, School of Public Health, University of Illinois at the Medical Center, PO Box 6998, Chicago, Illinois 60680, USA

R. Gingell, Assistant Professor, The Eppley Institute for Research in Cancer, University of Nebraska Medical Center, 42nd and Dewey Avenue, Omaha, Nebraska 68105, USA

K.S. Larsson, Laboratory of Teratology, Karolinska Institute, S-104 01 Stockholm, Sweden

J.A. Moore, Associate Director, Research Resources Program, National Institute of Environmental Health Sciences, PO Box 12233, Research Triangle Park, North Carolina 27709, USA

N. Nelson, Professor and Chairman, Institute of Environmental Medicine, New York University Medical Center, 550 First Avenue, New York, New York 10016, USA *(Chairman)*

K. Sankaranarayanan, Associate Professor, Department of Radiation Genetics and Chemical Mutagenesis, Sylvius Laboratories, State University of Leiden, Wassenaarseweg 72, Leiden, The Netherlands

B. Teichmann, Department of Chemical Carcinogenesis, Zentralinstitut für Krebsforschung, Akademie der Wissenschaften der DDR, Lindenberger Weg 80, 115 Berlin-Buch, German Democratic Republic

---

[1]Present address: Unit of Chemical Carcinogenesis, IARC, Lyon

B. Terracini, Epidemiologia dei Tumori, Istituto di Anatomia e Istologia
    Patologica dell'Università di Torino, Via Santena 7, 10126 Torino,
    Italy (*Vice-Chairman*)

R. Truhaut, Director, Centre de Recherches Toxicologiques, Faculté des
    Sciences pharmaceutiques et biologiques de l'Université René Descartes,
    4 Avenue de l'Observatoire, 75006 Paris, France

H. Uehleke, Chief Director, Toxicology, Department of Toxicology,
    Bundesgesundheitsamt, Thielallee 88/92, 1 Berlin 33-Postfach, Federal
    Republic of Germany

S. Venitt, Institute of Cancer Research, Pollards Wood Research Station,
    Nightingales Lane, Chalfont St Giles, Bucks HP8 4SP, UK

J.K. Wagoner, Special Assistant for Occupational Carcinogenesis, Office
    of the Assistant Secretary of Labor, US Occupational Safety and Health
    Administration, US Department of Labor, 200 Constitution Avenue NW,
    Washington DC 20210, USA

J.S. Wassom, Director, Environmental Mutagen and Teratology Information
    Centers, Oak Ridge National Laboratory, PO Box Y, Oak Ridge,
    Tennessee 37830, USA

F. Wiebel, Institute of Toxicology and Biochemistry, Gesellschaft für
    Strahlen- und Umweltforschung MBH München, Ingolstädter Landstrasse 1,
    Post Oberschleissheim, 8042 Neuherberg, Federal Republic of Germany

Observers

A.M. Kaplan, Chief, Oral Toxicology, Haskell Laboratory for Toxicology
    and Industrial Medicine, E.I. Du Pont de Nemours & Co., Inc.,
    Elkton Road, Newark, Delaware 19711, USA

L. Villemey, Délégué à l'Environnement, European Council of Chemical
    Manufacturers' Federations, Avenue Louise 250, 1050 Brussels, Belgium

Representative from SRI International

O.H. Johnson, Senior Industrial Economist, Chemical-Environmental Program,
    SRI International, 333 Ravenswood Avenue, Menlo Park, California 94025,
    USA (*Rapporteur sections 2.1 & 2.2*)

Representative from the Commission of the European Communities

M.-T. van der Venne, Commission of the European Communities, Health and
    Safety Directorate, Bâtiment Jean Monnet, Plateau du Kirchberg,
    Bôite Postale 1907, Luxembourg, Great Duchy of Luxembourg

Secretariat

C. Agthe[1], Chief Scientist, Responsible Officer (Food Safety), Environmental Health Criteria and Standards, Division of Environmental Health, WHO, Geneva

H. Bartsch, Unit of Chemical Carcinogenesis (*Rapporteur section 3.2*)

M. Castegnaro, Unit of Environmental Carcinogens

J. Cooper, Unit of Epidemiology and Biostatistics (*Co-rapporteur section 3.3*)

L. Griciute, Chief, Unit of Environmental Carcinogens

J.E. Huff, Unit of Chemical Carcinogenesis (*Co-secretary*)

T. Kuroki, Unit of Chemical Carcinogenesis

D. Mietton, Unit of Chemical Carcinogenesis (*Library assistant*)

R. Montesano, Unit of Chemical Carcinogenesis (*Rapporteur section 3.1*)

C. Partensky, Unit of Chemical Carcinogenesis (*Technical editor*)

I. Peterschmitt, Unit of Chemical Carcinogenesis, WHO, Geneva (*Bibliographic researcher*)

V. Ponomarkov, Unit of Chemical Carcinogenesis

R. Saracci, Unit of Epidemiology and Biostatistics (*Co-rapporteur section 3.3*)

L. Tomatis, Chief, Unit of Chemical Carcinogenesis (*Head of the Programme*)

E.A. Walker, Unit of Environmental Carcinogens (*Rapporteur sections 1 and 2.3*)

E. Ward, Montignac, France (*Editor*)

J.D. Wilbourn, Unit of Chemical Carcinogenesis (*Co-secretary*)

Secretarial assistance

A.V. Anderson

M.-J. Ghess

R.B. Johnson

J.A. Smith

---

[1]Present address: Director's Office, IARC, Lyon

The term 'carcinogenic risk' in the *IARC Monograph* series is taken to mean the probability that exposure to the chemical will lead to cancer in humans.

Inclusion of a chemical in the monographs does not imply that it is a carcinogen, only that the published data have been examined. Equally, the fact that a chemical has not yet been evaluated in a monograph does not mean that it is not carcinogenic.

Anyone who is aware of published data that may alter the evaluation of the carcinogenic risk of a chemical for humans is encouraged to make that information available to the Unit of Chemical Carcinogenesis, International Agency for Research on Cancer, Lyon, France, in order that the chemical may be considered for re-evaluation by a future Working Group.

Although every effort is made to prepare the monographs as accurately as possible, mistakes may occur. Readers are requested to communicate any errors to the Unit of Chemical Carcinogenesis, so that corrections can be reported in future volumes.

PREAMBLE

BACKGROUND

In 1971, the International Agency for Research on Cancer (IARC) initiated a programme on the evaluation of the carcinogenic risk of chemicals to humans with the object of producing monographs on individual chemicals*. The criteria established at that time to evaluate carcinogenic risk to humans were adopted by all the working groups whose deliberations resulted in the first 16 volumes of the *IARC Monograph* series. In October 1977, a joint IARC/WHO *ad hoc* Working Group met to re-evaluate these guiding criteria; this preamble reflects the results of their deliberations(1) and those of a subsequent IARC *ad hoc* Working Group which met in April 1978(2).

OBJECTIVE AND SCOPE

The objective of the programme is to elaborate and publish in the form of monographs critical reviews of data on carcinogenicity for groups of chemicals to which humans are known to be exposed, to evaluate these data in terms of human risk with the help of international working groups of experts in chemical carcinogenesis and related fields, and to indicate where additional research efforts are needed.

The monographs summarize the evidence for the carcinogenicity of individual chemicals and other relevant information. The critical analyses of the data are intended to assist national and international authorities in formulating decisions concerning preventive measures. No recommendations are given concerning legislation, since this depends on risk-benefit evaluations, which seem best made by individual governments and/or international agencies. In this connection, WHO recommendations on food additives(3), drugs(4), pesticides and contaminants(5) and occupational carcinogens(6) are particularly informative.

---

*Since 1972, the programme has undergone considerable expansion, primarily with the scientific collaboration and financial support of the US National Cancer Institute.

The *IARC Monographs* are recognized as an authoritative source of information on the carcinogenicity of environmental chemicals. The first users' survey, made in 1976, indicates that the monographs are consulted routinely by various agencies in 24 countries.

Since the programme began in 1971, 20 volumes have been published(7) in the *IARC Monograph* series, and 442 separate chemical substances have been evaluated (see also cumulative index to the monographs, p. 593). Each volume is printed in 4000 copies and distributed *via* the WHO publications service (see inside covers for a listing of IARC publications and back outside cover for distribution and sales services).

SELECTION OF CHEMICALS FOR MONOGRAPHS

The chemicals (natural and synthetic, including those which occur as mixtures and in manufacturing processes) are selected for evaluation on the basis of two main criteria: (a) there is evidence of human exposure, and (b) there is some experimental evidence of carcinogenicity and/or there is some evidence or suspicion of a risk to humans. In certain instances, chemical analogues were also considered.

Inclusion of a chemical in a volume does not imply that it is carcinogenic, only that the published data have been examined. The evaluations must be consulted to ascertain the conclusions of the Working Group. Equally, the fact that a chemical has not appeared in a monograph does not mean that it is without carcinogenic hazard.

The scientific literature is surveyed for published data relevant to the monograph programme. In addition, the IARC *Survey of Chemicals Being Tested for Carcinogenicity* (8) often indicates those chemicals that are to be scheduled for future meetings. The major aims of the survey are to prevent unnecessary duplication of research, to increase communication among scientists, and to make a census of chemicals that are being tested and of available research facilities.

As new data on chemicals for which monographs have already been prepared and new principles for evaluating carcinogenic risk receive acceptance, re-evaluations will be made at subsequent meetings, and revised monographs will be published as necessary.

WORKING PROCEDURES

Approximately one year in advance of a meeting of a working group, a list of the substances to be considered is prepared by IARC staff in consultation with other experts. Subsequently, all relevant biological data are collected by IARC; in addition to the published literature, US Public Health Service Publication No. 149(9) has been particularly

valuable and has been used in conjunction with other recognized sources
of information on chemical carcinogenesis and systems such as CANCERLINE,
MEDLINE and TOXLINE. The major collection of data and the preparation
of first drafts for the sections on chemical and physical properties, on
production, use, occurrence and on analysis are carried out by SRI
International under a separate contract with the US National Cancer
Institute. Most of the data so obtained on production, use and occurrence
refer to the United States and Japan; SRI International and IARC supplement this information with that from other sources in Europe. Biblio-
graphical sources for data on mutagenicity and teratogenicity are the
Environmental Mutagen Information Center and the Environmental Teratology
Information Center, both located at the Oak Ridge National Laboratory,
USA.

Six to nine months before the meeting, reprints of articles containing relevant biological data are sent to an expert(s), or are used by the
IARC staff, for the preparation of first drafts of the monographs. These
drafts are edited by IARC staff and are sent prior to the meeting to all
participants of the Working Group for their comments. The Working Group
then meets in Lyon for seven to eight days to discuss and finalize the
texts of the monographs and to formulate the evaluations. After the
meeting, the master copy of each monograph is verified by consulting the
original literature, then edited and prepared for reproduction. The
monographs are usually published within six months after the Working Group
meeting.

DATA FOR EVALUATIONS

With regard to biological data, only reports that have been published
or accepted for publication are reviewed by the working groups, although
a few exceptions have been made. The monographs do not cite all of the
literature on a particular chemical: only those data considered by the
Working Group to be relevant to the evaluation of the carcinogenic risk
of the chemical to humans are included.

Anyone who is aware of data that have been published or are in press
which are relevant to the evaluations of the carcinogenic risk to humans
of chemicals for which monographs have appeared is urged to make them
available to the Unit of Chemical Carcinogenesis, International Agency
for Research on Cancer, Lyon, France.

THE WORKING GROUP

The tasks of the Working Group are five-fold: (a) to ascertain that
all data have been collected; (b) to select the data relevant for the
evaluation; (c) to ensure that the summaries of the data enable the reader
to follow the reasoning of the committee; (d) to judge the significance
of the results of experimental and epidemiological studies; and (e) to

make an evaluation of the carcinogenic risk of the chemical.

Working Group participants who contributed to the consideration and evaluation of chemicals within a particular volume are listed, with their addresses, at the beginning of each publication (see p. 1). Each member serves as an individual scientist and not as a representative of any organization or government. In addition, observers are often invited from national and international agencies, organizations and industries.

GENERAL PRINCIPLES FOR EVALUATING THE CARCINOGENIC RISK OF CHEMICALS

The widely accepted meaning of the term 'chemical carcinogenesis', and that used in these monographs, is the induction by chemicals of neoplasms that are not usually observed, the earlier induction by chemicals of neoplasms that are usually observed, and/or the induction by chemicals of more neoplasms than are usually found - although fundamentally different mechanisms may be involved in these three situations. Etymologically, the term 'carcinogenesis' means the induction of cancer, that is, of malignant neoplasms; however, the commonly accepted meaning is the induction of various types of neoplasms or of a combination of malignant and benign tumours. In the monographs, the words 'tumour' and neoplasm' are used interchangeably (In scientific literature the terms 'tumourigen', 'oncogen' and 'blastomogen' have all been used synonymously with 'carcinogen', although occasionally 'tumourigen' has been used specifically to denote the induction of benign tumours).

Experimental Evidence

Qualitative aspects

Both the interpretation and evaluation of a particular study as well as the overall assessment of the carcinogenic activity of a chemical involve several qualitatively important considerations, including: (a) the experimental parameters under which the chemical was tested, including route of administration and exposure, species, strain, sex, age, etc.; (b) the consistency with which the chemical has been shown to be carcinogenic, e.g., in how many species and at which target organ(s); (c) the spectrum of neoplastic response, from benign neoplasia to multiple malignant tumours; (d) the stage of tumour formation in which a chemical may be involved: some chemicals act as complete carcinogens and have initiating and promoting activity, while others are promoters only; and (e) the possible role of modifying factors.

There are problems not only of differential survival but of differential toxicity, which may be manifested by unequal growth and weight gain in treated and control animals. These complexities should also be considered in the interpretation of data, or, better, in the experimental design.

Many chemicals induce both benign and malignant tumours; few instances are recorded in which only benign neoplasms are induced by chemicals that have been studied extensively. Benign tumours may represent a stage in the evolution of a malignant neoplasm or they may be 'end-points' that do not readily undergo transition to malignancy. If a substance is found to induce only benign tumours in experimental animals, the chemical should be suspected of being a carcinogen and requires further investigation.

Hormonal carcinogenesis

Hormonal carcinogenesis presents certain distinctive features: the chemicals involved occur both endogenously and exogenously; in many instances, long exposure is required; tumours occur in the target tissue in association with a stimulation of non-neoplastic growth, but in some cases, hormones promote the proliferation of tumour cells in a target organ. Hormones that occur in excessive amounts, hormone-mimetic agents and agents that cause hyperactivity or imbalance in the endocrine system may require evaluative methods comparable with those used to identify chemical carcinogens; particular emphasis must be laid on quantitative aspects and duration of exposure. Some chemical carcinogens have significant side effects on the endocrine system, which may also result in hormonal carcinogenesis. Synthetic hormones and anti-hormones can be expected to possess other pharmacological and toxicological actions in addition to those on the endocrine system, and in this respect they must be treated like any other chemical with regard to intrinsic carcinogenic potential.

Quantitative aspects

Dose-response studies are important in the evaluation of carcinogenesis: the confidence with which a carcinogenic effect can be established is strengthened by the observation of an increasing incidence of neoplasms with increasing exposure.

The assessment of carcinogenicity in animals is frequently complicated by recognized differences among the test animals (species, strain, sex, age), in route(s) of administration and in dose/duration of exposure; often, target organs at which a cancer occurs and its histological type may vary with these parameters. Nevertheless, indices of carcinogenic potency in particular experimental systems (for instance, the dose-rate required under continuous exposure to halve the probability of the animals remaining tumourless(10)) have been formulated in the hope that, at least among categories of fairly similar agents, such indices may be of some predictive value in other systems, including humans.

Chemical carcinogens differ widely in the dose required to produce a given level of tumour induction, although many of them share common biological properties which include metabolism to reactive (electrophilic (11-13)) intermediates capable of interacting with DNA. The reason for this variation in dose-response is not understood but may be due either to

differences within a common metabolic process or to the operation of
qualitatively distinct mechanisms.

Statistical analysis of animal studies

Tumours which would have arisen had an animal lived longer may not
be observed because of the death of the animal from unrelated causes, and
this possibility must be allowed for. Various analytical techniques have
been developed which use the assumption of independence of competing risks
to allow for the effects of intercurrent mortality on the final numbers
of tumour-bearing animals in particular treatment groups.

For externally visible tumours and for neoplasms that cause death,
methods such as Kaplan-Meier (i.e., 'life-table', 'product-limit' or
'actuarial') estimates(10), with associated significance tests(14,15),
are recommended.

For internal neoplasms which are discovered 'incidentally'(14) at
autopsy but which did not cause the death of the host, different estimates
(16) and significance tests(14,15) may be necessary for the unbiased study
of the numbers of tumour-bearing animals.

All of these methods(10,14-16) can be used to analyse the numbers of
animals bearing particular tumour types, but they do not distinguish
between animals with one or many such tumours. In experiments which end
at a particular fixed time, with the simultaneous sacrifice of many
animals, analysis of the total numbers of internal neoplasms per animal
found at autopsy at the end of the experiment is straightforward. However,
there are no adequate statistical methods for analysing the numbers of
particular neoplasms that kill an animal host.

Evidence of Carcinogenicity in Humans

Evidence of carcinogenicity in humans can be derived from three
types of study, the first two of which usually provide only suggestive
evidence: (1) reports concerning individual cancer patients (case reports),
including a history of exposure to the supposed carcinogenic agent; (2)
descriptive epidemiological studies in which the incidence of cancer in
human populations is found to vary (spatially or temporally) with exposure
to the agent; and (3) analytical epidemiological studies (e.g., case-
control or cohort studies) in which individual exposure to the agent is
found to be associated with an increased risk of cancer.

An analytical study that shows a positive association between an
agent and a cancer may be interpreted as implying causality to a greater
or lesser extent, if the following criteria are met: (a) there is no
identifiable positive bias (By 'positive bias' is meant the operation of
factors in study design or execution which lead erroneously to a more
strongly positive association between an agent and disease than in fact

exists. Examples of positive bias include, in case-control studies,
better documentation of exposure to the agent for cases than for controls,
and, in cohort studies, the use of better means of detecting cancer
in individuals exposed to the agent than in individuals not exposed);
(b) the possibility of positive confounding has been considered (By 'positive confounding' is meant a situation in which the relationship between
an agent and a disease is rendered more strongly positive than it truly
is as a result of an association between that agent and another agent
which either causes or prevents the disease. An example of positive
confounding is the association between coffee consumption and lung cancer,
which results from their joint association with cigarette smoking); (c)
the association is unlikely to be due to chance alone; (d) the association
is strong; and (e) there is a dose-response relationship.

In some instances, a single epidemiological study may be strongly
indicative of a cause-effect relationship; however, the most convincing
evidence of causality comes when several independent studies done under
different circumstances result in 'positive' findings.

Analytical epidemiological studies that show no association between
an agent and a cancer ('negative' studies) should be interpreted according
to criteria analogous to those listed above: (a) there is no identifiable
negative bias; (b) the possibility of negative confounding has been
considered; and (c) the possible effects of misclassification of exposure
or outcome have been weighed.

In addition, it must be recognized that in any study there are
confidence limits around the estimate of association or relative risk.
In a study regarded as 'negative', the upper confidence limit may indicate
a relative risk substantially greater than unity; in that case, the study
excludes only relative risks that are above this upper limit. This usually
means that a 'negative' study must be large to be convincing. Confidence
in a 'negative' result is increased when several independent studies
carried out under different circumstances are in agreement.

Finally, a 'negative' study may be considered to be relevant only to
dose levels within or below the range of those observed in the study and
is pertinent only if sufficient time has elapsed since first human exposure
to the agent. Experience with human cancers of known etiology suggests
that the period from first exposure to a chemical carcinogen to development
of clinically observed cancer is usually measured in decades and may be in
excess of 30 years.

Experimental Data Relevant to the Evaluation of Carcinogenic Risk to Humans

No adequate criteria are presently available to interpret experimental
carcinogenicity data directly in terms of carcinogenic potential for humans.
Nonetheless, utilizing data collected from appropriate tests in animals,
positive extrapolations to possible human risk can be approximated.

Information compiled from the first 17 volumes of the *IARC Monographs* (17-19) shows that of about 26 chemicals or manufacturing processes now generally accepted to cause cancer in humans, all but possibly two (arsenic and benzene) of those which have been tested appropriately produce cancer in at least one animal species. For several (aflatoxins, 4-aminobiphenyl, diethylstilboestrol, melphalan, mustard gas and vinyl chloride), evidence of carcinogenicity in experimental animals preceded evidence obtained from epidemiological studies or case reports.

In general, the evidence that a chemical produces tumours in experimental animals is of two degrees: (a) *sufficient evidence* of carcinogenicity is provided by the production of malignant tumours; and (b) *limited evidence* of carcinogenicity reflects qualitative and/or quantitative limitations of the experimental results.

For many of the chemicals evaluated in the first 20 volumes of the *IARC Monographs* for which there is *sufficient evidence* of carcinogenicity in animals, data relating to carcinogenicity for humans are either insufficient or nonexistent. In the absence of adequate data on humans, it is reasonable, for practical purposes, to regard such chemicals as if they presented a carcinogenic risk to humans.

Sufficient evidence of carcinogenicity is provided by experimental studies that show an increased incidence of malignant tumours: (i) in multiple species or strains, and/or (ii) in multiple experiments (routes and/or doses), and/or (iii) to an unusual degree (with regard to incidence, site, type and/or precocity of onset). Additional evidence may be provided by data concerning dose-response, mutagenicity or structure.

In the present state of knowledge, it would be difficult to define a predictable relationship between the dose (mg/kg bw/day) of a particular chemical required to produce cancer in test animals and the dose which would produce a similar incidence of cancer in humans. The available data suggest, however, that such a relationship may exist(20,21), at least for certain classes of carcinogenic chemicals. Data that provide *sufficient evidence* of carcinogenicity in test animals may therefore be used in an approximate quantitative evaluation of the human risk at some given exposure level, provided that the nature of the chemical concerned and the physiological, pharmacological and toxicological differences between the test animals and humans are taken into account. However, no acceptable methods are currently available for quantifying the possible errors in such a procedure, whether it is used to generalize between species or to extrapolate from high to low doses. The methodology for such quantitative extrapolation to humans requires further development.

Evidence for the carcinogenicity of some chemicals in experimental animals may be *limited* for two reasons. Firstly, experimental data may be restricted to such a point that it is not possible to determine a causal relationship between administration of a chemical and the development of a particular lesion in the animals. Secondly, there are certain neoplasms, including lung tumours and hepatomas in mice, which have been considered of lesser significance than neoplasms occurring at other sites for the purpose of evaluating the carcinogenicity of chemicals. Such tumours occur spontaneously in high incidence in these animals, and their malignancy is often difficult to establish. An evaluation of the significance of these tumours following administration of a chemical is the responsibility of particular Working Groups preparing individual monographs, and it has not been possible to set down rigid guidelines; the relevance of these tumours must be determined by considerations which include experimental design and completeness of reporting.

Some chemicals for which there is *limited evidence* of carcinogenicity in animals have also been studied in humans with, in general, inconclusive results. While such chemicals may indeed be carcinogenic to humans, more experimental and epidemiological investigation is required.

Hence, '*sufficient evidence*' of carcinogenicity and '*limited evidence*' of carcinogenicity do not indicate categories of chemicals: the inherent definitions of those terms indicate varying degrees of experimental evidence, which may change if and when new data on the chemicals become available. The main drawback to any rigid classification of chemicals with regard to their carcinogenic capacity is the as yet incomplete knowledge of the mechanism(s) of carcinogenesis.

In recent years, several short-term tests for the detection of potential carcinogens have been developed. When only inadequate experimental data are available, positive results in validated short-term tests (see p. 19) are an indication that the compound is a potential carcinogen and that it should be tested in animals for an assessment of its carcinogenicity. Negative results from short-term tests cannot be considered sufficient evidence to rule out carcinogenicity. Whether short-term tests will eventually be as reliable as long-term tests in predicting carcinogenicity in humans will depend on further demonstrations of consistency with long-term experiments and with data from humans.

EXPLANATORY NOTES ON THE MONOGRAPH CONTENTS

Chemical and Physical Data (Section 1)

The Chemical Abstracts Service Registry Number and the latest Chemical Abstracts Primary Name (9th Collective Index)(22) are recorded in section 1. Other synonyms and trade names are given, but no comprehensive list is provided. Further, some of the trade names are those of mixtures in which the compound being evaluated is only one of the ingredients.

The structural and molecular formulae, molecular weight and chemical and physical properties are given. The properties listed refer to the pure substance, unless otherwise specified, and include, in particular, data that might be relevant to carcinogenicity (e.g., lipid solubility) and those that concern identification. A separate description of the composition of technical products includes available information on impurities and formulated products.

Production, Use, Occurrence and Analysis (Section 2)

The purpose of section 2 is to provide indications of the extent of past and present human exposure to the chemical.

Synthesis

Since cancer is a delayed toxic effect, the dates of first synthesis and of first commercial production of the chemical are provided. In addition, methods of synthesis used in past and present commercial production are described. This information allows a reasonable estimate to be made of the date before which no human exposure could have occurred.

Production

Since Europe, Japan and the United States are reasonably representative industrialized areas of the world, most data on production, foreign trade and uses are obtained from those countries. It should not, however, be inferred that those nations are the sole or even the major sources or users of any individual chemical.

Production and foreign trade data are obtained from both governmental and trade publications by chemical economists in the three geographical areas. In some cases, separate production data on organic chemicals manufactured in the United States are not available because their publication could disclose confidential information. In such cases, an indication of the minimum quantity produced can be inferred from the number of companies reporting commercial production. Each company is required to report on individual chemicals if the sales value or the weight of the annual production exceeds a specified minimum level. These levels vary for chemicals classified for different uses, e.g., medicinals and plastics; in fact, the minimal annual sales value is between $1000 and $50,000 and the minimal annual weight of production is between 450 and 22,700 kg. Data on production in some European countries are obtained by means of general questionnaires sent to companies thought to produce the compounds being evaluated. Information from the completed questionnaires is compiled by country, and the resulting estimates of production are included in the individual monographs.

Use

Information on uses is meant to serve as a guide only and is not complete. It is usually obtained from published data but is often complemented by direct contact with manufacturers of the chemical. In the case of drugs, mention of their therapeutic uses does not necessarily represent current practice nor does it imply judgement as to their clinical efficacy.

Statements concerning regulations and standards (e.g., pesticide registrations, maximum levels permitted in foods, occupational standards and allowable limits) in specific countries are mentioned as examples only. They may not reflect the most recent situation, since such legislation is in a constant state of change; nor should it be taken to imply that other countries do not have similar regulations.

Occurrence

Information on the occurrence of a chemical in the environment is obtained from published data, including that derived from the monitoring and surveillance of levels of the chemical in occupational environments, air, water, soil, foods and tissues of animals and humans. When available, data on the generation, persistence and bioaccumulation of a chemical are also included.

Analysis

The purpose of the section on analysis is to give the reader an indication, rather than a complete review, of methods cited in the literature. No attempt is made to evaluate critically or to recommend any of the methods.

Biological Data Relevant to the Evaluation of Carcinogenic Risk to Humans (Section 3)

In general, the data recorded in section 3 are summarized as given by the author; however, comments made by the Working Group on certain shortcomings of reporting, of statistical analysis or of experimental design are given in square brackets. The nature and extent of impurities/contaminants in the chemicals being tested are given when available.

Carcinogenicity studies in animals

The monographs are not intended to cover all reported studies. Some studies are purposely omitted (a) because they are inadequate, as judged from previously described criteria(23-26) (e.g., too short a duration, too few animals, poor survival); (b) because they only confirm findings that have already been fully described; or (c) because they are judged irrelevant for the purpose of the evaluation. In certain cases, however, such studies are mentioned briefly, particularly when the information is considered to be a useful supplement to other reports or when it is the only data available. Their inclusion does not, however, imply acceptance of the adequacy of their experimental design and/or of the analysis and interpretation of their results.

Mention is made of all routes of administration by which the compound has been adequately tested and of all species in which relevant tests have been done(5,26). In most cases, animal strains are given (General characteristics of mouse strains have been reviewed(27)). Quantitative data are given to indicate the order of magnitude of the effective carcinogenic

doses. In general, the doses and schedules are indicated as they appear
in the original paper; sometimes units have been converted for easier
comparison. Experiments on the carcinogenicity of known metabolites,
chemical precursors, analogues and derivatives, and experiments on factors
that modify the carcinogenic effect are also reported.

Other relevant biological data

Lethality data are given when available, and other data on toxicity
are included when considered relevant. The metabolic data are restricted
to studies that show the metabolic fate of the chemical in animals and
humans, and comparisons of data from animals and humans are made when
possible. Information is also given on absorption, distribution, excretion
and placental transfer.

Embryotoxicity and teratogenicity

Data on teratogenicity from studies in experimental animals and from
observations in humans are also included. There appears to be no causal
relationship between teratogenicity(28) and carcinogenicity, but chemicals
often have both properties. Evidence of teratogenicity suggests transplacental transfer, which is a prerequisite for transplacental carcinogenesis.

Indirect tests (mutagenicity and other short-term tests)

Data from indirect tests are also included. Since most of these tests
have the advantage of taking less time and being less expensive than mammalian carcinogenicity studies, they are generally known as 'short-term'
tests. They comprise assay procedures which rely on the induction of
biological and biochemical effects in *in vivo* and/or *in vitro* systems.
The end-point of the majority of these tests is the production not of
neoplasms in animals but of changes at the molecular, cellular or multi-
cellular level: these include the induction of DNA damage and repair,
mutagenesis in bacteria and other organisms, transformation of mammalian
cells in culture, and other systems.

The short-term tests are proposed for use (a) in predicting potential
carcinogenicity in the absence of carcinogenicity data in animals, (b) as
a contribution in deciding which chemicals should be tested in animals,
(c) in identifying active fractions of complex mixtures containing carcinogens, (d) for recognizing active metabolites of known carcinogens in human
and/or animal body fluids and (e) to help elucidate mechanisms of carcinogenesis.

Although the theory that cancer is induced as a result of somatic
mutation suggests that agents which damage DNA *in vivo* may be carcinogens,
the precise relevance of short-term tests to the mechanism by which cancer
is induced is not known. Predictions of potential carcinogenicity are
currently based on correlations between responses in short-term tests and

data from animal carcinogenicity and/or human epidemiological studies.
This approach is limited because the number of chemicals known to be
carcinogenic in humans is insufficient to provide a basis for validation,
and most validation studies involve chemicals that have been evaluated
for carcinogenicity only in animals. The selection of chemicals is in
turn limited to those classes for which data on carcinogenicity are
available. The results of validation studies could be strongly influenced
by such selection of chemicals and by the proportion of carcinogens in the
series of chemicals tested; this should be kept in mind when evaluating
the predictivity of a particular test. The usefulness of any test is
reflected by its ability to classify carcinogens and noncarcinogens, using
the animal data as a standard; however, animal tests may not always
provide a perfect standard. The attainable level of correlation between
short-term tests and animal bioassays is still under investigation.

Since many chemicals require metabolism to an active form, tests
that do not take this into account may fail to detect certain potential
carcinogens. The metabolic activation systems used in short-term tests
(e.g., the cell-free systems used in bacterial tests) are meant to approximate the metabolic capacity of the whole organism. Each test has its
advantages and limitations; thus, more confidence can be placed in the
conclusions when negative or positive results for a chemical are confirmed
in several such test systems. Deficiencies in metabolic competence may
lead to misclassification of chemicals, which means that not all tests
are suitable for assessing the potential carcinogenicity of all classes of
compounds.

The present state of knowledge does not permit the selection of a
specific test(s) as the most appropriate for identifying potential carcinogenicity. Before the results of a particular test can be considered to be
fully acceptable for predicting potential carcinogenicity, certain criteria
should be met: (a) the test should have been validated with respect to
known animal carcinogens and found to have a high capacity for discrimin-
ating between carcinogens and noncarcinogens, and (b), when possible, a
structurally related carcinogen(s) and noncarcinogen(s) should have been
tested simultaneously with the chemical in question. The results should
have been reproduced in different laboratories, and a prediction of carcinogenicity should have been confirmed in additional test systems. Confidence
in positive results is increased if a mechanism of action can be deduced
and if appropriate dose-response data are available. For optimum usefulness,
data on purity must be given.

The short-term tests in current use that have been the most extensively
validated are the *Salmonella typhimurium* plate-incorporation assay(29-33),
the X-linked recessive lethal test in *Drosophila melanogaster*(34), unscheduled DNA synthesis(35) and *in vitro* transformation(33,36). Each is compa-
tible with current concepts of the possible mechanism(s) of carcinogenesis.

An adequate assessment of the genetic activity of a chemical depends
on data from a wide range of test systems. The monographs include, therefore, data not only from those already mentioned, but also on the induction

of point mutations in other systems(37-42), on structural(43) and numerical chromosome aberrations, including dominant lethal effects(44), on mitotic recombination in fungi(37) and on sister chromatid exchanges(45-46).

The existence of a correlation between quantitative aspects of muta-genic and carcinogenic activity has been suggested(5,44-50), but it is not sufficiently well established to allow general use.

Further information about mutagenicity and other short-term tests is given in references 45-53.

Case reports and epidemiological studies

Observations in humans are summarized in this section.

Summary of Data Reported and Evaluation (Section 4)

Section 4 summarizes the relevant data from animals and humans and gives the critical views of the Working Group on those data.

Experimental data

Data relevant to the evaluation of the carcinogenicity of a chemical in animals are summarized in this section. Results from validated muta-genicity and other short-term tests are reported if the Working Group considered the data to be relevant. Dose-response data are given when available. An assessment of the carcinogenicity of the chemical in animals is made on the basis of all of the available data.

The animal species mentioned are those in which the carcinogenicity of the substance was clearly demonstrated. The route of administration used in experimental animals that is similar to the possible human exposure is given particular mention. Tumour sites are also indicated. If the substance has produced tumours after prenatal exposure or in single-dose experiments, this is indicated.

Human data

Case reports and epidemiological studies that are considered to be pertinent to an assessment of human carcinogenicity are described. Human exposure to the chemical is summarized on the basis of data on production, use and occurrence. Other biological data which are considered to be relevant are also mentioned. An assessment of the carcinogenicity of the chemical in humans is made on the basis of all of the available evidence.

Evaluation

This section comprises the overall evaluation by the Working Group of the carcinogenic risk of the chemical to humans. All of the data in the monograph, and particularly the summarized information on experimental and human data, are considered in order to make this evaluation.

References

1. IARC (1977) IARC Monograph Programme on the Evaluation of the Carcinogenic Risk of Chemicals to Humans. Preamble. IARC intern. tech. Rep. No. 77/002

2. IARC (1978) Chemicals with *sufficient evidence* of carcinogenicity in experimental animals - *IARC Monographs* volumes 1-17. IARC intern. tech. Rep. No. 78/003

3. WHO(1961) Fifth Report of the Joint FAO/WHO Expert Committee on Food Additives. Evaluation of carcinogenic hazard of food additives. WHO tech. Rep. Ser., No. 220, pp. 5, 18, 19

4. WHO (1969) Report of a WHO Scientific Group. Principles for the testing and evaluation of drugs for carcinogenicity. WHO tech. Rep. Ser., No. 426, pp. 19, 21, 22

5. WHO (1974) Report of a WHO Scientific Group. Assessment of the carcinogenicity and mutagenicity of chemicals. WHO tech. Rep. Ser., No. 546

6. WHO (1964) Report of a WHO Expert Committee. Prevention of cancer. WHO tech. Rep. Ser., No. 276, pp. 29, 30

7. IARC (1972-1978) IARC Monographs on the Evaluation of the Carcinogenic Risk of Chemicals to Humans, Volumes 1-18, Lyon, France

    Volume 1 (1972) Some Inorganic Substances, Chlorinated Hydrocarbons, Aromatic Amines, *N*-Nitroso Compounds and Natural Products (19 monographs), 184 pages

    Volume 2 (1973) Some Inorganic and Organometallic Compounds (7 monographs), 181 pages

    Volume 3 (1973) Certain Polycyclic Aromatic Hydrocarbons and Heterocyclic Compounds (17 monographs), 271 pages

    Volume 4 (1974) Some Aromatic Amines, Hydrazine and Related Substances, *N*-Nitroso Compounds and Miscellaneous Alkylating Agents (28 monographs), 286 pages

    Volume 5 (1974) Some Organochlorine Pesticides (12 monographs), 241 pages

    Volume 6 (1974) Sex Hormones (15 monographs), 243 pages

    Volume 7 (1974) Some Anti-thyroid and Related Substances, Nitrofurans and Industrial Chemicals (23 monographs), 326 pages

Volume 8 (1975)   Some Aromatic Azo Compounds (32 monographs),
    357 pages

Volume 9 (1975)   Some Aziridines, *N*-, *S*- and *O*-Mustards and
    Selenium (24 monographs), 268 pages

Volume 10 (1976)   Some Naturally Occurring Substances (32 monographs),
    353 pages

Volume 11 (1976)   Cadmium, Nickel, Some Epoxides, Miscellaneous
    Industrial Chemicals and General Considerations on Volatile
    Anaesthetics (24 monographs), 306 pages

Volume 12 (1976)   Some Carbamates, Thiocarbamates and Carbazides
    (24 monographs), 282 pages

Volume 13 (1977)   Some Miscellaneous Pharmaceutical Substances
    (17 monographs), 255 pages

Volume 14 (1977)   Asbestos (1 monograph), 106 pages

Volume 15 (1977)   Some Fumigants, the Herbicides 2,4-D and
    2,4,5-T, Chlorinated Dibenzodioxins and Miscellaneous
    Industrial Chemicals (18 monographs), 354 pages

Volume 16 (1978)   Some Aromatic Amines and Related Nitro Compounds -
    Hair Dyes, Colouring Agents and Miscellaneous Industrial
    Chemicals (32 monographs), 400 pages

Volume 17 (1978)   Some *N*-Nitroso Compounds (17 monographs),
    365 pages

Volume 18 (1978)   Polychlorinated Biphenyls and Polybrominated
    Biphenyls (2 monographs), 140 pages

Volume 19 (1979)   Some Monomers, Plastics and Synthetic Elastomers,
    and Acrolein (17 monographs), 513 pages

Volume 20 (1979)   Some Halogenated Hydrocarbons (25 monographs),
    609 pages

8.   IARC (1973-1978)   Information Bulletin on the Survey of Chemicals
     Being Tested for Carcinogenicity, Numbers 1-7, Lyon, France

     Number 1 (1973) 52 pages
     Number 2 (1973) 77 pages
     Number 3 (1974) 67 pages
     Number 4 (1974) 97 pages
     Number 5 (1975) 88 pages
     Number 6 (1976) 360 pages
     Number 7 (1978) 460 pages
     Number 8 (1979) 604 pages

9.   PHS 149 (1951-1976) Public Health Service Publication No. 149,
      Survey of Compounds which have been Tested for Carcinogenic
      Activity, Washington DC, US Government Printing Office

      1951 Hartwell, J.L., 2nd ed., Literature up to 1947 on 1329
            compounds, 583 pages

      1957 Shubik, P. & Hartwell, J.L., Supplement 1, Literature for
            the years 1948-1953 on 981 compounds, 388 pages

      1969 Shubik, P. & Hartwell, J.L., edited by Peters, J.A.,
            Supplement 2, Literature for the years 1954-1960 on 1048
            compounds, 655 pages

      1971 National Cancer Institute, Literature for the years
            1968-1969 on 882 compounds, 653 pages

      1973 National Cancer Institute, Literature for the years
            1961-1967 on 1632 compounds, 2343 pages

      1974 National Cancer Institute, Literature for the years
            1970-1971 on 750 compounds, 1667 pages

      1976 National Cancer Institute, Literature for the years
            1972-1973 on 966 compounds, 1638 pages

10.   Pike, M.C. & Roe, F.J.C. (1963) An actuarial method of analysis
      of an experiment in two-stage carcinogenesis. Br. J. Cancer,
      17, 605-610

11.   Miller, E.C. & Miller, J.A. (1966) Mechanisms of chemical carcino-
      genesis: nature of proximate carcinogens and interactions with
      macromolecules. Pharmacol. Rev., 18, 805-838

12.   Miller, J.A. (1970) Carcinogenesis by chemicals: an overview -
      G.H.A. Clowes Memorial Lecture. Cancer Res., 30, 559-576

13.   Miller, J.A. & Miller, E.C. (1976) The metabolic activation of
      chemical carcinogens to reactive electrophiles. In:
      Yuhas, J.M., Tennant, R.W. & Reagon, J.D., eds, Biology of
      Radiation Carcinogenesis, New York, Raven Press

14.   Peto, R. (1974) Guidelines on the analysis of tumours rates and
      death rates in experimental animals. Br. J. Cancer, 29, 101-105

15.   Peto, R. (1975) Letter to the editor. Br. J. Cancer, 31, 697-699

16.   Hoel, D.G. & Walburg, H.E., Jr (1972) Statistical analysis of
      survival experiments. J. natl Cancer Inst., 49, 361-372

17.   Tomatis, L. (1977) The value of long-term testing for the implemen-
          tation of primary prevention. In: Hiatt, H.H., Watson, J.D.
          & Winsten, J.A., eds, Origins of Human Cancer, Book C, Cold
          Spring Harbour, N.Y., Cold Spring Harbor Laboratory, pp. 1339-
          1357

18.   IARC (1977) Annual Report 1977, Lyon, International Agency for
          Research on Cancer, p. 94

19.   Tomatis, L., Agthe, C., Bartsch, H., Huff, J., Montesano, R.,
          Saracci, R., Walker, E. & Wilbourn, J. (1978) Evaluation of
          the carcinogenicity of chemicals: a review of the IARC Monograph
          Programme, 1971-1977. Cancer Res., 38, 877-885

20.   Rall, D.P. (1977) Species differences in carcinogenesis testing.
          In: Hiatt, H.H., Watson, J.D. & Winsten, J.A., eds, Origins
          of Human Cancer, Book C, Cold Spring Harbor, N.Y., Cold Spring
          Harbor Laboratory, pp. 1383-1390

21.   National Academy of Sciences (NAS) (1975) Contemporary pest control
          practices and prospects: the report of the Executive Committee,
          Washington DC

22.   Chemical Abstracts Service (1978) Chemical Abstracts Ninth Collective
          Index (9CI), 1972-1976, Vols 76-85, Columbus, Ohio

23.   WHO (1958) Second Report of the Joint FAO/WHO Expert Committee on
          Food Additives. Procedures for the testing of intentional food
          additives to establish their safety and use. WHO tech. Rep.
          Ser., No. 144

24.   WHO (1967) Scientific Group. Procedures for investigating inten-
          tional and unintentional food additives. WHO tech. Rep. Ser.,
          No. 348

25.   Berenblum, I., ed. (1969) Carcinogenicity testing. UICC tech. Rep.
          Ser., 2

26.   Sontag, J.M., Page, N.P. & Saffiotti, U. (1976) Guidelines for
          carcinogen bioassay in small rodents. Natl Cancer Inst.
          Carcinog. tech. Rep. Ser., No. 1

27.   Committee on Standardized Genetic Nomenclature for Mice (1972)
          Standardized nomenclature for inbred strains of mice. Fifth
          listing. Cancer Res., 32, 1609-1646

28.   Wilson, J.G. & Fraser, F.C. (1977) Handbook of Teratology, New York,
          Plenum Press

29. Ames, B.N., Durston, W.E., Yamasaki, E. & Lee, F.D. (1973) Carcino-
     gens are mutagens: a simple test system combining liver homo-
     genates for activation and bacteria for detection. Proc. natl
     Acad. Sci. (Wash.), 70, 2281-2285

30. McCann, J., Choi, E., Yamasaki, E. & Ames, B.N. (1975) Detection
     of carcinogens as mutagens in the *Salmonella*/microsome test:
     assay of 300 chemicals. Proc. natl Acad. Sci. (Wash.), 72,
     5135-5139

31. McCann, J. & Ames, B.N. (1976) Detection of carcinogens as mutagens
     in the *Salmonella*/microsome test: assay of 300 chemicals:
     discussion. Proc. natl Acad. Sci. (Wash.), 73, 950-954

32. Sugimura, T., Sato, S., Nagao, M., Yahagi, T., Matsushima, T.,
     Seino, Y., Takeuchi, M. & Kawachi, T. (1977) Overlapping of
     carcinogens and mutagens. In: Magee, P.N., Takayama, S.,
     Sugimura, T. & Matsushima, T., eds, Fundamentals in Cancer
     Prevention, Baltimore, University Park Press, pp. 191-215

33. Purchase, I.F.M., Longstaff, E., Ashby, J., Styles, J.A.,
     Anderson, D., Lefevre, P.A. & Westwood, F.R. (1976) Evaluation
     of six short term tests for detecting organic chemical carcino-
     gens and recommendations for their use. Nature (Lond.), 264,
     624-627

34. Vogel, E. & Sobels, F.H. (1976) The function of *Drosophila* in
     genetic toxicology testing. In: Hollaender, A., ed.,
     Chemical Mutagens: Principles and Methods for Their Detection,
     Vol. 4, New York, Plenum Press, pp. 93-142

35. San, R.H.C. & Stich, H.F. (1975) DNA repair synthesis of cultured
     human cells as a rapid bioassay for chemical carcinogens.
     Int. J. Cancer, 16, 284-291

36. Pienta, R.J., Poiley, J.A. & Lebherz, W.B. (1977) Morphological
     transformation of early passage golden Syrian hamster embryo
     cells derived from cryopreserved primary cultures as a reliable
     in vitro bioassay for identifying diverse carcinogens. Int. J.
     Cancer, 19, 642-655

37. Zimmermann, F.K. (1975) Procedures used in the induction of mitotic
     recombination and mutation in the yeast *Saccharomyces cerevisiae*.
     Mutat. Res., 31, 71-86

38. Ong, T.-M. & de Serres, F.J. (1972) Mutagenicity of chemical
     carcinogens in *Neurospora crassa*. Cancer Res., 32, 1890-1893

39. Huberman, E. & Sachs, L. (1976) Mutability of different genetic
     loci in mammalian cells by metabolically activated carcinogenic
     polycyclic hydrocarbons. Proc. natl Acad. Sci. (Wash.), 73,
     188-192

40. Krahn, D.F. & Heidelburger, C. (1977) Liver homogenate-mediated
     mutagenesis in Chinese hamster V79 cells by polycyclic aromatic
     hydrocarbons and aflatoxins. Mutat. Res., 46, 27-44

41. Kuroki, T., Drevon, C. & Montesano, R. (1977) Microsome-mediated
     mutagenesis in V79 Chinese hamster cells by various nitrosamines.
     Cancer Res., 37, 1044-1050

42. Searle, A.G. (1975) The specific locus test in the mouse. Mutat.
     Res., 31, 277-290

43. Evans, H.J. & O'Riordan, M.L. (1975) Human peripheral blood lympho-
     cytes for the analysis of chromosome aberrations in mutagen
     tests. Mutat. Res., 31, 135-148

44. Epstein, S.S., Arnold, E., Andrea, J., Bass, W. & Bishop, Y. (1972)
     Detection of chemical mutagens by the dominant lethal assay in
     the mouse. Toxicol. appl. Pharmacol., 23, 288-325

45. Perry, P. & Evans, H.J. (1975) Cytological detection of mutagen-
     carcinogen exposure by sister chromatid exchanges. Nature
     (Lond.), 258, 121-125

46. Stetka, D.G. & Wolff, S. (1976) Sister chromatid exchanges as an
     assay for genetic damage induced by mutagen-carcinogens. I.
     In vivo test for compounds requiring metabolic activation.
     Mutat. Res., 41, 333-342

47. Bartsch, H. & Grover, P.L. (1976) Chemical carcinogenesis and muta-
     genesis. In: Symington, T. & Carter, R.L., eds, Scientific
     Foundations of Oncology, Vol. IX, Chemical Carcinogenesis,
     London, Heinemann Medical Books Ltd, pp. 334-342

48. Hollaender, A., ed. (1971a,b, 1973, 1976) Chemical Mutagens:
     Principles and Methods for Their Detection, Vols 1-4, New York,
     Plenum Press

49. Montesano, R. & Tomatis, L., eds (1974) Chemical Carcinogenesis
     Essays, Lyon (IARC Scientific Publications No. 10)

50. Ramel, C., ed. (1973) Evaluation of genetic risk of environmental
     chemicals: report of a symposium held at Skokloster, Sweden,
     1972. Ambio Spec. Rep., No. 3

51.   Stoltz, D.R., Poirier, L.A., Irving, C.C., Stich, H.F.,
      Weisburger, J.H. & Grice, H.C. (1974) Evaluation of short-term
      tests for carcinogenicity. Toxicol. appl. Pharmacol., 29,
      157-180

52.   Montesano, R., Bartsch, H. & Tomatis, L., eds (1976) Screening
      Tests in Chemical Carcinogenesis, Lyon (IARC Scientific
      Publications No. 12)

53.   Committee 17 (1976) Environmental mutagenic hazards. Science, 187,
      503-514

Introduction

This twentieth volume of the *IARC Monographs on the Evaluation of the Carcinogenic Risk of Chemicals to Humans* comprises monographs on 28 halogenated hydrocarbons (mainly organochlorine compounds), which are used as pesticides and microbicides, as industrial solvents and inter- mediates, or as flame retardants.

Of the chemicals considered in this volume, two are brominated com- pounds: the flame retardant, tris(2,3-dibromopropyl) phosphate, and the fumigant and nematocide, 1,2-dibromo-3-chloropropane, which is also an impurity in and a metabolite of tris(2,3-dibromopropyl) phosphate.

Polybrominated biphenyls were considered at the same time, but the resulting monograph has been combined with one on polychlorinated biphenyls which resulted from a previous meeting in October 1977; the two monographs have been published together as *IARC Monographs* Volume 18 (IARC, 1978a). The Working Group also considered a monograph on methyl bromide, but since no carcinogenicity studies on this compound had become available by the time of the meeting, publication of the monograph was postponed.

Several of the pesticides covered in this volume were considered previously: HCH and lindane, heptachlor, methoxychlor and mirex in Volume 5 of the *IARC Monographs*, (IARC, 1974); carbon tetrachloride and chloroform in Volume 1 (IARC, 1972); trichloroethylene in Volume 11 (IARC, 1976); and 1,2-dibromo-3-chloropropane in Volume 15 (IARC, 1977). Because new, relevant data on these compounds have since become available the monographs have been updated and the compounds re-evaluated.

Halogenated aromatic hydrocarbon pesticides and microbicides

Halogenated aromatic hydrocarbon pesticides and microbicides are or have been produced in vast quantities and have wide application. Their major uses are against insect pests (HCH and lindane, chlordane, chlordecone, 1,2-dibromo-3-chloropropane, dichlorvos, heptachlor, methoxychlor, mirex and toxaphene) and as microbicides (hexachlorobenzene, hexachlorobutadiene, hexachlorophene, pentachlorophenol and trichlorophenols).

Most of these chemicals, except the tri- and pentachlorophenols and dichlorvos (which also has an organophosphate grouping), are degraded slowly; the chlorophenols can, however, contain or form the highly toxic chlorinated aromatic hydrocarbon impurities, chlorinated dibenzo- *para*-dioxins and chlorinated dibenzofurans (IARC, 1978b), which are also degraded slowly. Such slow degradation and environmental persistence enhances potential chronic exposure. Other common characteristics of these chemicals are their lipid (fat) solubility and slow metabolism or limited excretion in vertebrate species, resulting in long-term persistence in body tissues. Environmental persistence combined with slow excretion strongly favours bioaccumulation in an ecosystem.

Human exposure to certain of the halogenated aromatic hydrocarbon pesticides and microbicides results in a body burden of long duration; preferential storage occurs in fat or in tissues with high lipid content. Blood levels are usually lower than those in fat but are proportional to the fat levels. Residues have also been observed in the skin months or years after dermal exposure (Kazen et al., 1974). Since these chemicals have an extended biological half-life, continuing exposure over a period of time is cumulative. Males typically retain higher levels than females (Burns & Miller, 1975; Wassermann et al., 1974a,b).

Body burdens of these pesticides have been reported in populations throughout the world: in Australia (Siyali, 1972; Siyali & Simson, 1973), the Federal Republic of Germany (Rappl & Waiblinger, 1975), France (Luquet et al., 1975), Israel (Wassermann et al., 1974a), Japan (Curley et al., 1973; Morita et al., 1975), Norway (Lunde & Bjørseth, 1977), Uganda (Wassermann et al., 1974b) and the US (Jonsson et al., 1977; Kutz et al., 1974).

The principal source of general human exposure is thought to be diet, although direct exposure is also likely to occur from the spraying of large geographic areas during insect control campaigns (Mughal & Rahman, 1973). Most of these compounds have also been detected in US drinking-water (US Environmental Protection Agency, 1978). Dietary exposure can result from consumption of contaminated vegetables and seeds, meat, fish, eggs, milk and dairy products. Occupational exposure to many of these chemicals results in body burdens that are higher than those of the general population (Burns et al., 1974; Lunde & Bjørseth, 1977). Populations geographically proximate to industrial chemical plants have also been found to have increased body burdens (Burns & Miller, 1975). Human infants are exposed transplacentally to chemicals stored in maternal tissues and subsequently through consumption of their mothers' milk (Rappl & Waiblinger, 1975; West et al., 1975).

Halogenated hydrocarbon solvents

The most widely used degreasing solvents among the compounds considered are tetrachloroethylene (also used in dry-cleaning textiles), 1,1,1-trichloroethane, trichloroethylene and dichloromethane. Trichloroethylene and dichloromethane have also been used in the extraction of caffeine, fats and hops; dichloromethane is used extensively as a paint remover. Carbon tetrachloride and chloroform have been used as fumigants and for the manufacture of fluorocarbons. 1,2-Dichloroethane is used as a fumigant, as a lead scavenger in petrol and in the manufacture of vinyl chloride. 1,1,1-Trichloroethane and 1,1,2-trichloroethane are used in the manufacture of vinylidene chloride. All of these compounds have been found in US drinking-water (US Environmental Protection Agency, 1978).

Unlike the halogenated aromatic hydrocarbon pesticides, these compounds are readily metabolized in vivo, and their degradation products are rapidly excreted, mainly in the urine. There is little long-term storage in fat tissues.

Flame retardant

The flame retardant, tris(2,3-dibromopropyl) phosphate, has been used widely in textiles, notably in those used to make sleeping apparel for children. It was considered here because the results of a National Cancer Institute Bioassay Report had become available, subsequent to its identification as a mutagen in bacterial systems.

Production volumes

The amounts of these compounds that are manufactured commercially and the year of their introduction into commerce are shown in Table 1. The year of first commercial production is given because it allows a reasonable estimation to be made of the time from which human exposure could have occurred. The total, worldwide annual production of these compounds was estimated on the basis of the latest available figures from three representative areas - Europe, Japan and the US.

Rebuttable presumption against registration of pesticides

The 1972 Federal Environmental Pesticide Control Act (amendments to the 1947 Federal Insecticide, Fungicide and Rodenticide Act) gives the US Environmental Protection Agency (EPA) additional authority for registering new pesticides and provides for re-authorization of currently registered pesticide uses. A pesticide is registered for use only if labelling re-quirements are satisfied and only if its use according to directions causes no 'unreasonable adverse effects on man or the environment'. The burden of providing evidence of safety is placed on the manufacturer.

In July 1975, the EPA implemented new regulations which further de-fined 'unreasonable adverse effects' in terms of chronic toxic, mutagenic or carcinogenic effects. Pesticides that produce such effects are subject to a 'rebuttable presumption' of being banned. If the EPA determines that the use of a pesticide meets or exceeds any of several published risk criteria that are designed to identify unreasonable adverse effects in the environment, a notice of a 'rebuttable presumption against registration' (RPAR) is issued. The prospective registrant is given 90 days to challenge this presumption by submitting information that the evidence supporting the RPAR is not valid, in that the risk is not real or that potential benefits exceed potential risks. If the notice is successfully rebutted, re-registration occurs without a hearing; if the new information is insufficient or if none is supplied, the EPA issues a notice of intent to deny, cancel or suspend registration, or to hold a public hearing. So far, the EPA has initiated RPARs against about 45 pesticides.

Experimental data

Evaluations of the carcinogenicity in experimental animals of several compounds considered in this volume are based largely on data obtained from the US National Cancer Institute Bioassay Program. The Working Group

TABLE 1

CHEMICAL	YEAR OF FIRST COMMERCIAL PRODUCTION	LATEST ESTIMATED ANNUAL WORLD PRODUCTION
Pesticides and microbicides		
Chlordane	1947	10 million kg
Chlordecone	1966	∿ 500,000 kg
1,2-Dibromo-3-chloropropane	1955	30 million kg
Dichlorvos	1961	12 million kg
Heptachlor and heptachlor epoxide	1953	3 million kg
Hexachlorobenzene	1933	2 million kg
Hexachlorobutadiene[a]	Unknown	Unknown
Hexachlorocyclohexane HCH	1945	∿100 million kg
Lindane	1950	8 million kg
Hexachlorophene	1951	Unknown
Methoxychlor	1946	2.5 million kg
Mirex	1958	225,000 kg
Pentachlorophenol	1950	20 million kg
Toxaphene	1947	∿ 20 million kg
2,4,5-Trichlorophenol	1950	Unknown, but >10 million kg
2,4,6-Trichlorophenol	1950	Unknown, but >120,000 kg

CHEMICAL	YEAR OF FIRST COMMERCIAL PRODUCTION	LATEST ESTIMATED ANNUAL WORLD PRODUCTION
Solvents		
Carbon tetrachloride	1907	806 million kg
Chloroform	1922	300 million kg
1,2-Dichloroethane	1922	5000 million kg
Dichloromethane	1934	>270 million kg
Hexachloroethane	1921	>730,000 kg
1,1,2,2-Tetrachloroethane	1921	20 million kg
Tetrachloroethylene	1925	950 million kg
1,1,1-Trichloroethane	1946	~ 600 million kg
1,1,2-Trichloroethane	1941-1943	Unknown, but >40 million kg
Trichloroethylene	1908	500 million kg
Flame retardant		
Tris(2,3-dibromopropyl) phosphate	1959	5 million kg

[a] Also a waste product in the manufacture of tetrachloroethylene, carbon tetrachloride, chlorine and trichloroethylene: ~ 6 million kg

recognized that in several instances these data had limitations, most
often due to the design of the test and partly to the incomplete reporting
of the results; in particular: (1) the limited number of concurrent
controls and the varying number of pooled controls do not permit, in
certain instances, a statistical analysis of the results; (2) the
initial doses used in tests on certain chemicals were in excess of the
maximum tolerated dose and caused early mortality among treated animals;
the dose levels and dosage schedules therefore had to be altered during
the course of the test; and (3) some of the reports were made available
in the form of preliminary drafts, and the results appearing on such
drafts will have to be compared with those in the final published reports.

With regard to the study involving intraperitoneal injection of
several of the compounds into mice (Theiss *et al*., 1977), the Working
Group noted that this test system was designed as a short-term, whole-
animal bioassay in which the development of lung tumours was used as an
indication of carcinogenicity. Negative results in this system were
considered to be insufficient evidence that a compound is not carcinogenic.

When the Working Group carried out statistical analyses of tumour
incidences in treated animals compared with those in controls, the χ^2
test (one-tailed) with the introduction of Yates' correction was normally
employed. When the incidence of tumours in controls was zero, a Fisher
exact analysis was done. The resulting P values have been inserted, in
square brackets, in the text of the monographs.

Among the chemicals considered in this volume that were evaluated
as having *sufficient evidence* of carcinogenicity in experimental animals
(see preamble, p. 14), the order of magnitude of the total doses of the
substances varied widely. On the other hand, adequate dose-response
experiments were not available for most substances, thus precluding any
indication of the lowest effective doses. For chemicals that caused
cancer in animals at relatively high dose levels, the possibility exists
that the effects were caused by impurities or additives; known carcinogens
that may occur, either as contaminants or additives, in several of the
chemicals evaluated (in parentheses) are: heptachlor (in chlordane);
2,3,7,8-tetrachlorodibenzo-*para*-dioxin, 2,4,5-trichloro- and pentachlorophen
(in hexachlorophene); epichlorohydrin (in trichloroethylene); and
1,2-dibromo-3-chloropropane [in tris(2,3-dibromopropyl) phosphate].
Human populations are exposed more often to such technical-grade products
or mixtures than they are to pure compounds. Another concern in evaluating
carcinogenic potential is the wide chemical variability and percentage
composition of certain commercial products, such as HCH and toxaphene.

For several of the chemicals considered in this volume, the data
available to the Working Group were considered inadequate to evaluate
carcinogenicity. The Working Group was aware, however, that carcinogenicity
studies are in progress on most of them (IARC, 1978c). For some,
further experimental studies using multiple doses would be desirable;

however, specific recommendations would necessitate extensive *ad hoc* discussions in each case.

The Working Group strongly supported the concept that negative results should be reported and disseminated with the same thoroughness and accuracy as are positive results. To satisfy the need to obtain results that are internationally acceptable and comparable, basic requirements for the conduct of long-term carcinogenicity and related short-term tests should be developed and followed.

In the section on mutagenicity and other related short-term tests, the variable results (or lack of concordance between carcinogenicity in experimental animals and results of short-term tests) for many of the compounds may indicate that these tests are of limited value for screening some halogenated hydrocarbons. Negative results may be attributable to low metabolic rates or to inappropriate pathways in *in vitro* metabolic systems, to limited solubility (which may prevent interaction with genetic targets) or to mutagen specificity (selective induction of genetic changes which are not scored in a particular test system).

Epidemiological data[1]

Results from epidemiological studies and/or case reports were available for only a limited number of chemicals considered in this volume; the scarcity of epidemiological studies on these compounds was stressed by the Working Group. A longitudinal study on exposed cohorts that were followed up for a reasonable period was available for only one substance, trichloroethylene; this careful, but relatively small study involved 518 individuals observed for a total of 7688 person-years (Axelson *et al.*, 1978).

Barthel (1976) reported a high incidence of lung cancer (10 cases *versus* 0.54 expected) among farm workers exposed to various pesticides (including DDT, HCH, toxaphene, phenoxyacetic acids, organophosphorous compounds and arsenic-containing agents). This study illustrates the difficulties of distinguishing between various concomitant, and therefore confounding, exposures. It would thus probably be difficult to undertake meaningful epidemiological studies for many of the compounds reviewed in this volume, since exposed individuals can be expected to have had contact with other carcinogenic substances; the detection of a carcinogenic risk due specifically to a particular chemical can rarely be assessed. This does not, however, rule out the usefulness of occupational health epidemiology related to work practices.

---

[1]The Working Group was aware of an epidemiological study in progress to evaluate the carcinogenic effects of pollutants in the general environment, including halogenated hydrocarbons in drinking-water (IARC, 1978d).

Reports of cases of cancer following exposure to a single chemical were available for HCH (Jedlicka *et al.*, 1958), carbon tetrachloride (Johnstone, 1948; Simler *et al.*, 1964; Tracey & Sherlock, 1968) and chlordane containing heptachlor (Infante & Newton, 1975).

Reports of medical surveys of workers exposed to particular chemicals were available for chlordane (Alvarez & Hyman, 1953; Fishbein *et al.*, 1964; Morgan & Roan, 1969; Princi & Spurbeck, 1951), chloroform (Bomski *et al.*, 1967) and dichloromethane (Kuzelova & Vlasak, 1966).

An epidemic of cutanea tarda porphyria in Turkey due to consumption of grain treated with hexachlorobenzene as a fungicide has been reported (Peters, 1976).

Other studies reported in the monographs, which do not relate directly to carcinogenicity in humans, include investigation of the concentrations of β-HCH and heptachlor in fat from terminal patients; there are case reports of aplastic anaemia following exposure to HCH and lindane (over 30 cases) and to pentachlorophenol plus tetrachlorophenol (1 case); lindane has been shown to induce inhibition of cell division in human peripheral blood lymphocytes *in vitro* and to increase the frequency of chromatid breaks; and a significant excess of chromosome aberrations has been observed in lymphocyte cultures from farm workers exposed to polychlorocamphene. The relevance of this information to evaluations of carcinogenicity for humans is unknown; nonetheless, it must be stressed that, although many of the chemicals considered in this volume are of industrial importance and are produced in considerable amounts in many parts of the world, very few investigations have been carried out on their long-term effects in humans.

References

Alvarez, W.C. & Hyman, S. (1953) Absence of toxic manifestations in
    workers exposed to chlordane. Arch. ind. Hyg. occup. Med., 8, 480-483

Axelson, O., Andersson, K., Hogstedt, C., Holmberg, B., Molina, G. &
    de Verdier, A. (1978) A cohort study on trichloroethylene exposure
    and cancer mortality. J. occup. Med., 20, 194-196

Barthel, E. (1976) High incidences of lung cancer in persons with chronic
    professional exposure to pesticides in agriculture (Ger.) Z. Erkrank.
    Atm.-Org., 146, 266-274

Bomski, H., Sobolewska, A. & Strakowski, A. (1967) Toxic effect of chloro-
    form on the liver of workers of the chemical industry (Ger.) Int.
    Arch. Gewerbepath. Gewerbehyg., 24, 127-134

Burns, J.E. & Miller, F.M. (1975) Hexachlorobenzene contamination: its
    effects in a Louisiana population. Arch. environ. Health, 30, 44-48

Burns, J.E., Miller, F.M., Gomes, E.D. & Albert, R.A. (1974) Hexachloro-
    benzene exposure from contaminated DCPA in vegetable spraymen. Arch.
    environ. Health, 29, 192-194

Curley, A., Burse, V.W., Jennings, R.W. & Villanueva, E.C. (1973)
    Chlorinated hydrocarbon pesticides and related compounds in adipose
    tissue from people of Japan. Nature (Lond.), 242, 338-340

Fishbein, W.I., White, J.V. & Isaacs, H.J. (1964) Survey of workers
    exposed to chlordane. Ind. Med. Surg., 33, 726-727

IARC (1972) IARC Monographs on the Evaluation of Carcinogenic Risk of
    Chemicals to Man, 1, Lyon, pp. 53-60, 61-65

IARC (1974) IARC Monographs on the Evaluation of Carcinogenic Risk of
    Chemicals to Man, 5, Some Organochlorine Pesticides, Lyon, pp. 47-74,
    173-191, 193-202, 203-210

IARC (1976) IARC Monographs on the Evaluation of Carcinogenic Risk of
    Chemicals to Man, 11, Cadmium, Nickel, Some Epoxides, Miscellaneous
    Industrial Chemicals and General Considerations on Volatile
    Anaesthetics, Lyon, pp. 263-276

IARC (1977) IARC Monographs on the Evaluation of the Carcinogenic Risk of
    Chemicals to Man, 15, Some Fumigants, the Herbicides 2,4-D and
    2,4,5-T, Chlorinated Dibenzodioxins and Miscellaneous Industrial
    Chemicals, Lyon, pp. 139-147

IARC (1978a) IARC Monographs on the Evaluation of the Carcinogenic Risk of Chemicals to Humans, 18, Polychlorinated Biphenyls and Polybrominated Biphenyls, Lyon

IARC (1978b) Long-term hazards of polychlorinated dibenzodioxins and poly-chlorinated dibenzofurans. IARC intern. tech. Rep., No. 78/001, Lyon

IARC (1978c) Information Bulletin on the Survey of Chemicals Being Tested for Carcinogenicity, No. 8, Lyon, pp. 269, 79, 121, 244, 127, 128, 266 242, 276, 326, 267, 25, 255, 277, 72, 250, 328, 226, 256, 272, 228, 241, 381, 243, 24, 270, 247, 271, 330, 256, 272, 277, 331, 382, 344

IARC (1978d) Directory of On-Going Research in Cancer Epidemiology, 1978 (IARC Scientific Publications No. 26), Lyon, p. 263 (Abstract no. 691)

Infante, P.F. & Newton, W.A., Jr (1975) Prenatal chlordane exposure and neuroblastoma. New Engl. J. Med., 293, 308

Jedlicka, V., Hermanska, Z., Smida, I. & Kouba, A. (1958) Paramyeloblastic leukaemia appearing simultaneously in two blood cousins after simultaneous contact with fammexane (hexachlorocyclohexane). Acta med scand., 161, 457-451

Johnstone, R.T. (1948) Occupational Medicine and Industrial Hygiene, St Louis, MO, C.V. Mosby Co., pp. 156-158

Jonsson, V., Liu, G.J.K., Armbruster, J., Kettelhut, L.L. & Drucker, B. (1977) Chlorohydrocarbon pesticide residues in human milk in greater St.Louis, Missouri, 1977. Am. J. clin. Nutr., 30, 1106-1109

Kazen, C., Bloomer, A., Welch, R., Oudbier, A. & Price, H. (1974) Persistence of pesticides on the hands of some occupationally exposed people. Arch. environ. Health, 29, 315-318

Kutz, F.W., Yobs, A.R., Johnson, W.G. & Wiersma, G.B. (1974) Mirex residues in human adipose tissue. Environ. Entomol., 3, 882-884

Kuzelova, M. & Vlasak, R. (1966) The effect of methylene-dichloride on the health of workers in production of film-foils and investigation of formic acid as the methylene-dichloride metabolite (Czech.) Pracov. Lek., 18, 167-170

Lunde, G. & Bjørseth, A. (1977) Human blood samples as indicators of occupational exposure to persistent chlorinated hydrocarbons. Sci. total Environ., 8, 241-246

Luquet, F.M., Goursaud, J. & Casalis, J. (1975) Pollution of human milk with organochlorine insecticide residues in France (Fr.). Lait, 55, 207-211

Morgan & Roan, C.C. (1969) Renal function in persons occupationally
    exposed to pesticides. Arch. environ. Health, 19, 633-636

Morita, M., Mimura, S., Ohi, G. & Yagyu, H. (1975) A systematic
    determination of chlorinated benzenes in human adipose tissue.
    Environ. Pollut., 9, 175-179

Mughal, H.A. & Rahman, M.A. (1973) Organochlorine pesticide content of
    human adipose tissue in Karachi. Arch. environ. Health, 27, 396-398

Peters, H.A. (1976) Hexachlorobenzene poisoning in Turkey. Fed. Proc.,
    35, 2400-2403

Princi, F. & Spurbeck, G.H. (1951) A study of workers exposed to the
    insecticides chlordane, aldrin, dieldrin. Arch. ind. Hyg. occup. Med.,
    3, 64-72

Rappl, A. & Waiblinger, W. (1975) Contamination of human milk with
    chlorinated hydrocarbon residues (Ger.). Dtsch. med. Wschr., 100,
    228-238

Simler, M., Maurer, M. & Mandard, J.C. (1964) Liver cancer and cirrhosis
    due to carbon tetrachloride (Fr.). Strasbourg Méd., December,
    pp. 910-918

Siyali, D.S. (1972) Hexachlorobenzene and other organochlorine pesticides
    in human blood. Med. J. Aust., 2, 1063-1066

Siyali, D.S. & Simson, R.E. (1973) Chlorinated hydrocarbon pesticides in
    human blood and fat. Med. J. Aust., 1, 212-213

Theiss, J.C. Stoner, G.D., Shimkin, M.B. & Weisburger, E.K. (1977) Test
    for carcinogenicity of organic contaminants of United States drinking
    waters by pulmonary tumor response in strain A mice. Cancer Res., 37,
    2717-2720

Tracey, J.P. & Sherlock, P. (1968) Hepatoma following carbon tetrachloride
    poisoning. New York State J. Med., 68, 2202-2204

US Environmental Protection Agency (1978) Chemical indications of indus-
    trial contamination. Fed. Regist., 43, 5773

Wassermann, M., Tomatis, L., Wassermann, D., Day, N.E., Groner, Y.,
    Lazarovici, S. & Rosenfeld, D. (1974a) Epidemiology of organochlorine
    insecticides in the adipose tissue of Israelis. Pest. Monit. J., 8,
    1-7

Wassermann, M., Tomatis, L., Wassermann, D., Day, N.E. & Djavaherian, M.
    (1974b) Storage of organochlorine insecticides in adipose tissue of
    Ugandans. Bull. environ. Contam. Toxicol., 12, 501-508

West, R.W., Wilson, D.J. & Schaffner, W. (1975) Hexachlorophene
     concentrations in human milk. <u>Bull. environ. Contam. Toxicol</u>., <u>13</u>,
     167-169

THE MONOGRAPHS

PESTICIDES AND MICROBICIDES

CHLORDANE

A review on chlordane is available (Mercier, 1975).

1.   Chemical and Physical Data

1.1   Synonyms and trade names

Chem. Abstr. Services Reg. No.: 57-74-9

Chem. Abstr. Name: 1,2,4,5,6,7,8,8-Octachloro-2,3,3a,4,7,7a-hexahydro-4,7-methano-1H-indene

Synonyms: Dichlorochlordene; 1,2,4,5,6,7,8,8-octachloro-2,3,3a,4,7,7a-hexahydro-4,7-methanoindene; 1,2,4,5,6,7,8,8-octachloro-4,7-methano-3a,4,7,7a-tetrahydroindane; octachloro-4,7-methanotetrahydroindane; 1,2,4,5,6,7,8,8-octachloro-3a,4,7,7a-tetrahydro-4,7-methanoindan

Trade names: 1068; Aspon; Belt; CD 68; Chlordan; Chlorindan; Chlor Kil; Chlorodane; Corodane; Cortilan-neu; Dowchlor; ENT-9932; HCS 3260; Kypchlor; M 140; M 410; Niran; Octachlor; Octa-Klor; Oktaterr; Ortho-Klor; Synklor; Tat Chlor 4; Topichlor 20; Topiclor; Toxichlor; Velsicol 1068

1.2   Structural and molecular formulae and molecular weight

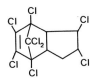

$C_{10}H_6Cl_8$ Mol. wt: 409.8

1.3   Chemical and physical properties

From Spencer (1973), unless otherwise specified

(a) Description: Viscous, amber-coloured liquid

(b) Melting-point: 106-107°C (*cis*-isomer); 104-105°C (*trans*-isomer) (Martin & Worthing, 1977)

(c) Density: d^{25} 1.59-1.63

(d) Refractive index: n_D^{25} 1.56-1.57

(e) Spectroscopy data: Infra-red, ultra-violet (Gore *et al.*, 1971) and Raman spectra (Nicholas *et al.*, 1976) have been tabulated.

(f) Solubility: Insoluble in water; soluble in most organic solvents, including petroleum hydrocarbons

(g) Viscosity: 75-120 centistokes at 55°C

(h) Volatility: Vapour pressure is 0.00001 mm at 25°C.

(i) Reactivity: Chlorine is lost in the presence of alkali.

1.4 Technical products and impurities

The approximate composition of technical chlordane is as follows: *trans*-chlordane (γ-chlordane), 24%; chlordene isomers, 21.5%; *cis*-chlordane (α-chlordane), 19%; heptachlor, 10%; nonachlor, 7%; Diels-Alder adduct of cyclopentadiene and pentachlorocyclopentadiene, 2%; hexachlorocyclopentadiene, 1%; octachlorocyclopentene, 1%; miscellaneous constituents, 15.5%.

Chlordane has been available in the US as dusts containing 5, 6 and 10% chlordane, as granules containing 5-33.3%, as wettable powders containing 25 and 40%, as oil solutions containing 2 and 20%, and as emulsifiable concentrates containing 4 and 8 lbs/gal (480 and 960 g/l) of the chemical (von Rumker *et al.*, 1975).

2. Production, Use, Occurrence and Analysis

2.1 Production and use

(a) Production

Chlordane was first prepared in the 1940s by exhaustive chlorination of the cyclopentadiene-hexachlorocyclopentadiene adduct (Hyman, 1949). For its commercial manufacture, hexachlorocyclopentadiene is condensed with cyclopentadiene to produce chlordene, which is then chlorinated to give chlordane.

Chlordane was first produced commercially in the US in 1947 (US Tariff Commission, 1949); in 1976, only one US company reported production of an undisclosed amount (see preamble, p. 16) (US International Trade Commission, 1977). US production in 1974 amounted to 9.5 million kg (US Environmental Protection Agency, 1976a). In 1972, US exports of chlordane were 2.3 million kg; none was imported (von Rumker *et al.*, 1975).

Chlordane is not produced in Europe and has never been manufactured or imported into Japan.

(b) Use

In the past, chlordane was registered in the US for insecticidal use on a wide variety of fruit, vegetable and grain crops, as well as for non-crop uses such as on agricultural premises, ditch banks and roadsides (US Environmental Protection Agency, 1971).

In 1974, 9.5 million kg chlordane were used in the US as follows: pest control (commercial), 34.7%; home, lawn and garden, 29.9%; corn, 20.4%; turf, 5.9%; potatoes, 5.2%; tomatoes, 1.6%; ornamental shrubs, 1.2%; strawberries, 0.8%; and other vegetables, 0.3% (US Environmental Protection Agency, 1976a).

On 6 March, 1978, a cancellation proceeding instituted by the US Environmental Protection Agency on heptachlor/chlordane was terminated, and a settlement was reached for the contested uses (US Environmental Protection Agency, 1978). The settlement allows for limited usage of chlordane by crop, location (in some cases), maximum time interval for permitted use and amount allowed for specific uses (technical chlordane), as follows: citrus, California and Texas, until 31 December 1979, a total of 36.3 thousand kg; grapes, California, until 1 July 1980, 40.9 thousand kg; flax, until 1 October 1978, 6.8 thousand kg; and strawberries, until 1 August 1979, 22.7 thousand kg. In addition, 159 thousand kg of technical chlordane may be used, until 31 December 1980, on fire ants in 9 US states; no more than 227 thousand kg may be used for nursery stock quarantine programs until 31 December 1979 (Anon. 1978a). After 1 July 1983, the only approved use for chlordane will be for underground termite control (Anon. 1978b).

A tolerance of 0.3 mg/kg has been established by the US Environmental Protection Agency for residues of chlordane (containing not more than 1% of the intermediate compound, hexachlorocyclopentadiene, as an impurity) in or on approximately 50 fruit and vegetable crops (US Environmental Protection Agency, 1976b).

The Joint Meeting of the FAO Working Party of Experts on Pesticide Residues and the WHO Expert Committee on Pesticide Residues, in November 1972, re-established residue tolerances ranging from 0.02-0.5 ppm (mg/kg) for the sum of the *cis*- and *trans*-isomers of chlordane and oxychlordane (WHO, 1973). An acceptable daily intake (ADI) for humans of 0-0.001 mg/kg bw was confirmed in December 1977 (FAO/WHO, 1978).

The US Occupational Safety and Health Administration's health standards require that an employee's dermal exposure to chlordane not exceed 0.5 mg/m^3 in the workplace in any 8-hr work shift of a 40-hr work week (US Occupational Safety & Health Administration, 1977).

2.2 Occurrence

Chlordane is not known to occur as a natural product.

Reviews on the occurrence of chlordane in fish and wildlife, air, soil, water, crops and food items have been published (Fairchild *et al.*, 1976; Fitzhugh *et al.*, 1976).

(a) Air

Chlordane was found in 10/13 air samples taken around Bermuda and between Bermuda and Rhode Island during February-June 1973; levels ranged from <0.005-0.90 ng/m^3 (Bidleman & Olney, 1974).

(b) Water and sediments

The occurrence of chlorinated cyclopentadiene pesticides, including chlordane, in US drinking-water has been reviewed (Safe Drinking Water Committee, 1977). Tabulations of the occurrence of chlordane in rain-water, river-water, drinking-water, land runoff and chemical plant effluent water in the US have also been published (Eurocop-Cost, 1976; Shackelford & Keith, 1976).

Rain, snow and lake water in Hawaii have been analysed for organo-chlorine pesticides: chlordane was found in 4 samples of rainwater in parts per trillion (ng/l) amounts (Bevenue, *et al.*, 1972).

Chlordane was found in two streams in Ontario at levels ranging from <1-21 ng/l (*trans*-chlordane) (Miles & Harris, 1973), in drainage ditches, wells, ponds and reservoirs in Nova Scotia at levels ranging from 0-31.3 µg/l (*cis*-chlordane) and 0-17.89 µg/l (*trans*-chlordane) (Burns *et al.*, 1975) and in the lower Mississippi River at concentrations which varied during the year from 0.4-1.2 ng/l (*trans*-chlordane) (Brodtmann, 1976).

cis-Chlordane was found in 89.9% of filtered samples and 42.7% of unfiltered samples of sea-water from a marina in Hawaii, and *trans*-chlordane in 67.7% of filtered and 67.7% of unfiltered samples. The authors suspected that organic particulate matter interfered with the determination of *cis*-chlordane in the unfiltered samples. Of samples of sediment from the same marina, 97.2% contained *cis*-chlordane, in a concentration range of 0.4-5.27 µg/kg (average, 3.0), and 92.7% contained *trans*-chlordane, in a concentration range of 1.33-5.12 µg/kg (average, 2.3) (Tanita *et al.*, 1976).

Chlordane was found in concentrations ranging from 4.3-8.0 µg/kg in bottom material from 36/39 streams tributary to San Francisco Bay (Law & Goerlitz, 1974), in 32.7% of 214 sediment samples from surface waters in southern Florida (Mattraw, 1975), in bottom mud from 2 streams in Ontario, at levels ranging from <0.1-3.1 µg/kg (*trans*-chlordane) (Miles & Harris, 1973), and in sediments from streambeds and drainage ditches in Nova Scotia, at levels ranging from 0-664 µg/kg (*cis*-chlordane) and 0-51 µg/kg (*trans*-chlordane) (Burns *et al.*, 1975).

(c) Soil

Residues of chlordane were found in 16-64% of 400 soil samples taken from 8 cities, at levels of 0.02-20.48 mg/kg (Wiersma *et al.*, 1972), and in 7.4-42.3% of 356 soil samples taken from 14 cities, at levels of 0.04-13.9 mg/kg (Carey *et al.*, 1976).

In 1970, as part of the National Soils Monitoring Program, data on soil and crop residues were collected from 1506 cropland sites in 35 states; chlordane was detected 165 times, in a range of 0.01-13.34 mg/kg (Crockett *et al.*, 1974).

The half-life of chlordane in soil when used at agricultural rates is approximately 1 year (Anon., 1976).

(d) Food and drink

In a continuing programme involving the monitoring of pesticide residues in food, the US Department of Health, Education, and Welfare found chlordane in a trace amount in one composite sample of garden fruits collected at retail outlets in the period July 1972-July 1973 (US Food & Drug Administration, 1975a), and in one composite sample of grains and cereals collected at retail outlets in the period August 1973-July 1974 (US Food & Drug Administration, 1977).

trans-Chlordane was found in 78% of chicken eggs, at an average concentration of 2 µg/kg, and *cis*-chlordane was found in 81% of eggs, at an average concentration of 1 µg/kg (Mes *et al.*, 1974).

Of 200 cow's milk samples analysed in the US, 87% were positive for chlordane, with levels ranging from 0.02-0.06 mg/l (Safe Drinking Water Committee, 1977).

Chlordane was found in Canadian meat samples at levels ranging from 0-106 µg/kg in beef, 0-32 µg/kg in pork and 0-70 µg/kg in fowl (Saschenbrecker, 1976).

One-third of small oysters sampled in Hawaii contained *cis*-chlordane
in a concentration range of 2.34-57.64 µg/kg (18.64 average), and 13% contained *trans*-chlordane in an average concentration of 8.17 µg/kg. All of
the large oysters sampled contained *cis*-chlordane in a concentration range
of 1.58-22.99 µg/kg (8.277 average), and 64% contained *trans*-chlordane in
a concentration range of 1.35-23.38 µg/kg (7.865 average) (Tanita *et al.*,
1976).

(e) Animals

cis-Chlordane was present in the carcasses of 10/37 bald eagles at
concentrations of 0.11-7.4 mg/kg (0.30 median) and in the brains of 7 of
the birds at concentrations of 0.05-1.7 mg/kg (0.11 median) (Cromartie
et al., 1975). Fish eggs taken from Iowa rivers in 1971 were found to
have chlordane residues of 24-350 µg/kg (Johnson & Morris, 1974).

(f) Occupational exposure

A 1974 National Occupational Hazard Survey in the US indicated that
workers primarily exposed to chlordane were those in gas and other service
industries, disinfecting and exterminating occupations and cigarette manufacture (National Institute for Occupational Safety & Health, 1977).

2.3 Analysis

A review of analytical methods for chlordane residues has been published (Fitzhugh *et al.*, 1976); extraction and clean-up methods have also
been evaluated (US Food & Drug Administration, 1975b). Methods used for
the analysis of chlordane in environmental samples are listed in Table 1.

Other analytical methods designed to isolate or identify chlordane include gel-permeation chromatography (Johnson *et al.*, 1976) and gas chroma-
tography/mass spectrometry (Keith *et al.*, 1976).

3.   Biological Data Relevant to the Evaluation
of Carcinogenic Risk to Humans

3.1 Carcinogenicity studies in animals

Oral administration

Mouse: Epstein (1976) reported a previously unpublished study by the
International Research and Development Corporation, carried out in 1973,
in which groups of 100 male and 100 female Charles River CD-1 mice, 6 weeks
of age, were fed technical-grade chlordane (purity not given) at three dose
levels, 5, 25 and 50 mg/kg diet, for 18 months. Excluding 10 animals sacrificed from each group for interim study at 6 months, mortality at 18 months
ranged from 27-49%, with the exception of males and females receiving the

TABLE 1. METHODS FOR THE ANALYSIS OF CHLORDANE

SAMPLE TYPE	ANALYTICAL METHOD			
	EXTRACTION/CLEAN-UP	DETECTION	LIMIT OF DETECTION	REFERENCE
Formulations				
Granules	Extract (acetone) in Soxhlet, evaporate to dryness, dissolve (carbon disulphide), evaporate, repeat dissolution in carbon disulphide and evaporation 4 times, dry, dissolve (carbon disulphide)	IR		Malina (1973)
Pesticides	Extract (acetone), filter or centrifuge	TLC		Bontoyan & Jung (1972)
Emulsifiable concentrates	Dilute (toluene), dechlorinate	Titration		Horwitz (1975)
Dusts, granular impregnates & wettable powders	Extract (benzene) in Soxhlet, dechlorinate	Titration		Horwitz (1975)
Liquids, high-concentration solids	Dilute (methanol-benzene)	Colorimetry		Horwitz (1975)
Low-concentration solids	Extract (pentane) in Soxhlet	Colorimetry		Horwitz (1975)
Soil	(a) Extract (hexane-acetone-methanol) in Soxhlet, transfer to hexane			Nash *et al.* (1973)

TABLE 1.   METHODS FOR THE ANALYSIS OF CHLORDANE (continued)

| SAMPLE TYPE | ANALYTICAL METHOD | | | |
	EXTRACTION/CLEAN-UP	DETECTION	LIMIT OF DETECTION	REFERENCE
	(b) Wet sample with ammonium chloride solution, extract (hexane-acetone), decant, repeat extraction	GC/ECD; TLC		
	(c) Prepare Florisil column, add soil, extract (hexane-acetone-methanol) on column, wash with water			
Foods				
Crops	Extract (acetonitrile), filter, liquid/liquid partition, CC	GC/ECD	0.005 mg/kg	Cochrane *et al*. (1975)
Unspecified	Extract (acetone), filter or centrifuge	TLC		Horwitz (1975)

Abbreviations: IR - infra-red spectrometry; TLC - thin-layer chromatography; CC - column chromatography;
               GC/ECD - gas chromatography/electron capture detection

50 mg/kg diet level, in which mortalities of 86 and 76%, respectively, were seen. In addition to high mortality, a relatively large number of animals were lost by autolysis. A dose-related increased incidence of liver nodules was reported in the 25 and 50 mg/kg diet test groups; a dose-related increased incidence of hepatocytomegaly was found in all test groups; and a dose-related increased incidence of nodular hyperplasia, which was statistically significant at the 25 and 50 mg/kg diet levels (P<0.01), was reported. Subsequent re-evaluation of the histology of this study, however, revealed a significant incidence of hepatocellular carcinomas compared with controls. In males receiving 0, 5, 25 or 50 mg/kg diet, hepatocellular carcinomas were found in 3/33, 5/55, 41/52 and 32/39 animals, respectively; in females, the respective incidences were 0/45, 0/61, 35/20 and 26/37.

Groups of 50 male and 50 female B6C3F1 hybrid mice, 5 weeks of age, were fed analytical-grade chlordane, consisting of 94.8% chlordane (71.7% *cis*-chlordane and 23.1% *trans*-chlordane), 0.3% heptachlor, 0.6% nonachlor, 1.1% hexachlorocyclopentadiene, 0.25% chlordene isomers and other chlorinated compounds for 80 weeks. Males received initial levels of 20 and 40 mg/kg diet, and females 40 and 80 mg/kg diet; time-weighted average dietary concentrations were 30 and 56 mg/kg diet for males and 30 and 64 mg/kg diet for females. There were 20 male and 10 female matched controls and 100 male and 80 female pooled controls. Survival in all groups was relatively high: over 60% in treated males and over 80% in treated females, and over 90% in male and female controls. A dose-related increase in the incidence of hepatocellular carcinomas was found in males and females in the high-dose group. The incidences were 43/49 and 34/49 in high-dose males and females, respectively, and 16/48 and 3/47 in low-dose males and females, respectively, compared with 2/18 and 0/19 in male and female matched controls, respectively (National Cancer Institute, 1977).

Rat: Groups of 50 male and 50 female, 5-week-old Osborne-Mendel rats were administered analytical-grade chlordane in the diet for 80 weeks, at initial dose levels of 400 and 800 mg/kg for males and 200 and 400 mg/kg for females. These were reduced during the experiment due to adverse toxic effects; the time-weighted average dietary concentrations were 407 and 203 mg/kg diet for males and 241 and 121 mg/kg diet for females. There were 10 male and 10 female matched controls and 60 male and 60 female pooled controls. Survivors were killed at 80 weeks, at which time approximately 50% of treated and control males and 60% of treated females and 90% of control females were still alive. In all treated animals combined there was an excess incidence of follicular-cell thyroid neoplasms (10/75 in treated females and 7/65 in treated males *versus* 0/10, 3/58, 0/6 and 4/51 in matched and pooled female and male controls); there was an excess of malignant fibrous histiocytomas in all treated males (8/88 *versus* 0/8 and 2/58 in matched and pooled controls) (National Cancer Institute, 1977).

3.2 Other relevant biological data

(a) Experimental systems

Toxic effects

The acute oral LD_{50} of chlordane is 335+ 40 mg/kg for male rats and 430+40 mg/kg bw for female rats (Gaines, 1960). The oral LD_{50} for mice is 430 mg/kg bw.

Commercial samples of chlordane may contain hexachlorocyclopentadiene (see section 1.4), whose toxicity has been described (WHO, 1968). When chlordane is given orally to rats at a dose of 25 mg/kg bw/day for 15 days it has no toxic effects, while 50 mg/kg bw or more result in toxic effects and death; it has cumulative toxic effects (Ambrose *et al.*, 1953). The toxic effects of chlordane in rats include stimulation of the central nervous system, stomach ulcers, inflammation of the intestine, nephritis, hepatitis, an increase in liver weight, coma and death (Boyd & Taylor, 1969).

Chlordane induces hepatic drug-metabolizing enzymes in all species examined (reviewed by Fouts, 1970). Oestradiol-17β and oestrone metabolism were also stimulated by chlordane pretreatment in mice and rats, respectively (Welch *et al.*, 1971).

Chlordane decreased fertility in female and male rats (Ambrose *et al.*, 1953) and in female mice (Welch *et al.*, 1971).

Embryotoxicity and teratogenicity

In an abstract, it was reported that mice maintained for 4 months on a diet containing 100 mg/kg diet chlordane had decreased viability of offspring (Deichmann & Keplinger, 1966). Ambrose *et al.* (1953) also reported reduced survival of offspring.

Absorption, distribution, excretion and metabolism

Rats excreted about 5% of an oral dose of chlordane in the urine and the rest in the faeces over 7 days. Only small amounts of unchanged chlordane were detected; the several metabolites have various degrees of dechlorination and ring hydroxylation (Barnett & Dorough, 1974). Oxychlordane (α-chloroepoxide) was the major residue in fat, liver and kidney (Barnett & Dorough, 1974; Street & Blau, 1972); it was also detected in the milk of cows administered chlordane (Lawrence *et al.*, 1970).

Both *cis*- and *trans*-chlordane were metabolized in rats *via* 1,2-dichlorochlordene (I) and oxychlordane (II) to 1-*exo*-hydroxy-2-chlorochlordene (III) and 1-*exo*-hydroxy-2-*endo*-chloro-2,3-*exo*-epoxychlordene (IV) (see

Fig. 1), which are not readily metabolized further, and to various other hydroxylated products. Another major metabolic route for the *cis* isomer involves more direct hydroxylation to form 1-*exo*-hydroxydihydrochlordene and 1,2-*trans*-dihydroxydihydrochlordene. The *cis* isomer was excreted as hydroxylated metabolites more readily than the *trans* isomer, which was more readily converted to oxychlordane. Heptachlor was a minor metabolite of both isomers (Tashiro & Matsumura, 1977).

Mutagenicity and other related short-term tests

Pure chlordane was not mutagenic in any strain of *Salmonella typhimurium* (TA1535, TA1537, TA1538, TA98, TA100) that was tested (Tardiff *et al.*, 1976). Chlordane induced gene conversions in *Saccharomyces cervisiae* strain D4 (Chambers & Dutta, 1976).

cis-Chlordane weakly inhibited sporulation in *Helminthosporium sativum* (Pero & Owens, 1971). Chlordane (60% pure) was not mutagenic in a spot test in the reverse mutation assay with *Escherichia coli* WP2 (try⁻) (Ashwood-Smith *et al.*, 1972).

A 0.01 mM concentration of chlordane induced ouabain-resistant mutants in Chinese hamster V79 cells (Ahmed *et al.*, 1977a).

Neither *cis*-chlordane (42, 58 and 290 mg/kg bw i.p., or 5 daily oral doses of 75 mg/kg bw) nor the *trans* isomer (5 daily oral doses of 50 mg/kg bw) had a significant effect in the dominant lethal assay in mice (Epstein *et al.*, 1972). Similar negative results were reported in dominant lethal studies with mice that were given single doses (50 or 100 mg/kg bw) of technical-grade chlordane either by oral intubation or by i.p. administration (Arnold *et al.*, 1977).

trans-Chlordane (99.8% pure) inhibited division of L-5178Y cells in culture but did not inhibit DNA synthesis (Brubaker *et al.*, 1970); *cis*-chlordane had no effect on DNA repair synthesis in HeLa cells (Brandt *et al.*, 1972). In concentrations of 1, 10, 100 and 1000 μM, chlordane induced unscheduled DNA synthesis (measured autoradiographically) in SV-40 transformed human cells (VA-4) in culture, but the effect disappeared when rat liver microsomes were added to the culture during treatment. The DNA repair kinetics and the size of the repaired regions resulting from chlordane treatment (studied by 313 nm photolysis of repaired regions containing bromodeoxyuridine) were similar to that after exposure to 254 nm ultra-violet radiation (Ahmed *et al.*, 1977b).

Technical-grade chlordane contains a volatile component (not specified) which causes mutations in *S. typhimurium* TA100, but not in TA1535, TA1537, TA1538 or TA98 (Tardiff *et al.*, 1976).

(b) Humans

Symptoms of acute chlordane poisoning in man include nervousness, convulsions and loss of coordination (Aldrich & Holmes, 1969). An oral

Figure 1.   Simplified metabolism of chlordane in rats (adapted from
            Tashira & Matsumura, 1977)

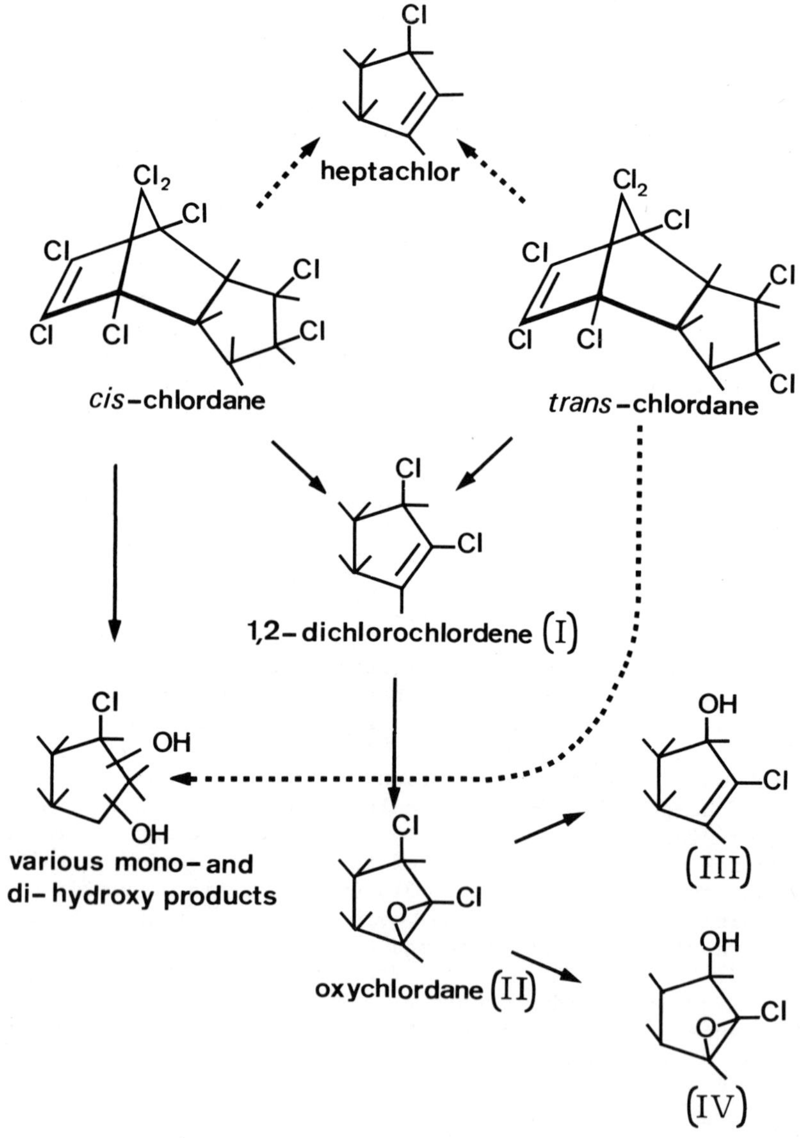

dose of 100 mg/kg bw was fatal (Derbes *et al.*, 1955).

In a case of acute chlordane poisoning in a 2-year-old child, the half-life of serum chlordane was about 21 days; 300 times more chlordane entered the fat than the urine (Curley & Garrettson, 1969).

In 1976, when a segment of a municipal water system was contaminated with chlordane, 13 persons showed gastrointestinal (nausea, vomiting) or neurological symptoms (Harrington *et al.*, 1978).

Metabolites of chlordane, *trans*-nonachlor and oxychlordane, have been found in the tissues of non-occupationally exposed people in the US (Sovocool & Lewis, 1975); 0.03-0.40 mg/kg oxychlordane have been found in adipose tissue in the general population (Biros & Enos, 1973).

3.3 Case reports and epidemiological studies

Several clinical studies have been made of men exposed to chlordane during its manufacture or during its use as a pesticide (Alvarez & Hyman, 1953; Fishbein *et al.*, 1964; Morgan & Roan, 1969; Princi & Spurbeck, 1951) [The Working Group noted that these studies were uninformative with regard to the carcinogenicity of chlordane, since each study had serious limitations, e.g., small numbers, disproportionate number of current employees, short follow-up time since first exposure].

Infante *et al.* (1978) reviewed 25 previously reported cases of blood dyscrasia associated with exposure to chlordane or heptachlor, either alone or in combination with other drugs, in conjunction with 3 newly diagnosed cases of aplastic anaemia and 3 of acute leukaemia associated with a prior history of exposure to technical-grade chlordane containing 3-7% heptachlor. During the period December 1974-February 1976, 5 of 14 children with neuroblastoma admitted to one paediatric hospital had a positive history of pre- or postnatal exposure to technical-grade chlordane containing 3-7% heptachlor; history of exposure to chlordane had not yet been ascertained for the remaining 9 cases.

4. Summary of Data Reported and Evaluation

4.1 Experimental data

Chlordane (analytical grade) was tested in one experiment in mice and in one in rats by oral administration. It produced hepatocellular carcinomas in mice of both sexes; in rats, the results were inconclusive. A re-evaluation of unpublished studies involving the oral administration of technical-grade chlordane to mice of another strain confirmed the hepatocarcinogenicity of chlordane for mice of both sexes.

Chlordane induced gene conversions in yeast but was not shown to be mutagenic in bacteria. It induced mutations in mammalian cells in culture but was negative in dominant lethal tests in mice.

4.2 Human data

Case reports suggest a relationship between exposure to chlordane or heptachlor (either alone or in combination with other compounds) and blood dyscrasias. Another publication has also suggested an association with acute leukaemia; an association between both pre- and postnatal exposure to technical-grade chlordane and the development of neuroblastomas in children was also suggested.

No epidemiological studies were available to the Working Group.

The extensive production and use of chlordane over the past several decades, together with the persistent nature of the compound, indicate that widespread human exposure occurs. This is confirmed by many reports of its occurrence in the general environment and in human tissues.

4.3 Evaluation

There is *sufficient evidence* that chlordane is carcinogenic in mice. A report of a number of cases of cancer in humans was also available, but these data do not allow an evaluation of the carcinogenicity of chlordane to humans to be made.

5. References

Ahmed, F.E., Lewis, N.J. & Hart, R.W. (1977a) Pesticide induced ouabain resistant mutants in Chinese hamster V79 cells. Chem.-biol. Interact., 19, 369-374

Ahmed, F.E., Hart, R.W. & Lewis, N.J. (1977b) Pesticide induced DNA damage and its repair in cultured human cells. Mutat. Res., 42, 161-174

Aldrich, F.D. & Holmes, J.H. (1969) Acute chlordane intoxication in a child. Case report with toxicological data. Arch. environ. Health, 19, 129-132

Alvarez, W.C. & Hyman, S. (1953) Absence of toxic manifestations in workers exposed to chlordane. Arch. ind. Hyg. occup. Med., 8, 480-483

Ambrose, A.M., Christensen, H.E., Robbins, D.J. & Rather, L.J. (1953) Toxicological and pharmacological studies on chlordane. Arch. ind. Hyg. occup. Med., 7, 197-210

Anon. (1976) Chlordane and heptachlor: second edition. Vet. Toxicol., 18, 217-221

Anon. (1978a) Heptachlor/chlordane settlement allows corn use until August 1, 1980. Pestic. Toxicol. chem. News, 6 (March 8), 17-19

Anon. (1978b) EPA, Velsicol agree on pesticide limits. Chem. Eng. News, 13 March, p. 15

Arnold, D.W., Kennedy, G.L., Jr, Keplinger, M.L., Calandra, J.C. & Calo, C.J. (1977) Dominant lethal studies with technical chlordane, HCS-3260, and heptachlor:heptachlor epoxide. J. Toxicol. environ. Health, 2, 547-555

Ashwood-Smith, M.J., Trevino, J. & Ring, R. (1972) Mutagenicity of dichlor-vos. Nature (Lond.), 240, 418-420

Barnett, J.R. & Dorough, H.W. (1974) Metabolism of chlordane in rats. J. agric. Food Chem., 22, 612-619

Bevenue, A., Ogata, N.J. & Hylin, J.W. (1972) Organochlorine pesticides in rainwater, Oahu, Hawaii, 1971-1972. Bull. environ. Contam. Toxicol., 8, 238-241

Bidleman, T.F. & Olney, C.E. (1974) Chlorinated hydrocarbons in the Sargasso Sea atmosphere and surface water. Science, 183, 516-518

Biros, F.J. & Enos, H.F. (1973) Oxychlordane residues in human adipose tissue. Bull. environ. Contam. Toxicol., 10, 257-260

Bontoyan, W.R., & Jung, P.D. (1972) Thin layer chromatographic detection of chlorinated hydrocarbons as cross-contaminants in pesticide formulations. J. Assoc. off. anal. Chem., 55, 851-856

Boyd, E.M. & Taylor, F.I. (1969) The acute oral toxicity of chlordane in albino rats fed for 28 days from weaning on a protein-deficient diet. Ind. Med., 38, 434-441

Brandt, W.N., Flamm, W.G. & Bernheim, N.J. (1972) The value of hydroxyurea in assessing repair synthesis of DNA in HeLa cells. Chem.-biol. Interact., 5, 327-339

Brodtmann, N.V., Jr (1976) Continuous analysis of chlorinated hydrocarbon pesticides in the lower Mississippi River. Bull. environ. Contam. Toxicol., 15, 33-39

Brubaker, P.E., Flamm, W.G. & Bernheim, N.J. (1970) Effect of γ-chlordane on synchronized lymphoma cells and inhibition of cell division. Nature (Lond.), 226, 548-549

Burns, B.G., Peach, M.E. & Stiles, D.A. (1975) Organochlorine pesticide residues in a farming area, Nova Scotia - 1972-73. Pestic. Monit. J., 9, 34-38

Carey, A.E., Wiersma, G.B. & Tai, H. (1976) Pesticide residues in urban soils from 14 United States cities, 1970. Pestic. Monit. J., 10, 54-60

Chambers, C. & Dutta, S.K. (1976) Mutagenic tests of chlordane on different microbial tester strains (Abstract). Genetics, 83, s13

Cochrane, W.P., Lawrence, J.F., Lee, Y.W., Maybury, R.B. & Wilson, B.P. (1975) Gas-liquid chromatographic determination of technical chlordane residues in food crops: interpretation of analytical data. J. Assoc. off. anal. Chem., 58, 1051-1061

Crockett, A.B., Wiersma, G.B., Tai, H., Mitchell, W.G., Sand, P.F. & Carey, A.E. (1974) Pesticide residue levels in soils and crops, FY-70 National Soils Monitoring Program (II). Pestic. Monit. J., 8, 69-97

Cromartie, E., Reichel, W.L., Locke, L.N., Belisle, A.A., Kaiser, T.E., Lamont, T.G., Mulhern, B.M., Prouty, R.M. & Swineford, D.M. (1975) Residues of organochlorine pesticides and polychlorinated biphenyls and autopsy data for bald eagles, 1971-72. Pestic. Monit. J., 9, 11-14

Curley, A. & Garrettson, L.K. (1969) Acute chlordane poisoning. Clinical and chemical studies. Arch. environ. Health, 18, 211-215

Deichmann, W.B. & Keplinger, M.L. (1966) Effect of combinations of pesticides on reproduction of mice (Abstract no. 11). Toxicol. appl. Pharmacol., 8, 337-338

Derbes, V.J., Dent, J.H., Forrest, W.W. & Johnson, M.F. (1955) Fatal chlor-
    dane poisoning. J. Am. med. Assoc., 158, 1367-1369

Epstein, S.S. (1976) Carcinogenicity of heptachlor and chlordane. Sci.
    total Environ., 6, 103-154

Epstein, S.S., Arnold, E., Andrea, J., Bass, W. & Bishop, Y. (1972)
    Detection of chemical mutagens by the dominant lethal assay in the
    mouse. Toxicol. appl. Pharmacol., 23, 288-325

Eurocop-Cost (1976) Cost-Project 64b. Analysis of Organic Micropollutants
    in Water, A Comprehensive List of Polluting Substances Which Have
    Been Identified in Various Fresh Waters, Effluent Discharges, Aquatic
    Animals and Plants, and Bottom Sediments, 2nd ed., EUCO/MDU/73/76,
    XII/476/76, Luxembourg, Commission of the European Communities, p. 29

Fairchild, H.E., Baer, L.J., Barfehenn, K.R., Beusch, G.J., Caswell, R.L.,
    Hageman, F.J., Markley, M.H., Payntee, O.E., Smith, K.K. & Spenser, R.
    (1976) Chlordane and Heptachlor in Relation to Man and the Environ-
    ment. A Further Pesticide Review 1972-1975, EPA-540/4-76-005, Spring-
    field, VA, National Technical Information Service, PB258339, pp. 33-72

FAO/WHO (1978) Pesticide residues in food - 1977. FAO Plant Production
    and Protection Paper, 10 Rev., pp. 18-19

Fishbein, W.I., White, J.V. & Isaacs, H.J. (1964) Survey of workers exposed
    to chlordane. Ind. med. Surg., 33, 726-727

Fitzhugh, O.G., Fairchild, H.E. et al. (1976) Pesticidal Aspects of
    Chlordane in Relation to Man and the Environment, EPA-540/4-76-006,
    Springfield, VA, National Technical Information Service, PB257107,
    pp.56-89

Fouts, J.R. (1970) Some effects of insecticides on hepatic microsomal
    enzymes in various animal species. Rev. Can. Biol., 29, 377-389

Gaines, T.B. (1960) The acute toxicity of pesticides to rats. Toxicol.
    appl. Pharmacol., 2, 88-99

Gore, R.C., Hannah, R.W., Pattacini, S.C. & Porro, T.J. (1971) Infrared
    and ultraviolet spectra of seventy-six pesticides. J. Assoc. off. anal.
    Chem., 54, 1040-1043, 1048-1049, 1082

Harrington, J.M., Baker, E.L., Jr, Folland, D.S., Saucier, J.W. &
    Sandifer, S.H. (1978) Chlordane contamination of a municipal water
    system. Environ. Res., 15, 155-159

Horwitz, W., ed. (1975) Official Methods of Analysis of the Association of
    Official Analytical Chemists, 12th ed., Washington DC, Association of
    Official Analytical Chemists, pp. 81-82, 105-107, 518-525

Hyman, J. (1949) Halogenated cyclopentadiene-hexachalocyclopentadiene
    adducts. British Patent 618,432, February 22 [Chem. Abstr., 43,
    57961]

Infante, P.F., Epstein, S.S. & Newton, W.A., Jr (1978) Blood dyscrasias
    and childhood tumors and exposure to chlordane and heptachlor.
    Scand. J. Work Environ. Health, 4, 137-150

Johnson. L.D., Waltz, R.H., Ussary, J.P. & Kaiser, F.E. (1976) Automated
    gel permeation chromatographic cleanup of animal and plant extracts
    for pesticide residue determination. J. Assoc. off. anal. Chem.,
    59, 174-187

Johnson, L.G. & Morris, R.L. (1974) Chlorinated insecticide residues in
    the eggs of some freshwater fish. Bull. environ. Contam. Toxicol.,
    11, 503-510

Keith, L.H., Garrison, A.W., Allen, F.R., Carter, M.H., Floyd, T.L.,
    Pope, J.D. & Thruston, A.D., Jr (1976) Identification of organic
    compounds in drinking water from thirteen US cities. In: Keith, L.H.,
    ed., First Chemical Congress of North America Continent, Identifica-
    tion and Analysis of Organic Pollutants in Water, 1975, Ann Arbor,
    Mich., Ann Arbor Science, pp. 329-373

Law, L.M. & Goerlitz, D.F. (1974) Selected chlorinated hydrocarbons in
    bottom material from streams tributary to San Francisco Bay.
    Pestic. Monit. J., 8, 33-36

Lawrence, J.H., Barron, R.P., Chen, J.-Y.T., Lombardo, P. & Benson, W.R.
    (1970) Note on identification of a chlordane metabolite found in
    milk and cheese. J. Assoc. off. anal. Chem., 53, 261-262

Malina, M.A. (1973) Collaborative study of methods for the analysis and
    control of AG-chlordane and its formulations. J. Assoc. off. anal.
    Chem., 56, 591-595

Martin, H. & Worthing, C.R., eds (1977) Pesticide Manual, 5th ed.,
    Malvern, Worcestershire, UK, British Crop Protection Council, p. 93

Mattraw, H.C., Jr (1975) Occurrence of chlorinated hydrocarbon insecticide
    Southern Florida - 1968-72. Pestic. Monit. J., 9, 106-114

Mercier, M. (1975) Preparatory Study for Establishing Criteria (Dose/
    Effect Relationships) For Humans on Organochlorine Compounds, i.e.
    Pesticides and their Metabolites, Doc. No. 1347/75e, Luxembourg,
    Commission of the European Communities, pp. 27, 58-59, 177a, 211-212

Mes, J., Coffin, D.E. & Campbell, D. (1974) Polychlorinated biphenyl and
    organochlorine pesticide residues in Canadian chicken eggs.
    Pestic. Monit, J., 8, 8-11

Miles, J.R.W. & Harris, C.R. (1973) Organochlorine insecticide residues in streams draining agricultural, urban-agricultural, and resort areas of Ontario, Canada - 1971. Pestic. Monit. J., 6, 363-368

Morgan, D.P. & Roan, C.C. (1969) Renal function in persons occupationally exposed to pesticides. Arch. environ. Health, 19, 633-636

Nash, R.G., Harris, W.G., Ensor, P.D. & Woolson, E.A. (1973) Comparative extraction of chlorinated hydrocarbon insecticides from soils 20 years after treatment. J. Assoc. off. anal. Chem., 56, 728-732

National Cancer Institute (1977) Bioassay of Chlordane for Possible Carcinogenicity, Technical Report Series No. 8, Washington DC, Department of Health, Education and Welfare, Publication No. DHEW (NIH) 77-808

National Institute for Occupational Safety & Health (1977) National Occupational Hazard Survey, Volume III, Survey Analyses and Supplemental Tables, Cincinnati, Ohio, Department of Health, Education, & Welfare, December, p. 2,749

Nicholas, M.L., Powell, D.L., Williams, T.R. & Bromund, R.H. (1976) Reference Raman spectra of DDT and five structurally related pesticides and of five pesticides containing the norbornene group. J. Assoc. off. anal. Chem., 59, 197-208

Pero, R.W. & Owens, R.G. (1971) Simple micromethod for detecting antifungal activity. Appl. Microbiol., 21, 546-547

Princi, F. & Spurbeck, G.H. (1951) A study of workers exposed to the insecticides chlordan, aldrin, dieldrin. Arch. ind. Hyg. occup. Med., 3, 64-72

von Rumker, R., Lawless, E.W., Meiners, A.F., Lawrence, K.A., Kelso, G.L. & Moray, F. (1975) Production, Distribution, Use and Environmental Impact Potential of Selected Pesticides, EPA 540/1-74-001, Washington DC, US Government Printing Office, pp. 149-156

Safe Drinking Water Committee (1977) Drinking Water and Health, Washington DC, National Academy of Sciences, pp. 556-561

Saschenbrecker, P.W. (1976) Levels of terminal pesticide residues in Canadian meat. Can. Vet. J., 17, 158-163

Shackelford, W.M. & Keith, L.H. (1976) Frequency of Organic Compounds Identified in Water, EPA-600/4-76-062, Athens, Georgia, US Environmental Protection Agency, p. 99

Sovocool, G.W. & Lewis R.G. (1975) The identification of trace levels of organic pollutants in human tissues: compounds related to chlordane/heptachlor exposure. Trace Subst. Environ. Health, 9, 265-280

Spencer, E.Y. (1973) Guide to the Chemicals Used in Crop Protection, Research Branch, Agriculture Canada, Publication 1093, 6th ed., London, Ontario, University of Western Ontario, pp. 94-95

Street, J.C. & Blau, S.E. (1972) Oxychlordane: accumulation in rat adipose tissue on feeding chlordane isomers or technical chlordane. J. agric. Food Chem., 20, 395-397

Tanita, R., Johnson, J.M., Chun, M. & Maciolek, J. (1976) Organochlorine pesticides in the Hawaii Kai Marina, 1970-74. Pestic. Monit. J., 10, 24-29

Tardiff, R.G., Carlson, G.P. & Simmon, V. (1976) Halogenated organics in tap water: A toxicological evaluation. In: Jolley, R.L., ed., Proceedings of the Conference on the Environmental Impact of Water Chlorination, Oak Ridge, Tennessee, 1975, CONF-751096, UC-11,41,48, available from Springfield, VA, National Technical Information Service, pp. 213-227

Tashiro, S. & Matsumura, F. (1977) Metabolic routes of cis- and trans-chlordane in rats. J. agric. Food Chem., 25, 872-880

US Environmental Protection Agency (1971) EPA Compendium of Registered Pesticides, Vol. III, Washington, DC, US Government Printing Office, pp. III-C-16.1-III-C-16.10

US Environmental Protection Agency (1976a). Consolidated heptachlor/chlordane hearing. Fed. Regist., 41, 7552-7572, 7584-7585

US Environmental Protection Agency (1976b) Protection of environment. US Code Fed. Regul., Title 40, part 180.122, p. 317

US Environmental Protection Agency (1978) Velsicol Chemical Co. et al. Consolidated heptachlor/chlordane cancellation proceedings. Fed. Regist., 43, 12372-12375

US Food & Drug Administration (1975a) Compliance Program Evaluation, Total Diet Studies: FY 1973 (7320.08), Washington DC, Bureau of Foods, Table 3

US Food & Drug Administration (1975b) Pesticide Analytical Manual, Volume I, Methods Which Detect Multiple Residues, Table 201-A, Rockville, MD, US Department of Health, Education, & Welfare

US Food & Drug Administration (1977) Compliance Program Evaluation, Total Diet Studies: FY74 (7320-08), Washington DC, Bureau of Foods, Tables 2 and 3

US International Trade Commission (1977) Synthetic Organic Chemicals, US Production and Sales, 1976, USITC Publication 833, Washington DC, US Government Printing Office, p. 276

US Occupational Safety & Health Administration (1977) Air contaminants.
    US Code Fed. Regul., Title 29, part 1910.1000, p. 28

US Tariff Commission (1949) Synthetic Organic Chemicals, US Production
    and Sales, 1947, Report No. 162, Second Series, Washington DC, US
    Government Printing Office, p. 138

Welch, R.M., Levin, W., Kuntzman, R., Jacobson, M. & Conney, A.H. (1971)
    Effect of halogenated hydrocarbon insecticides on the metabolism
    and uterotropic action of estrogens in rats and mice. Toxicol. appl.
    Pharmacol., 19, 234-246

WHO (1968) 1967 Evaluations of some pesticide residues in food. WHO/Food
    Add./68.30, Geneva, pp. 33-57

WHO (1973) 1972 Evaluations of some pesticide residues in food. WHO Pestic.
    Residues Ser., No. 2, pp. 101, 569

Wiersma, G.B., Tai, H. & Sand, P.F. (1972) Pesticide residues in soil
    from eight cities - 1969. Pestic. Monit. J., 6, 126-129

CHLORDECONE

Literature on the environmental effects of chlordecone has been reviewed recently (Black, 1977; Huff & Gerstner, 1978). A review on chlordecone is available (Epstein, 1978).

1. Chemical and Physical Data

1.1 Synonyms and trade names

Chem. Abstr. Services Reg. No.: 143-50-0

Chem. Abstr. Name: 1,1a,3,3a,4,5,5,5a,5b,6-Decachlorooctahydro-1,3,4-metheno-2H-cyclobuta[cd]pentalen-2-one

Synonyms: Decachloroketone; decachlorooctahydro-1,3,4-metheno-2H-cyclobuta[c,d]pentalen-2-one; decachloropentacyclo(5.2.1.0^{2,6}.0-^{3,9}.0^{5,8})decan-4-one; decachlorotetracyclodecanone

Trade names: Compound 1189; ENT 16391; GC 1189; Kepone; Merex

1.2 Structural and molecular formulae and molecular weight

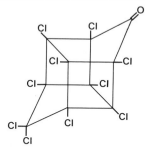

$C_{10}Cl_{10}O$ Mol. wt: 490.6

1.3 Chemical and physical properties of the pure substance

From Spencer (1973) unless otherwise specified

(a) Description: Tan-to-white solid

(b) Melting-point: Sublimes with some decomposition at about 350°C

(c) Solubility: Practically insoluble in water (0.4% at 100°C); soluble in strongly alkaline aqueous solutions; readily soluble in acetone, less soluble in benzene and light petroleum; soluble in alcohols, ketones and acetic acid (Windholz, 1976)

(d) Volatility: Vapour pressure is < 3×10^{-7} mm at 25°C (Allied Chemical Corp., undated).

(e) Stability: Stable to about 350°C

(f) Reactivity: Readily forms hydrates on exposure to standard temperatures and humidities; noncorrosive

1.4 Technical products and impurities

Chlordecone was available in the US until 1976 as a technical grade, typically containing 94.5% of the chemical (72.3% chlorine content), 0.30% methanol insolubles, 5.09% water, 0.01% sulphate and 0.10% hexachlorocyclopentadiene. Chlordecone was also available as a wettable powder containing 50% of the chemical, an emulsifiable concentrate containing 2 pounds per US gallon, ($\sim$ 200 g/l), and granules and dusts containing 5 or 10% (Spencer, 1973).

2. Production, Use, Occurrence and Analysis

A review on chlordecone has been published (Sterrett & Boss, 1977).

2.1 Production and use

(a) Production

Synthesis of chlordecone was first reported in 1952 (Gilbert & Giolito, 1952), by the dimerization of hexachlorocyclopentadiene catalysed by sulphur trioxide. This method has been used for its commercial production (Sterrett & Boss, 1977).

Commercial production of chlordecone in the US was first reported in 1966 (US Tariff Commission, 1968) and was last reported by a government agency in 1973 (US International Trade Commission, 1975). Production during that period was by a single company and is reported to have been intermittent; however, in 1974 continuous operation at the rate of 1350-2700 kg/day was initiated. Between 1968 and 1974, 720 thousand kg were produced (Epstein, 1978). Another plant, which operated for 18 months, produced 770 thousand kg chlordecone before it was closed down in late July 1975. Over 90% of the chemical produced during this period was exported to Latin America, Europe and Africa (Library of Congress, 1977; Sterrett & Boss, 1977).

Chlordecone is believed to be produced by one company in Europe (Epstein, 1978). It has never been produced or imported into Japan.

(b) Use

The only known use for chlordecone is as an insecticide. In the US, products containing this chemical are classified as 'accessible' or 'inaccessible' products: examples of 'inaccessible' products are household ant and roach traps containing a small amount of confined chlordecone; 'accessible' products are those which are applied to crops or structures for control of insects. Until 1 August 1976 (Epstein, 1978) chlordecone was registered in the US for use on bananas, non-bearing citrus trees, tobacco and ornamental shrubs and for control of insects that attack structures (US Environmental Protection Agency, 1973).

On 17 June 1976, the US Environmental Protection Agency (EPA) announced that it had notified the sole producer of chlordecone of the cancellation of the registration of their 12 products containing chlordecone (US Environmental Protection Agency, 1976). Cancellation was effective 45 days from the date of the notice. Agreement was reached in July 1977 between the EPA and the registrants of several inaccessible chlordecone products that the products would be voluntarily cancelled as of 1 May 1978. This agreement provides that all stocks of these inaccessible chlordecone products that were in existence before 1 May, 1978 may be sold, distributed and used indefinitely (Anon., 1977a). In October 1977, the EPA ruled that existing stocks of accessible products containing chlordecone could not be sold in the US (Anon., 1977b). On 27 January, 1978, the EPA revoked all residue tolerances for chlordecone in or on raw agricultural commodities. This action prevents the introduction of bananas containing residues of chlordecone into the US (US Environmental Protection Agency, 1978).

In February 1976, the US National Institute for Occupational Safety and Health recommended that chlordecone be controlled in the workplace so that its airborne concentration be no greater than 1 $\mu g/m^3$ of breathing zone air. This standard is part of a programme to protect workers during up to a 10-hr workday in a 40-hr work week over a working lifetime (Anon., 1976a).

2.2 Occurrence

Chlordecone is not known to occur as a natural product, but it is a degradation product of the insecticide mirex (Carlson *et al.*, 1976; see monograph, p. 283).

Chlordecone was detected in soil at a level of 0.02 $\mu g/g$ 12 years after application of 1 $\mu g/g$ mirex, and was found in a shallow pond at a level of 10 $\mu g/g$ 5 years after the crash of an aircraft containing mirex (Carlson *et al.*, 1976).

In the US, detectable levels of chlordecone have been found in 400 samples of air, drinking-water, plant life and municipal waste in a town where chlordecone was manufactured. Sludge near the town's sewage treatment plant contained 200-600 mg/kg chlordecone; waste-water at the sewage treatment plant contained levels of 0.1-10 mg/l of the chemical; fish and shellfish in a nearby river had 0.1-20 mg/kg; and water in the river, 0.1-4 μg/l. Studies showed that the air in a town about 16 miles from the plant had levels of 0.1-20 ng/m^3, while samples 100 metres from the plant showed 0.2-50 mg/m^3 during the 1-year sampling period. At that time, chlordecone comprised about 1-40% of the total suspended particulates in air in some areas (Anon., 1975).

Tests run by the state of Maryland in July 1976 on Chesapeake Bay water showed chlordecone levels of 0.04-0.08 mg/l (Anon., 1976b).

A single application of chlordecone as a wettable powder containing 50% of the chemical to apple trees at a rate of 2 pounds/acre (2.2 kg/ha) resulted in an initial residue level of 1.4 mg/kg, which decreased to 0.3 mg/kg after approximately 3 months. When treatment involved 8 fort- nightly applications over 3.5 months, residues fell from 5.0 mg/kg at the end of treatment to 1.4 mg/kg by harvest time 2 months later (Brewerton & Slade, 1964).

In February 1976, a study sponsored by the US Environmental Protection Agency reported chlordecone in 9 of 200 mother's milk samples taken in south- eastern US (Anon., 1976c).

Chlordecone was found at levels of 0.165-26 μg/ml in the blood of 32 workers who manufactured chlordecone (Epstein, 1978). A 1974 US National Occupational Hazard Survey determined that workers in the disinfecting and exterminating industries are exposed to chlordecone (National Institute for Occupational Safety & Health, 1977a).

2.3 Analysis

Methods used for the analysis of chlordecone in environmental samples are listed in Table 1.

Chromatographic methods, including thin-layer chromatography (Roscher & Onley, 1977) and gas chromatography/electron capture detection (Blanke et al., 1977), have also been used to separate and quantitate chlordecone.

3. Biological Data Relevant to the Evaluation

of Carcinogenic Risk to Humans

3.1 Carcinogenicity studies in animals

Oral administration

Mouse: Groups of 50 male and 50 female B6C3F1 hybrid mice, approximately 6 weeks of age, were fed technical-grade chlordecone (about 98% pure)

TABLE 1. METHODS FOR THE ANALYSIS OF CHLORDECONE

SAMPLE TYPE	ANALYTICAL METHOD			
	EXTRACTION/CLEAN-UP	DETECTION	LIMIT OF DETECTION	REFERENCE
Formulations				
Concentrates and wettable powders	Extract (acetone), decant, evaporate to dryness, dissolve (decane), boil, cool	IR (C = O band)		Allied Chemicals Corp. (1966)
Technical-grade	Extract (acetone-decane), heat to remove acetone, boil, cool	IR (C = O band)		Allied Chemicals Corp. (1966)
Air	Trap on filter and back-up impinger containing sodium hydroxide solution, extract filter (benzene-methanol), acidify extract (benzene), bulk extracts	GC/ECD	0.1 µg/m^3	National Institute for Occupational Safety & Health (1977b)
Food				
Apples	Extract (benzene), decant, filter	GC/ECD	0.08 mg/kg	Brewerton & Slade (1964)
Potatoes	Extract (methylene chloride), CC	TLC (revelation: silver nitrate/ultra-violet) GC/ECD	0.2 mg/kg 0.005 mg/kg	Proszynska (1977) Proszynska (1977)
Bananas	Extract (isopropanol-benzene), evaporate to dryness, dissolve (hexane), liquid/liquid partition, extract (benzene)	GC/microcoulo-metric detection	0.003 mg/kg	Allied Chemical Corp. (1963)

Abbreviations: IR - infra-red spectrometry; GC/ECD - gas chromatography/electron-capture detection; CC - column chromatography; TLC - thin-layer chromatography

at two levels in the diet for 80 weeks; there were 20 male and 10 female matched controls and 50 male and 40 female pooled controls. Males received initial levels of 40 mg/kg diet, and females 40 and 80 mg/kg diet; these levels were reduced during the experiment due to adverse toxic effects. The time-weighted average dietary concentrations were 20 and 23 mg/kg diet for males and 20 and 40 mg/kg diet for females. Survivors were sacrificed 90 weeks after the start of treatment; survival at that time was 58 and 50% in low- and high-dose male mice, respectively, in contrast with over 80% in all other groups (low- and high-dose females and controls). Well-differentiated hepatocellular carcinomas were found in over 80% of all treated males: in 39/48 low- and 43/49 high-dose males, compared with 6/19 matched male controls; and in 26/50 low- and 23/49 high-dose females, compared with none in female controls (National Cancer Institute, 1976).

Rat: Epstein (1978) reported a previously unpublished study by Larson *et al*., carried out in 1961, in which groups of 40 male and 40 female albino rats of an unspecified strain were administered technical chlordecone (approximately 94% pure) at 6 dose levels in the diet for 24 months, starting at an unspecified 'young age'. The dietary concentrations were 1, 5, 10, 25, 50 and 80 mg/kg diet for both males and females. Groups of 12-14 animals for each dose and for each sex were killed for interim histological examination at 13, 52 and 56 weeks. All remaining survivors were killed 24 months after the start of treatment. All males and females receiving 50 and 80 mg/kg diet had died by 25 weeks; mortality was also high in those given 25 mg/kg diet and in all males given more than 1 mg/kg diet; about 25% of controls were still alive at 2 years. Hepatocellular carcinomas were seen in 2/3 male survivors in the 25 mg/kg diet group, in 3/9 female survivors in the 10 mg/kg diet group and in 1/3 female survivors in the 25 mg/kg diet group. None were observed in other groups or in controls.

Groups of 50 male and 50 female Osborne-Mendel rats, approximately 6 weeks of age, were administered chlordecone (about 98% pure) in the diet for 80 weeks; there were 10 male and 10 female matched controls and 105 male and 100 female pooled controls. Initial dose levels were 15 and 30 mg/kg diet for males and 30 and 60 mg/kg diet for females; these levels were reduced during the experiment due to adverse toxic effects. The time-weighted average dietary concentrations were 8 and 24 mg/kg diet for males and 18 and 26 mg/kg diet for females. Survivors were killed 112 weeks after the start of treatment, at which time survival was low in all treated groups. An increased incidence of hepatocellular carcinomas was found in female rats given the high dose: 10/45 compared with 0/100 pooled controls (P<0.0001); and there were 3/44 hepatocellular carcinomas in high-dose males compared with 0/105 in pooled controls (P<0.05). Neoplastic nodules were diagnosed in 2 low-dose male rats, but none in the controls or in the high-dose group, and in 2 high-dose female rats, with 1 in the controls and none in the low-dose group. Extensive liver hyperplasia, fatty infiltration and degeneration were also found in rats of both sexes in both dose groups, while no such changes were seen in controls. Increased incidences of thyroid carcinomas and adenomas were observed in low-dose males and of reproductive tract tumours in both low- and high-dose females, but the differences were not statistically significant (National Cancer Institute, 1976).

3.2 Other relevant biological data

The toxicity of chlordecone (including its cumulative effects) has been reviewed (Epstein, 1978).

(a) Experimental systems

Toxic effects

The single oral LD_{50} of chlordecone in rats is 125 mg/kg bw; the LD_{50} by dermal application is > 2000 mg/kg bw (Gaines, 1969). The single oral LD_{50} for hens is 480 mg/kg bw and between 220 and 440 mg/kg bw when chlordecone is incorporated in the diet for longer periods (Sherman & Ross, 1961). The estimated maximum tolerated dose for a 6-week dietary exposure was 30 mg/kg diet for male rats, 60 mg/kg diet for female rats and 40 and 80 mg/kg diet for male and female mice, respectively (National Cancer Institute, 1976).

Both rats and mice administered high doses of chlordecone exhibited nervous tremors (National Cancer Institute, 1976). In mice fed diets containing 30-100 mg/kg diet chlordecone, the size of the liver was increased, and focal necrosis, cellular hypertrophy, hyperplasia and congestion were observed, depending on the length of treatment (Huber, 1965). Quail livers were also markedly enlarged by chlordecone exposure (Atwal, 1973; McFarland & Lacy, 1969).

Chicks, quail and fish showed neurotoxic symptoms on exposure to chlordecone (Couch et al., 1977; McFarland & Lacy, 1969; Sherman & Ross, 1961). A strong correlation was shown between the neurotoxic effects of chlordecone and the inhibition of Mg^{2+}-ATPases in fish brain (Desaiah & Koch, 1975; Yap et al., 1975) and rat liver (Desaiah et al., 1977).

Feeding mice and rats for 2 weeks with 50 mg/kg diet chlordecone induced hepatic mixed-function oxidase activity (Fabacher & Hodgson, 1976; Mehendale et al., 1977).

Female mice maintained on 40 mg/kg diet chlordecone failed to reproduce; the animals appeared to be in constant oestrus, and developed large ovarian follicles but no corpora lutea. The effects were consistent with a partial blockage of the release of luteinizing hormone from the pituitary (Huber, 1965). Chlordecone had an oestrogen-like effect on the oviducts of immature female quail and on the testes of males (Eroschenko & Wilson, 1975).

Embryotoxicity and teratogenicity

The size and numbers of litters were decreased in female mice fed doses as low as 10 mg/kg diet chlordecone for one month before mating (Good *et al.*, 1965).

Chlordecone was given by gastric intubation in doses of 2, 6 and 10 mg/kg bw/day to rats and 2, 4, 8 and 12 mg/kg bw/day to mice on days 7-16 of gestation. In rats, 19% of dams that received 10 mg/kg bw/day died; the foetuses of those which survived exhibited a variety of toxic effects, such as reduced body weight, reduced degree of ossification, oedema, undescended testes, enlarged renal pelvis and cerebral ventricles. Male rats showed no reproductive impairment. Lower dose levels only reduced foetal weight and degree of ossification. In mice, foetotoxicity occurred only in the highest dose group and was manifested by increased foetal mortality and clubfoot (Chernoff & Rogers, 1976).

In an abstract, it was reported that rats were exposed by gastric intubation to 1, 2 or 4 mg/kg bw/day chlordecone beginning on day 2 of gestation and ending at weaning. At parturition, all control animals and those receiving 1 mg/kg bw/day delivered healthy pups. Two-thirds of pregnant females that received 2 mg/kg bw/day and all those that received 4 mg/kg bw aborted or had stillbirths. Electroencephalograms and visual-evoked responses obtained in the offspring at 24 days of age indicated that chlordecone induces central nervous system impairment in the perinatal rat (Rosenstein *et al.*, 1977).

Chlordecone also decreased egg production in hens; and chicks of chlordecone-fed hens exhibited neurotoxic symptoms (Naber & Ware, 1965).

Absorption, distribution, excretion and metabolism

After mice were exposed to chlordecone for 5 months, maximum accumulati of residues occurred mainly in the liver; residues were also found in brair kidneys and body fat. On withdrawal of treatment, liver chlordecone levels decreased, and the neurotoxic effects were reversed. There was no evidence of metabolism (Huber, 1965).

Chlordecone was well absorbed and distributed throughout the body after its oral administration to rats. It had a long half-life and disappeared more slowly from the liver than from other tissues. By 84 days, 66% of the dose had been excreted in the faeces and less than 2% in the urine (Egle *et al.*, 1978). Faecal excretion of chlordecone in rats was increased by the administration of an anionic exchange resin, cholestyramine (Boylan *et al.*, 1977, 1978).

When chlordecone was fed to dairy cows in concentrations of 0.25-5.0 mg/kg in hay and in feed-concentrate for 60 days, the highest residue level in milk recorded from an individual cow was 0.44 mg/l. No measurable amounts of chlordecone were present in milk 83 days after treatment was discontinued (Smith & Arant, 1967).

Hens were fed 75 or 150 mg/kg diet chlordecone in their feed for 16 weeks. After 5 weeks of treatment, the chlordecone content of egg yolk was 163 and 336 mg/kg, respectively, for the two dosage levels. By the 13th week it was 100 and 214 mg/kg, respectively; and 3 weeks after treatment had ceased, the chlordecone content was 26 and 70 mg/kg, respectively (Naber & Ware, 1965).

Mutagenicity and other related short-term tests

It was reported in an abstract that no dominant lethal mutations were observed in male rats given 5 consecutive oral doses of 3.6 or 11.4 mg/kg bw/day chlordecone prior to mating (Simon *et al.*, 1978).

(b) Humans

Industrial workers exposed by inhalation, oral ingestion and skin contact to chlordecone showed signs of nervousness, tremors, visual deficiencies, pleural pain, weight loss, joint pain, tachycardia and hepatomegaly. Abnormal liver function tests, changes in electroencephalogram and electromyogram patterns, demyelination of peripheral nerves and oligospermia with decreased sperm mobility were noted. Dermatitis was seen in 60% of workers; skin rashes and nervous effects were also seen in family members of the workers. The severity of the symptoms was proportional to the blood levels of chlordecone (Cannon *et al.*, 1978; Cohn *et al.*, 1978; Epstein, 1978; Martinez *et al.*, 1978; Taylor *et al.*, 1978).

High concentrations of chlordecone were found in liver and body fat of workers exposed to the compound (Cohn *et al.*, 1978), and it has been determined in blood of workers (see section 2.2, p. 69). The serum half-life of chlordecone ranged from 63-148 days (Adir *et al.*, 1978).

Chlordecone undergoes extensive biliary excretion and enterohepatic circulation. Excretion in the faeces, unchanged and as the alcohol derivative, was the major route of elimination. Administration of cholestyramine, an anionic exchange resin which binds to chlordecone, increased faecal excretion, presumably by interfering with reabsorption from the intestine (Cohn *et al.*, 1976, 1978).

Most of a group of workers severely poisoned by chlordecone in Virginia in 1975 had severe neurological abnormalities, and some were reported to have become infertile (Whorton *et al.*, 1977).

3.3 Case reports and epidemiological studies

No data were available to the Working Group.

4. Summary of Data Reported and Evaluation

4.1 Experimental data

Chlordecone was tested in one experiment in mice and in two in rats by oral administration: it produced hepatocellular carcinomas in males and females of both species.

Chlordecone impairs fertility and is foetotoxic.

4.2 Human data

No case reports or epidemiological studies were available to the Working Group.

The extensive production and the widespread use of chlordecone and its persistence in the environment (where it may also occur as a result of degradation of the pesticide mirex) indicate that human exposure occurs. This is confirmed by many reports of its occurrence in human body fluids. A group of highly exposed workers is known to exist. Oligospermia with hypomobility of the sperm has been reported in heavily exposed workers.

4.3 Evaluation

There is *sufficient evidence* that chlordecone is carcinogenic in mice and rats. In the absence of adequate data in humans, it is reasonable, for practical purposes, to regard chlordecone as if it presented a carcinogenic risk to humans.

5. References

Adir, J., Caplan, Y.H. & Thompson, B.C. (1978) Kepone® serum half-life
    in humans. Life Sci., 22, 699-702

Allied Chemical Corporation (1963) Determination of Kepone (GC-1189)
    Residues in Crops, 26 June, Morristown, NJ

Allied Chemical Corporation (1966) Assay method for Kepone®, 8 March,
    Morristown, NJ

Allied Chemical Corporation (undated) Summary of Basic Information - Kepone®
    Insecticide, Morristown, NJ

Anon. (1975) End of line for Kepone. Chem. Week, 117, 10

Anon. (1976a) NIOSH recommends exposure limit of one microgram per cubic
    meter. Occup. Saf. Health Rep., 5, 1195

Anon. (1976b) Mandel says Kepone no problem in Bay. The News American,
    16 July, p. 5A

Anon. (1976c) EPA-sponsored study finds mirex in tissue samples taken in
    southeast. Environ. Rep., 7, 506

Anon. (1977a) Kepone settlement on inaccessible products results in May
    1978 cancellation. Pestic. Tox. Chem. News, 27 July, 17-18

Anon. (1977b) Kepone. Pestic. Tox. Chem. News, 2 November, 2

Atwal, O.S. (1973) Fatty changes and hepatic cell excretion in avian liver.
    An electron microscopical study of Kepone toxicity. J. comp. Pathol.,
    83, 115-124

Black, S.A. (1977) Kepone. II. An Abstracted Literature Collection. 1952-
    1977, ORNL/TIRC-76/3, Oak Ridge, TN, Oak Ridge National Laboratory

Blanke, R.V., Fariss, M.W., Griffith, F.D., Jr & Guzelian, P. (1977)
    Analysis of chlordecone (Kepone®) in biological specimens. J. anal.
    Toxicol., 1, 57-62

Boylan, J.J., Egle, J.L., Jr & Guzelian, P.S. (1977) Stimulation of chlor-
    decone (CD) (Kepone) excretion by cholestyramine in rats (Abstract
    no. 469). Pharmacologist, 19, 210

Boylan, J.J., Egle, J.L. & Guzelian, P.S. (1978) Cholestyramine: use as
    a new therapeutic approach for chlordecone (Kepone) poisoning.
    Science, 199, 893-895

Brewerton, H.V. & Slade, D.A. (1964) 'Kepone' residues on apples. N.Z.
    J. agric. Res., 7, 647-653

Cannon, S.B., Veazey, J.M., Jr, Jackson, R.S., Burse, V.W., Hayes, C.,
    Straub, W.E., Landrigan, P.J. & Liddle, J.A. (1978) Epidemic Kepone
    poisoning in chemical workers. Am. J. Epidemiol., 107, 529-537

Carlson, D.A., Konyha, K.D., Wheeler, W.B., Marshall, G.P. & Zaylskie, R.G.
    (1976) Mirex in the environment: its degradation to Kepone and
    related compounds. Science, 194, 939-941

Chernoff, N. & Rogers, E.H. (1976) Fetal toxicity of Kepone in rats and mic
    Toxicol. appl. Pharmacol., 38, 189-194

Cohn, W.J., Blanke, R.V., Griffith, F.D., Jr & Guzelian, P.S. (1976)
    Distribution and excretion of Kepone (KP) in humans (Abstract).
    Gastroenterology, 71, 901

Cohn, W.J., Boylan, J.J., Blanke, R.V., Fariss, M.W., Howell, J.R. &
    Guzelian, P.S. (1978) Treatment of chlordecone (Kepone) toxicity with
    cholestyramine. Results of a controlled clinical trial. New Engl. J.
    Med., 298, 243-248

Couch, J.A., Winstead, J.T. & Goodman, L.R. (1977) Kepone-induced scoliosis
    and its histological consequences in fish. Science, 197, 585-587

Desaiah, D. & Koch, R.B. (1975) Inhibition of ATPases activity in channel
    catfish brain by Kepone® and its reduction product. Bull. environ.
    Contam. Toxicol., 13, 153-158

Desaiah, D., Ho, I.K. & Mehendale, H.M. (1977) Effects of Kepone and mirex
    on mitochondrial Mg^{2+}-ATPase activity in rat liver. Toxicol. appl.
    Pharmacol., 39, 219-228

Egle, J.L., Jr, Fernandez, S.B., Guzelian, P.S. & Borzelleca, J.F. (1978)
    Distribution and excretion of chlordecone (Kepone) in the rat. Drug
    Metab. Disp., 6, 91-95

Epstein, S.S. (1978) Kepone - hazard evaluation. Sci. total Environ.,
    9, 1-62

Eroschenko, V.P. & Wilson, W.O. (1975) Cellular changes in the gonads,
    livers and adrenal glands of Japanese quail as affected by the insec-
    ticide Kepone. Toxicol. appl. Pharmacol., 31, 491-504

Fabacher, D.L. & Hodgson, E. (1976) Induction of hepatic mixed-function
    oxidase enzymes in adult and neonatal mice by Kepone and mirex.
    Toxicol. appl. Pharmacol., 38, 71-77

Gaines, T.B. (1969) Acute toxicity of pesticides. Toxicol. appl.
    Pharmacol., 14, 515-534

Gilbert, E.E. & Giolito, S.L. (1952) US Patent 2,616,825 & US Patent 2,616,928, 4 Nov., to Allied Chemical & Dye Corp.

Good, E.E., Ware, G.W. & Miller, D.F. (1965) Effects of insecticides on reproduction in the laboratory mouse. I. Kepone. J. econ. Entomol., 58, 754-757

Huber, J.J. (1965) Some physiological effects of the insecticide Kepone in the laboratory mouse. Toxicol. appl. Pharmacol., 7, 516-524

Huff, J.E. & Gerstner, H.B. (1978) Kepone: a literature summary. J. environ. Pathol. Toxicol., 1, 377-395

Library of Congress (1977) Water Contamination by Toxic Pollutants: An Assessment of Regulation, 95th Congress, 1st Session, Washington DC, US Government Printing Office, pp. 32-37

Martinez, A.J., Taylor, J.R., Dyck, P.J., Houff, S.A. & Isaacs, E. (1978) Chlordecone intoxication in man. II. Ultrastructure of peripheral nerves and skeletal muscle. Neurology, 28, 631-635

McFarland, L.Z. & Lacy, P.B. (1969) Physiologic and endocrinologic effects of the insecticide Kepone in the Japanese quail. Toxicol. appl. Pharmacol., 15, 441-450

Mehendale, H.M., Takanaka, A., Desaiah, D. & Ho, I.K. (1977) Kepone induction of hepatic mixed function oxidases in the male rat. Life Sci., 20, 991-997

Naber, E.C. & Ware, G.W. (1965) Effect of Kepone and mirex on reproductive performance in the laying hen. Poultry Sci., 44, 875-880

National Cancer Institute (1976) Report on Carcinogenesis Bioassay of Technical Grade Chlordecone (Kepone), Bethesda, MD, Carcinogenesis Program, Division of Cancer Cause & Prevention

National Institute for Occupational Safety & Health (1977a) National Occupational Hazard Survey, Vol. III, Survey Analyses and Supplemental Tables, Cincinnati, OH, Draft, December, p. 6,321

National Institute for Occupational Safety & Health (1977b) NIOSH Manual of Analytical Methods, Part I, NIOSH Monitoring Methods, Vol. 1, 2nd ed., Method No. P&CAM 225, DHEW (NIOSH), Pub. No. 77-157B, Washington DC, US Government Printing Office, pp. 225-1-256-6

Proszynska, B. (1977) Method for determining Despirol residues in potatoes (Pol.). Rocz. Panstew. Zakl. Hig., 28, 201-207 [Chem. Abstr., 87, 199267s].

Roscher, N.M. & Onley, J.H. (1977) Thin-layer chromatographic analysis of oxo and thio compounds. J. Chromatogr., 140, 109-113

Rosenstein, L., Brice, A., Rogers, N. & Lawrence, S. (1977) Neurotoxicity of Kepone in perinatal rats following in utero exposure (Abstract No. 28). Toxicol. appl. Pharmacol., 41, 142-143

Sherman, M. & Ross, E. (1961) Acute and subacute toxicity of insecticides to chicks. Toxicol. appl. Pharmacol., 3, 521-533

Simon, G.S., Kipps, B.R., Tardiff, R.G. & Borzelleca, J.F. (1978) Failure of Kepone and hexachlorobenzene to induce dominant lethal mutations in the rat (Abstract No. 260). Toxicol. appl. Pharmacol., 45, 330-331

Smith, J.C. & Arant, F.S. (1967) Residues of Kepone in milk from cows receiving treated feed. J. econ. Entomol., 60, 925-927

Spencer, E.Y. (1973) Guide to the Chemicals Used in Crop Protection, 6th ed., Research Branch, Agriculture Canada, Publication 1093, London, Ontario, University of Western Ontario, p. 96

Sterrett, F.S. & Boss, C.A. (1977) Careless Kepone. Environment, 19, 30-37

Taylor, J.R., Selhorst, J.B., Houff, S.A. & Martinez, A.J. (1978) Chlordecone intoxication in man. I. Clinical observations. Neurology, 28, 626-630

US Environmental Protection Agency (1973) EPA Compendium of Registered Pesticides, Washington, DC, US Government Printing Office, pp. III-D-2.1-III-D-2.5

US Environmental Protection Agency (1976) Cancellation of registration of pesticide products containing chlordecone (Kepone). Fed. Regist., 41, 24624

US Environmental Protection Agency (1978) Tolerances and exemptions from tolerances for pesticide chemicals in or on raw agricultural commodities. Fed. Regist., 43, 3708-3709

US International Trade Commission (1975) Synthetic Organic Chemicals, US Production and Sales, 1973, ITC Publication 728, Washington DC, US Government Printing Office, p. 192

US Tariff Commission (1968) Synthetic Organic Chemicals, US Production and Sales, 1966, TC Publication 248, Washington DC, US Government Printing Office, p. 164

Whorton, D., Krauss, R.M., Marshall, S. & Milby, T.H. (1977) Infertility in male pesticide workers. Lancet, ii, 1259-1261

Windholz, M., ed (1976) The Merck Index, 9th ed., Rahway, NJ, Merck & Co., Inc., pp. 263-264

Yap, H.H., Desaiah, D., Cutkomp, L.K. & Koch, R.B. (1975) _In vitro_ inhibition of fish brain ATPase activity by cyclodiene insecticides and
related compounds. _Bull. environ. Contam. Toxicol._, _14_, 163-167

1,2-DIBROMO-3-CHLOROPROPANE

This substance was considered by a previous Working Group, in
February 1977 (IARC, 1977). Since that time new data have become available
and these have been incorporated into the monograph and taken into account
in the present evaluation.

1.   Chemical and Physical Data

1.1   Synonyms and trade names

Chem. Abstr. Services Reg. No.:   96-12-8

Chem. Abstr. Name: 1,2-Dibromo-3-chloropropane

Synonyms: 3-Chloro-1,2-dibromopropane; DBCP; dibromochloropropane

Trade names: BBC 12; Fumagon; Fumazone; Fumazone 86; Fumazone
86E; Nemabrom; Nemafume; Nemagon; Nemagon 20; Nemagon 90;
Nemagon 20G; Nemagon Soil Fumigant; Nemanax; Nemapaz; Nemaset;
Nematox; OS 1897

1.2   Structural and molecular formulae and molecular weight

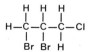

$C_3H_5Br_2Cl$ Mol. wt: 236.3

1.3   Chemical and physical properties of the pure substance

From Spencer (1973), unless otherwise specified

(a) Description: Dark-amber to dark-brown liquid with pungent odour

(b) Boiling-point: 196°C

(c) Density: d_{20}^{20} 2.08 (Martin & Worthing, 1977)

(d) Spectroscopy data: Infra-red, nuclear magnetic resonance
     and mass spectral data have been tabulated (Grasselli & Ritchey,
     (1975).

(e) Refractive index: n_D^{25} 1.5518

(f) Solubility: Slightly soluble in water (0.1% w/w); miscible with liquid hydrocarbons, ethanol, methanol, isopropanol and halogenated hydrocarbons

(g) Volatility: Vapour pressure is 0.8 mm at 21°C.

(h) Stability: Stable in neutral and acidic media; hydrolysed by alkali to 2-bromoallyl alcohol; dehalogenated by soil bacteria to n-propanol (Castro, 1977)

(i) Reactivity: Corrodes aluminium, magnesium, tin and alloys containing these metals; attacks rubber materials and coatings (US Occupational Safety & Health Administration, 1977a)

(j) Conversion factor: 1 ppm in air is equivalent to approximately 10 mg/m^3.

1.4 Technical products and impurities

1,2-Dibromo-3-chloropropane is available in the US as a technical grade containing not less than 95% of the pure chemical (Johnson & Lear, 1969), as emulsifiable concentrates containing 70.7-87.8%, as solutions containing 47.2%, as granules containing 5.25-34%, and in fertilizer mixtures containing 0.6-5% (US Environmental Protection Agency, 1974).

A technical grade available in the USSR contains 97-98% of the pure chemical and 1-3% of other halogenated hydrocarbons. A technical grade available in Japan contains at least 99% of the pure chemical.

2. Production, Use, Occurrence and Analysis

2.1 Production and use

(a) Production

1,2-Dibromo-3-chloropropane was first prepared by Oppenheim in 1833 by the addition of bromine to allyl chloride (Prager *et al.*, 1918); this is the method used currently for its production in the US and Japan.

1,2-Dibromo-3-chloropropane was first produced commercially in the US in 1955 (US Tariff Commission, 1956). In 1969, US production was 3.9 million kg (US Tariff Commission, 1971); in 1974, estimated production

by one source was 9 million kg (Kelso *et al.*, 1976). In 1976, 3 US
companies reported commercial production of an undisclosed amount (see
preamble, p. 16) (US International Trade Commission, 1977); by 1977,
only 2 US companies were producing it (US Environmental Protection
Agency, 1977a). 1,2-Dibromo-3-chloropropane has been imported into the
US from the Federal Republic of Germany and Israel (US Occupational
Safety & Health Administration, 1977a) and from Mexico and Japan (US
Occupational Safety & Health Administration, 1978).

Production in the Benelux, France, Italy, Spain, Switzerland and
the UK has been estimated to be 3-30 million kg annually.

1,2-Dibromo-3-chloropropane was first produced commercially in
Japan in 1960. In 1974, the single Japanese producer manufactured 496
thousand kg; in 1975, production dropped to 159 thousand kg and in 1976
to 154 thousand kg.

(b) Use

The only known use for 1,2-dibromo-3-chloropropane is as a soil
fumigant for control of nematodes. Its nematocidal activity was first
reported in 1955 (McBeth & Bergeson, 1955). About 5.4 million kg
were used in 1972 in the US (US Occupational Safety & Health
Administration, 1978), where it is used mainly for soil treatment
for soya beans, pineapples, peaches, grapes and citrus fruits; minor
uses are for turf, ornamental shrubs and vegetable crops. Some of
these uses, particularly on vegetables, may be discontinued due to
recent suspension actions (US Environmental Protection Agency, 1977a).
In 1971, US farmers used 1.6 million kg on crops (US Department of
Agriculture, 1974); and in 1977, a total of 378 thousand kg were used
in California alone, mostly on grapes and tomatoes (California Department
of Food & Agriculture, 1978).

On 22 September 1977, the US Environmental Protection Agency (EPA)
issued a notice of rebuttable presumption against renewal of registration
(RPAR) (see General Remarks on Substances Considered, p. 31) of all
pesticide products containing 1,2-dibromo-3-chloropropane, on the basis
of carcinogenic and reproductive effects (US Environmental Protection
Agency, 1977a). Four days later, the EPA issued an order suspending
registration of those pesticide products containing 1,2-dibromo-3-
chloropropane which were found to pose an 'imminent hazard' to humans or to
the environment. The suspended products were those intended for use on
19 food crops in which residues are likely to occur in edible portions.
Conditional suspensions were declared for those products used on other
crops, pending label changes to restrict use to certified applicators
wearing protective clothing and respirators (US Environmental Protection
Agency, 1977b).

The US Food and Drug Administration has established maximum residue
levels of 1.5 mg/l in raw milk and 0.05 mg/kg in all other raw agricultural

commodities (Anon., 1977). Tolerance levels of 5-130 mg/kg had previously
been established on some 30 food crops (US Environmental Protection
Agency, 1974).

On 9 September 1977, the US Occupational Safety and Health Administration established an emergency temporary health standard for exposure
to 1,2-dibromo-3-chloropropane as an air contaminant. This requires
that an employee's exposure to the chemical not exceed an 8-hr time-
weighted average of 100 $\mu g/m^3$ (10 ppb) in the workplace air in any
8-hr work shift of a 40-hr week, with a ceiling level of 500 $\mu g/m^3$
(50 ppb) for any 15-min period during the 8-hr day. The emergency
temporary standard was to be superseded by a permanent standard within
6 months (US Occupational Safety & Health Administration, 1977a). A
proposed permanent standard was issued on 1 November, 1977. This proposal
reduced the time-weighted average from 10 ppb to 1 ppb and the ceiling
from 50 ppb to 10 ppb (US Occupational Safety & Health Administration,
1977b). The proposed time-weighted average of 1 ppb became a permanent
standard, effective 17 April, 1978. In the final ruling, the ceiling
exposure requirement of 10 ppb was eliminated since it was judged to be
adequately covered by the time-weighted average standard (US Occupational
Safety & Health Administration, 1978).

No data were available on use of 1,2-dibromo-3-chloropropane in Japan;
it is used as a soil fumigant in Europe.

2.2 Occurrence

1,2-Dibromo-3-chloropropane is not known to occur as a natural
product. It is present at a level of 0.05% or 0.002% in the flame retardant
tris(2,3-dibromopropyl) phosphate (see monograph, p. 575) (Prival *et al.*,
1977).

(a) Soil

1,2-Dibromo-3-chloropropane has been applied to various types of
agricultural soils in California by injection, flooding and sprinkling.
The chemical was still present 40 weeks after application; and its
distribution in soil was proportional to the size of soil particles,
with the greatest concentration found in sandy soils and the lowest in
clay (Hodges, 1972).

In field experiments, 1,2-dibromo-3-chloropropane was detected in
soil at levels in the mean range of 0.008-1.64 mg/kg from 1 day to 16
weeks after application at the rate of 13.75 kg/ha (Newsome *et al.*,
1977).

(b) Food

The US Environmental Protection Agency has estimated that human
dietary exposure to 1,2-dibromo-3-chloropropane is in the range of 2.2-
61.0 x 10^{-6} mg/kg/day (US Environmental Protection Agency, 1977b).

1,2-Dibromo-3-chloropropane was detected in carrots in the range of 0.009-1.5 mg/kg and in radishes in the range of 0.03-0.194 mg/kg after application of 13.75 kg/ha to soil. In the same study, the compound was detected in carrot peel and pulp in concentrations of 0.339 and 0.607 mg/kg, respectively. After unpeeled carrots were boiled for 5 min, they still contained 0.251 mg/kg 1,2-dibromo-3-chloropropane (Newsome *et al.*, 1977).

(c) Occupational exposure

Occupational exposure to 1,2-dibromo-3-chloropropane in production or formulation plants at levels which caused physiological changes has been reported for: (1) 41 employees in California; (2) 86 employees in Arkansas; and (3) a total of 50 employees in Colorado and Alabama. One US manufacturer of 1,2-dibromo-3-chloropropane estimated that employee exposure ranged from < 1-6 mg/m^3 (100-600 ppb) over 3 years. The US Occupational Safety and Health Administration has estimated that 2000-3000 employees have recently been or may currently be exposed during the manufacture and formulation of 1,2-dibromo-3-chloropropane (US Occupational Safety & Health Administration, 1977a,b).

Whorton *et al.* (1977) have detected an average of 4 mg/m^3 (0.4 ppm) 1,2-dibromo-3-chloropropane over an 8-hr day in a manufacturing plant. In another factory, levels of 1-6 mg/m^3 (0.1-0.6 ppm) have been estimated during the past 3 years (US Occupational Safety & Health Administration, 1977a).

2.3 Analysis

Methods used for the analysis of 1,2-dibromo-3-chloropropane in environmental samples are listed in Table 1.

3.   Biological Data Relevant to the Evaluation of Carcinogenic Risk to Humans

3.1 Carcinogenicity studies in animals[1]

Oral administration

Mouse: Two groups of 50 male and 50 female B6C3F1 hybrid mice, 5-6 weeks old, were fed technical-grade 1,2-dibromo-3-chloropropane (minimum 90% purity) in corn oil by gavage on 5 consecutive days per week. Approximate time-weighted average doses were 114 and 219 mg/kg bw for males and 110 and 209 mg/kg bw for females. Two groups, each of 20

---

[1]The Working Group was aware of a completed but as yet unpublished study involving the i.p. administration of 1,2-dibromo-3-chloropropane to mice and of studies in progress by inhalation exposure in rats and mice and by skin application in mice (IARC, 1978).

TABLE 1. METHODS FOR THE ANALYSIS OF 1,2-DIBROMO-3-CHLOROPROPANE

SAMPLE TYPE	EXTRACTION/CLEAN-UP	ANALYTICAL METHOD DETECTION	LIMIT OF DETECTION	REFERENCE
Formulations				
Liquids	Dilute (chloroform)	GC/TCD		US Environmental Protection Agency (1976)
Dry formulations	Extract (chloroform), filter	GC/TCD		US Environmental Protection Agency (1976)
Emulsifiable concentrates	Dilute (carbon disulphide), dry	IR		US Environmental Protection Agency (1976)
Granules	Extract (acetone), filter, evaporate to dryness (with care), take up in carbon disulphide	IR		US Environmental Protection Agency (1976)
Air	Trap in dimethyl sulphoxide	Polarography	7 mg/m^3	Novik & Flyngyu (1973)
Water	Extract (petroleum ether)	Polarography		Novik & Kozlova (1971)
	Extract (hexane)	GC/ECD		Johnson & Lear (1969)
Soil	Extract (acetone), decant	GC/ECD	1 mg/kg	Gutenmann & Lisk (1968)
	Extract (hexane)	CC/ECD	1 mg/kg	Johnson & Lear (1969)
	Extract (ether-water)	Polarography	0.1 mg/kg	Novik & Kozlova (1973)
Food				
Root crops	Extract (absolute ethanol) in blender, filter, add sodium chloride solution, extract (hexane), dry, CC	GC/ECD	2 µg/kg	Newsome et al. (1977)

Abbreviations: GC/TCD - gas chromatography/thermal conductivity detection; IR - infra-red spectrometry; ECD - electron capture detection; CC - column chromatography

males and 20 females, were used as vehicle-treated and untreated controls.
Low-dose animals and vehicle controls had to be killed at 60 and 59
weeks and high-dose animals at 47 weeks because of high mortality related
to tumours; untreated male and female controls were sacrificed at 78
and 90 weeks. Animals dying with tumours were observed in high-dose
groups as early as 27 weeks. In males, 40/50 of the high-dose group had
died by the end of week 47, and 42/50 of the low-dose group had died by
week 59. In females, 30/50 of the high-dose group had died by the end
of week 47, and 41/50 of the low-dose group had died by week 60. Squamous-
cell carcinomas of the forestomach occurred in 43/46 low-dose males, 47/49
high-dose males, 50/50 low-dose females and 47/48 high-dose females.
This lesion occurred with frequent metastases to the abdominal viscera
and the lungs. No gastric neoplasms occurred in either vehicle or
untreated controls (National Cancer Institute, 1978).

Rat: Two groups of 50 male and 50 female Osborne-Mendel rats, 6-7
weeks old, were fed 1,2-dibromo-3-chloropropane (minimum 90% pure) in
corn oil by gavage at approximately time-weighted average dosages of 15
and 29 mg/kg bw on 5 consecutive days per week. Two groups, each of 20
males and 20 females, were used as vehicle-treated and untreated controls.
Low- and high-dose females were treated for 73 and 64 weeks, respectively,
and then killed because of high mortality related to tumours. High-dose
males were treated for 64 weeks and then killed; low-dose males were
treated for 78 weeks and killed at 83 weeks. Vehicle-treated controls
were killed after 83 weeks, and untreated controls at 109 weeks. Animals
dying with tumours were observed in high-dose groups as early as 33
weeks. Of males, 40/50 in the high-dose group had died by week 62,
and 45/50 in the low-dose group had died by week 83; of females, 47/50
in the high-dose group had died by week 61, and 42/50 in the low-dose
group had died by week 73. Squamous-cell carcinomas of the forestomach
occurred in 47/50 both low- and high-dose males, 38/50 low-dose females
and 29/49 high-dose females. These lesions occurred with frequent
metastases to the abdominal viscera and the lungs. No gastric carcinomas occurred in either vehicle or untreated controls. In females,
adenocarcinomas of the mammary gland occurred in 24/50 of the low-dose
group, in 31/50 of the high-dose group, in 2/20 untreated controls and
in none of the vehicle controls (National Cancer Institute, 1978).

3.2 Other relevant biological data

(a) Experimental systems

Toxic effects

The LD_{50} of 1,2-dibromo-3-chloropropane by oral intubation is 150-
370 mg/ kg bw in male rats, 260-620 mg/kg bw in female rats and 150-300
mg/kg bw in male guinea-pigs (Torkelson et al., 1961). The percutaneous
LD_{50} in rabbits is 1400 mg/kg bw (Kodama & Dunlap, 1956).

Daily oral administration of 70 mg/kg bw (20% of the acute LD_{50}) to rats was lethal after 3 weeks of dosing. Degenerative effects were noted in the vascular system and in all internal organs (Faidysh *et al.*, 1970).

1,2-Dibromo-3-chloropropane (97% pure) was given by gavage to 190 rats either in a dose of 100 mg/kg bw (single dose), or in repeated doses of 10 mg/kg bw for 5 months. After the single dose, the animals developed symptoms of acute poisoning - mostly nervous system depression - and weight loss. Following repeated treatment, an effect on spermatogenesis was observed in males, and the number and viability of spermatozoa were decreased; oestrus was inhibited in females (Reznik & Sprinchan, 1975). Severe atrophy and degeneration of the testes were observed in rats, guinea-pigs and rabbits (Torkelson *et al.*, 1961). Testicular atrophy was also observed in rats during the long-term oral carcinogenicity study reported in section 3.1 (National Cancer Institute, 1978).

1,2-Dibromo-3-chloropropane induced skin irritation and irritation of the eyes in rabbits (Kodama & Dunlap, 1956). Inhalation of concentrations of over 600 mg/m^3 (60 ppm) in air caused irritation of the skin, eyes, mucous membranes and respiratory tract, hepatic degeneration, neurotoxicity and nephrotoxicity in rats (Torkelson *et al.*, 1961).

No data on the embryotoxicity, teratogenicity, absorption, distribution, excretion or metabolism of 1,2-dibromo-3-chloropropane were available to the Working Group.

Mutagenicity and other related short-term tests

1,2-Dibromo-3-chloropropane was mutagenic in *Salmonella typhimurium* TA100, TA1530 and TA1535, but not in TA1538, both in the presence and absence of a liver microsomal activation system (Blum & Ames, 1977; Prival *et al.*, 1977; Rosenkranz, 1975).

(b) Humans

Sperm counts were determined for 36 workers potentially exposed to 1,2-dibromo-3-chloropropane (the extent of exposure to other pesticides is not clear). Of these, 11 were found to be vasectomized. Of the remaining 25, 3 had sperm counts between 10 and 30 million/ml; 11 who had normal counts (>40 million/ml) had had a short duration of exposure (less than 3 months); 11 who had significantly decreased sperm counts (<1 million/ml) had been exposed for at least 3 years. Of the latter, 9 had no detectable sperm cells (Whorton *et al.*, 1977). In a later report (Whorton *et al.*, 1979), among 142 non-vasectomized workers (including the ones mentioned above) providing semen samples, the median sperm count was 46 million/ml for 107 men exposed to 1,2-dibromo-3-chloropropane and 79 million/ml for 35 men never exposed.

Glass *et al.* (1979) found that 24 pesticide applicators who were exposed to 1,2-dibromo-3-chloropropane for 2 months or more during the year in which they were studied had a mean sperm count of 22 million/ml. Thirty-one applicators who were exposed for less than 2 months but more than 2 weeks had a mean sperm count of 39 million/ml, while the mean count for 19 men exposed for less than 2 weeks was 46 million/ml. Twenty-two applicators who reported no exposure to 1,2-dibromo-3-chloropropane had a mean count of 62 million/ml. This trend was statistically significant ($P = 0.018$); however, only the men exposed for 2 months or more had counts which were significantly lower ($P < 0.01$) than the rest. Serum levels of follicle stimulating hormone (FSH) increased with increasing period of exposure ($P < 0.05$). Neither the depression of sperm counts nor the increased FSH levels were associated with exposure in prior years, suggesting that these effects develop quickly after exposure to the chemical and are apparently reversible when exposure to the chemical is removed.

Of 86 other workers examined, 24% had aspermia and 46% had oligospermia. Of workers from two other factories, 7/11 and 20/27 had sperm counts of 40 million/ml or less (US Occupational Safety & Health Administration, 1977a).

Of 18 workers exposed to 1,2-dibromo-3-chloropropane for 6-18 months, 16 had abnormal incidences (greater than 2%) of Y-chromosomal nondisjunction (Kapp *et al.*, 1979).

Spermatogenic activity was either significantly decreased or absent in 7/10 men with a history of exposure to 1,2-dibromo-3-chloropropane (Biava *et al.*, 1978).

3.3 Case reports and epidemiological studies

No data were available to the Working Group.

4. Summary of Data Reported and Evaluation

4.1 Experimental data

1,2-Dibromo-3-chloropropane was tested in one experiment in mice and one in rats by oral administration: it produced squamous-cell carcinomas of the forestomach in animals of both species and adenocarcinomas of the mammary gland in female rats.

1,2-Dibromo-3-chloropropane is mutagenic in *Salmonella typhimurium*.

4.2 Human data

No case reports or epidemiological studies were available to the Working Group.

The extensive production of 1,2-dibromo-3-chloropropane and its use as a pesticide over the past two decades indicate that widespread human exposure occurs. This is confirmed by reports of its presence in soils and vegetables following experimental application and by the observation of increased sterility in identified industrial groups.

4.3 Evaluation

There is *sufficient evidence* that 1,2-dibromo-3-chloropropane is carcinogenic in mice and rats. In the absence of adequate data in humans, it is reasonable, for practical purposes, to regard 1,2-dibromo-3-chloropropane as if it presented a carcinogenic risk to humans.

5. References

Anon. (1977) Shell, NCCA defend continued use of DBCP with worker precau-
tions. Pestic. Tox. chem. News, 5, 31-32

Biava, C.G., Smuckler, E.A. & Whorton, D. (1978) The testicular
morphology of individuals exposed to dibromochloropropane. Exp.
mol. Pathol., 29, 448-458

Blum, A. & Ames, B.N. (1977) Flame-retardant additives as possible cancer
hazards. The main flame retardant in children's pajamas is a mutagen
and should not be used. Science, 195, 17-23

California Department of Food & Agriculture (1978) Pesticide Use Report,
1977, Sacramento, pp. 51-52

Castro, C.E. (1977) Biodehalogenation. Environ. Health Perspect., 21,
279-283

Faidysh, E.V., Rakhmatullaev, N.N. & Varshavskii, V.A. (1970) Cytotoxic
action of Nemagon in a subacute experiment (Russ.). Med. Zh. Uzb., (1),
64-65 [Chem. Abstr., 73, 108692y]

Glass, R.I., Lyness, R.N., Mengle, D.C., Powell, K.E. & Kahn, E. (1979)
Sperm count depression in pesticide applicators exposed to
dibromochloropropane. Am. J. Epidemiol., 109, 346-351

Grasselli, J.G. & Ritchey, W.M., eds (1975) CRC Atlas of Spectral Data and
Physical Constants for Organic Compounds, 2nd ed., Vol. IV, Cleveland,
OH, Chemical Rubber Co., p. 206

Gutenmann, W.H. & Lisk, D.J. (1968) Gas chromatographic analysis of
Nemagon fumigant in extracts of soil on porous polymer beads. J. Gas
Chromatogr., 6, 124-125

Hodges, L.R. (1972) Distribution and persistence of 1,2-dibromo-3-chloro-
propane in soil (Abstract). Diss. Abstr. Int., 32, 4968B

IARC (1977) IARC Monographs on the Evaluation of the Carcinogenic Risk
of Chemicals to Man, 15, Some Fumigants, the Herbicides 2,4-D and
2,4,5-T, Chlorinated Dibenzodioxins and Miscellaneous Industrial
Chemicals, Lyon, pp. 139-147

IARC (1978) Information Bulletin on the Survey of Chemicals Being Tested
for Carcinogenicity, No. 7, Lyon, pp. 242, 276, 326

Johnson, D.E. & Lear, B. (1969) 1,2-Dibromo-3-chloropropane: recovery from
soil and analysis by GLC. J. chromatogr. Sci., 7, 384-385

Kapp, R.W., Jr, Picciano, D.J. & Jacobson, C.B. (1979) Y-Chromosomal
    nondisjunction in dibromochloropropane-exposed workmen. Mutat. Res.,
    64, 47-51

Kelso, G.L., Wilkinson, R.R., Ferguson, T.L., Malone, J.R., Jr & Oestreich,
    D.K. (1976) Development of Information on Pesticides Manufacturing
    for Source Assessment, EPA Contract No. 68-02-1324, Task 43,
    US Environmental Protection Agency, Washington DC, US Governmer.t
    Printing Office, p. 75

Kodama, J.K. & Dunlap, M.K. (1956) Toxicity of 1,2-dibromo-3-chloropropane
    (Abstract No. 1459). Fed. Proc., 15, 448

Martin, H. & Worthing, C.R., eds. (1977) Pesticide Manual, Basic Informatio
    on the Chemicals Used as Active Components of Pesticides, 5th ed.,
    Malvern, Worcestershire, UK, British Crop Protection Council, p. 162

McBeth, C.W. & Bergeson, G.B. (1955) 1,2-Dibromo-3-chloropropane - A new
    nematocide. Plant Dis. Rep., 39, 223-225

National Cancer Institute (1978) Bioassay of Dibromochloropropane for
    Possible Carcinogenicity (Carcinogenesis Technical Report Series,
    No. 28), National Institutes of Health, US Department of Health,
    Education, & Welfare, DHEW Publication No. (NIH) 78-828

Newsome, W.H., Iverson, F., Panopio, L.G. & Hierlihy, S.L. (1977) Residues
    of dibromochloropropane in root crops grown in fumigated soil. J.
    agric. Food Chem., 25, 684-685

Novik, R.M. & Kozlova, I.V. (1971) Polarographic method of determining
    the insecticide Nemagon in water (Russ.) Fiz.-Khim. Metody Anal.,
    84-91 [Chem. Abstr., 78, 140273b]

Novik, R.M. & Kozlova, I.V. (1973) Possibility of determining Nemagon in
    soil (Russ.). In: Lyalikov, Y.S. & Novik, R.M., eds, Theory and
    Practice of Methods of Polarographic Analyses, Kishinev, USSR,
    Shtiintsa, pp. 71-76 [Chem. Abstr., 83, 2015w]

Novik, R.M. & Plyngyu, N.I. (1973) Use of a.c. polarography to determine
    the insecticide Nemagon in air (Russ.) In: Lyalikov, Y.S. & Novik,
    R.M., eds, Theory and Practice of Methods of Polarographic Analyses,
    Kishinev, USSR, Shtiintsa, pp. 19-24 [Chem. Abstr., 83, 1609f]

Prager, B., Jacobson, P., Schmidt, P. & Stern, D., eds (1918) Beilsteins
    Handbuch der Organischen Chemie, 4th ed., Vol. 1, Syst. no. 10,
    Berlin, Springer, p. 111

Prival, M.J., McCoy, E.C., Gutter, B. & Rosenkranz, H.S. (1977) Tris(2,3-
    dibromopropyl)phosphate: mutagenicity of a widely used flame retar-
    dant. Science, 195, 76-78

Reznik, J.B. & Sprinchan, G.K. (1975) Experimental data on gonadotoxic action of Nemagon (Russ.). Gig. Sanit., 6, 101-102

Rosenkranz, H.S. (1975) Genetic activity of 1,2-dibromo-3-chloropropane, a widely-used fumigant. Bull. environ. Contam. Toxicol., 14, 8-12

Spencer, E.Y. (1973) Guide to the Chemicals Used in Crop Protection, Research Branch, Agriculture Canada, Publication 1093, 6th ed., London, Ontario, University of Western Ontario, p. 172

Torkelson, T.R., Sadek, S.E., Rowe, V.K., Kodama, J.K., Anderson, H.H., Loquvam, G.S. & Hine, C.H. (1961) Toxicologic investigations of 1,2-dibromo-3-chloropropane. Toxicol. appl. Pharmacol., 3, 545-559

US Department of Agriculture (1974) Farmers' Use of Pesticides in 1971... Quantities, Agricultural Economic Report No. 252, Washington DC, Economic Research Service, p. 54

US Environmental Protection Agency (1974) EPA Compendium of Registered Pesticides, Vol. II, Fungicides and Nematicides, Part II, Washington DC, US Government Printing Office, pp. D-25-00.01-D-25-00.13

US Environmental Protection Agency (1976) Manual of Chemical Methods for Pesticides and Devices, Washington DC, Association of Official Analytical Chemists

US Environmental Protection Agency (1977a) Rebuttable presumption against registration and continued registration of pesticide products containing dibromochloropropane (DBCP). Fed. Regist., 42, 48026-48031

US Environmental Protection Agency (1977b) Intent to suspend and conditionally suspend registrations of pesticide products. Fed. Regist., 42, 48915-48922

US International Trade Commission (1977) Synthetic Organic Chemicals, US Production and Sales, 1976, USITC Publication 833, Washington DC, US Government Printing Office, p. 280

US Occupational Safety & Health Administration (1977a) Occupational exposure to 1,2-dibromo-3-chloropropane (DBCP). Emergency temporary standard, hearing. Fed. Regist., 42, 45536-45549

US Occupational Safety & Health Administration (1977b) Occupational exposure to 1,2-dibromo-3-chloropropane (DBCP). Proposed standard, hearing. Fed. Regist., 42, 57266-57283

US Occupational Safety & Health Administration (1978) Occupational exposure to 1,2-dibromo-3-chloropropane (DBCP). Occupational safety and health standards. Fed. Regist., 43, 11514-11533

US Tariff Commission (1956) Synthetic Organic Chemicals, US Production
     and Sales, 1955, Report No. 198, Second Series, Washington DC, US
     Government Printing Office, p. 138

US Tariff Commission (1971) Synthetic Organic Chemicals, US Production
     and Sales, 1969, TC Publication 412, Washington DC, US Government
     Printing Office, p. 191

Whorton, D., Krauss, R.M., Marshall, S. & Milby, T.H. (1977) Infertility
     in male pesticide workers. Lancet, ii, 1259-1261

Whorton, D., Milby, T.H., Krauss, R.M. & Stubbs, H.A. (1979) Testicular
     function in DBCP exposed pesticide workers. J. occup. Med., 21,
     161-166

DICHLORVOS

1. Chemical and Physical Data

1.1 Synonyms and trade names

Chem. Abstr. Services Reg. No.   62-73-7

Chem. Abstr. Name: 2,2-Dichloroethenyl phosphoric acid dimethyl ester

Synonyms: Chlorvinphos; DDVP; dichlorophos; 2,2-dichlorovinyl dimethyl phosphate; 2,2-dichlorovinyl dimethyl phosphoric acid ester; dichlorovos; dimethyl 2,2-dichloroethenyl phosphate; dimethyl dichlorovinyl phosphate; dimethyl 2,2-dichlorovinyl phosphate; vinylophos

Trade names: Atgard; Atgard V; Bibesol; Brevinyl; Brevinyl E50; Canogard; Dedevap; Dichlorman; ENT-20738; Equigard; Equigel; Estrosel; Estrosol; Herkol; Mafu Strip; Mopari; Nerkol; Nogos; Nogos 50; Nogos G; No-Pest Strip; Nuvan; Nuvan 100 EC; OMS 14; SD 1750; Szklarniak; TAP 9VP; Task; Unifos; Unifos 50 EC; Vapona; Vapona Insecticide; Vaponite

1.2 Structural and molecular formulae and molecular weight

$C_4H_7Cl_2O_4P$ Mol. wt: 221.0

1.3 Chemical and physical properties of the pure substance

From Spencer (1973), unless otherwise specified

(a) Description: Colourless-to-amber liquid

(b) Boiling-point: 140°C at 20 mm; 84°C at 1 mm (Windholz, 1976)

(c) Density: $d_4^{25} 1.1415$

(d) Refractive index: n_D^{25} 1.4523

(e) Spectroscopy data: Infra-red, ultra-violet (Gore *et al.*, 1971)
     and Raman spectral data (Nicholas *et al.*, 1976) have been
     tabulated.

(f) Solubility: Soluble in water (1 g/100 ml), glycerol (0.5 g/100
     ml) (Windholz, 1976) and kerosene (2-3 g/100 g); miscible with
     aromatic and chlorinated hydrocarbon solvents and alcohols
     (Hawley, 1977)

(g) Volatility: Vapour pressure is 1.2 x 10^{-2} mm at 20°C.

(h) Stability: Practically nonflammable (Windholz, 1976). A satu-
     rated aqueous solution is hydrolysed at the rate of 3% per day.

(i) Reactivity: Hydrolyses rapidly in alkali. Corrosive to
     iron and mild steel but noncorrosive to stainless steel, alumi-
     nium, nickel, Hastelloy 13 and Teflon

1.4 Technical products and impurities

Dichlorvos is available in the US as a technical grade containing not
less than 93 wt % of the pure chemical and not more than 7 wt % of insec-
ticidally active related compounds (Shell Chemical Company, 1973). Technical grade dichlorvos can contain trichlorphon (*O,O*-dimethyl 2,2,2-trichlo-
ro-1-hydroxyethylphosphonate), *O,O*-dimethyl 2-chlorovinyl phosphate, *O,O*-
dimethyl methylphosphonate, *O,O,O*-trimethyl phosphate and chloral (trichlo-
roacetaldehyde) (Gillett *et al.*, 1972a).

Dichlorvos is formulated as solutions (fogging concentrates), emulsifiable concentrates, dilute spray solutions, baits and resin strips (Shell
Chemical Company, 1973).

2. Production, Use, Occurrence and Analysis

2.1 Production and use

(a) Production

Dichlorvos was prepared independently in several laboratories in the
period 1951-1955. It can be prepared by the reaction of trimethyl phos-
phite and chloral (the commercial process) or by the dehydrochlorination of
trichlorphon (Spencer, 1973).

Commercial production of dichlorvos in the US was first reported in 1961 (US Tariff Commission, 1962). In the period 1961-1972, only one US company reported commercial production of an undisclosed amount (see preamble, p. 16) (US International Trade Commission, 1977). Kelso *et al.* (1976) estimated that 0.9 million kg dichlorvos were produced in the US in 1974.

Six companies in Benelux, the Federal Republic of Germany, Spain and Switzerland produce an estimated 1-10 million kg dichlorvos annually. Imports and exports are in the range of 100-1000 thousand kg for most of these regions. Production in the eastern European countries is estimated to be less than 100 thousand kg dichlorvos annually, and imports and exports are each less than 100 thousand kg.

In Japan, dichlorvos was first produced commercially in 1963. In 1976, 3 companies produced a total of 1.1 million kg, of which 573 thousand kg were exported; 4000 kg were imported.

(b) Use

The only known uses of dichlorvos are as an insecticide and as an anthelminthic for swine and dogs. It is registered for use in flea collars for pets; in the control of external parasites on livestock, insects in buildings and outdoor areas, insects affecting certain greenhouse crops and insects on harvested tomatoes; and on mushrooms in mushroom houses (US Environmental Protection Agency, 1973). It is also used for mosquito and fly control (US Environmental Protection Agency, 1976a).

In 1971, 16 thousand kg were used on crops in the US and 1.1 million kg on livestock and in livestock buildings (US Department of Agriculture, 1974). In 1975, 80% of the dichlorvos produced in the US was formulated into resin strips containing 20% of the compound and used primarily in households. Aerosol sprays containing dichlorvos are also used by pest control operators in households and elsewhere (US Environmental Protection Agency, 1976a).

Use of dichlorvos in Europe in 1968 was reviewed (WHO, 1968), but no data on its use in Japan were available.

In November 1970, the Joint Meeting of the FAO Working Party of Experts on Pesticide Residues and the WHO Expert Committee on Pesticide Residues recommended tolerances for preharvest and postharvest treatment of many commodities: the range was from 0.02 mg/kg for milk to 5 mg/kg for cocoa beans; 0.5 mg/kg was recommended for fresh vegetables and tomatoes (WHO, 1971). Residue tolerances established on commodities in the US are generally in the range of 0.02 mg/kg in meat and milk to 1 mg/kg on lettuce (US Environmental Protection Agency, 1976b).

The US Environmental Protection Agency reported on 20 January 1978 that dichlorvos may qualify as a candidate for issuance of a notice of a rebuttable presumption against renewal of registration (RPAR) (see

General Remarks on the Substances Considered, p. 31) on the basis of mutagenic, reproductive and foetotoxic effects and possible carcinogenicity. A decision on this possible course of action awaits the recommendations of the Carcinogen Assessment Group of the US Environmental Protection Agency (Anon., 1978).

A maximum acceptable daily intake of dichlorvos for humans of 0-0.004 mg/kg bw was established at the Joint Meeting of the FAO Working Group of Experts on Pesticide Residues and the WHO Expert Committee on Pesticide Residues in December 1974 (WHO, 1975). This was confirmed in December 1977 (FAO/WHO, 1978).

The US Occupational Safety and Health Administration standards for exposure to air contaminants require that an employee's exposure to dichlorvos not exceed an 8-hr time-weighted average of 1 mg/m^3 (about 0.1 ppm) in the working atmosphere in any 8-hr work shift of a 40-hr work week (US Occupational Safety & Health Administration, 1977). The corresponding standard in the Federal Republic of Germany is also 1 mg/m^3 (about 0.1 ppm), and the acceptable ceiling concentration in the USSR is 0.2 mg/m^3 (about 0.02 ppm) (Winell, 1975).

2.2 Occurrence

Although dichlorvos is not known to occur as a natural product, it does occur in organs and muscles of cattle as a residue after its application as a pesticide and as a conversion product of the insecticide trichlorphon (*O,O*-dimethyl 2,2,2-trichloro-1-hydroxyethyl phosphonate) (Nepoklonov & Metelitsa, 1971). In the US, over 600 thousand kg trichlorphon were used on livestock in 1971.

Dichlorvos has been found in mouse brain after i.p. injection of trichlorphon (Nordgren *et al.*, 1978); it is formed by heating trichlorphon at 70°C (Holmstedt *et al.*, 1978).

(a) Air and food

Dichlorvos has been detected in: (1) stored wheat, at levels of 2.4-6.0 mg/kg, which decreased to 0.5 mg/kg or less during 6 weeks of storage (Vardell *et al.*, 1973); (2) cereal products and flour, at levels of 0-5.8 mg/kg (Raffke & Wirthgen, 1976); (3) crude soya bean oil and meal, at levels of < 1 mg/kg (La Hue *et al.*, 1975); and (4) malt and worts, at levels of 0-2 mg/kg (Leuzinger, 1975). Dichlorvos has also been detected in: (1) mushrooms and the air above them (< 0.2 mg/m^3) 8 hrs after spraying (Gruebner, 1972); (2) raspberries, at levels of 0.2-7 mg/kg (Romaniuk, 1976); (3) milk and milk products (Konrad *et al.*, 1975); and (4) vegetable food products (0.24 mg/kg) (Lyubenko *et al.*, 1973).

Dichlorvos has been found in prepared foods at concentrations of 0.005-1.653 mg/kg after experimental exposure to air containing dichlorvos in concentrations ranging from 0.035-0.577 mg/m^3 (0.003-0.06 ppm) (Dale et al., 1973).

Dichlorvos has been found in households in which commercial pest strips were used, in concentrations of 0-0.24 mg/m^3 (0-0.026 ppm) in ambient air and <0.01-0.12 mg/kg in the foods prepared therein (Collins & DeVries, 1973; Elgar & Steer, 1972; Elgar et al., 1972a; Leary et al., 1974). It has also been detected in the air of food shops where the strips were used, at mean concentrations of <0.01-0.03 mg/m^3 (<0.001-0.003 ppm), and in the foods in the shops, at concentrations of <0.05 mg/kg (Elgar et al., 1972b).

Seven days after application of trichlorphon, dichlorvos was found in sheep organs, at concentrations of 0.8-1.2 mg/kg (Nepoklonov & Bukshtynov, 1971); in the tissue of cattle, 15-22 days after application (Nepoklonov & Metelitsa, 1971); and in the leaves of cabbages and onion plants, at low levels during the first 7 days after application (Baida, 1975).

(b) Water

Dichlorvos has been detected in: (1) a water reservoir and a water supply-irrigation system in the USSR (Akimov & Babich, 1975); (2) the polluted waters of 4 rivers (Drevenkar et al., 1975); and (3) the waste-water from a dichlorvos production plant in Bulgaria (16 g/l) (Andreeva et al., 1973).

(c) Occupational exposure

Dichlorvos has been detected in the workplace environment: (1) in concentrations of 0.7 mg/m^3 (0.077 ppm) in air, during the production and processing of a dichlorvos-releasing vaporizer (Menz et al., 1974); and (2) in average concentrations of 1.19 mg/m^3 (0.13 ppm) in air during the spraying of an orchard. In the latter case, the rate of skin contamination was 0.072 mg/100 cm^2/hr (Sawinsky et al., 1973).

2.3 Analysis

Methods used for the analysis of dichlorvos in environmental samples are listed in Table 1.

Other analytical methods used to isolate and identify dichlorvos include: gel-permeation chromatography (Johnson et al., 1976); gas chromatography on packed columns (Thompson et al., 1975) or on capillary columns (Krijgsman & Van De Kamp, 1976); gas chromatography/mass spectrometry (Rosen & Pareles, 1974); high-pressure liquid chromatography (Szalontai, 1976); thin-layer chromatography (Štefanac et al., 1976); polarography (Seifert & Davidek, 1974); and spectrophotometry (Fitak & Gwiazda, 1975; Mukherjee et al., 1973; Ogata et al., 1975; Rajak & Krishnamurthy, 1974; Turner, 1974).

TABLE 1. METHODS FOR THE ANALYSIS OF DICHLORVOS

SAMPLE TYPE	EXTRACTION/CLEAN-UP	ANALYTICAL METHOD DETECTION	LIMIT OF DETECTION	REFERENCE
Formulations	Dissolve (chloroform), centrifuge, filter	IR		Goza (1972)
Fly bait	Extract (chloroform) on CC	IR		Horwitz (1975)
Spray in hydrocarbon solvents	Wash (alkali)	IR (on hydrocarbon phase)		Horwitz (1975)
Air	Trap in acetone	Spectrophotometry of resorcinol complex at 490 nm	0.14 mg/m^3	Leo & Suwalska (1977)
Water	Extract (benzene or chloroform)	Spectrophotometry of ortho-tolidine complex at 400-500 nm; or TLC (revelation: sodium carbonate/resorcinol)	50 µg/l	Babina et al. (1972)
			30 µg/l	Babina et al. (1972)
	Extract (dichloromethane)	Spectrophotometry of resorcinol derivative of dichlorvos dichloroacetaldehyde adduct at 487 nm	40 µg/l	Novikova & Mel'tser (1973)
Food & drinks				
Whole meals	Blend, absorb on Celite, extract (acidified ethyl acetate/hexane), filter, CC	GC/flame photometry	5 µg/kg	Dale et al. (1973)

TABLE 1. METHODS FOR THE ANALYSIS OF DICHLORVOS (continued)

SAMPLE TYPE	ANALYTICAL METHOD			
	EXTRACTION/CLEAN-UP	DETECTION	LIMIT OF DETECTION	REFERENCE
Beverages	Acidify, extract (hexane)	GC/flame photometry	5 µg/kg	Dale *et al.* (1973)
Margarine	Dissolve (ethyl acetate-hexane), CC	GC/flame photometry	5 µg/kg	Dale *et al.* (1973)
Cereals & pulses	Extract (hexane) in Soxhlet, liquid/liquid partition, CC	GC/flame photometry	0.008-1.01 ng/sample	Aoki *et al.* (1975)
Grain	Grind, homogenize (methanol), concentrate, add acetone	GC/flame photometry or thermionic detection	20 µg/kg	Panel on Malathion & Dichlorvos Residues in Grain (1973)
Vegetables	Extract (acetonitrile)	TLC (revelation: sodium carbonate-resorcinol)	0.25 µg/ml	Kavetskii (1974)
Mixed feed	Extract (acetone), transfer to water, filter, extract (chloroform)	TLC (revelation:sodium carbonate-resorcinol)	0.5-0.8 mg/kg	Konyukhov (1974)
Vegetables & fruit	Extract (chloroform), purify (activated charcoal)	TLC (revelation: enzymatic technique)	0.01 mg/kg	Zadrozinska (1973)
Milk	Coagulate (acetone), extract supernatant (petroleum ether)	Spectrophotometry of resorcinol derivative of dichlorvos dichloro-acetaldehyde adduct at 487 nm	0.1 mg/1	Novika & Mel'tser (1973)
Vegetables	Homogenize (acetone), liquid/liquid partition, gel permeation chromatography	GC/thermionic detection	50 µg/kg	Pflugmacher & Ebing (1974)

TABLE 1. METHODS FOR THE ANALYSIS OF DICHLORVOS (continued)

| SAMPLE TYPE | ANALYTICAL METHOD | | | |
	EXTRACTION/CLEAN-UP	DETECTION	LIMIT OF DETECTION	REFERENCE
Biological				
Blood	Extract (petroleum ether-ethyl ether), CC	TLC (revelation: 4-nitrobenzylpyridine)	15-20 µg	Becsey (1974)
Human tissues	Extract (hexane or acetone), slurry of sodium sulphate, liquid/liquid partition	TLC (revelation: silver nitrate or palladium chloride reagents)	10 µg/kg	Tewari & Harpalani (1977)
Animal organs & tissues	Extract (chloroform or acetone), liquid/liquid partition	TLC (revelation: silver nitrate)	1-5 µg	Kazanovskii (1975)

Abbreviations: IR - infra-red spectrometry; CC - column chromatography; GC - gas chromatography;
TLC - thin-layer chromatography

3. Biological Data Relevant to the Evaluation
of Carcinogenic Risk to Humans

3.1 Carcinogenicity studies in animals

(a) Oral administration

Mouse: Groups of 50 male and 50 female 5-7-week-old B6C3F1 hybrid mice were fed technical-grade dichlorvos (94% minimum purity) in their diet. Initially, high-dose animals received 2000 mg/kg diet, and low-dose animals received 1000 mg/kg diet; however, after 2 weeks these doses were reduced to 600 mg/kg and 300 mg/kg diet, respectively, because of severe toxicity. Test animals were maintained at these dietary levels for 78 weeks, followed by 12-14 weeks on dichlorvos-free diets, after which time (90-94 weeks) the animals were killed and necropsied. The measured, time-weighted, average doses were 635 (high dose) and 318 (low dose) mg/kg diet. Groups of 10 male and 10 female mice that served as matched controls were maintained on dichlorvos-free diets for 92 weeks. Further control data were obtained from pooled control animals (100 males and 80 females), in order to increase the scope of the statistical analysis. In the female low-dose groups, 13/50 animals died before week 90; survival to 90 weeks was greater than 84% in all other groups. Histopathology was performed on all organ systems in 94% or more of animals entered into the experiment. Average weights of high-dose mice of both sexes were generally lower than those of low-dose and control groups, but the differences never exceeded 10%. In male mice, 29/92 in the pooled control group that were examined histopathologically developed tumours, compared with 1/10 in matched controls, 21/50 of the low-dose group and 14/50 in the high-dose group. In female mice, the respective tumour incidences were 14/79 in pooled controls, 1/9 in matched controls, 11/49 in low-dose animals and 8/50 in high-dose animals. There were no significant differences between test and control groups in the age at observation of any tumours. The only unusual findings were 2 squamous-cell carcinomas (in 1 low-dose male and 1 high-dose female), 1 papilloma of the oesophagus (high-dose female), and 3 cases of focal hyperplasia of the oesophageal epithelium (2 low-dose males and 1 high-dose female) (National Cancer Institute, 1977).

Rat: Groups of 50 male and 50 female 5-7-week-old Osborne-Mendel rats were fed diets containing technical-grade dichlorvos (94% minimum purity). High-dose animals received 1000 mg/kg diet for 3 weeks; this level was reduced to 300 mg/kg diet for the rest of the study after severe toxicity was observed. Low-dose animals received 150 mg/kg diet. Both groups were fed dichlorvos for 80 weeks and were maintained for a further 30 weeks on a dichlorvos-free diet. Time-weighted average doses were 326 mg/kg and 150 mg/kg diet, respectively. Groups of 10 animals of each sex were used as matched controls, and groups of 60 animals of each sex as pooled controls. Weight gain was consistently lower in high-dose groups compared with low-dose and control groups: 76% of high-dose males, 84% of high-dose females, 64% of low-dose males and 80% of low-dose females survived for more than 105 weeks. There was no evidence of dose-related mortality and no significant difference in survival between treated and control groups. Histopathology of all organ systems was performed on 94% or more of the animals entered into the study. The numbers of tumour-bearing males, excluding those with tumours of the reproductive tract, were: pooled controls, 37/58; matched controls, 6/10; low-dose, 20/48; high-dose, 33/50; males with tumours of the reproductive tract were: 2/58, 0/10, 3/48 and 2/50, respectively. The numbers of tumour-bearing females, excluding those with tumours of the reproductive tract, were: pooled controls, 38/60; matched controls, 8/10; low-dose, 34/48; high-dose, 30/50; females with tumours of the reproductive tract were: 19/60, 5/10, 17/48 and 10/50, respectively. The incidence of malignant fibrous histiocytomas in male rats was the only one that showed a statistically significant trend (2/58 pooled controls; 4/48 low-dose; 8/50 high-dose; P = 0.018); however, the occurrence of malignant fibrous histiocy-toma in 1/10 animals in the matched-control group does not support the suggestion of a treatment-related effect. Furthermore, on the basis of the variability of both incidence and type of spontaneous lesions and the lack of significant increases in tumour yield or decreases in time to first tumour in dosed groups, no significance could be attached to the trend in tumours seen in dichlorvos-fed rats (National Cancer Institute, 1977).

(b) Inhalation and/or intratracheal administration

Rat: Groups of 50 male and 50 female 5-week-old Carworth Farm E strain rats were exposed continuously to atmospheres containing 0 (control), 0.05, 0.5 or 5 mg/m^3 (0.0055, 0.05 or 0.55 ppm) technical-grade dichlor-vos (purity greater than 97%) for 104 weeks. The mean values for the en-tire test period were 0.05, 0.48 and 4.7 mg/m^3, all $\pm$ 20%. All treated groups showed decreases in weight gain compared with controls, this being most marked in those given 5 mg/m^3. The numbers of males still alive at 104 weeks were 11/50 controls, 21/50 given 0.05 mg/m^3, 15/50 given 0.5 mg/m^3, and 32/50 given 5 mg/m^3; females still alive at that time were 22/47 controls, 27/47 given 0.05 mg/m^3, 26/47 given 0.5 mg/m^3 and 34/47 given 5 mg/m^3. Complete necropsy and histopathology were performed on 20-32% of male rats and 20-36% of females, reducing the effective numbers of animals per group to between 10 and 18. No significantly increased risk of tumour incidence could be attributed to treatment with dichlorvos (Blair et al., 1976) [The Working Group noted the very low doses used, the small number of animals submitted for complete necropsy and the high incidence of tumours in control groups].

3.2 Other relevant biological data

The toxicology, biochemistry and possible health hazards of dichlorvos have been reviewed (Anon, 1974; Attfield & Webster, 1966; Gillett et al., 1972a,b; WHO, 1971; Wright et al., 1979).

(a) Experimental systems

Toxic effects

The LD_{50} by inhalation is 75-108 mg/kg bw in mice, 56-65 mg/kg bw in rats, and 25 mg/kg bw in rabbits; the LD_{100} for cats is 50 mg/kg bw (Sasinovich, 1967). The oral LD_{50} for chicks is 15 mg/kg bw (Sherman & Ross, 1961); for rats, 56-80 mg/kg bw (Durham et al., 1957); and for mice, about 140-275 mg/kg bw (Anon, 1974; Holmstedt et al., 1978). The dermal LD_{50} for rats is 75-900 mg/kg, depending on the solvent (Jones et al., 1968). In mice, the i.p. LD_{50} is 28-41 mg/kg bw; the s.c. LD_{50}, 20-26 mg/kg bw; and the i.v. LD_{50}, 8-10 mg/kg bw (Holmstedt et al., 1978).

The LC_{100} for rats was exposure to more than 30 mg/m^3 (3.3 ppm) dichlorvos in air for 5-83 hrs (Durham et al., 1957).

Feeding dichlorvos at up to 1000 mg/kg diet for 90 days caused no signs of intoxication in rats, but dietary levels as low as 50 mg/kg diet produced definite reductions of plasma and erythrocyte cholinesterase levels. Rats exposed to dichlorvos vapours in air [6.0 decreasing to 0.1 mg/m^3 (0.66-0.011 ppm) over 2 weeks] showed no signs of organic phosphate poisoning, but slight reductions in plasma and erythrocyte cholinesterase levels were observed. The erythrocyte and plasma cholinesterase levels in monkeys similarly exposed fell rapidly during exposure but recovered after exposure was discontinued. Three monkeys treated daily with dermal doses of 50, 75 and 100 mg/kg bw dichlorvos in xylene for 5 days per week died after 8, 10 and 4 doses, respectively. The erythrocyte cholinesterase activity fell rapidly and remained depressed for the period of the experiment; plasma cholinesterase levels fell, then returned to normal (Durham et al., 1957).

In 48 male rats that received daily topical applications of 21.4 mg/kg bw dichlorvos in ethanol on 5 days/week for 90 days, no gross or histological changes associated with dichlorvos exposure were seen in the skin or testes (Dikshith et al., 1976).

In male rats fed dichlorvos, non-neoplastic lesions were observed, including aggregates of alveolar macrophages in the lungs, interstitial fibrosis of the myocardium and focal follicular-cell hyperplasia of the thyroid. Focal hepatocytomegaly and chronic nephritis were also observed (National Cancer Institute, 1977).

Cholinesterase activity in the plasma and brains of male and female rats exposed to 0.5 and 5 mg/m^3 in air was reduced significantly compared with control values. The cholinesterase activity of erythrocytes was reduced significantly in males and females exposed to 5 mg/m^3 and in females exposed to 0.5 and 0.05 mg/m^3. No dichlorvos-related changes were seen in brain acetylcholine or choline levels after 2 years' exposure. Respiratory tissues showed no ultrastructural changes attributable to exposure to 5 mg/m^3 dichlorvos for 2 years (Blair et al., 1976).

Nursing female rats were given repeated oral doses of 30 mg/kg bw dichlorvos. Their litters showed normal plasma and erythrocyte cholinesterase activities and normal weight-gain curves. Two cows suckling calves showed normal erythrocyte cholinesterase levels while ingesting 200 mg dichlorvos/kg diet daily; however at 500 mg/kg diet, a severe depression in these levels occurred, and a single dose of 27 mg/kg bw caused cholinergic collapse, followed by recovery. The cholinesterase levels of the calves remained normal throughout the 78-day test. Five horses exposed continuously to vapours of 0.5 mg dichlorvos/ft^3 of air [17.7 mg/m^3 (2 ppm)], giving a range of 0.24-1.5 mg/m^3 (0.026-0.16 ppm), in a closed barn for 22 days showed mild erythrocyte cholinesterase depression after 7 days, which returned to normal at 11-22 days. Plasma cholinesterase levels remained normal during the experiment (Tracy *et al.*, 1960).

Dogs, cats and rabbits were exposed continuously for 8 weeks to dichlorvos atmospheres in air ranging from 0.05-0.3 mg/m^3 (0.0055-0.033 ppm). No effects were found on general health, behaviour, plasma or erythrocyte cholinesterase activities or electroencephalographic patterns (Walker *et al.*, 1972).

Thirty-two rhesus monkeys were given pellets of polyvinyl chloride resin formulations containing dichlorvos orally at doses ranging from 5-80 mg/kg bw, daily or twice daily for 10-21 days. Plasma and erythrocyte cholinesterase activities were significantly inhibited in all treated animals (Hass *et al.*, 1972).

Embryotoxicity and teratogenicity

When dichlorvos was given by i.p. injection to rats on day 11 of pregnancy at a dose of 15 mg/kg bw, 3 of 41 foetuses developed malformations (omphaloceles) (Kimbrough & Gaines, 1968).

Groups of 15 rats were exposed to atmospheres containing 0.25, 1.25 and 6.25 mg/m^3 (0.027-0.69 ppm) for 23 hrs, daily, from days 1 to 20 of pregnancy. The treatment had no effect on the pregnancies, number of foetal resorptions or late foetal deaths, litter size or mean weight per foetus. The observation of only one malformed foetus in the group given 0.25 mg/m^3 (skeletal defects and gastroschisis) was regarded as unrelated to exposure of the dam to dichlorvos (Thorpe *et al.*, 1972).

In studies reported as abstracts, concentrations of up to 500 mg/kg diet dichlorvos given to rats through 3 generations and 12 mg/kg bw given orally to rabbits during the period of major organogenesis had no teratogenic effects (Vogin *et al.*, 1971; Witherup *et al.*, 1971). Mean foetal weight was slightly depressed in offspring of rabbits that inhaled 4 mg/m^3 (0.44 ppm) dichlorvos in air from days 1-28 of gestation; this was considered to be the result of toxic effects on the mother (Thorpe *et al.*, 1972).

In two abstracts, it was reported that doses of 800 mg/animal
dichlorvos fed daily to pigs through gestation, or from 18-56 days
before parturition, did not interfere with development of the offspring
(Batte et al., 1969); reproduction was not impaired when male and
female swine were fed for up to 37 months on a diet containing up to
500 mg/kg diet dichlorvos (Collins et al., 1971).

No abortions or malformations were induced in a pregnant cow fed
6.2 mg/kg bw/day dichlorvos for 134 days before parturition (Macklin &
Ribelin, 1971).

A single oral dose of 40 µg/kg bw induced a drastic reduction in
germinal epithelium of mouse testis (Krause & Homola, 1972).

[The Working Group noted that the low doses used in many of the above
studies might explain the lack of embryotoxicity or teratogenicity
reported].

Absorption, distribution, excretion and metabolism

Studies using ^{32}P-, ^{36}Cl-, [vinyl-^{14}C]- and [methyl-^{14}C]-dichlor-
vos in pigs, rats and mice, have shown that dichlorvos is degraded
rapidly, whether it is administered orally or by inhalation (reviewed by
Blair et al., 1975). After oral administration of [vinyl-1-^{14}C]-dichlorvos
to male rats, 42% of the radioactivity was recovered as metabolites
during the first 24 hrs. After 4 days, 39% of the radioactivity was
recovered as ^{14}C-carbon dioxide, 13% was excreted in the urine and 3.4% in
the faeces, and 16% was found in the carcass. At least 9 metabolites
were detected in the urine; ^{14}C-labelled metabolites were dichloroethyl
β-D-glucopyranosiduronic acid, demethyldichlorvos, hippuric acid, N-
benzoyl glycine and urea. Four days after dosing, 5% of the radioactivity
of the administered dose was associated with liver, largely in the
protein fraction as ^{14}C-glycine and ^{14}C-serine. Similar results were
obtained in rats exposed by inhalation to ^{14}C-dichlorvos (Hutson et al.,
1971a,b).

Exposure of rats to 10 mg/m^3 (1.1 ppm) for 4 hrs was required before
dichlorvos could be detected reliably, and then only in kidneys; the half-
life of dichlorvos in kidneys of animals exposed to 50 mg/m^3 (5.5 ppm)
for 4 hrs was 13.5 min. With 90 mg/m^3 (10 ppm), which is equivalent to 60%
of full air saturation, dichlorvos could be detected in most tissues. In
mice similarly exposed, dichlorvos was found in most tissues, but at 1/10 of
the levels found in rats (Blair et al., 1975).

The metabolism of dichlorvos has been reviewed (Hathway, 1975;
Wright et al., 1979); it is metabolized via two major pathways: (1)
hydrolysis and (2) O-demethylation. (1) The primary products of the
esterase-catalysed hydrolysis of the P-O (vinyl) bond are dimethyl
phosphate, which is excreted in the urine, and dichloroacetaldehyde,
which is rapidly degraded to dichloroethanol. This may be glucuronidated

and excreted in the urine or dehalogenated to a 2-carbon fragment,
which may then enter pathways of intermediary metabolism. (2) *O*-Demethyl-
ation of dichlorvos can proceed *via* (a) oxidative demethylation catalysed
by microsomal mono-oxygenases, with formation of formaldehyde and demethyldichlorvos, or (b) *S*-methyl transferase-catalysed monomethylation, to
yield *S*-methylglutathione and demethyldichlorvos. Of the two major
metabolic routes (1) and (2), esterase-catalysed hydrolysis is quantita-
tively more important and occurs in a wide range of tissues. The tissue
distribution of methyl transferases is less well defined, but such
activities have been demonstrated in liver and kidney.

Reaction with macromolecules

Dichlorvos alkylates bacteriophage and bacterial and mammalian
nucleic acids *in vitro* (Lawley *et al.*, 1974; Löfroth, 1970; Löfroth
et al., 1969; Shooter, 1975; Wennerberg & Löfroth, 1974).

When [methyl-^{14}C]-dichlorvos (36.6 Ci/mol) was reacted with salmon
sperm DNA, *Escherichia coli* DNA, *E. coli* cells and HeLa cells, it was
found that dichlorvos broadly resembles methyl methanesulphonate (MMS)
in its pattern of alkylation. In DNA, 7-methylguanine was the major
product (63-93%), and 3-methyladenine was the principle minor product
(8.8-13.7%) (except in *E. coli* cells, where there was rapid excision of
3-methyladenine); O^6-methylguanine was detected only in trace amounts.
This pattern of methylation is ascribed to the S$_N$2 mechanism of alkylation
characteristic of agents such as MMS and dimethylsulphate; however, dichlorvos methylated DNA at about 1/4 the rate of MMS and to 1/15 the
extent per unit time under comparable conditions. Dichlorvos methylated
cellular proteins more rapidly than it did the nucleic acids of *E. coli*
cells and HeLa cells (Lawley *et al.*, 1974). Studies of the effect of
dichlorvos on the survival of bacteria and Chinese hamster cells suggest
that dichlorvos caused DNA-strand breakage by an indirect mechanism
(probably by alkylation of cellular protein and subsequent uncontrolled
nuclease activity), and to a lesser extent by direct methylation of DNA
(Green *et al.*, 1974; Lawley *et al.*, 1974).

Mice were exposed to [^{14}C-methyl]- or [^{3}H-methyl]-dichlorvos (3.2
Ci/mol or 0.7 Ci/mol, respectively), by inhalation or intraperitoneally,
at doses ranging from about 5-45 mg/kg bw. Peaks of radioactivity (10-
30 cpm/ml) coincident with markers of hypoxanthine and 7-methylguanine,
together with peaks for unidentified material, were detected in column
chromatograms of 24-hr urine samples collected from exposed mice. The
most probable explanation for these results was said to be a chemical,
non-enzymatic methylation of guanine moieties by dichlorvos. No data
showing levels of alkylation of tissue macromolecules of exposed mice
were given (Wennerberg & Löfroth, 1974).

Twenty male rats were exposed to atmospheres containing 0.064 mg/m^3
(0.007 ppm) ('practical use concentration') [methyl-^{14}C]-dichlorvos (113
Ci/mol) for 12 hrs, giving a total inhaled dose of 6 µg/rat (∿0.03 mg/kg
bw). Traces of radioactivity were detected in RNA, DNA and protein of

major soft-tissue organs;   these ranged, in DNA, from 0.83 dpm/mg (testis)
to 9.9 dpm/mg (spleen);   in RNA, from 1.46 dpm/mg (brain) to 5.54 dpm/mg
(heart/lung);   and in protein, from 1.93 dpm/mg (brain) to 20.8 dpm/mg
(heart/lung).   Analysis of the DNA and RNA from total soft tissues
revealed no 7-methylguanine, the limits of detection of methylation
being 1 methyl group per 6×10^{11} nucleotides DNA and 2×10^9 nucleotides
RNA.   Chromatographic analysis of urine from exposed rats revealed no
radioactivity associated with added marker 7-methylguanine (Wooder *et
al.*, 1977).

Mutagenicity and other related short-term tests

The mutagenicity of dichlorvos has been reviewed (Wild, 1975).

Dichlorvos induced reverse mutations to streptomycin-independence
in *E. coli* B (Sd-4) (Löfroth *et al.*, 1969).   In plate tests with *E. coli*
WP2, dichlorvos induced *trp* reversions (Ashwood-Smith *et al.*, 1972;
Nagy *et al.*, 1975);   although, in the same system, negative (Dean, 1972a)
and variable results (Bridges *et al.*, 1973) have also been reported.   In
liquid tests with the same bacterial strain, a time-dependent increase
in *trp* reversions was observed with 1-3 hrs' treatment with   13 mM dichlorvos
(Bridges *et al.*, 1973).   Also in liquid tests, Wild (1973, 1975) recorded
a time- and concentration-dependent increase in the frequency of forward
mutations to streptomycin-resistance in a streptomycin-sensitive *E. coli*
B strain with up to 10 hrs' treatment with 5-25 mM dichlorvos.   Similar
results were obtained by Mohn (1973) with much lower concentrations,
i.e., up to 6 hrs' treatment with 0.3-3.2 mM dichlorvos, for the induction
of forward mutations to 5-methyltryptophan resistance in *E. coli* K12.

Positive results have also been obtained (i) in plate tests with
Serratia marcescens (Dean, 1972a), *Streptomyces coelicolor* (Carere *et
al.*, 1976) and *Salmonella typhimurium* strains TA1535, 1537 and 1538
(Shirasu *et al.*, 1976);   (ii) in liquid tests with *Pseudomonas aeruginosa*
strain PAO38 and *S. typhimurium* strains C117 and TA1535 (Carere *et al.*,
1978a,b;   Dyer & Hanna, 1973);   (iii) in fluctuation tests with *Klebsiella
pneumoniae*, *E. coli* K12, *Citrobacter freundii* and *Enterobacter aerogenes*
(Voogd *et al.*, 1972);   and (iv) in *rec* assays (disc assays on nutrient
agar plates) with *Bacillus subtilis* strain M45 *rec⁻* (Shirasu *et al.*,
1976).   An *E. coli* strain deficient in DNA polymerase (*pol A*) was more
susceptible than the wild type to the lethal and mutagenic actions of
dichlorvos (Bridges *et al.*, 1973;   Rosenkranz, 1973).

The results with bacteria (Bridges *et al.*, 1973;   Mohn, 1973;
Shirasu *et al.*, 1976) suggest that dichlorvos induces base-pair substitution type mutations.   The mutation process is largely error-prone
(i.e., *exrA+-* and *recA+-*dependent).   The pattern of response of strains
of *E. coli* WP2 that are deficient at 4 different loci concerned with DNA
repair (*polA, uvrA, recA, exrA*) is   qualitatively similar with dichlorvos
and with the methylating agent MMS, with regard both to survival and

mutation induction. Thus, the mutagenic action of dichlorvos is most
probably a result of DNA alkylation (Bridges *et al.*, 1973).

Dichlorvos induced point mutations, mitotic crossing-over and non-
disjunction in *Aspergillus nidulans* (Bignami *et al.*, 1977). It was not
mutagenic to conidia of *Neurospora crassa* exposed to an atmosphere
containing dichlorvos, but the actual concentration of dichlorvos in the
cell environment was unknown (Michalek & Brockman, 1969). In *Saccharomyces
cerevisiae* strain D4, dichlorvos produced a concentration-dependent increase
in the frequency of mitotic gene convertants at the *ade* and *trp* loci,
with exposure for 5 hrs to 5-40 mM (Dean *et al.*, 1972; Fahrig, 1973).
Host-mediated assays, involving *S. typhimurium* and *Serratia marcescens*
bacteria as indicator organisms and mice injected subcutaneously with 25
mg/kg bw dichlorvos as hosts, were negative (Buselmaier *et al.*, 1972;
Voogd *et al.*, 1972).

In those microbial systems in which positive results have been
recorded, dichlorvos is much less effective than 'reference' alkylating
agents such as MMS or *N*-nitrosomethylguanidine, i.e., the concentration
of dichlorvos that produced a given mutagenic effect was 20-50 times
higher than for MMS and about 100 times higher than for the nitrosamine
(Bridges *et al.*, 1973; Fahrig, 1973; Wild, 1973).

Dichlorvos induced chromosome aberrations in onion root tips (Sax &
Sax, 1968). When barley seeds were treated with 0.25-0.75 nM dichlorvos
for 6 or 18 hrs, there was an increased frequency of chromosome aberrations
in the root-tip preparations of the seedlings, but no chlorophyll mutations were observed in the M2 generation (Bhan & Kaul, 1975).

No significant effects were noted in tests for sex-linked lethal
mutations in male *Drosophila melanogaster* raised in a medium containing
0.009-0.09 mg/kg dichlorvos (Jayasuriya & Ratnayake, 1973; Kramers &
Knaap, 1978). The observation by Gupta & Singh (1974) of a high incidence
(10%) of aberrations in the salivary gland chromosome of third instar
larvae grown in food containing 1 mg/kg dichlorvos is difficult to
interpret, since it is very unlikely that a chemical would produce such
a high frequency of chromosome aberrations but no sex-linked lethal
mutations.

A significant increase in the frequency of autosomal lethal mutations in flies reared in a dichlorvos-containing medium was found in
studies in which populations were exposed continuously to a dichlorvos-
containing medium over about 30 generations (Hanna & Dyer, 1975).
During this period, larvae developed increasing resistance to dichlorvos,
and its concentration had to be raised from 0.1 mg/kg to 0.75 mg/kg in
the course of the experiment. The results of this study are therefore
not directly comparable with those from standard recessive lethal tests.

No induction of 8-azaguanine-resistant mutations was detected in
V79 Chinese hamster cells that had been treated in serum-containing
culture medium for 2 hrs with up to 1 mM dichlorvos (Wild, 1975). In

another study with human peripheral blood lymphocytes treated *in vitro*
with up to 0.18 mM dichlorvos for different durations, no significant
cytogenetic changes were observed (Dean, 1972b).

No significant effect of dichlorvos was found in any *in vivo* mammalian
study. Negative results were reported in dominant lethal studies: (1)
with male mice that received 5 x 10 mg/kg bw dichlorvos orally or 13
and 16.5 mg/kg bw by i.p. injection (Epstein *et al.*, 1972) or were
exposed to atmospheres containing dichlorvos at concentrations of 30 and
55 mg/m^3 of air for 16 hrs or to 2.1 and 5.8 mg/m^3 for 23 hrs, daily for
4 weeks (Dean & Thorpe, 1972a); and (2) with female mice that received
25 and 50 mg/kg bw dichlorvos orally or were exposed to atmospheres
containing up to about 8 mg/m^3 dichlorvos in air (Dean & Blair, 1976).
In cytogenetic studies, no effects were seen when male mice were exposed
to dichlorvos by inhalation of 64-72 mg/m^3 of air for 16 hrs or of 5
mg/m^3 of air for 21 days; and none were seen in male Chinese hamsters
exposed by inhalation and orally to high concentrations of dichlorvos.
In chromosome preparations made from bone marrow and spermatocytes of
exposed mice and hamsters, the incidence of chromosome abnormalities did
not differ from that in controls (Dean & Thorpe, 1972b). The incidence
of sperm abnormalities in dichlorvos-treated male mice was increased
slightly (Wyrobek & Bruce, 1975).

Dichloroacetaldehyde, a metabolite of dichlorvos, was positive in
the dominant lethal test when given intraperitoneally to mice at a dose
of 176 mg/kg bw saline (Fischer *et al.*, 1977).

Trimethyl phosphate, an impurity of dichlorvos, was also positive
in the dominant lethal assay in mice when given as 5 oral doses of 500
mg/kg bw or as a single i.p. dose of 700-2000 mg/kg bw (Epstein *et al.*,
1972).

(b) Humans

The numerous studies of the effects of dichlorvos on human subjects
have been reviewed (Cavagna & Vigliani, 1970; Gillett *et al.*, 1972a,b;
WHO, 1965, 1967, 1968, 1971).

Toxic effects

In a study of household exposure to dichlorvos, families were
exposed intermittently to maximum concentrations of approximately 0.1
mg/m^3 (0.01 ppm) for periods ranging from 2-6 months in their homes.
Other volunteers were exposed cutaneously to dichlorvos for 30 min daily
for 5 days. No significant degree of inhibition of plasma and erythrocyte
cholinesterase resulted from either exposure (Zavon & Kindel, 1966).

Plasma and erythrocyte cholinesterase activities were measured in
groups of hospital patients exposed to dichlorvos concentrations ranging
from 0.02-0.28 mg/m^3 (0.002-0.03 ppm), for 16-24 hrs per day, for periods

ranging from 3-29 days. Control values for plasma and erythrocyte
cholinesterase activities were established for 250 healthy male and 100
healthy female subjects not exposed to dichlorvos. Of 66 adult males
without liver disease, 5 who were exposed for 24 hrs/day to levels of
over 0.1 mg/m^3 (0.01 ppm) had plasma cholinesterase levels that were 35-
72% lower than the control value; there was no depression of erythrocyte
cholinesterase. Depression of plasma cholinesterase was seen only in
those sick babies and children exposed to clothes disinfected with
dichlorvos vapour and in healthy women exposed during labour or post-partum
when the dichlorvos level was more than 0.1 mg/m^3 (0.001 ppm). All of 6
patients with liver disease showed a 25-66% reduction in plasma cholinesteras
when exposed to <0.1 mg/m^3 (<0.01 ppm) and above. None of these subjects
showed clinical symptoms of organophosphate poisoning. The amount of
inhaled dichlorvos that caused a reduction in plasma cholinesterase was
about the same for children and adults, i.e., 0.028-0.030 mg/kg bw/day
(corresponding to a daily inhalation of 0.2 mg in children and to 1.7 mg
in adults) (Cavagna *et al*., 1969).

It was reported in an abstract that plasma and erythrocyte cholinesterase levels were normal in 22 healthy babies, at birth and after 5
days' exposure for 18 hrs/day to a time-weighted concentration of 0.05
mg/m^3 (0.005 ppm) dichlorvos. Another group of 22 babies exposed to
0.152-0.159 mg/m^3 (0.017 ppm) dichlorvos also showed no acute adverse
effects (Vigliani, 1971).

Eleven male and 2 female factory workers producing and processing a
dichlorvos-releasing product were monitored for haematology, blood
chemistry (including plasma and erythrocyte cholinesterase) and urinalysis
throughout an 8-month exposure period and for 4 months after exposure
had ceased. Plasma cholinesterase activity was inhibited by approximately
60%, and erythrocyte cholinesterase by 35%, as a result of repeated
exposure to an average dichlorvos concentration of 0.7 mg/m^3 (0.077 ppm)
for up to 216 hrs/month for 8 months. One month after exposure had
ceased both esterases had returned to normal levels. No other effects,
in the blood picture, blood chemistry, urinalysis or general health,
attributable to dichlorvos exposure were noted (Menz *et al*., 1974).
Chow & Bellin (1975) challenged both the statistical analysis and the
conclusions of Menz *et al*. and surmised that '... the observed large
decreases in blood cholinesterases [following dichlorvos] exposure may
well be injurious to the health of workers even in the absence of overt
clinical symptoms....'

Absorption, distribution, excretion and metabolism

In one man who ingested 5 mg [^{14}C-vinyl]-dichlorvos, a large proportion
of the dose was excreted as ^{14}C-CO_2; 8 hrs after administration the
yield of ^{14}C-CO_2 was 27%. A total of 9% of the dose was excreted in the
urine over a period of 48 hrs. The rates and routes of excretion of
radioactivity from rats, mice, hamsters and humans after oral ingestion
of [^{14}C-vinyl]-dichlorvos suggest that the metabolic fate of the compound
in these species is similar (Hutson & Hoadley, 1972).

Two male subjects were exposed for 10 and 20 hrs to atmospheres containing 0.25 mg/m^3 (0.027 ppm) and 0.7 mg/m^3 (0.077 ppm) dichlorvos, respectively. Blood samples taken within 1 min after exposure contained no detectable dichlorvos (detection limit, 0.1 μg/g; 4.5 x 10^{-7}M). The half-life of dichlorvos (5 x 10^{-6}M) added to human blood *in vitro* was found to range from 7-11 min at 37°C (data from 4 subjects), and the degradation was shown to be enzyme-catalysed, with a K_m of the order of 3.2 x 10^{-6}M (Blair *et al.*, 1975).

3.3 Case reports and epidemiological studies

No data were available to the Working Group.

4. Summary of Data Reported and Evaluation

4.1 Experimental data

Dichlorvos was tested in one experiment in mice and in one in rats by oral administration: no statistically significant excess of tumours was observed. However, in mice, a few oesophageal tumours, rarely seen in untreated animals, were found. Dichlorvos was also tested by inhalation in a small number of rats, using low exposure levels; no conclusive evaluation of this study could be made.

Dichlorvos is an alkylating agent and binds to bacterial and mammalian nucleic acids. It is a mutagen in a number of microbial systems; but there is no evidence of its mutagenicity in mammals, in which it is rapidly degraded.

4.2 Human data

No case reports or epidemiological studies were available to the Working Group.

The extensive production and the widespread use of dichlorvos since the early 1960s in agricultural, veterinary and household products indicate that widespread human exposure occurs. This is confirmed by a number of reports of its occurrence in the general environment. A group of people intentionally exposed to specific levels of dichlorvos is known to exist.

4.3 Evaluation

The available data do not allow an evaluation of the carcinogenicity of dichlorvos to be made.

5. References

Akimov, A.M & Babich, A.I. (1975) Hygienic problems of contamination of
    Volgograd water reservoir and the water supply-irrigation system of
    Saratov channel with organochlorine and organophosphorus compounds
    and 2,4-D (Russ.). Gig. Sanit., 6, 110 [Chem. Abstr., 83, 91991b]

Andreeva, K., Trayanova, M., Dimitrova, L. & Stroichkova, A. (1973) Char-
    acteristics of the waste water from the production of the organophos-
    phorus insecticide chlorvinphos (Bulg.). God Nauchnoizsled. Inst.
    Khim. Prom-st., 12, 311-319 [Chem. Abstr., 86, 21422e]

Anon. (1974) Studies on dichlorvos. Food Cosmet. Toxicol., 28, 765-772

Anon. (1978) OSPR updates and expands RPAR actions summary to add post
    RPAR status. Pestic. Tox. Chem. News, 6, 20-21

Aoki, Y., Takeda, M. & Uchiyama, M. (1975) Comparative study of methods
    for the extraction of eleven organophosphorus pesticide residues in
    rice. J. Assoc. off. anal. Chem., 58, 1286-1293

Ashwood-Smith, M.J., Trevino, J. & Ring, R. (1972) Mutagenicity of dichlor-
    vos. Nature (Lond.), 240, 418-420

Attfield, J.G. & Webster, D.A. (1966) Dichlorvos. Chem. Ind., 12
    February, pp. 272-278

Babina, Y. K., Vershinin, P.V., Kucherova, A.I. & Parfenov, A.I. (1972)
    Determination of the total chlorophos and DDVP in industrial waste
    waters and natural water (Russ.). Probl. Anal. Khim., 2, 9-13
    [Chem. Abstr., 79, 62442k]

Baida, T.A. (1975) Dynamics and metabolism of chlorophos in cabbage and
    onion plants (Russ.). Khim. Sel'sk. Khoz., 13, 67-68 [Chem. Abstr.,
    82, 119816d]

Batte, E.G., Robison, O.W. & Moncol, D.J. (1969) Influence of dichlorvos
    on swine reproduction and performance of offspring to weaning (Abstract
    no. 105). J. Am. vet. med. Assoc., 154, 1397

Becsey, T. (1974) Rapid semiquantitative chromatographic method for the
    determination of phosphoric acid ester insecticides in blood (Hung.).
    Gyogyszereszet, 18, 50-52 [Chem. Abstr., 83, 54015r]

Bhan, A.K. & Kaul, B.L. (1975) Cytogenic activity of dichlorvos in barley.
    Indian J. exp. Biol. 13, 403-405

Bignami, M., Aulicino, F., Velcich, A., Carere, A. & Morpurgo, G. (1977)
    Mutagenic and recombinogenic action of pesticides in Aspergillus
    nidulans. Mutat. Res., 46, 395-402

Blair, D., Hoadley, E.C. & Hutson, D.H. (1975) The distribution of di-
    chlorvos in the tissues of mammals after its inhalation or intra-
    venous administration. Toxicol. appl. Pharmacol., 31, 243-253

Blair, D., Dix, K.M., Hunt, P.F., Thorpe, E., Stevenson, D.E. & Walker,
    A.I.T. (1976) Dichlorvos - a 2-year inhalation carcinogenesis study
    in rats. Arch. Toxikol., 35, 281-294

Bridges, B.A., Mottershead, R.P., Green, M.H.L & Gray, W.J.H. (1973) Muta-
    genicity of dichlorvos and methyl methanesulphonate for *Escherichia
    coli* WP2 and some derivatives deficient in DNA repair. Mutat. Res.,
    19, 295-303

Buselmaier, W., Röhrborn, G. & Propping, P. (1972) Mutagenicity investi-
    gation with pesticides in the host-mediated assay and the dominant
    lethal test in mice (Germ.). Biol. Zbl., 91, 311-325

Carere, A., Cardamone, G., Ortali, V., Bruzzone, M.L. & Di Giuseppe, G.
    (1976) Mutational studies with some pesticides in *Streptomyces
    coelicolor* and *Salmonella typhimurium* (Abstract no. 60). Mutat. Res.,
    38, 136

Carere, A., Ortali, V.A., Cardamone, G. & Morpurgo, G. (1978a) Mutageni-
    city of dichlorvos and other structurally related pesticides in
    Salmonella and *Streptomyces*. Chem.-biol. Interact., 22, 297-308

Carere, A., Ortali, V.A., Cardamone, G., Torracca, A.M. & Raschetti, R.
    (1978b) Microbiological mutagenicity studies of pesticides *in vitro*.
    Mutat. Res., 57, 277-286

Cavagna, G. & Vigliani, E.C. (1970) Health and safety problems in the
    use of Vapona as insecticide in domestic places (Fr.). Med. Lav.,
    61, 409-423

Cavagna, G., Locati, G. & Vigliani, E.C. (1969) Clinical effects of expo-
    sure to DDVP (Vapona) insecticide in hospital wards. Arch. environ.
    Health, 19, 112-123

Chow, I. & Bellin, J. (1975) Long-term exposure of factory workers to
    dichlorvos (DDVP) insecticide [Letter to the Editor]. Arch. environ.
    Health, 30, 111-112

Collins, J.A., Schooley, M.A. & Singh, V.K (1971) The effect of dietary
    dichlorvos on swine reproduction and viability of their offspring.
    (Abstract no. 41). Toxicol. appl. Pharmacol., 19, 377

Collins, R.D. & DeVries, D.M. (1973) Air concentrations and food residues
    from use of Shell's No-Pest[®] insecticide strip. Bull. environ.
    Contam. Toxicol., 9, 227-233

Dale, W.E., Miles, J.W. & Weathers, D.B. (1973) Measurement of residues
    of dichlorvos absorbed by food exposed during disinsection of aircraft.
    J. agric. Food Chem., 21, 858-860

Dean, B.J. (1972a) The mutagenic effects of organophosphorus pesticides on
    micro-organisms. Arch. Toxikol., 30, 67-74

Dean, B.J. (1972b) The effect of dichlorvos on cultured human lymphocytes.
    Arch. Toxikol., 30, 75-85

Dean, B.J. & Blair, D. (1976) Dominant lethal assay in female mice after
    oral dosing with dichlorvos or exposure to atmospheres containing di-
    chlorvos. Mutat. Res., 40, 67-72

Dean, B.J. & Thorpe, E. (1972a) Studies with dichlorvos vapour in dominant
    lethal mutation tests on mice. Arch. Toxikol., 30, 51-59

Dean, B.J. & Thorpe, E. (1972b) Cytogenic studies with dichlorvos in mice
    and Chinese hamsters. Arch. Toxikol., 30, 39-49

Dean, B.J., Doak, S.M.A. & Funnell, J. (1972) Genetic studies with di-
    chlorvos in the host-mediated assay and in liquid medium using
    Saccharomyces cerevisiae. Arch. Toxikol., 30, 61-66

Dikshith, T.S.S., Datta, K.K. & Chandra, P. (1976) 90 Day dermal toxicity
    of DDVP in male rats. Bull. environ. Contam. Toxicol., 15, 574-580

Drevenkar, V., Fink, K., Stipcevic, M. & Stengl, B. (1975) The fate of
    pesticides in aquatic environment. I. The persistence of some organo-
    phosphorus pesticides in river water. Arh. Hig. Toksikol., 26,
    257-266 [Chem. Abstr., 85, 197827j]

Durham, W.F., Gaines, T.B., McCauley, R.H., Jr, Sedlak, V.A., Mattson, A.M.
    & Hayes, W.J., Jr (1957) Studies on the toxicity of O,O-dimethyl-2,2-
    dichlorovinyl phosphate (DDVP). Arch. ind. Health, 15, 340-349

Dyer, K.F. & Hanna, P.J. (1973) Comparative mutagenic activity and toxi-
    city of triethylphosphate and dichlorvos in bacteria and Drosophila.
    Mutat. Res., 21, 175-177

Elgar, K.E. & Steer, B.D. (1972) Dichlorvos (2,2-dichlorovinyl dimethyl
    phosphate) concentrations in the air of houses arising from the use of
    dichlorvos PVC [poly(vinyl chloride)] strips. Pestic. Sci., 3,
    591-600 [Chem. Abstr., 78, 25330f]

Elgar, K.E., Mathews, B.L. & Bosio, P. (1972a) Dichlorvos (2,2-dichloro-
    vinyl dimethyl phosphate) residue in food arising from the domestic
    use of dichlorvos PVC [poly(vinyl chloride)] strips. Pestic. Sci.,
    3, 601-607 [Chem. Abstr., 78, 28044b]

Elgar, K.E., Mathews, B.L & Bosio, P. (1972b) Vapona strips in shops -
    residues in foodstuffs. Environ. Qual. Saf., 1, 217-221

Epstein, S.S., Arnold, E., Andrea, J., Bass, W. & Bishop, Y. (1972) Detec-
    tion of chemical mutagens by the dominant lethal assay in the mouse.
    Toxicol. appl. Pharmacol., 23, 288-325

Fahrig, R. (1973) Observation of a genetic effect of organophosphorus insec-
    ticide (Germ.). Naturwissenschaffen, 60, 50-51

FAO/WHO (1978) Pesticide residues in food - 1977. FAO Plant Production &
    Protection Paper, 10 Rev., p. 24

Fischer, G.W., Schneider, P. & Scheufler, H. (1977) Mutagenicity of
    dichloroacetaldehyde and 2,2-dichloro-1,1-dihydroxy-ethane-
    phosphoric acid methyl ester, possible metabolites of the organo-
    phosphorus pesticide trichlorphon (Germ.). Chem.-biol. Interact.,
    19, 205-213

Fitak, B. & Gwiazda, J. (1975) Determination of DDVP by colorimetric and
    fluorometric methods in high-concentration and partly decomposed pre-
    parations (Pol). Rocz. Panstw. Zakl. Hig., 26, 93-99 [Chem. Abstr.,
    83, 38610a]

Gillett, J.W., Harr, J.R., Lindstrom, F.T., Mount, D.A., St Clair, A.D. &
    Weber, L.J. (1972a) Evaluation of human health hazards on use of di-
    chlorvos (DDVP), especially in resin strips. Residue Rev., 44,
    115-159

Gillett, J.W., Harr, J.R., St Clair, A.D. & Weber, L.J. (1972b) Comment
    on the distinction between hazard and safety in evaluation of human
    health hazards on use of dichlorvos, especially in resin strips.
    Residue Rev., 44, 161-184

Gore, R.C., Hannah, R.W., Pattacini, S.C. & Porro, T.J. (1971) Infrared and
    ultraviolet spectra of seventy-six pesticides. J. Assoc. off. anal.
    Chem., 54, 1040-1043, 1080-1082

Goza, S.W. (1972) Infrared analysis of pesticide formulations. J. Assoc.
    off. anal. Chem., 55, 913-917

Green, M.H.L., Medcalf, A.S.C., Arlett, C.F., Harcourt, S.A. & Lehmann, A.R.
    (1974) DNA strand breakage caused by dichlorvos, methyl methanesul-
    phonate and iodoacetamide in Escherichia coli and cultured Chinese
    hamster cells. Mutat. Res., 24, 365-378

Gruebner, P. (1972) Residue problems in the use of phosphoric acid ester
    insecticides in mushroom cultures (Germ.). Nachrichtenbl. Pflanzen-
    schutzdienst DDR, 26, 245-247 [Chem. Abstr., 78, 157943t]

Gupta, A.K. & Singh, J. (1974) Dichlorvos (DDVP) induced breaks in the salivary gland chromosomes of *Drosophila melanogaster*. Curr. Sci., 43, 661-662

Hanna, P.J. & Dyer, K.F. (1975) Mutagenicity of organophosphorus compounds in bacteria and *Drosophila*. Mutat. Res., 28, 405-420

Hass, D.K., Collins, J.A. & Kodama, J.K. (1972) Effects of orally administered dichlorvos in rhesus monkeys. J. Am. vet. med. Assoc., 161, 714-719

Hathway, D.E. (1975) Chronic toxicity testing and metabolic considerations. In: Foreign Compound Metabolism in Mammals, Vol. 3, London, The Chemical Society, pp. 370-373

Hawley, G.G., ed. (1977) The Condensed Chemical Dictionary, 9th ed., New York, Von Nostrand-Reinhold, p. 282

Holmstedt, B., Nordgren, I., Sandoz, M. & Sundwall, A. (1978) Metrifonate. Summary of toxicology and pharmacological information available. Arch. Toxikol., 41, 3-29

Horwitz, W., ed. (1975) Official Methods of Analysis of the Association of Analytical Chemists, 12th ed., Washington DC, Association of Official Analytical Chemists, pp. 115-116

Hutson, D.H. & Hoadley, E.C. (1972) The comparative metabolism of [^{14}C-vinyl]-dichlorvos in animals and man. Arch. Toxikol., 30, 9-18

Hutson, D.H., Blair, D., Hoadley, E.C. & Pickering, B.A. (1971a) The metabolism of ^{14}C Vapona® in rats after administration by oral and inhalation routes (Abstract no. 45). Toxicol. appl. Pharmacol., 19, 378-379

Hutson, D.H., Hoadley, E.C. & Pickering, B.A. (1971b) The metabolic fate of [vinyl-1-^{14}C]dichlorvos in the rat after oral and inhalation exposure. Xenobiotica, 1, 593-611

Jayasuriya, V.U. de S. & Ratnayake, W.E. (1973) Screening of some pesticides on *Drosophila melanogaster* for toxic and genetic effects. Drosophila Inf. Serv., 50, 184-186

Johnson, L.D., Waltz, R.H., Ussary, J.P. & Kaiser, F.E. (1976) Automated gel permeation chromatographic cleanup of animal and plant extracts for pesticide residue determination. J. Assoc. off. anal. Chem., 59, 174-187

Jones, K.H., Sanderson, D.M. & Noakes, D.N. (1968) Acute toxicity data for pesticides (1968). World Rev. Pestic. Control, 7, 135-143

Kavetskii, V.N. (1974) Chromatographic determination of some organophosphorus pesticides and study of their transformation in plants (Ukr.). Zashch. Rast. (Kiev), 19, 101-108 [Chem. Abstr., 82, 133718x]

Kazanovskii, E.S. (1975) Determination of residues of organophosphorus insecticides in animal organs and tissues (Russ.). Veterinariya (Moscow), 3, 105-106 [Chem. Abstr., 83, 54028x]

Kelso, G.L., Wilkinson, R.R., Ferguson, T.L., Malone, J.R., Jr & Oestreich, D.K. (1976) Development of Information on Pesticides Manufacturing for Source Assessment, EPA Contract No. 68-02-1324, Task 43, US Environmental Protection Agency, Washington DC, US Government Printing Office, p. 75

Kimbrough, R.D. & Gaines, T.B. (1968) Effect of organic phosphorus compounds and alkylating agents on the rat fetus. Arch. environ. Health, 16, 805-808

Konrad, H., Gabrio, T. & Penner, G. (1975) Pesticide contamination of milk and milk products. 4. (Germ.). Milchforsch.-Milchprax., 17, 67-69 [Chem. Abstr., 84, 103926v]

Konyukhov, A.F. (1974) Determination of pesticides in mixed feeds (Russ.). Veterinariya (Moscow), 6, 101-102 [Chem. Abstr., 81, 167888e]

Kramers, P.G.N. & Knaap, A.G.A.C. (1978) Absence of a mutagenic effect after feeding dichlorvos to larvae of Drosophila melanogaster. Mutat. Res., 57, 103-105

Krause, W. & Homola, S. (1972) Effect of DDVP (dichlorvos) on spermatogenesis (Germ.). Arch. Dermatol. Forsch., 244, 439-441

Krijgsman, W. & Van De Kamp, C.G. (1976) Analysis of organophosphorus pesticides by capillary gas chromatography with flame photometric detection. J. Chromatogr., 117, 201-205

La Hue, D.W., Kirk, L.D. & Mustakas, G.C. (1975) Fate of dichlorvos residues during milling and oil extraction of soybeans. Environ. Entomol., 4, 11-14

Lawley, P.D., Shah, S.A. & Orr, D.J. (1974) Methylation of nucleic acids by 2,2-dichlorovinyl dimethyl phosphate (dichlorvos, DDVP). Chem.-biol. Interact., 8, 171-182

Leary, J.S., Keane, W.T., Fontenot, C., Feichtmeir, E.F., Schultz, D., Koos, B.A., Hirsch, L., Lavor, E.M., Roan, C.C. & Hine, C.H. (1974) Safety evaluation in the home of polyvinyl chloride resin strip containing dichlorvos (DDVP). Arch. environ. Health, 29, 308-314

Leo, E. & Suwalska, D. (1977) Modification of a colorimetric method for
    determination of dimethyl dichlorovinyl phosphate (DDVP) in the air
    (Pol.). Bromatol. Chem. Toksykol., 10, 97-99 [Chem. Abstr., 87,
    43474w]

Leuzinger, S. (1975) Brew testing with NUVAN-7-treated malts (Germ.).
    Schweiz. Brau.-Rundsch., 86, 160-161 [Chem. Abstr., 84, 41915e]

Löfroth, G. (1970) Alkylation of DNA by dichlorvos. Naturwissenschaften,
    57, 393-394

Löfroth, G., Kim, C. & Hussain, S. (1969) Alkylating property of 2,2-
    dichlorovinyl dimethyl phosphate: a disregarded hazard. EMS News
    Lett., 2, 21-26

Lyubenko, N., Sasinovich, L.M. & Zor'yeva, T.D. (1973) Effects of various
    food processing treatments on organophosphate pesticide residue
    levels (Russ.) (Abstract). Khim. Sel. Kholz., 11, 439-440

Macklin, A.W. & Ribelin, W.E. (1971) The relation of pesticides to abor-
    tion in dairy cattle. J. Am. vet. med. Assoc., 159, 1743-1748

Menz, M., Luetkemeier, H. & Sachsse, K. (1974) Long-term exposure of fac-
    tory workers to dichlorvos (DDVP) insecticide. Arch. environ. Health,
    28, 72-76

Michalek, S.M. & Brockman, H.E. (1969) A test for mutagenicity of Shell
    'No-Pest Strip Insecticide' in Neurospora crassa. Neurospora News-
    lett., 14, 8

Mohn, G. (1973) 5-Methyltryptophan resistance mutations in Escherichia
    coli K-12. Mutagenic activity of monofunctional alkylating agents
    including organophosphorus insecticides. Mutat. Res., 20, 7-15

Mukherjee, G., Banerjee, T.S., Mukherjee, A.K. & Mathew, T.V. (1973) Col-
    orimetric estimation of dichlorvos (DDVP). J. Food Sci. Technol.,
    10, 126

Nagy, Z., Mile, I. & Antoni, F. (1975) The mutagenic effect of pesticides
    on Escherichia coli WP2 try⁻. Acta microbiol. acad. sci. hung.,
    22, 309-314

National Cancer Institute (1977) Bioassay of Dichlorvos for Possible
    Carcinogenicity (Carcinogenesis Technical Report Series, No. 10),
    DHEW Publication No. (NIH) 77-810, Washington DC, US Government
    Printing Office

Nepoklonov, A.A. & Bukshtynov, V.I. (1971) Chlorophos release time from
    sheep after aerosol treatment (Russ.). Tr., Vses. Nauch.-Issled.
    Inst. Vet. Sanit., 39, 200-202 [Chem. Abstr., 81, 2465b]

Nepoklonov, A.A. & Metelitsa, V.K. (1971) Metabolism and retention of
    chlorophos in cattle (Russ.). Tr., Vses. Nauch.-Issled. Inst. Vet.
    Sanit., 39, 155-164 [Chem. Abstr., 82, 81416h]

Nicholas, M.L., Powell, D.L., Williams, T.R. & Huff, S.R. (1976) Reference
    Raman spectra of ten phosphorus-containing pesticides. J. Assoc. off.
    anal. Chem., 59, 1071-1080

Nordgren, I., Bergström, M., Holmstedt, B. & Sandoz, M. (1978) Transfor-
    mation and action of metrifonate. Arch. Toxikol., 41, 31-41

Novikova, K.F. & Mel'tser, F.R. (1973) Colorimetric determination of trace
    amounts of DDVP in milk and water (Russ.). Khim. Sel. Khoz., 11,
    607-609 [Chem. Abstr., 80, 664w]

Ogata, H., Saito, E., Murata, H. Shibazaki, T. & Inoue, T. (1975) A new
    colorimetric method of determination of 0,0-dimethyl 2,2-dichloro-
    vinyl phosphate in insecticidal preparations (Jap.). Yakugaku Zasshi,
    95, 1483-1491 [Chem. Abstr., 84, 85390j]

Panel on Malathion & Dichlorvos Residues in Grain (1973) The determination
    of malathion and dichlorvos residues in grain. Analyst, 98, 19-24

Pflugmacher, J. & Ebing, W. (1974) Clean-up of organophosphorus insecticide
    residues in vegetable extracts by gel chromatography on Sephadex LH-20
    (Germ.). J. Chromatogr., 93, 457-463

Raffke, W. & Wirthgen, B. (1976) On the formation of dichlorvos residues
    in cereal products (Germ.). Nahrung, 20, 37-40 [Chem. Abstr., 85,
    19199y]

Rajak, R.L. & Krishnamurthy, K. (1974) Use of dichlorvos for disinfes-
    tation of foodgrains. I. Determination of microquantities of dichlor-
    vos. Bull. Grain Technol., 12, 89-94 [Chem. Abstr., 83, 162271e]

Romaniuk, J. (1976) Study of the disappearance dynamics of dichlorphos
    residues from raspberries (Pol.). Rocz. Nauk Roln., Ser. E., 6,
    137-142 [Chem. Abstr., 86, 87795k]

Rosen, J.D. & Pareles, S.R. (1974) Mass fragmentography as applied to some
    organophosphate insecticides. In: Haque, R., ed., Proceedings of a
    Symposium on Mass Spectrometry, NMR Spectroscopy in Pesticides
    Chemistry, 1973, New York, Plenum, pp. 91-98 [Chem. Abstr., 82,
    81536x]

Rosenkranz, H.S. (1973) Preferential effect of dichlorvos (Vapona) on bac-
    teria deficient in DNA polymerase. Cancer Res., 33, 458-459

Sasinovich, L.M. (1967) Toxicology of DDVP (Russ.). Gig. Toksikol.
    Pestits. Klin. Otravlenii, 5, 361-372 [Chem. Abstr., 71, 122775t]

Sawinsky, A., Pasztor, G. & Sandor, E. (1973) Exposure examination of
    spraying performed with Vapona 48 EC (Hung.). Egeszsegtudomany, 17,
    285-288 [Pestic. Abstr., 7, 74-0772]

Sax, K. & Sax, H.J. (1968) Possible mutagenic hazards of some food addi-
    tives, beverages and insecticides. Jpn. J. Genet., 43, 89-94

Seifert, J. & Davidek, J. (1974) Indirect polarographic determination of
    trichlorfon and dichlorvos. Z. Lebensm.-Unters. Forsch., 155, 266-270
    [Chem. Abstr., 82, 26991s]

Shell Chemical Company (1973) Summary of Basic Data for Vapona® Insec-
    ticide, Technical Data Bulletin ACD: 67-110, San Ramon, CA

Sherman, M. & Ross, E. (1961) Acute and subacute toxicity of insecticides
    to chicks. Toxicol. appl. Pharmacol., 3, 521-533

Shirasu, Y., Moriya, M., Kato, K., Furuhashi, A. & Kada, T. (1976) Muta-
    genicity screening of pesticides in the microbial system. Mutat. Res.
    40, 19-30

Shooter, K.V. (1975) Assays for phosphotriester formation in the reaction
    of bacteriophage R17 with a group of alkylating agents. Chem.-biol.
    Interact., 11, 575-588

Spencer, E.Y. (1973) Guide to the Chemicals Used in Crop Protection,
    Research Branch, Agriculture Canada, Publication 1093, 6th ed.,
    London, Ontario, University of Western Ontario, p. 194

Štefanac, Z., Štengl, B. & Vasilić, Ž. (1976) Quantitative determination
    of organophosphorous pesticides by thin-layer densitometry. J.
    Chromatogr., 124, 127-133

Szalontai. G. (1976) High-performance liquid chromatography of organo-
    phosphorus insecticides. J. Chromatogr., 124, 9-16

Tewari, S.N. & Harpalani, S.P (1977) Detection and determination of
    organophosphorus insecticides in tissues by thin-layer chromatography.
    J. Chromatogr., 130, 229-236

Thompson, J.F., Mann, J.B., Apodaca, A.O. & Kantor, E.J. (1975) Relative
    retention ratios of ninety-five pesticides and metabolites on nine
    gas-liquid chromatographic columns over a temperature range of 170
    to 204°C in two detection modes. J. Assoc. off. anal. Chem., 58,
    1037-1050

Thorpe, E., Wilson, A.B., Dix, K.M. & Blair, D. (1972) Teratological
    studies with dichlorvos vapour in rabbits and rats. Arch. Toxikol.,
    30, 29-38

Tracy, R.L., Woodcock, J.G. & Chodroff, S. (1960) Toxicological aspects
    of 2,2-dichlorovinyl dimethyl phosphate (DDVP) in cows, horses, and
    white rats. J. econ. Entomol., 53, 593-601

Turner, C.R. (1974) Spectrophotometric determination of organophosphorus
    pesticides with 3-(4-nitrobenzyl)pyridine. Analyst, 99,
    431-434

US Department of Agriculture (1974) Farmers' Use of Pesticides in 1971...
    Quantities (Agricultural Economic Report, No. 252), Economic Research
    Service, Washington DC, US Government Printing Office, p. 13

US Environmental Protection Agency (1973) EPA Compendium of Registered
    Pesticides, Vol. III, Insecticides, Acaricides, Molluscicides and
    Antifouling Compounds, Washington DC, US Government Printing Office,
    pp. III-D-23.1-III-D-23.4

US Environmental Protection Agency (1976a) Investigation of Selected
    Potential Environmental Contaminants, Haloalkyl Phosphates, PB-
    257 910, Springfield, VA, National Technical Information Service,
    pp. 55-56

US Environmental Protection Agency (1976b) Protection of environment.
    US Code Fed. Regul., Title 40, part 180.235, p. 341

US International Trade Commission (1977) Synthetic Organic Chemicals, US
    Production and Sales, 1976, USITC Publication 833, Washington DC,
    US Government Printing Office, p. 280

US Occupational Safety & Health Administration (1977) Occupational
    Safety and Health Standards, Subpart Z - Toxic and Hazardous Substances.
    US Code Fed. Regul., Title 29, part 1910.93, p. 60

US Tariff Commission (1962) Synthetic Organic Chemicals, US Production and
    Sales, 1961, TC Publication 72, Washington DC, US Government
    Printing Office, p. 167

Vardell, H.H., Gillenwater, H.B., Whitten, M.E., Cagle, A., Eason, G. &
    Cail, R.S. (1973) Dichlorvos degradation on stored wheat and resul-
    ting milling fractions. J. Econ. Entomol., 66, 761-763

Vigliani, E.C. (1971) Exposure of newborn babies to Vapona® insecticide
    (Abstract No. 48). Toxicol. appl. Pharmacol., 19, 379-380

Vogin, E.E., Carson, S. & Slomka, M.B. (1971) Teratology studies with di-
    chlorvos in rabbits (Abstract no. 42). Toxicol. appl. Pharmacol.,
    19, 377-378

Voogd, C.E., Jacobs, J.J.J.A.A. & Van der Stel, J.J. (1972) On the muta-
    genic action of dichlorvos. Mutat. Res., 16, 413-416

Walker, A.I.T., Blair, D., Stevenson, D.E. & Chambers, P.L. (1972) An inhalational toxicity study with dichlorvos. Arch. Toxikol., 30, 1-7

Wennerberg, R. & Löfroth, G. (1974) Formation of 7-methylguanine by dichlorvos in bacteria and mice. Chem.-biol. Interact., 8, 339-348

WHO (1965) 1965 Evaluation of some pesticide residues in food. The Monographs. WHO/Food Add./27.65, pp. 84-88

WHO (1967) 1966 Evaluation of some pesticide residues in food. The Monographs. WHO/Food Add./67.32, pp. 69-81

WHO (1968) 1967 Evaluations of some pesticide residues in food. The Monographs. WHO/Food Add./68.30, pp. 90-102

WHO (1971) 1970 Evaluations of some pesticide residues in food. The Monographs. WHO/Food Add./71.42, pp. 123-174

WHO (1975) 1974 Evaluations of some pesticide residues in food. WHO Pestic. Residue Ser., No. 4, p. 539

Wild, D. (1973) Chemical induction of streptomycin-resistant mutations in Escherichia coli. Dose and mutagenic effects of dichlorvos and methylmethanesulfonate. Mutat. Res., 19, 33-41

Wild, D. (1975) Mutagenicity studies on organophosphorus insecticides. Mutat. Res., 32, 133-150

Windholz, M., ed. (1976) The Merck Index, 9th ed., Rahway, NJ, Merck & Co., p. 407

Winell, M. (1975) An international comparison of hygienic standards for chemicals in the work environment. Ambio, 4, 34-36

Witherup, S., Jolley, W.J., Stemmer, K. & Pfitzer, E.A. (1971) Chronic toxicity studies with 2,2-dichlorovinyl dimethyl phosphate (DDVP) in dogs and rats including observations on rat reproduction (Abstract no. 40). Toxicol. appl. Pharmacol., 19, 377

Wooder, M.F., Wright, A.S. & King, L.J. (1977) In vivo alkylation studies with dichlorvos at practical use concentrations. Chem.-biol. Interact. 19, 25-46

Wright, A.S., Hutson, D.H. & Wooder, M.F. (1979) The chemical and biochemical reactivity of dichlorvos. Arch. Toxikol., 42, 1-18

Wyrobek, A.J. & Bruce, W.R. (1975) Chemical induction of sperm abnormalities in mice. Proc. natl Acad. Sci. (Wash.), 72, 4425-4429

Zadrozinska, J. (1973) Enzymic method combined with thin-layer chroma-
    tography for determination of organophosphorus insecticides in veg-
    etables and fruits (Pol.). Rocz. Panstw. Zakl. Hig., 24, 297-308
    [Chem. Abstr., 80, 46572t]

Zavon, M.R. & Kindel, E.A., Jr (1966) Potential hazard in using dichlor-
    vos insecticide resin. Adv. Chem. Ser., 60, 177-186

HEPTACHLOR AND HEPTACHLOR EPOXIDE

These substances were considered by a previous Working Group, in October 1973 (IARC, 1974). Since that time new data have become available, and these have been incorporated into the monograph and taken into account in the present evaluation.

A review is available (Mercier, 1975).

1. Chemical and Physical Data

1.1 Synonyms and trade names

Heptachlor

Chem. Abstr. Services Reg. No.: 76-44-8

Chem. Abstr. Name: 1,4,5,6,7,8,8-Heptachloro-3a,4,7,7a-tetrahydro-4,7-methano-1*H*-indene

Synonyms: 3-Chlorochlordene; 3,4,5,6,7,8,8a-heptachlorodicyclopenta-diene; 1,4,5,6,7,8,8-heptachloro-3a,4,7,7a-tetrahydro-4,7-endo-methanoindene; 1,4,5,6,7,8,8-heptachloro-3a,4,7,7a-tetrahydro-4,7-methanoindene; 1(3a),4,5,6,7,8,8-heptachloro-3a(1),4,7,7a-tetrahydro-4,7-methanoindene; 3a,4,5,6,7,8,8-heptachloro-3a,4,7,-7a-tetrahydro-4,7-methanoindene; 1,4,5,6,7,8,8-heptachloro-3a,4,7,7a-tetrahydro-4,7-methylene indene; 1,4,5,6,7,10,10-hepta-chloro-4,7,8,9-tetrahydro-4,7-methyleneindene; 1,4,5,6,7,10,10-heptachloro-4,7,8,9-tetrahydro-4,7-*endo*methyleneindene

Trade names: Aahepta; Agroceres; Drinox; E 3314; ENT 15,152; GPKh; H34; Heptachlorane; Heptagran; Heptamul; Rhodiachlor; Velsicol 104

Heptachlor epoxide

Chem. Abstr. Services Reg. No.: 1024-57-3

Chem. Abstr. Name: 2,3,4,5,6,7,7-Heptachloro-1a,1b,5,5a,6,6a-hexahydro-2,5-methano-2*H*-indeno(1,2-b)oxirene

Synonyms: Epoxyheptachlor; HCE; 1,4,5,6,7,8,8-heptachloro-2,3-epoxy-3a,4,7,7a-tetrahydro-4,7-methanoindan

Trade names: ENT 25,584; Velsicol 53-CS-17

1.2 Structural and molecular formulae and molecular weights

Heptachlor

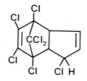

$C_{10}H_5Cl_7$ Mol. wt: 373.5

Heptachlor epoxide

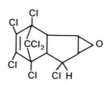

$C_{10}H_5Cl_7O$ Mol. wt: 389.4

1.3 Chemical and physical properties of the substances

From Fairchild et al. (1976a), unless otherwise specified

Heptachlor (99% pure)

(a) Description: White, crystalline solid

(b) Boiling-point: 135–145°C at 1–1.5 mm

(c) Melting-point: 93°C

(d) Spectroscopy data: λ_{max} 236 nm (E_1^1 = 1611), 309 nm (E_1^1 = 270), 328 nm (E_1^1 = 203) (in ethanol) (Grasselli & Ritchey, 1975); infra-red (Gore et al., 1971) and Raman spectral data (Nicholas et al., 1976) have also been published.

(e) Solubility: Practically insoluble in water (0.056 mg/l); soluble in ethanol (4.5 g/100 ml), xylene (102 g/100 ml), carbon tetrachloride (112 g/100 ml), acetone (75 g/100 ml) and benzene (106 g/100 ml)

(f) Volatility: Vapour pressure is 0.0003 mm at 25°C.

(g) Stability: Stable in daylight, air, moisture and moderate heat
     (160°C); oxidized biologically to heptachlor epoxide (Whetstone,
     1964)

Heptachlor epoxide (99.5% pure)

(a) Melting-point: 160-161.5°C

(b) Solubility: Insoluble in water

1.4 Technical products and impurities

Heptachlor

Technical heptachlor available in the US has the following specifications: waxy solid; assay, 72% min; related compounds, 28% max;
hexachlorocyclopentadiene content, 1% max; melting range, 46.1-73.9°C
(typical); density at 68.9°C, 1.61 (typical); and storage stability,
one year minimum. It is available as dusts, dust concentrates, emulsifiable concentrates, wettable powders and oil solutions (Berg, 1978).

Heptachlor epoxide

Heptachlor epoxide is not available as a commercial product in the
US. It is not normally present in commercial heptachlor but is apparently
formed by biological and chemical transformation of heptachlor in the
environment.

2. Production, Use, Occurrence and Analysis

2.1 Production and use

(a) Production

Heptachlor was isolated in about 1946 as a constituent of chlordane
(Lawless *et al.*, 1972). It is manufactured by the chlorination of
chlordene in the presence of a catalyst such as Fuller's earth (Whetstone,
1964).

Commercial production of heptachlor in the US was first reported in 1953
(US Tariff Commission, 1954). In 1976, only one US company reported
production of an undisclosed amount (see preamble, p. 16). US production
in 1971 has been estimated at 2.7 million kg (Johnson, 1972); on the basis
of the manufacturer's estimated production figures for the last 6 months
of 1975, a total of approximately 4.5 million kg heptachlor (for uses

other than subsurface ground insertion for termite control and the dipping of roots and tops of nonfood plants) were to be produced during the 18-month period from July 1975-December 1976 (US Environmental Protection Agency, 1976a).

No data on its production in Europe were available. It has never been produced commercially in Japan and was last imported in 1972, in a quantity of about 71 thousand kg.

(b) Use

The only known use of heptachlor is as an insecticide. As of 4 June 1971, it was registered for use in the US on 22 agricultural crops, involving both foliar and seed treatment (US Environmental Protection Agency, 1971). An estimated 930 thousand kg were used in the US in 1974, as follows: on corn, 58%; by pest control operators, 26.8%; as a seed treatment, 13.2%; and for miscellaneous other uses (including use to control fire ants, use on pineapple and possibly on citrus), 2% (US Environmental Protection Agency, 1976a).

On 6 March 1978, the US Environmental Protection Agency's heptachlor/chlordane cancellation proceeding was terminated and a settlement reached for the contested uses (US Environmental Protection Agency, 1978). The settlement allows for use of technical heptachlor on corn cutworms until 1 August 1980. A maximum of 2.27 million kg heptachlor may be produced for this use from the date of the settlement. A total of 443 thousand kg may be used until 1 July 1983 for sorghum seed treatment and until 1 September 1982 for barley, oats, wheat, rye and corn seed treatment. The settlement allows for use of smaller amounts of technical heptachlor for other purposes. These are listed below by crop, location (in some cases), maximum time interval for permitted use and amount allowed for specific uses: (1) citrus, Florida, until 31 December 1979, 18.2 thousand kg; (2) pineapples, Hawaii, 31 December 1982, 68.1 thousand kg; and (3) narcissus bulbs, 31 December 1980, 204.3 kg (Anon., 1978a). After 1 July 1983, the only approved use for heptachlor will be for underground termite control (Anon., 1978b).

No data on use of heptachlor in Europe were available. It has been used in Japan as an insecticide; however, its registration was cancelled in 1972 and it is no longer used there.

In November 1971, the Joint Meeting of the FAO Working Party of Experts on Pesticide Residues and the WHO Expert Committee on Pesticide Residues recommended practical residue limits in 15 commodities, ranging from 0.01 mg/kg for citrus fruit to 0.5 mg/kg for crude soya bean oil, with a limit of 0.05 mg/kg for vegetables and 0.15 mg/kg for milk and milk products (WHO, 1972).

Tolerances for total residues of heptachlor and heptachlor epoxide in or on raw agricultural commodities have been established by the US Environmental Protection Agency as follows: 0.1 mg/kg in or on cabbage, lettuce, rutabagas (yellow turnips) and snap beans; and none in or on a variety of about 30 vegetable, fruit and field crops, and in meat and milk (US Environmental Protection Agency, 1976b).

The Joint Meeting of the FAO Working Party of Experts on Pesticide Residues and the WHO Expert Committee on Pesticide Residues in 1970 established an acceptable daily intake (ADI) for humans of 0-0.0005 mg/kg bw (WHO, 1972).

The US Occupational Safety and Health Administration's health standards require that an employee's dermal exposure to heptachlor not exceed 0.5 mg/m^3 in the workplace in any 8-hr work shift of a 40-hr week (US Occupational Safety & Health Administration, 1977). The corresponding standard in the Federal Republic of Germany is also 0.5 mg/m^3, and the acceptable ceiling concentration in the USSR is 0.01 mg/m^3 (Winell, 1975).

2.2 Occurrence

Heptachlor

Heptachlor is not known to occur as a natural product. It is a contaminant of technical chlordane (about 10%) (see monograph, p. 45).

A review of the environmental distribution of heptachlor is available (Fairchild et al., 1976b).

(a) Air

Air was sampled in 9 US cities (representative of both urban and agricultural areas) for pesticides and their metabolites during 2 weeks of each month over 6 months. Heptachlor was detected in 37 samples of air from 1 city (maximum level, 19.2 ng/m^3) and in 7 air samples from another (maximum level, 2.3 ng/m^3) (Stanley et al., 1971).

Weekly air samples were taken in the middle of a primary cotton-growing area during 1972, 1973 and 1974. The maximum level of heptachlor found was 0.8 ng/m^3 (Arthur et al., 1976).

(b) Water

Heptachlor has been found in drinking-water, ground-water, chemical plant effluents, river-water (Shackelford & Keith, 1976) and in sediments, lakes and rivers at 18 US and European locations (Eurocop-Cost, 1976).

In a 1958-1965 survey of US rivers, heptachlor was found in 17% of the samples at average concentrations up to 3 ng/l (Safe Drinking Water Committee, 1977). It has been detected in ambient water in Nova Scotia at levels up to 0.46 µg/l (Burns *et al.*, 1975).

In 1977, a study was conducted in 2 US counties on the effects of agricultural practices on the pesticide residue levels in rural drinking-water samples from 1 out of 100 households. Heptachlor was detected in 62.5% of samples from one county, at a mean level of 15 µg/l, and in 45.5% of those from the other, at a mean level of 9 µg/l (Sandhu *et al.*, 1978).

(c) Soil

The half-life of heptachlor in soil is 9–10 months when used at agricultural rates (Anon., 1976).

Pesticide residues were measured in cropland soils from 43 states and in noncropland soils from 11 states during fiscal year 1969, as part of the US National Pesticide Monitoring Program. Heptachlor was detected in 68 of 1729 samples analysed; levels ranged from 0.01-0.97 mg/kg in soil used for corn, cotton, general farming and hay and in irrigated land and vegetable fruit cropping regions. Heptachlor was not detected in noncropland soil samples (Wiersma *et al.*, 1972a). It was also detected in soil samples from 7/8 US cities taken in 1969; levels ranged from 0.01-0.53 mg/kg (Wiersma *et al.*, 1972b).

Heptachlor residues in the soil of 7/16 farms ranged from trace amounts to 0.24 mg/kg (Harris & Sans, 1971). Residues were also detected in soil samples from 6 of the 12 states in the Corn Belt region of the US, in an average of 5.7% of the sites, at levels ranging from 0.01-0.84 mg/kg (Carey *et al.*, 1973).

In 1973, a study was performed to determine the persistence of pesticides in tobacco fields. Heptachlor was applied to 3 plots of soil at a rate of 2.24 kg/ha active ingredient; the soil was rototilled to a depth of 15 cm; soil samples were taken at 0-15 cm depth; and tobacco plants were planted 6 days later. When soil samples were taken at 0-15 cm and 15-23 cm nearly 3 months later, slightly more heptachlor was found in the later 0-15 cm sample (0.37 mg/kg) than in the earlier one (0.34 mg/kg) (1 day after planting); 0.04 mg/kg was found in the later 15-23 cm samples. The authors suggested that, due to soil compaction during the 3 months, some of the insecticide that was initially deposited below 15 cm appeared in the 0-15 cm samples (Townsend & Specht, 1975).

Heptachlor was detected in sediments from stream beds and natural drainage ditches, at maximum levels of 174 and 4.8 µg/kg, respectively (Burns *et al.*, 1975).

(d) Food

Samples of raw oil and oil in various stages of processing (neutralized, hydrogenated, decolourized and deodorized oils and shortenings) were

taken at 7 cooking-oil processing factories. Heptachlor was present at
9 µg/kg in raw oil and at 2 µg/kg in neutralized oil, but none was found
in the remaining samples (Hashemy-Tonkabony & Soleimani-Amiri, 1976).

Heptachlor residues were not found in any food composites collected
during the 9th year (August 1972-July 1973) of the Total Diet Study of
the US Food and Drug Administration (Johnson & Manske, 1976).

(e) Animals

Heptachlor was found in 3/15 seals at levels of 0.003, 0.017 and
0.039 mg/kg, respectively (Clausen *et al*., 1974).

Heptachlor epoxide

Heptachlor epoxide is not known to occur as a natural product.

(a) Air

Heptachlor epoxide was detected at a maximum level of 9.3 ng/m^3
in weekly air samples taken in the middle of a primary cotton-growing
area (Arthur *et al*., 1976).

(b) Water and sediments

Heptachlor epoxide has been found in drinking-water, ground-water,
land-runoff effluent and river-water at 7 US and European locations
(Shackelford & Keith, 1976) and in sediments, lakes, rivers, tap-water
and effluent water from a biological sewage treatment plant at 28 US and
European locations (Eurocop-Cost, 1976).

In a 1958-1965 survey of US rivers, heptachlor epoxide was found in
25% of the samples at average concentrations of <1-8 ng/l (Safe Drinking
Water Committee, 1977).

Heptachlor epoxide levels in tributary streams of Lake Michigan
averaged <0.6, 2.1 and 2.9 ng/l in 1970, 1971 and 1972, respectively,
and annual ranges were <0.2-1.0, 0-5.4 and 1.2-4.5 ng/l. Average concentrations of heptachlor epoxide in sewage treatment plant effluents were
<0.3, 5.4 and 2.8 ng/l, respectively, and annual ranges were 0.2-0.7, 0.3-
17.2 and 1.2-7.8 ng/l (Schacht, 1974).

Heptachlor epoxide was detected in 57% of water samples in Nova
Scotia, at levels up to 6.1 µg/l (Burns *et al*., 1975). In a study of water
supplies in 2 US counties, heptachlor epoxide was detected in 41.7% of
samples from 1 county, at a mean level of 8 ng/l, and in 63.6% of those
from the other, at a mean level of 18 ng/l (Sandhu *et al*., 1978).

(c) Soil

Heptachlor epoxide was detected in the soil of 7/16 farms at levels ranging from trace amounts to 0.24 mg/kg (Harris & Sans, 1971). It was also found in 139 of 1729 samples of cropland soil analysed as part of the US National Pesticide Monitoring Program in fiscal year 1969; levels ranged from 0.01-1.08 mg/kg in all the cropping regions sampled. It was also detected at a level of 0.01 mg/kg in 2/199 samples of noncropland soil (Wiersma et al., 1972a).

In a study of organochlorine pesticide residues in soil in the US Corn Belt region, heptachlor epoxide was detected in 7 of the 12 states in the region, at levels ranging from 0.01-0.31 mg/kg at an average of 8% of sites (Carey et al., 1973). It was also detected in hayfield soils in 9 US states at 1.1% of sites, at a maximum level of 0.15 mg/kg, on a dry-weight basis (Gowen et al., 1976).

In a study of pesticide residues in tobacco fields, no heptachlor epoxide was found in the soil immediately after application of heptachlor. After nearly 3 months, heptachlor epoxide was detected at levels of 0.03 and 0.01 mg/kg at depths of 0-15 cm and 15-23 cm, respectively (Townsend & Specht, 1975).

(d) Food

During the period August 1972-July 1973, market basket surveys were carried out in 30 US cities, which ranged in population from less than 50,000 to 1,000,000 or more, to measure pesticide residues by food class. Heptachlor epoxide was found in 21 samples of dairy products at levels from trace amounts to 2 µg/kg; in 24 samples of meat, fish and poultry, from trace amounts to 2 µg/kg; and in one sample of potatoes in trace amounts (Johnson & Manske, 1976). It has been found in soya bean oil at levels up to 0.01 mg/kg (Yang et al., 1976).

(e) Animals

Heptachlor epoxide was found in muscle tissue of fish collected from a river in British Columbia, in 14 of 61 samples at levels of up to 86.6 µg/kg, and in 4 of 11 samples of shellfish collected from the estuary at levels up to 23 µg/kg (Albright et al., 1975). The edible portions of four species of fish were found to contain 0.1 mg/kg bw or less (Schacht, 1974).

In breast muscle samples from doves from 15 US states, levels of heptachlor epoxide ranged from 0.14-8.7 mg/kg lipid weight (<0.006-0.17 mg/kg wet weight) (Kreitzer, 1974). It was detected in starlings from approximately 97% of 126 collection sites, at levels ranging from trace amounts to 0.31 mg/kg wet weight (White, 1976).

Heptachlor epoxide was found in most species of arctic mammals: levels ranged from 0.005 mg/kg in a ringed seal to 0.49 mg/kg in a polar bear (Clausen *et al.*, 1974).

(f) Humans

Trace amounts of heptachlor epoxide have been found in fat in the general population in most countries (Abbott *et al.*, 1968, 1972; Curley *et al.*, 1973; Davies *et al.*, 1971; Edwards, 1970; Fournier *et al.*, 1972; Hayes *et al.*, 1965; Wassermann *et al.*, 1970, 1972a,b,c). Maximum levels were reported in 1970 in France (0.28-0.36 mg/kg) (Fournier *et al.*, 1972). In the US, levels of 0.24 mg/kg were found in 1964 (Hayes *et al.*, 1965), which had decreased to 0.05 mg/kg by 1969 (Davies *et al.*, 1971).

2.3 Analysis

Analytical methods used to determine heptachlor and its epoxide have been reviewed (Fairchild *et al.*, 1976b). Methods used for the analysis of heptachlor and its epoxide in environmental samples are listed in Table 1.

More than 80% of heptachlor and heptachlor epoxide is recovered in the method of the Association of Official Analytical Chemists (US Food & Drug Administration, 1975). Other analytical investigations designed to isolate and identify heptachlor include paper chromatography (Dyatlovitiskaya *et al.*, 1972), thin-layer chromatography (Yurkova & Klisenko, 1970) and gas chromatography/electron capture detection (Arthur *et al.*, 1976).

3. Biological Data Relevant to the Evaluation
of Carcinogenic Risk to Humans

3.1 Carcinogenicity studies in animals

Oral administration

Mouse: Epstein (1976) reported a previously unpublished study by the Food & Drug Administration, carried out in 1965, in which 3 groups of 100 male and 100 female C3H mice were fed heptachlor or heptachlor epoxide at a concentration of 10 mg/kg diet for 24 months or received a standard diet. Data were reported for males and females combined in a summary memorandum form. The numbers of mice still alive at 24 months were 62 controls, 60 given heptachlor and 19 given heptachlor epoxide. The incidences of hepatic hyperplasia and benign hepatomas were doubled in mice treated with heptachlor and heptachlor epoxide in comparison with control animals. The incidence of hepatic carcinomas, diagnosed on the basis of pulmonary metastases or extrahepatic invasion, was the same in heptachlor-treated and control groups, but doubled in the group given heptachlor epoxide. When all malignant tumours were combined, their incidence in

TABLE 1. METHODS FOR THE ANALYSIS OF HEPTACHLOR AND HEPTACHLOR EPOXIDE

SAMPLE TYPE	ANALYTICAL METHOD			
	EXTRACTION/CLEAN-UP	DETECTION	LIMIT OF DETECTION	REFERENCE
Formulations				
Emulsifiable concentrates	Dechlorinate	Titration		Horwitz (1970)
Granules and dusts	Dechlorinate	Titration		Horwitz (1970)
Liquids	Extract (carbon disulphide)	GC/FID		Horwitz (1970)
Solids	Extract (pentane) in Soxhlet	GC/FID		Horwitz (1970)
Air				
Ambient	Trap in ethylene glycol	GC/ECD	0.1 ng/m^3	Arthur et al. (1976)
Soil				
Sediments and sewage sludge	Centrifuge, extract solid (acetone), liquid/liquid partition, transfer into trimethylpentane, treat to remove sulphur, isolate in trimethylpentane	GC/ECD	1-10 µg/kg	Jensen et al. (1977)
Soil	Add acetone, extract (petroleum ether or hexane), filter, wash (water) to remove acetone, CC	GC/ECD	1 µg/kg	Harris & Sans (1971)
Soil	Extract (hexane-isopropanol), filter, wash (water) to remove isopropanol, filter, dry	GC/ECD	10 µg/kg	Wiersma et al. (1972a,b)

TABLE 1. METHODS FOR THE ANALYSIS OF HEPTACHLOR AND HEPTACHLOR EPOXIDE (continued)

SAMPLE TYPE	ANALYTICAL METHOD			
	EXTRACTION/CLEAN-UP	DETECTION	LIMIT OF DETECTION	REFERENCE
Soil	Extract (acetone-hexane), add benzene to extract, evaporate to dryness, dissolve in hexane, CC	GC/ECD		Townsend & Specht (1975)
Soil	Wet sample, extract (hexane-isopropanol), filter, wash (water) to remove isopropanol, dry	GC/ECD	10 µg/kg	Carey et al. (1973)
Food				
Fruits, vegetables, dairy products, vegetable oils	Extract (acetonitrile), dilute (water), extract (petroleum ether), CC	GC/ECD, thermionic detection TLC, PC		Horwitz (1975)
Fish, crabs, shellfish	Extract (hexane-acetone), dry, filter, wash filtrate (water), distill, CC	GC/ECD	4 µg/kg	Albright et al. (1975)
Molasses	Dilute (water), add hexane, shake, add isopropanol, shake, wash (water), separate hexane layer, dry, filter	GC/ECD	10 µg/kg	Yang et al. (1976)
Crops	Blend with water-acetonitrile, decant, separate liquid, concentrate, extract (hexane), transfer to hexane, liquid/liquid partition, transfer to hexane, CC	GC/ECD	10 µg/kg	Carey et al. (1973)
Corn fodder	Extract (hexane)	TLC/oscillo-polarography on TLC plate	20 µg/kg	Kosmatyi & Bǔblik (1974)

TABLE 1. METHODS FOR THE ANALYSIS OF HEPTACHLOR AND HEPTACHLOR EPOXIDE (continued)

SAMPLE TYPE	ANALYTICAL METHOD			
	EXTRACTION/CLEAN-UP	DETECTION	LIMIT OF DETECTION	REFERENCE
Water				
Rural potable	Extract (hexane), CC	GC/ECD	10 ng/l	Sandhu *et al.* (1978)
Biological				
Adipose tissue	Extract (hexane), re-extract (petroleum ether, chloroform-methanol, acetonitrile or acetone-hexane), dry, dissolve (hexane), CC	GC/ECD and TLC		Clausen *et al.* (1974)
Wildlife tissues	Grind with sodium sulphate, extract (ethyl ether-petroleum ether) in Soxhlet, CC	GC/ECD	5 μg/kg	White (1976)
Plant tissues	Blend in acetonitrile, extract (hexane), wash (water), evaporate to dryness, dissolve (hexane), CC	GC/ECD		Townsend & Specht (1975)

Abbreviations: GC/FID - gas chromatography/flame-ionization detection; GC/ECD - gas chromatography/electron capture
detection; CC - column chromatography; TLC - thin-layer chromatography; PC - paper chromatography

controls was approximately double that in the two test groups. Following histological reevaluation, however, a significant excess (P<0.001) of liver carcinomas was found in males and females treated with heptachlor and heptachlor epoxide when compared with controls, as shown below in Table 2.

TABLE 2.   NUMBER OF LIVER CARCINOMAS
IN UNTREATED MICE AND IN THOSE RECEIVING 10 MG/KG DIET
HEPTACHLOR AND HEPTACHLOR EPOXIDE FOR 2 YEARS

	Controls	Heptachlor	Heptachlor Epoxide
Males	22/73	64/87	73/79
Females	2/54	57/78	77/81

Epstein (1976) also reviewed and reevaluated unpublished studies carried out in 1973 by the International Research and Development Corporation, in which groups of 100 male and 100 female Charles River CD-1 mice were each fed a mixture of 75% heptachlor epoxide and 25% heptachlor at levels of 1, 5 and 10 mg/kg diet, for 18 months starting at 7 weeks of age. Excluding groups of 10 mice from each group that were sacrificed for interim histology at 6 months, mortality at 18 months in all groups ranged from 34-49%, with the exception of the males and females given 10 mg/kg diet, which had mortalities of approximately 70%; in addition, comparatively large numbers of animals from all groups were lost to histology by autolysis. A dose-related incidence of 'compound-related liver masses' and 'compound-related nodular hyperplasia' was reported in test groups; the incidence in those receiving 1 mg/kg diet decreased to the level of negative controls. Histological reevaluation revealed an excess of liver carcinomas in both sexes given the 10 mg/kg diet level and in males given 5 mg/kg diet (P<0.01; see Table 3). The pathology of these liver carcinomas was reported by Reuber (1977).

TABLE 3.   NUMBER OF LIVER CARCINOMAS
IN UNTREATED MICE AND IN THOSE RECEIVING 1, 5 AND 10 MG/KG DIET
OF A MIXTURE OF 75% HEPTACHLOR EPOXIDE AND 25% HEPTACHLOR

	Controls	1 mg/kg	5 mg/kg	10 mg/kg
Males	0/62	2/61	18/68	52/80
Females	6/76	1/70	6/65	30/57

Groups of 50 male and 50 female B6C3F1 hybrid mice, 5 weeks of age, were fed technical-grade heptachlor (72% heptachlor, 18% *trans*-chlordane and 2% *cis*-chlordane) in the diet for 80 weeks. Males received initial dietary concentrations of 10 and 20 mg/kg diet and time-weighted average concentrations of 6 and 14 mg/kg diet; females received initial concentrations of 20 and 40 mg/kg diet and time-weighted average concentrations of 9 and 18 mg/kg diet. Initial dose levels were reduced during the experiment due to adverse toxic effects. Matched controls consisted of 20 males and 10 females; and pooled controls consisted of 100 males and 80 females. Survival in all groups was relatively high: over 70% of test and control males and 60% of test and control females were still alive at 90 weeks. Liver carcinomas were found in 34/47 males (P<0.001) and 30/42 females (P<0.01) that received the higher dose, and in 11/46 males and 3/47 females in the lower dose group, compared with 5/19 male and 2/10 female matched controls (National Cancer Institute, 1977).

Rat: Epstein (1976) reported a previously unpublished study by Kettering Laboratories, carried out in 1955, in which heptachlor of unspecified purify was administered to groups of 20 male and 20 female CF rats, 10 weeks of age, at concentrations of 1.5, 3, 5, 7 and 10 mg/kg diet, by spraying alcoholic solutions onto Purina Chow Pellets, for 100 weeks. Mortality in all test groups was stated to be random, although it was generally elevated in male test groups (50-75%). Liver-cell abnormalities were reported in males and females of the 7 and 10 mg/kg diet test groups. In addition, an excess of heterogenous, multiple-site tumours was reported in all females, particularly in those given 5 and 7 mg/kg; these data were interpreted as insignificant. Subsequent statistical analysis revealed a significant incidence of all tumours combined in female groups given the higher levels of heptachlor (P<0.01).

Epstein (1976) also reported another unpublished study by Kettering Laboratories, carried out in 1959, in which groups of 25 male and 25 female CFN rats, 7 weeks of age, were fed heptachlor epoxide at concentrations of 0.5, 2.5, 5.0, 7.5 and 10.0 mg/kg diet, by spraying alcoholic solutions on Purina Chow pellets, for 108 weeks. Survival at that time was over 45% in test and control groups. The following changes were noted in test groups: hepatic-cell vacuolization (which was centrilobular in those given lower test doses and irregular in those on higher doses), an excess of hepatomas and a spectrum of unusual malignant tumours. Subsequent analysis revealed an excess of all tumours in all test groups combined (P<0.001). Histological reevaluation revealed an excess of hepatic carcinomas in females given 5 and 10 mg/kg diet (P<0.05); males given 10 mg/kg diet also showed an excess when hepatic carcinomas and hyperplastic nodules were combined.

A group of 95 male and female suckling Wistar rats were administered 10 mg/kg bw heptachlor (97% pure) in corn oil by gavage on 5 successive occasions at 2-day intervals starting at 10 days of age; 19 male and 27 female controls received corn oil alone. Excluding 9 male and 20 female test animals sacrificed for interim histology at 60 weeks, survival in test and control groups was high and comparable. While the numbers of total tumours in test and control groups were comparable, 'lipomatous' renal tumours were noted in two females treated with heptachlor (Cabral *et al.*, 1972) [The Working Group noted the small number of doses administered and the short duration of treatment].

Groups of 50 male and 50 female 5-week-old Osborne-Mendel rats were fed technical-grade heptachlor (72% heptachlor, 18% *trans*-chlordane and 2% *cis*-chlordanc) in the diet for 80 weeks. Males received initial concentrations of 80 and 160 mg/kg diet and time-weighted concentrations of 40 and 78 mg/kg diet; females received initial concentrations of 40 and 80 mg/kg diet and time-weighted concentrations of 26 and 51 mg/kg diet. Initial dose levels were reduced during the experiment due to adverse toxic effects. Matched controls consisted of 10 males and 10 females; pooled controls consisted of 60 males and 60 females. Survival in all groups was high: approximately 60% of all test and control groups were still alive at 110 weeks. An excess of follicular-cell thyroid neoplasms was noted in females that received the low dose (3/43) and in those that received the high dose (14/38) (P<0.01), compared with pooled female controls (3/58) (National Cancer Institute, 1977).

3.2   Other relevant biological data

(a)   Experimental systems

Toxic effects

The oral LD_{50} for heptachlor in rats is 100 mg/kg bw in males and 160 mg/kg bw in females (Gaines, 1969), the i.v. LD_{50} in mice is about 20 mg/kg bw (Radomski & Davidow, 1953). The oral LD_{50} of the epoxide in rats is 62 mg/kg bw (Sperling & Ewinike, 1969).

Daily oral administration of 2 or 5 mg/kg bw heptachlor for 78-86 days to pigs, sheep and rats induced hepatic necrosis and synthesis of smooth endoplasmic reticulum. Rats were the most sensitive species (Halačka *et al.*, 1975). Chronic i.m. treatment of rats with daily doses of 3 and 15 mg/kg bw heptachlor and 1 and 5 mg/kg bw heptachlor epoxide decreased liver size but had no effect on other tissues. Certain hepatic and renal gluconeogenic enzymes were stimulated (Kacew *et al.*, 1973).

Embryotoxicity and teratogenicity

Injection of 1.5 mg/egg heptachlor resulted in a 12% reduction in hatchability but no abnormal chicks (Smith *et al.*, 1970). It was toxic to sea urchins and induced greatly abnormal embryos (Bresch & Arendt, 1977).

Absorption, distribution, excretion and metabolism

Rats metabolize intravenously administered C^{14}-labelled heptachlor to the epoxide (found in the tissues, faeces and urine) and to 4,5,6,7,8,8-hexachloro-1-*exo*-hydroxy-6,7-*exo*-epoxy-1,2,3a,4,7,7a-hexahydro-1,4-*endo*-methyleneindene (1,2,3,4,8,8-hexachloro-5-*exo*-hydroxy-6,7-*exo*-epoxy-1,4,4a,7a,5,6-hexahydro-1,4-*endo*-methyleneindene), a hydrophilic metabolite which is excreted in the urine. In rabbits, the radioactive label was found mainly in the urine (20% epoxide, 80% hydrophilic metabolite) (Klein *et al.*, 1968). Another faecal metabolite (a dehydrogenated derivative of 1-hydroxy-2,3-epoxychlordene) was isolated from rats fed 10 mg/kg diet heptachlor epoxide for 30 days (Matsumura & Nelson, 1971).

Rats fed 30 mg/kg diet heptachlor had maximum concentrations of heptachlor epoxide in fat within 2-4 weeks; 12 weeks after exposure was discontinued, heptachlor epoxide had completely disappeared from adipose tissue (Radomski & Davidow, 1953). Heptachlor is also stored as heptachlor epoxide in the fat of steers (Bovard *et al.*, 1971) and dogs (Davidow & Radomski, 1953).

Mutagenicity and other related short-term tests

Heptachlor showed no activity in the *rec* assay with *Bacillus subtilis* (Shirasu *et al.*, 1976), and both heptachlor and heptachlor epoxide were nonmutagenic to *Salmonella typhimurium* strains TA1535, TA1536, TA1537 and TA1538 in the presence or absence of a rat liver microsomal activation system (Marshall *et al.*, 1976).

In *Drosophila melanogaster* injected with aqueous solutions of 5 µg/ml heptachlor or 2.5 µg/ml heptachlor epoxide, there was no evidence of induction of X-linked recessive lethals in post-meiotic germ-cell stages (Benes & Sram, 1969).

Male albino mice that received single doses of heptachlor:heptachlor epoxide (25:75) either by oral intubation or by i.p. injection (7.5 or 15 mg/kg bw) were mated with untreated females (1 male:3 females) sequentially for 6 successive weeks. There was no evidence of an increase in dominant lethality (relative to controls) as measured by pregnancy rates, early deaths and number of live implants/female (Arnold *et al.*, 1977).

In a study reported as an abstract, rats were fed on diets containing 1 and 5 mg/kg diet heptachlor for 3 generations, and treated males were then used in dominant lethal tests. There was a statistically significant increase in the number of resorbed foetuses, relative to controls. Investigation of chromosomal damage in bone-marrow cells of the test animals of the second and third generations showed an increased incidence of abnormal mitosis relative to controls (Čerey *et al.*, 1973).

An increase in the frequency of chromosome aberrations was found in the bone-marrow cells of mice 21 hrs after i.p. injection of 5.2 mg/kg bw heptachlor (4% of the LD_{50} dose) (Markarjan, 1966).

In SV40 transformed human cells (VA-4) *in vitro*, both heptachlor and heptachlor epoxide induced unscheduled DNA synthesis (measured autoradiographically) at all concentrations tested - 8 hrs' exposure to 100 and 1000 μM heptachlor; 8 hrs' exposure to 10, 100 and 1000 μM heptachlor epoxide - but only in the presence of a rat liver microsomal activation system (Ahmed *et al.*, 1977).

(b) Humans

Heptachlor epoxide has been found in human fat [see section 2.2 (f)]. It has also been found in the blood and fat of stillborn infants (levels of 0.01-0.3 mg/kg were found in fat; 0.001 mg/1 in blood), indicating transplacental transfer to the foetus (Curley *et al.*, 1969; Wassermann *et al.*, 1972a,c; Zavon *et al.*, 1969). It is excreted in human milk (0.001-0.003 mg/1) (Curley & Kimbrough, 1969).

In a clinical study, it was demonstrated that the sera of pregnant women in a rural agricultural area in the Mississippi Delta contained levels of residues of chlorinated hydrocarbon insecticides, including heptachlor epoxide (0.08-0.1 μg/1), that were comparable to those found in occupationally exposed men. Cordblood of offspring also contained significant residue levels (0.02 μg/1) (D'Ercole *et al.*, 1976).

Chlorinated insecticides were found in the blood of all 35 mothers and 35 newborn infants examined in two Italian provinces. Heptachlor was found in 62/70 blood samples in high concentrations (up to 0.06 mg/1); heptachlor epoxide (up to 0.015 mg/1) was found in only 4 cases (Grasso *et al.*, 1973).

3.3 Case reports and epidemiological studies

Infante *et al.* (1978) reviewed 25 previously reported cases of blood dyscrasia associated with exposure to chlordane or heptachlor, either alone or in combination with other drugs, in conjunction with 3 newly diagnosed cases of aplastic anaemia and 3 of acute leukaemia associated with a prior history of exposure to technical- grade chlordane containing 3-7% heptachlor. During the period December 1974-February 1976, 5 of 14 children with neuroblastoma admitted to one paediatric hospital had a positive history of pre- or postnatal exposure to technical-grade chlordane containing 3-7% heptachlor; history of exposure to chlordane/heptachlor had not yet been ascertained for the remaining 9 cases.

4. Summary of Data Reported and Evaluation

4.1 Experimental data

Heptachlor containing about 20% chlordane was tested in one experiment
in mice and in one in rats by oral administration. It produced liver
carcinomas in mice of both sexes. In rats, the results suggest a
carcinogenic effect on the thyroid in females. Heptachlor (97% pure)
was also inadequately tested in one experiment in rats by oral administration. A reevaluation of unpublished studies involving the oral administration of heptachlor of unspecified purity to mice and rats of other
strains confirms the hepatocarcinogenicity of heptachlor for mice and
suggests a carcinogenic effect in female rats.

The latter studies also suggested that heptachlor epoxide produced
liver carcinomas in mice of both sexes and hepatomas in rats of both
sexes.

Heptachlor and heptachlor epoxide were not mutagenic in *Salmonella
typhimurium* or *Drosophila melanogaster* and were negative in dominant
lethal tests in mice.

4.2 Human data

Case reports suggest a relationship between exposure to heptachlor
or chlordane (either alone or in combination with other compounds) and
blood dyscrasias. Another publication has also suggested an association
with acute leukaemia; an association between both pre- and postnatal
exposure to technical-grade chlordane containing heptachlor and the
development of neuroblastomas in children was also suggested.

No epidemiological studies were available to the Working Group.

The extensive production of heptachlor and its use over the past
several decades, together with the persistent nature of the compound,
indicate that widespread human exposure occurs. This is confirmed by
many reports of its occurrence in the general environment and by the
finding of its epoxide in the fat and body fluids of human adults and
stillborn infants.

4.3 Evaluation

There is *sufficient evidence* that heptachlor (containing chlordane)
is carcinogenic in mice. There is *limited evidence* that heptachlor
epoxide is carcinogenic in experimental animals. A report of a series
of cases of human cancer associated with exposure to heptachlor was
also available, but these data do not allow an evaluation of the carcinogenicity of heptachlor or heptachlor epoxide to humans to be made.

5. References

Abbott, D.C., Goulding, R. & Tatton, J.O'G. (1968) Organochlorine
    pesticide residues in human fat in Great Britain. Br. med. J.,
    iii, 146-149

Abbott, D.C., Collins, G.B. & Goulding, R. (1972) Organochlorine
    pesticide residues in human fat in the United Kingdom 1969-71.
    Br. med. J., ii, 553-556

Ahmed, F.E., Hart, R.W. & Lewis, J.J. (1977) Pesticide induced DNA
    damage and its repair in cultured human cells. Mutat. Res., 42,
    161-174

Albright, L.J., Northcote, T.G., Oloffs, P.C. & Szeto, S.Y. (1975)
    Chlorinated hydrocarbon residues in fish, crabs, and shellfish
    of the Lower Fraser River, its estuary, and selected locations in
    Georgia Strait, British Columbia - 1972-73. Pestic. Monit. J., 9,
    134-140

Anon. (1976) Chlordane and heptachlor: second edition. Vet. Toxicol.
    18, 217-221

Anon. (1978a) Heptachlor/chlordane settlement allows corn use until
    August 1, 1980. Pestic. Tox. Chem. News, 6, 17-19

Anon. (1978b) EPA, Velsicol agree on pesticide limits. Chem. Eng.
    News, March 13, p. 15

Arnold, D.W., Kennedy, G.L., Jr, Keplinger, M.L., Calandra, J.C. & Calo,
    C.J. (1977) Dominant lethal studies with technical chlordane, HCS-
    3260, and heptachlor:heptachlor epoxide. J. Toxicol. environ. Health,
    2, 547-555

Arthur, R.D., Cain, J.D. & Barrentine, B.F. (1976) Atmospheric levels
    of pesticides in the Mississippi delta. Bull. environ. Contam. Toxicol.,
    15, 129-134

Benes, V. & Sram, R. (1969) Mutagenic activity of some pesticides in
    Drosophila melanogaster. Ind. Med., 38, 50-52

Berg, G.L., ed. (1978) Farm Chemicals Handbook 1978, Willoughby, OH,
    Meister Publishing Co., p. D-137

Bovard, K.P., Fontenot, J.P. & Priode, B.M. (1971) Accumulation and
    dissipation of heptachlor residues in fattening steers. J. Anim. Sci.,
    33, 127-132

Bresch, H. & Arendt, U. (1977) Influence of different organochlorine
    pesticides on the development of the sea urchin embryo. Environ. Res.,
    13, 121-128

Burns, B.G., Peach, M.E. & Stiles, D.A. (1975) Organochlorine pesticide residues in a farming area, Nova Scotia - 1972-73. Pestic. Monit. J., 9, 34-38

Cabral, J.R., Testa, M.C. & Terracini, B. (1972) Lack of long-term effects of the administration of heptachlor to suckling rats (Ital.). Tumori, 58, 49-53

Carey, A.E., Wiersma, G.B., Tai, H. & Mitchell, W.G. (1973) Organochlorine pesticide residues in soils and crops of the Corn Belt region, United States - 1970. Pestic. Monit. J., 6, 369-376

Cerey, K., Izakovič, V. & Ruttkay-Nedecká, J. (1973) Effect of heptachlor on dominant lethality and bone marrow in rats (Abstract no. 10). Mutat. Res., 21, 26

Clausen, J., Braestrup, L. & Berg, O. (1974) The content of polychlorinate hydrocarbons in Arctic mammals. Bull. environ. Contam. Toxicol., 12, 529-534

Curley, A. & Kimbrough, R. (1969) Chlorinated hydrocarbon insecticides in plasma and milk of pregnant and lactating women. Arch. environ. Health, 18, 156-164

Curley, A., Copeland, M.F. & Kimbrough, R.D. (1969) Chlorinated hydrocarbon insecticides in organs of stillborn and blood of newborn babies. Arch. environ. Health, 19, 628-632

Curley, A., Burse, V.W., Jennings, R.W., Villanueva, E.C., Tomatis, L. & Akazaki, K. (1973) Chlorinated hydrocarbon pesticides and related compounds in adipose tissue from people of Japan. Nature (Lond.), 242, 338-340

Davidow, B. & Radomski, J.L. (1953) Isolation of an epoxide metabolite from fat tissues of dogs fed heptachlor. J. Pharmacol. exp. Ther., 107, 259-265

Davies, J.E., Edmundson, W.F., Maceo, A., Irvin, G.L., III, Cassady, J. & Barquet, A. (1971) Reduction of pesticide residues in human adipose tissue with diphenylhydantoin. Food Cosmet. Toxicol., 9, 413-423

D'Ercole, A.J., Arthur, R.D., Cain, J.D. & Barrentine, B.F. (1976) Insecticide exposure of mothers and newborns in a rural agricultural area. Pediatrics, 57, 869-874

Dyatlovitiskaya, F.G., Gladenko, E.F. & Kruchinina, A.A. (1972) Determination of organochlorrine insecticides in reservoir water (Russ.). Probl. anal. Khim., 2, 43-46 [Chem. Abstr., 79, 62445p]

Edwards, C.A. (1970) Persistent Pesticides in the Environment, London, Butterworths, pp. 49-50

Epstein, S.S. (1976) Carcinogenicity of heptachlor and chlordane. Sci. total Environ., 6, 103-154

Eurocop-Cost (1976) A Comprehensive List of Polluting Substances Which Have Been Identified in Various Fresh Waters, Effluent Discharges, Aquatic Animals and Plants, and Bottom Sediments, 2nd ed., EUCO/-MDU/73/76, XII/476/76, Luxembourg, Commission of the European Communities, pp. 46-47

Fairchild, H.E., Dale, L.B., Baron, R.L., Carver, T., Cummings, J.G., Duvall, A.J., Kolojeski, J.C., Menzie, C.M., Payntec, O.E., Tschirley, F.H., Williams, C.H., Yobs, A.R., Hartwell, W.V. & Billings, S.C. (1976a) Heptachlor in Relation to Man and the Environment, EPA-540/4-76-007, Washington DC, US Environmental Protection Agency, pp. 24-26

Fairchild, H.E., Baer, L.J., Barfehenn, K.R., Beusch, G.J., Caswell, R.L., Hageman, F.J., Markley, M.H., Payntec, O.E., Smith, K.K. & Spenser, R. (1976b) Chlordane and Heptachlor in Relation to Man and the Environment. A Further Pesticide Review, 1972-1975, EPA-540/4-76-005, Washington DC, US Environmental Protection Agency

Fournier, E., Treich, I., Campagne, L. & Capelle, N. (1972) Organochloride pesticide residues in human adipose tissue in France (Fr.). Eur. J. Toxicol., 5, 11-26

Gaines, T.B. (1969) Acute toxicity of pesticides. Toxicol. appl. Pharmacol., 14, 515-534

Gore, R.C., Hannah, R.W., Pattacini, S.C. & Porro, T.J. (1971) Infrared and ultraviolet spectra of seventy-six pesticides. J. Assoc. off. anal. Chem., 54, 1040-1043, 1060-1061, 1082

Gowen, J.A., Wiersma, G.B., Tai, H. & Mitchell, W.G. (1976) Pesticide levels in hay and soils from nine states, 1971. Pestic. Monit. J. 10, 114-116

Grasselli, J.G. & Ritchey, W.M., eds (1975) CRC Atlas of Spectral Data and Physical Constants for Organic Compounds, 2nd ed., Vol. III, Cleveland, OH, Chemical Rubber Co., p. 190

Grasso, C., Bernardi, G. & Martinelli, F. (1973) The significance of the presence of chlorinated insecticides in the blood of newborns and their mothers (Ital.). Ig. Mod., 66, 362-371

Halačka, K., Dvorák, M., Ryšánek, K., Jagoš, P. & Černý, E. (1975) The effect of small orally administered doses of heptachlor on ultrastructure of hepatocytes and their enzyme systems in experimental animals (Czech.) Cesk. Hyg., 20, 286-291

Harris, C.R. & Sans, W.W. (1971) Insecticide residues in soils on 16
    farms in southwestern Ontario - 1964, 1966, and 1969. Pestic. Monit.
    J., 5, 259-267

Hashemy-Tonkabony, S.E. & Soleimani-Amiri, M.J. (1976) Detection and
    determination of chlorinated pesticide residues in raw and various
    stages of processed vegetable oil. J. Am. Oil Chem. Soc., 53,
    752-753

Hayes, W.J., Jr, Dale, W.E. & Burse, V.W. (1965) Chlorinated hydro-
    carbon pesticides in the fat of people in New Orleans. Life Sci.,
    4, 1611-1615

Horwitz, W., ed. (1970) Official Methods of Analysis of the Association
    of Official Analytical Chemists, 11th ed., Washington DC,
    Association of Official Analytical Chemists, pp. 107-109

Horwitz, W., ed. (1975) Official Methods of Analysis of the Association
    of Official Analytical Chemists, 12th ed., Washington DC,
    Association of Official Analytical Chemists, pp. 475-484

IARC (1974) IARC Monographs on the Evaluation of Carcinogenic Risk of
    Chemicals to Man, 5, Some Organochloride Pesticides, Lyon,
    pp. 173-191

Infante, P.F., Epstein, S.S. & Newton, W.A., Jr (1978) Blood dyscrasias
    and childhood tumors and exposure to chlordane and heptachlor.
    Scand. J. Work Environ. Health, 4, 137-150

Jensen, S., Renberg, L. & Reutergårdh, L. (1977) Residue analysis of
    sediment and sewage sludge for organochlorines in the presence of
    of elemental sulfur. Anal. Chem., 49, 316-318

Johnson, O. (1972) Pesticides '72. Part 2. Chem. Week, 111 (4), 19

Johnson, R.D. & Manske, D.D. (1976) Pesticide residues in total diet
    samples (IX). Pestic. Monit. J., 9, 157-169

Kacew, S., Sutherland, D.J.B. & Singhal, R.L. (1973) Biochemical
    changes following chronic administration of heptachlor, heptachlor
    epoxide and endrin to male rats. Environ. Physiol. Biochem., 3,
    221-229

Klein, W., Korte, F., Weisgerber, I., Kaul, R., Müller, W. & Djirsarai,
    A. (1968) Metabolism of endrin, heptachlor and telodrin (Germ.).
    Qual. Plant Mater. Veg., 15, 225-238

Kosmatyi, E.S. & Bublik, L.I. (1974) Use of a chromatopolarographic
    method in pesticide analysis (Russ.). Ukr. Khim. Zh., 40, 1316-1318
    [Chem. Abstr., 82, 137835p]

Kreitzer, J.F. (1974) Residues of organochlorine pesticides, mercury,
    and PCB's in mourning doves from eastern United States - 1970-1971.
    Pestic. Monit. J., 7, 195-199

Lawless, E.W., von Rumker, R. & Ferguson, T.L. (1972) The Pollution
    Potential In Pesticide Manufacturing, Technical Studies Report:
    TS-00-72-04, US Environmental Protection Agency, Washington DC, US
    Government Printing Office, pp. 7, 14, 26, 44, 65, 224, 236

Markarjan, D.S. (1966) Cytogenetic effect of some chlororganic insecticides
    on the nuclei of mouse bone-marrow cells (Russ.). Genetika, 1,
    132-137

Marshall, T.C., Dorough, H.W. & Swim, H.E. (1976) Screening of pesticides
    for mutagenic potential using Salmonella typhimurium mutants.
    J. agric. Food Chem., 24, 560-563

Matsumura, F. & Nelson, J.O. (1971) Identification of the major
    metabolic product of heptachlor epoxide in rat feces. Bull. environ.
    Contam. Toxicol., 5, 489-492

Mercier, M. (1975) Preparatory Study for Establishing Criteria (Dose/
    Effect Relationships) for Humans on Organochlorine Compounds, i.e.
    Pesticides and their Metabolites, Doc. No. 1347/75 e, Luxembourg,
    Commission of the European Communities, pp. 24-26, 63-66, 176-177,
    219-220

National Cancer Institute (1977) Bioassay of Heptachlor for Possible
    Carcinogenicity, Technical Report Series No. 9, DHEW
    Publication No. (NIH) 77-809, Washington DC, US Government Printing
    Office

Nicholas, M.L., Powell, D.L., Williams, T.R. & Bromund, R.H. (1976)
    Reference Raman spectra of DDT and five structurally related pesticides
    and of five pesticides containing the norbornene group. J. Assoc. off.
    anal. Chem., 59, 197-208

Radomski, J.L. & Davidow, B. (1953) The metabolite of heptachlor, its
    estimation, storage, and toxicity. J. Pharmacol. exp. Ther., 107,
    266-272

Reuber, M.D. (1977) Histopathology of carcinomas of the liver in mice
    ingesting heptachlor or heptachlor epoxide. Exp. Cell Biol., 45,
    147-157

Safe Drinking Water Committee (1977) Drinking Water and Health,
    Washington DC, National Academy of Sciences, pp. 556-561

Sandhu, S.S., Warren, W.J. & Nelson, P. (1978) Pesticidal residue in
    rural potable water. J. Am. Water Works Assoc., 70, 41-45

Schacht, R.A. (1974) Pesticides in the Illinois Waters of Lake Michigan, EPA-660/3-74-002, Washington DC, US Government Printing Office

Shackelford, W.M. & Keith, L.H. (1976) Frequency of Organic Compounds Identified in Water, EPA-600/4-76-062, Athens, GA, US Environmental Protection Agency, pp. 140-141

Shirasu, Y., Moriya, M., Kato, K., Furuhashi, A. & Kada, T. (1976) Mutagenicity screening of pesticides in the microbial system. Mutat. Res., 40, 19-30

Smith, S.I., Weber, C.W. & Reid, B.L. (1970) The effect of injection of chlorinated hydrocarbon pesticides on hatchability of eggs. Toxicol. appl. Pharmacol., 16, 179-185

Sperling, F. & Ewinike, H. (1969) Changes in LD_{50} of parathion and heptachlor after turpentine pretreatment (Abstract no. 24). Toxicol. appl. Pharmacol., 14, 622

Stanley, C.W., Barney, J.E., II, Helton, M.R. & Yobs, A.R. (1971) Measurement of atmospheric levels of pesticides. Environ. Sci. Technol., 5, 430-435

Townsend, L.R. & Specht, H.B. (1975) Organophosphorus and organochlorine pesticide residues in soils and uptake by tobacco plants. Can. J. Plant Sci., 55, 835-842

US Environmental Protection Agency (1971) EPA Compendium of Registered Pesticides, Vol. III, Washington DC, US Government Printing Office, pp. III-H-1.1 - III-H-1.4

US Environmental Protection Agency (1976a) Velsicol Chemical Co. et al. Consolidated heptachlor/chlordane hearing. Fed. Regist., 41, 7552-757

US Environmental Protection Agency (1976b) Heptachlor and heptachlor epoxide; tolerances for residues. US Code Fed. Regul., Title 40, part 180.104, p. 312

US Environmental Protection Agency (1978) Velsicol Chemical Co. et al. Consolidated heptachlor/chlordane cancellation proceedings. Fed. Regist., 43, 12372-12375

US Food & Drug Administration (1975) Pesticide Analytical Manual, Vol. I, Foods and Feeds, Rockville, MD, Table 201-A

US Occupational Safety & Health Administration (1977) Occupational safety and health standards, subpart Z - Toxic and hazardous substances. US Code Fed. Regul., Title 40, part 1910-1000, p. 27

US Tariff Commission (1954) Synthetic Organic Chemicals, US Production and
    Sales, 1953, Report No. 194, Second Series, Washington DC, US Govern-
    ment Printing Office, p. 134

Wassermann, M., Wassermann, D., Lazarovici, S., Coetzee, A.M. & Tomatis, L.
    (1970) Present state of the storage of the organochlorine insecticides
    in the general population of South Africa. S. Afr. med. J., 44, 646-648

Wassermann, M., Nogueira, D.P., Tomatis, L., Athie, E., Wassermann, D.,
    Djavaherian, M. & Guttel, C. (1972a) Storage of organochlorine insecti-
    cides in people of Sao Paulo, Brazil. Ind. Med., 41, 22-25

Wassermann, M., Rogoff, M.G., Tomatis, L., Day, N.E., Wassermann, D.,
    Djavaherian, M. & Guttel, C. (1972b) Storage of organochlorine insecti-
    cides in the adipose tissue of people in Kenya. Ann. Soc. belge Méd.
    trop., 52, 509-514

Wassermann, M., Sofoluwe, G.O., Tomatis, L., Day, N.E., Wassermann, D.
    & Lazarovici, S. (1972c) Storage of organochlorine insecticides in
    people of Nigeria. Environ. Physiol. Biochem., 2, 59-67

Whetstone, R.R. (1964) Chlorocarbons and chlorohydrocarbons. Heptachlor.
    In: Kirk, R.E. & Othmer, D.F., eds, Encyclopedia of Chemical Technology,
    2nd ed., Vol. 5, New York, John Wiley and Sons, p. 249

White, D.H. (1976) Nationwide residues of organochlorines in starlings,
    1974. Pestic. Monit. J., 10, 10-17

WHO (1972) 1971 Evaluations of Some Pesticide Residues in Food.
    WHO Pestic. Residues Ser., No. 1, Geneva, p. 314

Wiersma, G.B., Tai, H., & Sand, P.F. (1972a) Pesticide residue levels in
    soils, FY 1969 - National Soils Monitoring Program. Pestic. Monit. J.,
    6, 194-228

Wiersma, G.B., Tai, H., & Sand, P.F. (1972b) Pesticide residues in soil
    from eight cities - 1969. Pestic. Monit. J., 6, 126-129

Winell, M. (1975) An international comparison of hygienic standards for
    chemicals in the work environment. Ambio, 4, 34-36

Yang, H.S.C., Wiersma, G.B. & Mitchell, W.G. (1976) Organochlorine
    pesticide residues in sugarbeet pulps and molasses from 16 states,
    1971. Pestic. Monit. J., 10, 41-43

Yurkova, Z.F. & Klisenko, M.A. (1970) Use of thin-layer chromatography
    for detecting chloroorganic pesticides in foods and in water (Russ.)
    In: Lyalikoy, Y.S., ed., Methods of Analysis of Pesticides,
    Kishinev, Department of Edition & Publication of the Academy of
    Science of the Moldavian Republic of the USSR, pp. 112-115
    [Chem. Abstr., 76, 23871t]

Zavon, M.R., Tye, R. & Latorre, L. (1969) Chlorinated hydrocarbon
    insecticide content of the neonate. Ann. N.Y. Acad Sci., 160, 196-200

HEXACHLOROBENZENE

1. Chemical and Physical Data

1.1 Synonyms and trade names

Chem. Abstr. Services Reg. No.: 118-74-1

Chem. Abstr. Name: Hexachlorobenzene

Synonyms: HCB; pentachlorophenyl chloride; perchlorobenzene

Trade names: Amatin; Anticarie; Bunt-cure; Bunt-no-more;
Co-op Hexa; Granox NM; Julin's carbon chloride; No Bunt; No
Bunt 40; No Bunt 80; No Bunt Liquid; Sanocide; Snieciotox

1.2 Structural and molecular formulae and molecular weight

C_6Cl_6 Mol. wt: 284.8

1.3 Chemical and physical properties of the pure substance

From Weast (1976), unless otherwise specified

(a) Description: White needles (Hawley, 1977)

(b) Boiling-point: Sublimes at 322°C

(c) Melting-point: 230°C

(d) Spectroscopy data: λ_{max} 291, 301 nm (E_i^1 = 7.7, 7.9) in
isooctane; infra-red, ultra-violet and mass spectral data
have been tabulated (Grasselli & Ritchey, 1975).

(e) Solubility: Insoluble in water, sparingly soluble in cold
ethanol and soluble in ether, benzene, chloroform and boiling
ethanol (Hawley, 1977)

(f) Volatility: Vapour pressure is 1.089×10^{-5} mm at 20°C
(Mumma & Lawless, 1975).

(g) Stability: Very stable; nonreactive; inflammable, with a
flash-point at 242°C (Hawley, 1977)

(h) Reactivity: Not broken down by physical or chemical processes
in the environment (Mumma & Lawless, 1975); photolysis in
methanol or hexane (λ_{max} >260 or 220 nm) is rapid, giving
penta- and tetrachlorobenzenes (Plimmer & Klingebiel, 1976)

1.4 Technical products and impurities

Hexachlorobenzene is available in the US as a technical grade,
containing 98% hexachlorobenzene, 1.8% pentachlorobenzene and 0.2%
1,2,4,5-tetrachlorobenzene. Some commercial hexachlorobenzene is
derived from residual tar obtained as a byproduct in the production
of tetrachloroethylene. Since this tar also contains hexachlorobutadiene, it is a potential impurity in commercial hexachlorobenzene
derived from this source.

Hepta- and octachlorodibenzofurans and octachlorodibenzo-*para*-
dioxin have been found in commercial hexachlorobenzene (Villanueva *et
al*., 1974).

Formulations include wettable powders containing 40 or 80%, liquids
containing 12.4-33% and a flowable product containing 35.1% of the
chemical (US Environmental Protection Agency, 1972). Other commercial
dust formulations for fungicidal use contain 10-40% hexachlorobenzene.

2. Production, Use, Occurrence and Analysis

2.1 Production and use

(a) Production

Hexachlorobenzene was prepared by Lorentz in 1893 by heating carbon
with chlorine in the presence of boric oxide (Prager *et al*., 1922). It
can be produced commercially by reacting benzene with excess chlorine in
the presence of ferric chloride at 150-200°C. However, at least one US
producer isolates hexachlorobenzene from the distillation residues
obtained as a byproduct in the manufacture of tetrachloroethylene.

Commercial production of hexachlorobenzene in the US was first
reported in 1933 (US Tariff Commission, 1934). Three US producers made

it up to the end of 1973 (with an estimated total production of 300 thousand kg in 1973); but there was only one US producer in 1974, and only one company reported commercial production of an undisclosed amount in 1975 (see preamble, p. 16) (US International Trade Commission, 1977a). That company is believed to have discontinued production in early 1978.

Hexachlorobenzene is a byproduct or waste material in the production of many chemicals. The quantities produced in 1972 have been estimated in relation to various end-products: tetrachloroethylene, 0.8-1.6 million kg; trichloroethylene, 104-203 thousand kg; carbon tetra- chloride, 90-181 thousand kg; chlorine, 90-176 thousand kg; dimethyl tetrachloroterephthalate, 36-45 thousand kg; vinyl chloride, 0-12 thousand kg; atrazine, propazine and simazine, as a group, 2-4 thousand kg; pentachloronitrobenzene, 1-3 thousand kg; and mirex, 0.5-0.9 thousand kg.

In 1975, imports through the principal US customs districts of Grannox NM Seed Treatment, a formulation of hexachlorobenzene in combi- nation with maneb, were 100 thousand kg (US International Trade Commission, 1977b).

One company in Spain produces an estimated 150 thousand kg hexachloro- benzene annually. In Japan, about 300 thousand kg were obtained in 1977 as a byproduct in the production of tetrachloroethylene; almost all was incinerated.

(b) Use

In 1972, the principal use of hexachlorobenzene in the US was as a fungicide to control wheat bunt and smut fungi on other grains. Other applications in 1972 were as an additive for pyrotechnic compositions for military uses, as a porosity controller in the manufacture of electrodes, as a chemical intermediate in dye manufacture and organic synthesis and use as a wood preservative.

Minor amounts have been used as an additive for polymers and as a raw material for synthetic rubber. It has been used as a plasticizer for polyvinyl chloride (Plimma & Klingebiel, 1976). In 1974, the largest US producer reported that all of its production for several years had been committed for use as a rubber peptizing agent in the manufacture of nitroso and styrene-type rubbers.

Hexachlorobenzene is registered by the US Environmental Protection Agency as a treatment for control of fungi which infect the seeds of onions, sorghum and wheat. It is also used in combination with captan or maneb for the treatment of seeds of barley, beans, corn, flax, oats, peanuts, rye and soya beans (US Environmental Protection Agency, 1972). It is reported to be a candidate for the issuance of a notice of a rebuttable presumption against renewal of registration (RPAR) (see

General Remarks on the Substances Considered, p. 31) because of
possible carcinogenicity, teratogenicity and mutagenicity (Anon., 1978).

From 1 August 1974, the use on lettuce and on seed-potatoes of
pentachloronitrobenzene containing more than 0.1% hexachlorobenzene was
prohibited in The Netherlands.   From 1 May 1975, the same restriction
was applied to its use on flower bulbs and to all other uses (WHO, 1975).

In December 1974, the Joint Meeting of the FAO Working Party of
Experts on Pesticide Residues and the WHO Expert Committee on Pesticide
Residues established a value of 0-0.0006 mg/kg bw as a conditional
acceptable daily intake in man (WHO, 1975).

2.2 Occurrence

Hexachlorobenzene is not known to occur as a natural product.
It is a contaminant of various pesticides, including dimethyl tetrachloroterephthalate (Dacthal) and pentachloronitrobenzene (Cabral *et
al.*, 1977).

The distribution of hexachlorobenzene as a byproduct of the petro-
chemical industry has been reviewed (Laska *et al.*, 1976).   Reviews
have been published on the occurrence of hexachlorobenzene residues in
the environment in Italy (Leoni & D'Arca, 1976) and in Czechoslovakia
(Mahelova *et al.*, 1977).

(a) Water

Hexachlorobenzene has been found in 4 river-water samples, 8
finished drinking-water samples, 1 sample from a sewage treatment plant
and in the effluent water from 7 chemical plants in various US and
European locations (Shackelford & Keith, 1976).   It has also been
detected in urban rainwater runoff in the US, at levels of 0-339 ng/1
(Dappen, 1974);   in the Rhine River (Greve, 1972);   in 108 samples of
surface waters in Italy, at average levels of 2.5 ng/1 (Leoni & D'Arca,
1976);   and in most river-water residues in an industrialized region of
the US, at levels of less than 2 µg/1, but as high as 90 µg/1 in one
sample (Laska *et al.*, 1976).

(b) Soil and sediments

Hexachlorobenzene has been detected in: (1) greenhouse soil in
the US, 19 months after application, at levels of 0.19 mg/kg in the top
2 cm of soil and of 0.11 mg/kg in the 2-4 cm layer (Beall, 1976);
(2) soil in Belgium, at average levels of 0.44 and 0.85 mg/kg (Dejonckheere *et al.*, 1976);   (3) untreated and treated greenhouse and field
soil in the Federal Republic of Germany, at levels of 0.002-1.03 mg/kg
(Haefner, 1975, 1977);   (4) the soil in farming areas in Italy, at levels
of 40 µg/kg (Leoni & D'Arca, 1976);   and (5) levee and ditch soil in an

industrialized region of the US, at levels ranging from 0 to nearly
900 µg/kg (wet-weight basis) and 1677 µg/kg (dry-weight basis) (Laska
et al., 1976).

(c) Food and drink

In the Total Diet Program of the US Food and Drug Administration,
hexachlorobenzene was detected in food composites in 30 US cities, at
levels of 0.006-0.041 mg/kg (Johnson & Manske, 1976). As part of the
same study, the average daily intake of hexachlorobenzene was calculated
to be 0.3978 µg/day in fiscal year 1973 and 0.0725 µg/day in fiscal year
1974 (US Food & Drug Administration, 1977).

The average intake of hexachlorobenzene from cooked food samples
taken from an Italian Navy mess was reported to be 4.11 µg/man/day
(Leoni *et al.*, 1975).   In Japan, hexachlorobenzene residues were
detected at low levels in 16 foods, e.g., beef, 12 µg/kg; pike, 11 µg/kg;
salmon, 9 µg/kg; carp, 8 µg/kg; and pork, 7 µg/kg (Morita *et al.*,
1975a,b).   Residues of pesticides, including hexachlorobenzene, have
been detected in foods representing an average Canadian diet, at levels
of 0.001-0.085 mg/kg (Smith *et al.*, 1975).

The contamination of milk and dairy products by organochlorine
pesticides, including hexachlorobenzene, in The Netherlands between 1967
and 1973 has been reviewed (Tuinstra, 1974).   Hexachlorobenzene residues
have been detected in: (1) milk and milk products in the Federal Republic
of Germany, at levels of up to 0.5 mg/kg (Heeschen *et al.*, 1976) and
0-2 mg/l (Knöppler, 1976) on a fat basis; (2) whole cow's milk in Italy,
at an average level of 4.2 µg/l (Leoni & D'Arca, 1976);   (3) some Italian
grating cheeses (Corvi *et al.*, 1976);   (4) milk in Spain, at a mean level
of 0.654 mg/l (Pozo Lora *et al.*, 1977);   (5) butter from 5 Spanish
regions, with a mean level of 0.15 mg/kg on a fat basis (Polo Villar *et
al.*, 1977);   and (6) dairy products in France (Richou-Bac *et al.*, 1974).

Hexachlorobenzene has also been detected in tinned vegetables and
fruits (Biston *et al.*, 1975) and in meat at mean levels of 0.08-0.064 mg/
kg (Knöppler, 1976).

(d) Animals

Hexachlorobenzene has been detected in: (1) starlings from 126 US
sites, at levels of 0-9.11 mg/kg (White, 1976); (2) wild ducks, at levels
of 0-0.24 mg/kg (White & Kaiser, 1976); (3) eggs of common terns, at a
level of 7.67 mg/kg (dry weight) (Gilbertson & Reynolds, 1972); (4)
captive and free pheasants, at levels of 1.2-3.8 and 2.3-2.8 µg/kg,
respectively (Mikulik *et al.*, 1977); (5) the livers of birds, at levels
of up to 7.2 mg/kg (Leoni & D'Arca, 1976); (6) wild foxes, boars and
does, at levels of 0.02-3.11 mg/kg (Koss & Manz, 1976); and (7) swine,
at an average level of 0.616 mg/kg, with 67% of the samples containing
residues of more than 0.5 mg/kg (Lohse, 1975).

It has also been detected in: (1) fish in Lake Superior, at concentrations of < 0.1 mg/kg (Veith et al., 1977); (2) aquatic animals in Australia, at levels of 1-2 µg/kg (Thomson & Davie, 1974); (3) 8 species of fish, at mean levels of < 1 µg/kg to 16 mg/kg (Johnson et al., 1974); and (4) mosquito fish, at levels of 71.8-379.8 µg/kg, and commercial fish, at a level of 88 µg/kg, from an industrialized region of the US (Laska et al., 1976).

(e) Humans

Hexachlorobenzene residues have been detected in human milk in: (1) Ghana, at a level of 0.086 mg/l (Polishuk et al., 1977); (2) Australia, at levels of 0.012-0.034 mg/l (Stacey & Thomas, 1975); (3) Norway (Bakken & Seip, 1977); (4) Austria, at a mean concentration of 1.24 mg/l (Pesendorfer, 1975); (5) France, at average levels of 0.98 mg/l (Luquet et al., 1975); and (6) Spain, at levels of up to 0.08 mg/l (Trigo Lorenzo & Fernandez Garcia, 1976).

It has also been detected in human adipose tissue in: (1) Japan, at levels of <0.003-0.77 µg/g (Curley et al., 1973) and at a level of 0.21 µg/g (Morita et al., 1975a,b); (2) New Zealand, at a mean level of 0.31 µg/g (Solly & Shanks, 1974); (3) Canada, at levels of 0.001-0.520 µg/g (Mes et al., 1977); and (4) Italy, at an average level of 491 ng/g (Leoni & D'Arca, 1976).

Hexachlorobenzene has been detected in the blood of the umbilical cord in newborn infants and of their mothers in Argentina, at levels of up to 19 ng/l (Astolfi et al., 1974), and in the blood of children 1-18 years old in the Federal Republic of Germany at a maximum of 22 ng/l in boys and 17 ng/l in girls (Richter & Schmid, 1976).

(f) Occupational exposure

Hexachlorobenzene has been detected in: workplace air during the production of pentachlorophenol (Mel'nikova et al., 1975); the blood of workers in a factory making chlorinated solvents, at levels of 14-233 µg/l (Burns & Miller, 1975); and the blood of vegetable spraymen, at levels of 0-310 µg/l (Burns et al., 1974).

(g) Other

Hexachlorobenzene has been detected in: animal feeds (Richou-Bac et al., 1975); various grain samples, at mean levels of 0.27 mg/kg or less (Arrifai & Acker, 1975); and laboratory plastic wash bottles, at levels of 0.16-2.7 µg/bottle (Rourke et al., 1977).

2.3 Analysis

A review of methods of analysis for hexachlorobenzene is available (Li *et al*., 1976).

Determination and confirmation of low levels of hexachlorobenzene residues is hampered by the presence of other organochlorine pesticides and polychlorinated biphenyls. Methods for analysing residual hexachlorobenzene include separation and clean-up procedures, specific gas-chromatographic columns and formation of chemical derivatives. Methods used for the analysis of hexachlorobenzene in environmental samples are listed in Table 1.

Other analytical methods to isolate and identify hexachlorobenzene include: gel-permeation chromatography (Johnson *et al*., 1976), gas chromatography/electron capture detection on various columns (Di Muccio *et al*., 1972; Szokolay *et al*., 1975) and gas chromatography/mass spectrometry (Lunde & Baumann Ofstad, 1976).

Recovery of hexachlorobenzene from a magnesium silicate (Florisil) column, eluted with methylene chloride-hexane-acetonitrile, has been investigated for use with fatty and non-fatty foods (US Food & Drug Administration, 1975).

3. Biological Data Relevant to the Evaluation
of Carcinogenic Risk to Humans

3.1 Carcinogenicity studies in animals[1]

(a) Oral administration

Mouse: Groups of 30-50 male and 30-50 female 6-7 week-old Swiss mice were fed diets containing 0, 50, 100 or 200 mg/kg diet hexachlorobenzene (> 99.5% pure) until the animals were 120 weeks old, at which time all survivors were killed. Another group of 30 male and 30 female mice were fed 300 mg/kg diet hexachlorobenzene for 15 weeks. At 90 weeks of age, the percentage survival rates in males and females in the five different groups were: 50 and 48, 30 and 40, 27 and 30, 4 and 0, 13 and 57, respectively. The incidence of lymphomas and lung tumours was not increased in treated animals; no liver-cell tumours were found

---

[1]The Working Group was aware of studies in progress to assess the carcinogenicity of hexachlorobenzene in mice and rats by oral administration (IARC, 1978).

TABLE 1. METHODS FOR THE ANALYSIS OF HEXACHLOROBENZENE

| SAMPLE TYPE | ANALYTICAL METHOD | | | |
	EXTRACTION/CLEAN-UP	DETECTION	LIMIT OF DETECTION	REFERENCE
Formulations	Acidify, extract (hexane), CC, form pentachlorophenol derivative, liquid/liquid partition, acidify, extract (dichloromethane), evaporate to dryness, acetylate, dilute (ethyl acetate)	GC/colorimetric detection	0.3 mg/l	Alam (1977)
Air	Trap on GC packing, desorb by heating	GC/FID	10 $\mu g/m^3$	Russell (1975)
	Trap on chromosorb 101, extract (hexane)	GC/ECD	28 ng/m^3	Mann *et al.* (1974)
Soil	Extract (hexane-acetone), liquid/liquid partition	GC/ECD	7 $\mu g/kg$	Babkina *et al.* (1976)
Sediments and sewage sludge	Centrifuge, extract solid (acetone), liquid/liquid partition, transfer into trimethylpentane, treat to remove sulphur, isolate in trimethylpentane	GC/ECD	1-10 $\mu g/kg$	Jensen *et al.* (1977)
Food				
Fat and oil	Mix sample with Florisil, extract (acetonitrile), liquid/liquid partition, CC	GC/ECD		Bong (1977)
Fish	Grind with sodium sulphate, extract (hexane), CC	GC/ECD		Holden (1973)

TABLE 1. METHODS FOR THE ANALYSIS OF HEXACHLOROBENZENE (continued)

SAMPLE TYPE	EXTRACTION/CLEAN-UP	ANALYTICAL METHOD		REFERENCE
		DETECTION	LIMIT OF DETECTION	
Dairy products, meat, fat	Melt and filter if necessary, GC	GC/ECD TLC	2 µg/kg	Smyth (1972)
Eggs	Grind with sodium sulphate, extract (hexane), filter, CC	GC/ECD TLC	2 µg/kg	Smyth (1972)
Milk	Extract (petroleum ether-ether), CC	GC/ECD	5 µg/l	Goursaud et al. (1976)
Biological				
Adipose tissues	Dissolve (hexane), CC, form bisisopropoxytetrachlorobenzene derivative	GC/ECD	5 µg/kg	Crist et al. (1975)
Faeces	Grind, homogenize (benzene), extract (benzene-methanol-water) in Soxhlet, CC	TLC LC/UV GC/ECD		Yang et al. (1975)
Miscellaneous				
Plastic wash bottles	Extract (hexane), CC	GC/MS		Rourke et al. (1977)

Abbreviations: CC - column chromatography; GC - gas chromatography; FID - flame-ionization detection; ECD - electron capture detection; TLC - thin-layer chromatography; LC/UV - liquid chromatography/ultra-violet spectrometry; MS - mass spectrometry

in the controls or in the group receiving 50 mg/kg diet.   In the groups
receiving 100, 200 and 300 mg/kg diet, the incidences of liver-cell
tumours in the survivors (males and females) at the time the first
liver-cell tumour was observed were: 3/12 and 3/12, 7/29 and 14/26, 1/3
and 1/10.   The effective intake of hexachlorobenzene that induced liver-
cell tumours was 12-24 mg/kg bw/day (Cabral *et al.*, 1978, 1979[1]).

Hamster: A total of 159 female and 157 male Syrian golden hamsters,
6 weeks of age, were administered dietary concentrations of 0, 50, 100
and 200 mg/kg diet hexachlorobenzene (> 99.5% pure) for lifespan,
equivalent to 0, 4, 8 and 16 mg/kg bw/day.   The incidences of hepatomas,
liver haemangioendotheliomas and thyroid adenomas were increased by
exposure to hexachlorobenzene.   In females and males given 0, 50, 100
and 200 mg/kg diet hexachlorobenzene, hepatomas occurred in 0/39 and
0/40, 14/30 and 14/30, 17/30 and 26/30 and 51/60 and 49/57 animals,
respectively;   the first hepatoma (with multiple nodules, largest
diameter 7 mm) was found in one female hamster after 18 weeks of treatment.   The incidences of liver haemangioendotheliomas in males and
females receiving the highest dose were 20/57 and 7/60;   3 of these gave
metastases;   no liver haemangioendotheliomas were found in the controls.
Alveolar thyroid adenomas were found in treated animals, and a significant increase (P < 0.05) was found in males treated with 200 mg/kg diet
(8/57 *versus* 0/40 controls);   these tumours also occurred in 2/30 females
given 50 mg, in 1/30 males and 1/30 females given 100 mg and in 3/60
females given 200 mg (Cabral *et al.*, 1977).

(b)   Intraperitoneal administration

Mouse: Groups of 20 male A/St mice, 6-8 weeks old, were given
thrice weekly i.p. injections of 8, 20 or 40 mg/kg bw hexachlorobenzene
in tricaprylin for 8 weeks.   All survivors were killed 24 weeks after
the first injection.   The average numbers of lung tumours per mouse
were 0.68, 0.28 and 0.75 in the treated groups, which were not significantly different from that in controls injected with tricaprylin (Theiss
et al., 1977)   [The Working Group noted the limitations of a negative
result obtained with this test system;   see General Remarks on the
Substances Considered, p. 34].

---

[1]It was also reported in this article that an increased incidence
of liver-cell tumours was observed in a small group of MRC rats fed
100 mg/kg diet hexachlorobenzene (5 mg/kg bw/day) for 75 weeks.

3.2 Other relevant biological data

(a) Experimental systems

The toxicity and metabolism of hexachlorobenzene have been reviewed (Cooper, 1976, 1978).

Toxic effects

The oral LD_{50} of hexachlorobenzene in rats varies from 3500-10,000 mg/kg bw; death is due to neurotoxic effects (Booth & McDowell, 1975).

The LD_{50} of technical hexachlorobenzene (93-95% pure) in female rats given repeated administrations in the diet over 4 months was about 500 mg/kg diet, which was lower than for males.   Effects of such chronic feeding included hepatocellular hypertrophy and necrosis, spleen enlargement and porphyria (Kimbrough & Linder, 1974).   Porphyrins accumulate in urine, liver, kidney and spleen, suggesting an effect on the activity of uroporphyrinogen decarboxylase (Doss *et al.*, 1976; Goerz *et al.*, 1978; Kuiper-Goodman *et al.*, 1977).   Mice given 167 mg/kg diet hexachlorobenzene for 6 weeks became immunosuppressed, as indicated by decreased serum globulin levels and a decreased response of spleen lymphocytes to sheep red blood cells (Loose *et al.*, 1977).   In rats fed hexachlorobenzene for 4 weeks, subsequent food deprivation appeared to enhance the toxic response, implying decreased mobilization of hexachlorobenzene residues into fat and resulting in a higher plasma, liver, brain and adrenal accumulation of hexachlorobenzene (Villeneuve *et al.*, 1977).

Doses ranging from 0.05-50 mg/kg bw/day hexachlorobenzene were administered to pigs for 90 days.   Porphyria and death occurred in animals given the highest dose level.   Increased urinary excretion of coproporphyrin was observed in groups receiving 0.5 and 5 mg/kg bw/day after 8 weeks; in those receiving 5 mg/kg bw, induction of microsomal liver enzymes, accompanied by increased liver weight, was also observed (den Tonkelaar *et al.*, 1978).

Low dietary doses of hexachlorobenzene induced various hepatic mixed-function oxidases in rats (Grant *et al.*, 1974; Mehendale *et al.*, 1975; Stonard, 1975).

Hexachlorobenzene enhanced the hepatocarcinogenicity of polychlorinated terphenyls (PCT) in ICR mice: 0/28 animals had hepatocellular carcinomas with 250 mg/kg diet PCT, while 8/26 had these tumours with the same dose of PCT plus 50 mg/kg diet hexachlorobenzene (Shirai *et al.*, 1978).

Embryotoxicity and teratogenicity

Placental transfer of hexachlorobenzene has been reported in mice and rats (Andrews & Courtney, 1976; Villeneuve & Hierlihy, 1975). A minimal teratogenic effect of hexachlorobenzene observed in Wistar rats could not be reproduced in the same laboratory with doses up to 120 mg/kg bw administered during organogenesis (Khera, 1974). In other studies with 100 mg/kg bw hexachlorobenzene and with pentachloronitrobenzene (PCNB) contaminated by hexachlorobenzene, cleft palate and some kidney malformations were found in mice (Courtney *et al.*, 1976).

In a 4-generation test, groups of 10 male and 20 female Sprague-Dawley rats were treated with 0, 10, 20, 40, 80, 160, 320 or 640 mg/kg diet hexachlorobenzene from weaning. Suckling pups in the F1 generation were particularly sensitive, and many died prior to weaning when the mothers were fed concentrations of 320 or 640 mg/kg diet. No gross abnormalities were found (Grant *et al.*, 1977).

Hexachlorobenzene decreased survival of chicks of Japanese quail treated with 20 mg/kg diet for 90 days (Schwetz *et al.*, 1974). These results confirmed those of another study in which administration of 80 mg/kg diet for 90 days reduced egg production and hatchability (Vos *et al.*, 1971).

Absorption, distribution, excretion and metabolism

Hexachlorobenzene administered orally to rats was absorbed slowly from the gut, mainly *via* the lymphatic system, and was stored extensively in the fat after 48 hrs (Iatropoulos *et al.*, 1975). The quantitative recovery of intraperitoneally and orally administered ^{14}C-hexachlorobenzene in rats was dose-dependent, but more ^{14}C was recovered from faeces than from the urine. The major urinary metabolites were pentachlorophenol, tetrachlorohydroquinone and pentachlorothiophenol. The other urinary metabolites were tetrachlorobenzene, pentachlorobenzene, 2,4,5- and 2,4,6-trichlorophenols and 2,3,4,6- and 2,3,5-6-tetrachlorophenols; 2,3,4-trichlorophenol and other tetrachlorophenols were present in traces. These metabolites were excreted as conjugates or in free form in the urine. Unchanged hexachlorobenzene was found in the faeces and in fat (Engst *et al.*, 1976; Koss *et al.*, 1976; Mehendale *et al.*, 1975; Renner & Schuster, 1977).

When 110 µg/day ^{14}C-hexachlorobenzene were given orally to *Macaca mulatta* monkeys for 11-15 months, 50% of the radioactivity found in the urine was in pentachlorophenol and 25% in pentachlorobenzene, the remainder being in unidentified metabolites and unchanged hexachlorobenzene. In the faeces, 99% of the radioactivity was in unchanged hexachlorobenzene. During the last 10 days of the experiment, males excreted 7.2% of the administered dose in the urine and 52% in the faeces; females excreted 4.6 and 42.2%, respectively (Rozman *et al.*, 1977).

Hexachlorobenzene was found in the milk of cows administered hexa-chlorobenzene (Fries & Marrow, 1976), and in organs of 18-day-old rats whose mothers were fed a diet containing hexachlorobenzene (Mendoza *et al.*, 1975).

Mutagenicity and other related short-term tests

Hexachlorobenzene did not significantly increase the frequency of reversions to histidine and methionine auxotrophy in *Saccharomyces cerevisiae* (strain 632/4) in the absence of a metabolic activation system (Guerzoni *et al.*, 1976).

In a dominant lethal test, male rats that received 20, 40 or 60 mg/kg bw hexachlorobenzene orally for 10 days were mated sequentially with un-treated females (1 male × 2 females;   14 mating periods, each of 5-days' duration).   There were no significant differences between the test and control groups with regard to the incidence of pregnancies, corpora lutea, live implants or deciduomas, at any dose level or in any of the mating periods (Khera, 1974).

(b)   Humans

The occurrence of hexachlorobenzene in human tissues is described in section 2.2 (e).

An epidemic of 4000 cases of porphyria cutanea tarda occurred in Turkey between 1955 and 1959 as a result of human consumption of grain that had been treated with hexachlorobenzene.   The estimated daily in-take was 50-200 mg/day hexachlorobenzene over a relatively long period before the disease became apparent (Mazzei & Mazzei, 1973;   Peters, 1976;   Peters *et al.*, 1966, 1978).   The majority of the patients were children, mostly boys, aged 4-14 years old (Cam & Nigogosyan, 1963). A mortality rate of 14% was reported within several years (Peters *et al.*, 1966, 1978).   Children under the age of 4 rarely developed porphyria, but in breast-fed infants a condition known as 'pink-sore' was reported, with a mortality rate greater than 95% (Cam, 1960;   Peters, 1976). Samples of breast milk from the mothers of these infant were shown to contain hexachlorobenzene (Peters *et al.*, 1966).   Follow-up studies of 32 of the patients have shown that abnormal porphyrin metabolism and active symptomatology persist 20 years after hexachlorobenzene ingestion (Peters *et al.*, 1978).

Hexachlorobenzene levels in plasma of people living near a hexachloro-benzene manufacturing plant but not exposed occupationally averaged 3.6 µg/l;   there was no evidence of porphyria, but plasma coproporphyrin levels were abnormally high (Burns & Miller, 1975).

Farm workers exposed occupationally to hexachlorobenzene-contaminated Dacthal (dimethyl-tetrachloroterephthalate) had average blood hexachlorobenzene concentrations of 0.040 mg/l, but no evidence of porphyria was found in this group (Burns *et al.*, 1974).

3.3 Case reports and epidemiological studies

No data were available to the Working Group.

4. Summary of Data Reported and Evaluation

4.1 Experimental data

Hexachlorobenzene was tested by oral administration in one experiment in mice and in one in hamsters. In mice, it produced liver-cell tumours in animals of both sexes. In hamsters of both sexes, it produced hepatomas, liver haemangiotheliomas and thyroid adenomas. An experiment involving intraperitoneal administration in mice was considered to be inadequate.

Hexachlorobenzene is foetotoxic and produces some teratogenic effects. It was not mutagenic in yeast and did not induce dominant lethal effects in male rats.

4.2 Human data

No case reports or epidemiological studies were available to the Working Group.

The production and use of hexachlorobenzene as a fungicide over the past several decades and its occurrence as a byproduct in the manufacture of other chemicals indicate that widespread human exposure occurs in both the general and working environments. This is confirmed by many reports of its occurrence in the general environment and in human body fluids.

A group of people who were accidentally exposed over a period of time is known to exist; many of these showed toxic manifestations, some lasting for as long as 20 years. No data on carcinogenic effects have been reported.

4.3 Evaluation

There is *sufficient evidence* that hexachlorobenzene is carcinogenic in mice and hamsters. In the absence of adequate data in humans, it is reasonable, for practical purposes, to regard hexachlorobenzene as if it presented a carcinogenic risk to humans.

5. References

Alam, M. (1977) Analytical method for traces of hexachlorobenzene in
    formulations of other pesticides. Pestic. Sci., 8, 167-171

Andrews, J.E. & Courtney, K.D. (1976) Inter- and intralitter variation
    of hexachlorobenzene (HCB) deposition in fetuses (Abstract No. 87).
    Toxicol. appl. Pharmacol., 37, 128

Anon. (1978) EPA plans to list pesticides accepted and rejected as RPAR
    candidates. Pestic. Tox. Chem. News, 8 February, pp. 3-4

Arrifai, K. & Acker, L. (1975) The contamination of grain with polychlori-
    nated biphenyls and hexachlorobenzene (Ger.). Ber. Getreidechem.-Tag.,
    Detmold, 103-110 [Chem. Abstr., 84, 178344n]

Astolfi, E., Alonso, A.H., Mendizabal, S. & Zubizarreta, E. (1974) Chlori-
    nated pesticides in mothers and in the umbilical cord of newborns (Fr.).
    Eur. J. Toxicol. environ. Hyg., 7, 330-338 [Chem. Abstr., 83, 1877s]

Babkina, E.I., Bobovnikova, T.I., Mironyuk, G.V. & Dibtseva, A.V. (1976)
    Determination of organochlorine pesticides and their metabolites in
    different types of soils (Russ.). Khim. Sel'sk. Khoz., 14, 68-70
    [Chem. Abstr., 85, 138391q]

Bakken, A.F. & Seip, M. (1977) Insecticides in human breast milk. Obstet.
    Gynecol. Surv., 32, 283-285 [Chem. Abstr., 87, 63726h]

Beall, M.L., Jr (1976) Persistence of aerially applied hexachlorobenzene
    on grass and soil. J. environ. Qual., 5, 367-369 [Chem. Abstr., 86,
    26902w]

Biston, R., Zenon-Roland, L. & Martens, P.H. (1975) Level of chlorinated
    hydrocarbon residues in canned vegetables (Fr.). Meded. Fac.
    Landbouwwet., Rijksuniv. Gent, 40, 1095-1106 [Chem. Abstr., 84,
    88109k]

Bong, R.L. (1977) Collaborative study of the recovery of hexachlorobenzene
    and mirex in butterfat and fish. J. Assoc. off. anal. Chem., 60,
    229-232

Booth, N.H. & McDowell, J.R. (1975) Toxicity of hexachlorobenzene and
    associated residues in edible animal tissues. J. Am. Vet. med. Assoc.,
    166, 591-595

Burns, J.E. & Miller, F.M. (1975) Hexachlorobenzene contamination: its
    effects in a Louisiana population. Arch. environ. Health, 30, 44-48

Burns, J.E., Miller, F.M., Gomes, E.D. & Albert, R.A. (1974) Hexachloro-
    benzene exposure from contaminated DCPA in vegetable spraymen. Arch.
    environ. Health, 29, 192-194

Cabral, J.R.P., Shubik, P., Mollner, T. & Raitano, F. (1977) Carcinogenic activity of hexachlorobenzene in hamsters. Nature (Lond.), 269, 510-511

Cabral, J.R.P., Mollner, T., Raitano, F. & Shubik, P. (1978) Carcinogenesis study in mice with hexachlorobenzene (Abstract No. 242). Toxicol. appl. Pharmacol., 45, 323

Cabral, J.R.P., Mollner, T., Raitano, F. & Shubik, P. (1979) Carcinogenesis of hexachlorobenzene in mice. Int. J. Cancer, 23, 47-51

Cam, C. (1960) A new epidemic dermatosis of children (Fr.). Ann. Derm. Syph. (Paris), 87, 393-397

Cam, C. & Nigogosyan, G. (1963) Acquired toxic porphyria cutanea tarda due to hexachlorobenzene. Report of 348 cases caused by this fungicide. J. Am. med. Assoc., 183, 88-91

Cooper, P. (1976) More light on hexachlorobenzene. Food Cosmet. Toxicol., 14, 351-353

Cooper, P. (1978) Hexachlorobenzene metabolism - mainly in the rat. Food Cosmet. Toxicol., 16, 287-288

Corvi, C., Vogel, J., Yter, C. & Dallmayr, I. (1976) Change in the organo-chlorinated pesticide content of Italian hard cheese (Fr.). Mitt. Geb. Lebensmittelunters. Hyg., 67, 147-153 [Chem. Abstr., 85, 61530z]

Courtney, K.D., Copeland, M.F. & Robbins, A. (1976) The effects of penta-chloronitrobenzene, hexachlorobenzene, and related compounds on fetal development. Toxicol. appl. Pharmacol., 35, 239-256

Crist, H.L., Moseman, R.F. & Noneman, J.W. (1975) Rapid determination and confirmation of low levels of hexachlorobenzene in adipose tissues. Bull. environ. Contam. Toxicol., 14, 273-280

Curley, A., Burse, V.W., Jennings, R.W., Villanueva, E.C., Tomatis, L. & Akazaki, K. (1973) Chlorinated hydrocarbon pesticides and related compounds in adipose tissue from people of Japan. Nature (Lond.), 242, 338-340

Dappen, G. (1974) Pesticide Analysis From Urban Storm Runoff, Department of the Interior, Office of Water Resources Research, Report No. PB-238 593, Springfield, VA, National Technical Information Service

Dejonckheere, W., Steurbaut, W. & Kips, R.H. (1976) Residues of quintozene, its contaminants and metabolites in soil, lettuce, and witloof-chicory, Belgium - 1969-74. Pestic. Monit. J., 10, 68-73

Di Muccio, A., Boniforti, L. & Monacelli, R. (1972) Gas chromatographic separation of hexachlorobenzene and the α-, β-, γ- and δ-isomers of hexachlorocyclohexane. J. Chromatogr., 71, 340-346

Doss, M., Schermuly, E. & Koss, G. (1976) Hexachlorobenzene porphyria in rats as a model for human chronic hepatic porphyrias. Ann. clin. Res., 8, 171-181

Engst, R., Macholz, R.M. & Kujawa, M. (1976) The metabolism of hexachlorobenzene (HCB) in rats. Bull. environ. Contam. Toxicol., 16, 248-252

Fries, G.F. & Marrow, G.S. (1976) Hexachlorobenzene retention and excretion by dairy cows. J. Dairy Sci., 59, 475-480

Gilbertson, M. & Reynolds, L.M. (1972) Hexachlorobenzene (HCB) in the eggs of common terns in Hamilton Harbour, Ontario. Bull. environ. Contam. Toxicol., 7, 371-373

Goerz, G., Vizethum, W., Bolsen, K., Krieg, T. & Lissner, R. (1978) Hexachlorobenzene (HCB) induced porphyria in rats. Influence of HCB-metabolites on the biosynthesis of heme (Ger.). Arch. dermatol. Res., 263, 189-196

Goursaud, J., Luquet, F. & Casalis, J. (1976) Method for the determination of hexachlorobenzene, pentachloronitrobenzene, and pentachloroaniline residues in milk (Fr.). Ann. Falsif. Expert. Chim., 69, 327-336 [Chem. Abstr., 87, 51709s]

Grant, D.L., Iverson, F., Hatina, G.V. & Villeneuve, D.C. (1974) Effects of hexachlorobenzene on liver porphyrin levels and microsomal enzymes in the rat. Environ. physiol. Biochem., 4, 159-165

Grant, D.L., Phillips, W.E.J. & Hatina, G.V. (1977) Effect of hexachlorobenzene on reproduction in the rat. Arch. environ. Contam. Toxicol., 5, 207-216

Grasselli, J.G. & Ritchey, W.M., eds (1975) CRC Atlas of Spectral Data and Physical Constants for Organic Compounds, 2nd ed., Vol. 11, Cleveland, OH, Chemical Rubber Co., p. 308

Greve, P.A. (1972) Potentially hazardous substances in surface waters. I. Pesticides in the river Rhine. Sci. total environ., 1, 173-180 [Chem. Abstr., 79, 118193z]

Guerzoni, M.E., Del Cupolo, L. & Ponti, I. (1976) Mutagenic activity of pesticides (Ital.). Riv. Sci. Tecnol. Aliment. Nutr. Um., 6, 161-165

Haefner, M. (1975) Contamination of garden soil and agriculturally useful soil with hexachlorobenzene and pentachloronitrobenzene (Ger.). Gesunde Pflanz., 27, 81-84, 86, 88-95 [Chem. Abstr., 84, 39579e]

Haefner, M. (1977) The metabolism of quintozene in vegetables and soils, part 2 (Ger.). Anz. Schaedlingskd., Pflanz.-Umweltschutz, 50, 1-8 [Chem. Abstr., 86, 184537k]

Hawley, G.G., ed. (1977) The Condensed Chemical Dictionary, 9th ed.,
    New York, Van Nostrand-Reinhold, p. 436

Heeschen, W., Bluethgen, A. & Tolle, A. (1976) Residues of chlorinated
    hydrocarbons in milk and milk products - situation and evaluation (Ger.)
    Zbl. Bakteriol., Parasitenkd., Infektionskr. Hyg., Abt. 1: Orig.,
    Reihe B, 162, 188-197 [Chem. Abstr., 85, 107575y]

Holden, A.V. (1973) Mercury and organochlorine residue analysis of fish
    and aquatic mammals. Pestic. Sci., 4, 399-408

IARC (1978) Information Bulletin on the Survey of Chemicals Being Tested
    for Carcinogenicity, No. 7, Lyon, pp. 25, 121

Iatropoulos, M.J., Milling, A., Müller, W.F., Nohynek, G., Rozman, K.,
    Coulston, F. & Korte, F. (1975) Absorption, transport and organo-
    tropism of dichlorobiphenyl (DCB), dieldrin, and hexachlorobenzene
    (HCB) in rats. Environ. Res., 10, 384-389

Jensen, S., Renberg, L. & Reutergardh, L. (1977) Residue analysis of sedi-
    ment and sewage sludge for organochlorines in the presence of elemental
    sulfur. Anal. Chem., 49, 316-318

Johnson, J.L., Stalling, D.L. & Hogan, J.W. (1974) Hexachlorobenzene (HCB)
    residues in fish. Bull. environ. Contam. Toxicol., 11, 393-398

Johnson, L.D., Waltz, R.H., Ussary, J.P. & Kaiser, F.E. (1976) Automated gel
    permeation chromatographic cleanup of animal and plant extracts for
    pesticide residue determination. J. Assoc. off. anal. Chem., 59, 174-18

Johnson, R.D. & Manske, D.D. (1976) Pesticide residues in total diet samples
    (IX). Pestic. Monit. J., 9, 157-169

Khera, K.S. (1974) Teratogenicity and dominant lethal studies on hexachloro-
    benzene in rats. Food Cosmet. Toxicol., 12, 471-477

Kimbrough, R.D. & Linder, R.E. (1974) The toxicity of technical hexachloro-
    benzene in the Sherman strain rat. A preliminary study. Res. Commun.
    chem. Path. Pharmacol., 8, 653-664

Knöppler, H.-O. (1976) Pesticide residues in food of animal origin (Ger.).
    Fleischwirtschaft, 56, 1643-1646

Koss, G. & Manz, D. (1976) Residues of hexachlorobenzene in wild mammals of
    Germany. Bull. environ. Contam. Toxicol., 15, 189-191

Koss, G., Koransky, W. & Steinback, K. (1976) Studies on the toxicology
    of hexachlorobenzene. II. Identification and determination of
    metabolites. Arch. Toxikol., 35, 107-114

Kuiper-Goodman, T., Grant, D.L., Moodie, C.A., Korsrud, G.O. & Munro, I.C. (1977) Subacute toxicity of hexachlorobenzene in the rat. Toxicol. appl. Pharmacol., 40, 529-549

Laska, A.L., Bartell, C.K. & Laseter, J.L. (1976) Distribution of hexachlorobenzene and hexachlorobutadiene in water, soil, and selected aquatic organisms along the lower Mississippi River, Louisiana. Bull. environ. Contam. Toxicol., 15, 535-542

Leoni, V. & D'Arca, S.U. (1976) Experimental data and critical review of the occurrence of hexachlorobenzene in the Italian environment. Sci. total environ., 5, 253-272

Leoni, V., d'Alessandro de Luca, E. & Puccetti, G. (1975) Chlorinated organic pesticides of the total diet in Italy. V. Hexachlorobenzene in prepared and ready-to-eat foods. Update of data on some chlorinated pesticides (Ital.). Nuovi Ann. Ig. Microbiol., 26, 44-56

Li, R.T., Spigarelli, J.L. & Going, J.E. (1976) Sampling and Analysis of Selected Toxic Substances, Task 1A-Hexachlorobenzene, EPA-560/6-76/001, US Environmental Protection Agency, Office of Toxic Substances, Report No. PB-253794, available from, Springfield, VA, National Technical Information Service

Lohse, H. (1975) Chlorinated hydrocarbon residues in animal matter (Ger.). Mitteilungsbl. GDCh-Fachgruppe Lebensmittelchem. Gerichtl. Chem., 29, 227-229 [Chem. Abstr., 83, 158815t]

Loose, L.D., Pittman, K.A., Benitz, K.-F. & Silkworth, J.B. (1977) Polychlorinated biphenyl and hexachlorobenzene induced humoral immunosuppression. J. Reticuloendothel. Soc., 22, 253-271

Lunde, G. & Baumann Ofstad, E. (1976) Determination of fat-soluble chlorinated compounds in fish. Fresenius' Z. Anal. Chem., 282, 395-399 [Chem. Abstr., 86, 66339z]

Luquet, F.M., Goursaud, J. & Casalis, J. (1975) Pollution of human milk in France with organochlorine insecticide residues (Fr.). Pathol.-Biol., 23, 45-49 [Chem. Abstr., 83, 1880n]

Mahelova, E., Uhnak, J. & Sackmauerova, M. (1977) Hexachlorobenzene residues in the environment (Slo.). Cesk. Hyg., 22, 279-285 [Chem. Abstr., 88, 16714p]

Mann, J.B., Enos, H.F., Gonzalez, J. & Thompson, J.F. (1974) Development of sampling and analytical procedure for determining hexachlorobenzene and hexachloro-1,3-butadiene in air. Environ. Sci. Technol., 8, 584-585

Mazzei, E.S. & Mazzei, C.M. (1973) Intoxication by a fungicide, hexachlorobenzene, contaminating wheat grains (Fr.). Sem. Hôp. Paris, 49, 63-67

Mehendale, H.M., Fields, M. & Matthews, H.B. (1975) Metabolism and effects of hexachlorobenzene on hepatic microsomal enzymes in the rat. J. agric. Food Chem., 23, 261-265

Mel'nikova, L.V., Belyakov, A.A., Smirnova, V.G. & Kurenko, L.T. (1975) Sanitary-chemical methods for determination of noxious substances encountered in the production of sodium pentachlorophenolate (Russ.). Gig. Tr. Prof. Zabol., 7, 37-39 [Chem. Abstr., 84, 94734b]

Mendoza, C.E., Grant, D.L. & Shields, J.B. (1975) Body burden of hexachlorobenzene in suckling rats and its effects on various organs and on liver porphyrin accumulation. Environ. physiol. Biochem., 5, 460-464

Mes, J., Campbell, D.S., Robinson, R.N. & Davies, D.J.A. (1977) Polychlorinated biphenyl and organochlorine pesticide residues in adipose tissue of Canadians. Bull. environ. Contam. Toxicol., 17, 196-203

Mikulik, A., Vavrova, M., Dobes, M., Krul, J. & Svojanovska, S. (1977) Residues of chlorinated hydrocarbons in pheasant meat (Czech.). Veterinarstvi, 27, 314-316 [Chem. Abstr., 87, 166170b]

Morita, M., Nishizawa, T. & Mimura, S. (1975a) Environmental pollution by hexachlorobenzene (Jap.). Tokyo Toritsu Eisei Kenkyusho Kenkyu Nempo, 26-1, 333-335 [Chem. Abstr., 85, 51355g]

Morita, M., Ushio, F., Nishizawa, T., Fukano, S., Doguchi, M. & Mimura, S. (1975b) Hexachlorobenzene in foods (Jap.). Shokuhin Eiseigaku Zasshi, 16, 53-54 [Chem. Abstr., 83, 56836h]

Mumma, C.E. & Lawless, E.W. (1975) Survey of Industrial Processing Data, Task 1 - Hexachlorobenzene and Hexachlorobutadiene Pollution from Chlorocarbon Processing, EPA 560/3-75-003, US Environmental Protection Agency, Report No. PB-243641, available from Springfield, VA, National Technical Information Service, p. 107

Pesendorfer, H. (1975) Organochlorine pesticide (DDT etc.) and polychlorinated biphenyl (PCB) residues in human milk (from the area of Vienna and Lower Austria) (Ger.). Wien. Klin. Wschr., 87, 732-736

Peters, H.A. (1976) Hexachlorobenzene poisoning in Turkey. Fed. Proc., 35, 2400-2403

Peters, H.A., Johnson, S.A.M., Cam, S., Oral, S., Müftü, Y. & Ergene, T. (1966) Hexachlorobenzene-induced porphyria: effect of chelation on the disease, porphyrin and metal metabolism. Am. J. med. Sci., 251, 314-322

Peters, H.A., Cripps, D.J. & Gocmen, A. (1978) Porphyria 20 years after hexachlorobenzene exposure (Abstract No. PP 10). Neurology, 28, 333

Plimmer, J.R. & Klingebiel, U.I. (1976) Photolysis of hexachlorobenzene.
    J. agric. Food Chem., 24, 721-723

Polishuk, Z.W., Ron, M., Wassermann, M., Cucos, S., Wassermann, D. &
    Lemesch, C. (1977) Organochlorine compounds in human blood plasma
    and milk. Pestic. Monit. J., 10, 121-129

Polo Villar, L.M., Herrera Marteache, A., Lopez Gimenez, R.,
    Jodral Villarejo, M., Iglesias Perez, J. & Pozo Lora, R. (1977)
    Study into hexachlorobenzene (HCB) fungicide contamination in Spanish
    butter (Span.). Arch. Zootec., 26, 89-95 [Chem. Abstr., 87, 199310a]

Pozo Lora, R., Herrera Marteache, A., Polo Villar, L.M., Lopez Gimenez, R.,
    Jodral Villarejo, M. & Iglesias Perez, J. (1977) Studies on hexachloro-
    benzene (HCB) contamination in natural cow's milk in the south of
    Spain (Span.). Arch. Zootec., 26, 45-63 [Chem. Abstr., 87, 199309g]

Prager, B., Jacobson, P., Schmidt, P. & Stern, D., eds (1922) Beilsteins
    Handbuch der Organischen Chemie, 4th ed., Vol. 5, Syst. No. 464,
    Berlin, Springer, p. 205

Renner, G. & Schuster, K.P. (1977) 2,4,5-Trichlorophenol, a new urinary
    metabolite of hexachlorobenzene. Toxicol. appl. Pharmacol., 39,
    355-356

Richou-Bac, L., Mollet, M.F., Restuit, A. & Pantaleon, J. (1974) Contamin-
    ation of French dairy products by organochlorine compounds (Fr.).
    Bull. Acad. Vet. Fr., 47, 379-390 [Chem. Abstr., 83, 56880t]

Richou-Bac, L., Restuit, A. & Pantaleon, J. (1975) Pesticide residues in
    animal feeds. Evaluation of tolerance standards (Fr.). Bull. Acad.
    Vet. Fr., 48, 483-498 [Chem. Abstr., 85, 61521x]

Richter, E. & Schmid, A. (1976) Hexachlorobenzene content in the whole
    blood of children (Ger.). Arch. Toxikol., 35, 141-147

Rourke, D.R., Mueller, W.F. & Yang, R.S.H. (1977) Identification of hexa-
    chlorobenzene as a contaminant in laboratory plastic wash bottles.
    J. Assoc. off. anal. Chem., 60, 233-235

Rozman, K., Mueller, W., Coulston, F. & Korte, F. (1977) Long-term feeding
    study of hexachlorobenzene in rhesus monkeys. Chemosphere, 6, 81-84

Russell, J.W. (1975) Analysis of air pollutants using sampling tubes and
    gas chromatography. Environ. Sci. Technol., 9, 1175-1178

Schwetz, B.A., Norris, J.M., Kociba, R.J., Keeler, P.A., Cornier, R.F. &
    Gehring, P.J. (1974) Reproduction study in Japanese quail fed hexa-
    chlorobutadiene for 90 days. Toxicol. appl. Pharmacol., 30, 255-265

Shackelford, W.M. & Keith, L.H. (1976) Frequency of Organic Compounds Identified in Water, EPA-600/4-76-062, Athens, GA, US Environmental Protection Agency, p. 69

Shirai, T., Miyata, Y., Nakanishi, K., Murasaki, G. & Ito, N. (1978) Hepatocarcinogenicity of polychlorinated terphenyl (PCT) in ICR mice and its enhancement by hexachlorobenzene (HCB). Cancer Lett., 4, 271-275

Smith, D.C., Leduc, R. & Tremblay, L. (1975) Pesticide residues in the total diet in Canada. IV. 1972 and 1973. Pestic. Sci., 6, 75-82

Smyth, R.J. (1972) Detection of hexachlorobenzene residues in dairy products, meat fat, and eggs. J. Assoc. off. anal. Chem., 55, 806-808

Solly, S.R.B. & Shanks, V. (1974) Polychlorinated biphenyls and organochlorine pesticides in human fat in New Zealand. N.Z. J. Sci., 17, 535-544

Stacey, C.I. & Thomas, B.W. (1975) Organochlorine pesticide residues in human milk, Western Australia - 1970-71. Pestic. Monit. J., 9, 64-66

Stonard, M.D. (1975) Mixed type hepatic microsomal enzyme induction by hexachlorobenzene. Biochem. Pharmacol., 24, 1959-1963

Szokolay, A., Uhnák, J., Sackmauerová, M. & Maďarič, A. (1975) Analysis of HCB and BHC isomer residues in food. J. Chromatogr., 106, 401-404

Theiss, J.C., Stoner, G.D., Shimkin, M.B. & Weisburger, E.K. (1977) Test for carcinogenicity of organic contaminants of United States drinking waters by pulmonary tumor response in strain A mice. Cancer Res., 37, 2717-2720

Thomson, J.M. & Davie, J.D.S. (1974) Pesticide residues in the fauna of the Brisbane River estuary. Search, 5, 152 [Chem. Abstr., 81, 115611q]

den Tonkelaar, E.M., Verschuuren, H.G., Bankovska, J., de Vries, T., Kroes, R. & van Esch, G.J. (1978) Hexachlorobenzene toxicity in pigs. Toxicol. appl. Pharmacol., 43, 137-145

Trigo Lorenzo, D. & Fernandez Garcia, M.I. (1976) Determination of organochlorine pesticide residues in human milk (Span.). Quim. Anal., 30, 319-321 [Chem. Abstr., 86, 184211z]

Tuinstra, L.G.M.T. (1974) Contamination of milk and dairy products by organochlorinated pesticides in the past 5-6 years (Neth.). Bedrijfsontwikkel 5, 215-222 [Chem. Abstr., 83, 41644v]

US Environmental Protection Agency (1972) EPA Compendium of Registered Pesticides, Washington DC, US Government Printing Office, p. I-H-03-00.0

US Food & Drug Administration (1975) Pesticide Analytical Manual, Vol. I, Methods which Detect Multiple Residues, Rockville, MD, Table 201-A

US Food & Drug Administration (1977) Compliance Program Evaluation, FY 74 Total Diet Studies (7320.08), Washington DC, US Government Printing Office, Table 6

US International Trade Commission (1977a) Synthetic Organic Chemicals, US Production and Sales, 1976, USITC Publication 833, Washington DC, US Government Printing Office, p. 57

US International Trade Commission (1977b) Imports of Benzenoid Chemicals and Products, 1975, USITC Publication 806, Washington DC, US Government Printing Office, p. 99

US Tariff Commission (1934) Production and Sales of Dyes and Other Synthetic Organic Chemicals, 1933, Report No. 89, Second Series, Washington DC, US Government Printing Office, p. 11

Veith, G.D., Kuehl, D.W., Puglisi, F.A., Glass, G.E. & Eaton, J.G. (1977) Residues of PCB's and DDT in the western Lake Superior ecosystem. Arch. environ. Contam. Toxicol., 5, 487-499 [Chem. Abstr., 87, 189021t]

Villanueva, E.C., Jennings, R.W., Burse, V.W. & Kimbrough, R.D. (1974) Evidence of chlorodibenzo-p-dioxin and chlorodibenzofuran in hexachlorobenzene. J. agric. Food Chem., 22, 916-917

Villeneuve, D.C. & Hierlihy, S.L. (1975) Placental transfer of hexachlorobenzene in the rat. Bull. environ. Contam. Toxicol., 13, 489-491

Villeneuve, D.C., van Logten, M.J., den Tonkelaar, E.M., Greve, P.A., Vos, J.G., Speijers, G.J.A. & van Esch, G.J. (1977) Effect of food deprivation on low level hexachlorobenzene exposure in rats. Sci. total Environ., 8, 179-186

Vos, J.G., van der Maas, H.L., Musch, A. & Ram, E. (1971) Toxicity of hexachlorobenzene in Japanese quail with special reference to porphyria, liver damage, reproduction, and tissue residues. Toxicol. appl. Pharmacol., 18, 944-957

Weast, R.C., ed. (1976) CRC Handbook of Chemistry and Physics, 57th ed., Cleveland, Ohio, Chemical Rubber Co., p. C-165

White, D.H. (1976) Nationwide residues of organochlorines in starlings, 1974. Pestic. Monit. J., 10, 10-17

White, D.H. & Kaiser, T.E. (1976) Residues of organochlorines and heavy metals in ruddy ducks from the Delaware River, 1973. Pestic. Monit. J., 9, 155-156

WHO (1975) 1974 Evaluations of some pesticide residues in food. WHO Pestic. Residues Ser., No. 4, pp. 397-405

Yang, R.S.H., Coulston, F. & Golberg, L. (1975) Chromatographic methods for the analysis of hexachlorobenzene and possible metabolites in monkey fecal samples. J. Assoc. off. anal. Chem., 58, 1197-1201

HEXACHLOROBUTADIENE

1. Chemical and Physical Data

1.1 Synonyms and trade names

Chem. Abstr. Services Reg. No.: 87-68-3

Chem. Abstr. Name: 1,1,2,3,4,4-Hexachloro-1,3-butadiene

Synonyms: HCBD; hexachloro-1,3-butadiene; perchlorobutadiene

Trade names: C 46; Dolen-Pur

1.2 Structural and molecular formulae and molecular weight

$$Cl_2C=CCl-CCl=CCl_2$$

C_4Cl_6 Mol. wt: 260.7

1.3 Chemical and physical properties of the substance

From Hawley (1977), unless otherwise specified

(a) Description: Clear, colourless liquid

(b) Boiling range: 210 to 220°C

(c) Freezing range: -19 to -22°C

(d) Density: $d_{15.5}^{15.5}$ 1.675

(e) Refractive index: n_D^{20} 1.552

(f) Spectroscopy data: λ max 249 nm (E_1^1 = 168); 220 nm (E_1^1 = 704); infra-red, nuclear magnetic resonance and mass spectral data have been tabulated (Grasselli & Ritchey, 1975).

(g) Solubility: Insoluble in water; soluble in ethanol and diethyl ether

(h) Volatility: Vapour pressure is 22 mm at 100°C.

(i) Stability: Nonflammable; stable

1.4 Technical products and impurities

No data were available to the Working Group.

2. Production, Use, Occurrence and Analysis

A review on hexachlorobutadiene has been published (US Environmental Protection Agency, 1975a).

2.1 Production and use

(a) Production

Hexachlorobutadiene was first prepared in 1877 by the chlorination of hexyl iodide (Prager *et al.*, 1918). The production of commercial quantities of hexachlorobutadiene in the US has never been reported (but see General Remarks on the Substances Considered, p. 16); however, until about 1974, it was recovered as a by-product in the production of tetrachloroethylene (US Environmental Protection Agency, 1975a).

In 1972, 3.3-6.6 million kg hexachlorobutadiene were present in US industrial wastes and as by-products of the following chemical products (percent of total hexachlorobutadiene produced): tetrachloroethylene (60), trichloroethylene (21), carbon tetrachloride (19) and chlorine (< 1) (US Environmental Protection Agency, 1975a).

Since 1974, all hexachlorobutadiene used commercially in the US has been imported from the Federal Republic of Germany; 91-227 thousand kg hexachlorobutadiene have been imported annually since then (US Environmental Protection Agency, 1975a). It is believed that all hexachlorobutadiene now produced as a by-product in the US is disposed of, mostly by incineration, although landfill has been used in the past and may still be used at some plants.

No data on its production in Europe were available; and no evidence has been found that hexachlorobutadiene has ever been produced or imported in Japan.

(b) Use

In 1975, hexachlorobutadiene was used in the US for recovery of chlorine-containing gas in chlorine plants, as a fluid for gyroscopes, as a chemical intermediate to produce lubricants, and as an intermediate in the manufacture of rubber compounds. No information was available on the quantities used.

The largest use of hexachlorobutadiene in the US in 1975 was for recovery of 'snift' (chlorine-containing) gas in chlorine plants. This gas occurs at the liquefaction unit and is cleaned by passing it through hexachlorobutadiene or carbon tetrachloride. Many US chlorine producers were reported to have changed to hexachlorobutadiene from carbon tetrachloride in recent years (US Environmental Protection Agency, 1975a).

It is used as a solvent for elastomers, as a heat-transfer liquid, in transformers and as hydraulic fluid (Hawley, 1977); it has been used by at least one US manufacture in the production of high-temperature fluorinated lubricants.

The USSR is believed to be one of the major users of hexachlorobutadiene; 600-800 thousand kg are used annually, mainly as a fumigant against *Phylloxera* on grapes (US Environmental Protection Agency, 1975a). It is also used as a fumigant in vineyards in France, Italy, Greece, Spain and Argentina.

2.2 Occurrence

Hexachlorobutadiene is not known to occur as a natural product.

(a) Air

The air over cultivated fields within a radius of $\geq$ 100 m of vineyards in which hexachlorobutadiene had been applied to the soil was found to have been contaminated with hexachlorobutadiene (Gul'ko *et al.*, 1972).

Hexachlorobutadiene was found in air samples collected upwind and downwind from a tetrachloroethylene manufacturing plant and from the vicinity of a landfill area used by the plant for disposal of waste chemicals (Mann *et al.*, 1974). In another study of 9 chemical manufacturing factories, the highest levels of hexachlorobutadiene were present in air samples associated with production of tetrachloroethylene and trichloroethylene (highest level reported, 463 $\mu g/m^3$); low levels were encountered at plants associated with production of chlorine and triazine herbicide; and none was detected in samples from the pentachloronitrobenzene production plant (Li *et al.*, 1976).

(b) Water

The highest concentration of hexachlorobutadiene found in US drinking-water up to 1975 was 0.07 $\mu g/l$ (US Environmental Protection Agency, 1975b). It has been detected in the effluent water from a US chemical manufacturing plant (Shackelford & Keith, 1976); in the effluent from a European chemical manufacturing plant, at a concentration of 6.4 $\mu g/l$; in the Rhine River, at 5 $\mu g/l$; and in European drinking-water at 0.27 $\mu g/l$ (Eurocop-Cost, 1976).

Hexachlorobutadiene was found at a level of 0.13 µg/l in the Rhine and at levels of 0.13-0.20 µg/l and 0.05-0.07 µg/l in lakes fed by the Rhine (Goldbach et al., 1976).   In a UK study, an average concentration of 0.004 µg/l and a maximum concentration of 0.03 µg/l hexachlorobutadiene were reported in sea-water (Pearson & McConnell, 1975).   Mississippi River water contained 0.9-1.9 µg/l hexachlorobutadiene; water at sites removed from a transect of the levees contained < 0.7-1.5 µg/l (Laska et a 1976).   In another US study, highest levels of hexachlorobutadiene were detected in water at the sites of factories associated with the production of tetrachloroethylene and trichloroethylene (highest reported concentration, 244 µg/l) (Li et al., 1976).

(c)   Soil and sediments

Concentrations of hexachlorobutadiene in sediments from Liverpool bay ranged from < 0.02 - > 8 mg/kg (Pearson & McConnell, 1975).   Levee soil in Louisiana contained levels ranging from undetectable to 800 µg/ kg, ditch mud levels ranged from undetectable to 500 µg/kg and soil samples collected from sites removed from a transect of the levees contained levels ranging from < 0.7-321.5 µg/kg (433.0 µg/kg corrected to dry weight) (Laska et al., 1976).   In a US study, highest levels were detected in soil around factories associated with the production of tetrachloroethylene and trichloroethylene (highest reported concentration, 980 µg/g) (Li et al., 1976).

(d)   Food and drink

Hexachlorobutadiene residues have been detected in must wine (< 0.01-0.45 µg/l) and grape juice in the USSR; however, no residues were detected in fermented wine or in pasteurized grape juices (Gorenshtein, 1973).

Hexachlorobutadiene residues were found in the following foods and feeds (µg/kg): evaporated milk (4), egg yolk (42), vegetable-oil margarine (33), chicken grain feed (39) and chicken laying rations (20) (Kotzias et al., 1975).   In a study of foods collected within a 25-mile (40-km) radius of factories producing tetrachloroethylene or trichloro-ethylene, no hexachlorobutadiene residues were found in any of 15 egg samples or 20 samples of a variety of vegetables; of 20 milk samples collected, only one contained hexachlorobutadiene residues (1.32 mg/kg on a fat basis); in a later follow-up sample, no residues were detected (Yip, 1976).

Hexachlorobutadiene residues were reported in the following foods in the UK (µg/kg): fresh milk (0.08), butter (2), vegetable cooking oil (0.2), light ale (0.2), tomatoes (0.8) and black grapes (3.7) (McConnell et al., 1975).

(e) Marine organisms

     Eight of 16 fish samples were found to contain hexachlorobutadiene
residues ranging from traces (< 0.005 mg/kg) to 4.65 mg/kg (Yurawecz *et
al*., 1976).   Residues were also found in 10 samples from 28 fish
collected from within 25 miles (40 km) of tetrachloroethylene or trichloroethylene production plant sites, at levels ranging from 0.01-1.2 mg/kg
(Yip, 1976).   The mean concentration of hexachlorobutadiene residues
detected in mosquito fish in Louisiana ranged from 112.8-827.3 µg/kg
and that in crayfish from 10.6-70.1 µg/kg (Laska *et al*., 1976).

     Thirty fish from lakes fed by the Rhine River contained 0.11-2.04
mg/kg hexachlorobutadiene on a wet weight basis, and 3 species of invertebrates and detritus contained 0.03-2.41 mg/kg;   20 sea fish contained
0.008-0.136 mg/kg (Goldbach *et al*., 1976).

     In a UK study, 14 species of invertebrates were found to contain
hexachlorobutadiene residues at levels ranging from 0-7 µg/kg by weight
of wet tissue;   5 species of marine algae, 0-8.9 µg/kg;   various organs
of 15 species of fish, 0-2.6 µg/kg;   eggs or organs of 8 species of sea
and freshwater birds, 0-9.9 µg/kg;   and organs of 2 species of mammals,
0-3.6 µg/kg (Pearson & McConnell, 1975).

(f) Humans

     Hexachlorobutadiene has been detected in post-mortem human tissue
samples, at levels of 0.8-13.7 µg/kg (wet tissue) (McConnell *et al*., 1975).

2.3 Analysis

     Methods used for the analysis of hexachlorobutadiene in environmental
samples are listed in Table 1.

     Other methods using spectrophotometry (Simonov *et al*., 1971) and
gas chromatography/electron capture detection (Yip, 1976) have been
proposed.

TABLE 1. METHODS OF ANALYSIS FOR HEXACHLOROBUTADIENE

SAMPLE TYPE	ANALYTICAL METHOD			
	EXTRACTION/CLEAN-UP	DETECTION	LIMIT OF DETECTION	REFERENCE
Air				
	Trap on Chromosorb 101, extract (hexane)	GC/ECD		Mann et al. (1974)
Ambient	Trap on Tenax GC, extract (hexane) in ultra-sound	GC/ECD		Li et al. (1976)
Ambient	Trap on silica gel, extract (ether), prepare derivative with pyridine	Colorimetry	5 mg/m^3	Lebedeva & Klisenko (1970)
	Trap on silica gel or in solvent (cyclohexane-hexane-petroleum ether)	UV	0.2 mg/m^3	Gul'ko et al. (1972)
Water				
Grab water	Extract (hexane)	GC/ECD		Li et al. (1976)
	Extract (benzene)	GC/ECD		Laseter et al. (1976)
	Extract (ether), prepare derivative with pyridine	Colorimetry	0.2 mg/l	Lebedeva & Klisenko (1970)
Food & drink				
Fish	Homogenize with sodium sulphate and acetone, filter, add sodium chloride to filtrate, extract (hexane), evaporate, take up in hexane, CC, transfer to benzene	GC/ECD		Laseter et al. (1976)
Vegetable	Extract (petroleum ether), CC	GC/ECD	5 µg/kg	Yurawecz et al. (1976)

TABLE 1. METHODS OF ANALYSIS FOR HEXACHLOROBUTADIENE (continued)

SAMPLE TYPE	ANALYTICAL METHOD		LIMIT OF DETECTION	REFERENCE
	EXTRACTION/CLEAN-UP	DETECTION		
Fish, eggs	Grind, extract (petroleum ether), CC	GC/ECD	5 µg/kg	Yurawecz et al. (1976)
Milk	Extract fat solution (petroleum ether saturated with acetonitrile)	GC/ECD	40 µg/kg	Yurawecz et al. (1976)
Wine	Extract (hexane), purify with potassium dichromate	UV		Podolenko & Timofeeva (1970)
Wine	Extract (petroleum ether), purify with potassium dichromate	TLC (revelation: silver nitrate)	5 µg/l	Vaintraub (1970)
Biological				
Blood	Extract (heptane), prepare derivative with pyridine	Colorimetry	5 mg/l	Gauntley et al. (1975)
Urine	Extract (heptane), prepare derivative with pyridine	UV	0.05 mg/l	Gauntley et al. (1975)
Soil	Extract (hexane) in Soxhlet	GC/ECD		Li et al. (1976)
	Extract (acetone), add benzene	GC/ECD		Laseter et al. (1976)

Abbreviations: GC/ECD – gas chromatography/electron capture detection; UV – ultra-violet spectrometry; CC – column chromatography; TLC – thin-layer chromatography

3. Biological Data Relevant to the Evaluation
of Carcinogenic Risk to Humans

3.1 Carcinogenicity studies in animals[1]

(a) Oral administration

Rat: Groups of 39 or 40 male and 40 female SPF Sprague-Dawley rats,
8-weeks old at the start of treatment, were fed diets containing hexachlorobutadiene (99% pure) at concentrations providing intakes of 0.2,
2.0 or 20 mg/kg bw/day. Ninety males and 90 females served as untreated
controls. All male survivors were killed after 22 months, and all females
after 24 months of test diet; median survival times were 17-19 months for
males and 20-23 months for females. In males, tumour incidences were
39/90 controls, 24/40 low-dose, 13/40 mid-dose and 15/39 high-dose. In
females, the tumour incidences were 82/90 controls, 35/40 low-dose, 37/40
mid-dose and 39/40 high-dose. A statistically significant increase
($P < 0.05$) of kidney tumours was observed in male and female rats fed
the highest dose level (9/39 males *versus* 0/40 and 0/40 at lower doses
and 1/90 in controls; 6/40 females *versus* 0/40, 0/40, 0/90). Six of
the 39 high-dose males had adenocarcinomas (some bilateral); 2 developed
adenomas only (another had an adenoma as well as adenocarcinomas); and
1 male had an undifferentiated carcinoma in one kidney and an adenocarcinoma with metastases to the lung in the other kidney. One control
male had an adenoma; 3 females had kidney adenomas (uni- or bilateral),
1 developed an adenocarcinoma, 1 had an adenocarcinoma with metastases
to the lung and 1 developed an undifferentiated, unilateral carcinoma
(Kociba *et al.*, 1977).

(b) Intraperitoneal administration

Mouse: Two groups of male A/St mice, 6-8 weeks of age, were given
thrice weekly i.p. injections of 4 or 8 mg/kg bw hexachlorobutadiene in
tricaprylin for a total of 12-13 injections (total doses, 52 and 96 mg/kg
bw). All surviving mice (19 and 14 animals) were killed 24 weeks after
the first injection and examined for lung tumours. The incidence of
lung tumours per mouse was not increased compared with that in tricaprylin-
injected controls (Theiss *et al.*, 1977) [The Working Group noted the
limitations of a negative result obtained with this test system; see
General Remarks on Substances Considered, p. 34].

---

[1]The Working Group was aware of studies in progress to assess the
carcinogenicity of hexachlorobutadiene in mice by skin and oral administration (IARC, 1978).

3.2 Other relevant biological data

(a) Experimental systems

Toxic effects

The single oral LD_{50}s of hexachlorobutadiene in male and female mice and rats are 80, 65, 250 and 270 mg/kg bw, respectively; the i.p. LD_{50}s are 105, 76, 216 and 175 mg/kg bw, respectively (Gradiski *et al.*, 1975). The oral LD_{50} in neonatal rats is 1/4 that in adult animals. Female rats are more sensitive to hexachlorobutadiene than males (Schwetz *et al.*, 1977).

Hexachlorobutadiene is toxic to experimental animals when inhaled, ingested, injected intraperitoneally or absorbed through the skin (Gage, 1970; Gradiski *et al.*, 1975; Poteryaeva, 1972, 1973). It has a moderate acute toxicity but is more toxic after chronic exposure, indicating a cumulative effect. It affects the central nervous system and causes hepatic disorders (Gradiski *et al.*. 1975). A major target organ appears to be the kidney (Gage, 1970; Gradiski *et al.*, 1975; Kociba *et al.*, 1977; Schwetz *et al.*, 1977). Feeding of 30-100 mg/kg bw/day to rats for 30 days caused renal tubular degeneration, necrosis and regeneration (Schwetz *et al.*, 1977). Renal necrosis also occurred after a single dose of 10 mg/kg bw (Shroit *et al.*, 1972).

Male and female Sprague-Dawley rats were fed a diet providing an intake of 0, 0.2, 2 or 20 mg hexachlorobutadiene/kg bw/day for up to 2 years. Doses of 2 and 20 mg/kg bw/day caused renal tubular hyperplasia. Urinary excretion of coproporphyrin was increased in males and females receiving the highest dose and in females receiving 2 mg/kg bw/day (Kociba *et al.*, 1977).

Embryotoxicity and teratogenicity

All newborn rats from mothers that received a single s.c. dose of 20 mg/kg bw hexachlorobutadiene before mating died during the next 3 months, compared with only 21.3% in a control group (Poteryaeva, 1966). Schwetz *et al.* (1977) observed no significantly deleterious effects on fertility or health of pups when adult male and female rats were maintained on a diet that contained up to 20 mg/kg bw/day hexachlorobutadiene for 90 days prior to mating.

Adult male and female Japanese quails were fed diets containing 0.3, 3, 10 or 30 mg/kg diet hexachlorobutadiene for 90 days. These dose levels had no effect on body weight, demeanour, food consumption, egg production, percent fertility and hatchability of eggs, survival of hatched chicks or eggshell thickness (Schwetz *et al.*, 1974).

Absorption, distribution, excretion and metabolism

In rats, hexachlorobutadiene was found in lung, blood, liver, brain, kidney, spleen and mesentery after a single injection (unspecified) and was excreted with the urine for 7 days (Gul'ko & Dranovskaya, 1972). In the kidney, the highest concentration was observed in the proximal section of the nephron (Shroit et al., 1972).

Mutagenicity and other related short-term tests

Hexachlorobutadiene was reported to be mutagenic in spot tests with *Salmonella typhimurium* TA100 (Tardiff et al., 1976), but no data were given.

(b) Humans

A group of 205 vineyard workers who were exposed seasonally to hexachlorobutadiene and polychlorobutane-80 (0.8-30 mg/m^3 and 0.12-6.7 mg/m^3, respectively, in the air over the fumigated zones) showed multiple toxic effects contributing to the development of hypotension, cardiac disease, chronic bronchitis, disturbances of nervous function and chronic hepatitis (Krasniuk et al., 1969).

For the occurrence of hexachlorobutadiene in human tissues see section 2.2 (f).

3.3 Case reports and epidemiological studies

No data were available to the Working Group.

4. Summary of Data Reported and Evaluation

4.1 Experimental data

Hexachlorobutadiene was tested in one experiment in rats by oral administration: it produced benign and malignant tumours in the kidneys of animals of both sexes. It was tested inadequately in one experiment in mice by intraperitoneal injection.

4.2 Human data

No case reports or epidemiological studies were available to the Working Group.

The occurrence of hexachlorobutadiene as a by-product in the production of various chlorinated hydrocarbons for over 50 years and its use in some areas as a pesticide indicate that widespread human exposure in both the occupational and general environment occurs. This is confirmed by reports of its occurrence in the environment.

4.3 Evaluation

There is *limited evidence* that hexachlorobutadiene is carcinogenic in rats.

5. References

Eurocop-Cost (1976)   A Comprehensive List of Polluting Substances Which Have Been Identified in Various Fresh Waters, Effluent Discharges, Aquatic Animals and Plants, and Bottom Sediments, 2nd ed., EUCO/MDU/-73/76, XII/476/76, Luxembourg, Commission of the European Communities, p. 48

Gage, J.C. (1970)   The subacute inhalation toxicity of 109 industrial chemicals. Brit. J. ind. Med., 27, 1-15

Gauntley, P., Magadur, J.L., Morel, G., Chaumont, P. & Canel, F. (1975) Determination of hexachlorobutadiene in biological media (Fr.). Eur. J. Toxicol., 8, 152-158 [Chem. Abstr., 83, 158607b]

Goldbach, R.W., van Genderen, H. & Leeuwangh, P. (1976) Hexachlorobutadiene residues in aquatic fauna from surface water fed by the river Rhine. Sci. Total Environ., 6, 31-40

Gorenshtein, R.S. (1973) Hexachlorobutadiene residues in wine and grape juice (Russ.). Zashch. Rast. (Moscow), 12, 27 [Chem. Abstr., 81, 48484k]

Gradiski, D., Duprat, P., Magadur, J.-L. & Fayein, E. (1975) Experimental toxicological study of hexachlorbutadiene (Fr.). Eur. J. Toxicol., 8, 180-187

Grasselli, J.G. & Ritchey, W.M., eds (1975) CRC Atlas of Spectral Data and Physical Constants for Organic Compounds, 2nd ed., Vol. II, Cleveland, OH, Chemical Rubber Co., p. 566

Gul'ko, A.G. & Dranovskaya, L.M. (1972) Distribution and excretion of hexachlorobutadiene from rats (Russ.). Aktual. Vop. Gig. Epidemiol., 58-60 [Chem. Abstr., 81, 346q]

Gul'ko, A.G., Dranovskaya, L.M. & Chernokan, V.F. (1972) Contamination of atmospheric air by hexachlorobutadiene (Russ.). Vliyanie Yadokhim. Vnesh. Sredy, 39-40 [Chem. Abstr., 79, 82953f]

Hawley, G.G., ed. (1977) The Condensed Chemical Dictionary, 9th ed., New York, Van Nostrand-Reinhold, p. 436

IARC (1978) Information Bulletin on the Survey of Chemicals Being Tested for Carcinogenicity, No. 7, Lyon, p. 277

Kociba, R.J., Keyes, D.G., Jersey, G.C., Ballard, J.J., Dittenber, D.A., Quast, J.F., Wade, C.E., Humiston, C.G. & Schwetz, B.A. (1977) Results of a two year chronic toxicity study with hexachlorobutadiene in rats. Am. ind. Hyg. Assoc. J., 38, 589-602

Kotzias, D., Lay, J.P., Klein, W. & Korte, F. (1975) Ecological chemistry. CIV. Residue analysis of hexachlorobutadiene in food and poultry feed (Germ.). Chemosphere, 4, 247-250 [Chem. Abstr., 83, 176818a]

Krasniuk, E.P., Zaritskaya, L.A., Boiko, V.G., Voitenko, G.A. & Matokhnyuk, L.A. (1969) Health condition of vine-growers contacting with fumigants hexachlorobutadien and polychlorbutan-80 (Russ.) Vrach. Delo, 7, 111-115

Laseter, J.L., Bartell, C.K., Laska, A.L., Holmquist, D.G., Condie, D.B., Brown, J.W. & Evans, R.L. (1976) An Ecological Study of Hexachloro-butadiene (HCBD), EPA-560/6-76-010, US Environmental Protection Agency, Report No. PB-252671, available from Springfield, VA, National Technical Information Service

Laska, A.L., Bartell, C.K. & Laseter, J.L. (1976) Distribution of hexachlorobenzene and hexachlorobutadiene in water, soil, and selected aquatic organisms along the lower Mississippi River, Louisiana. Bull. environ. Contam. Toxicol., 15, 535-542

Lebedeva, T.A. & Klisenko, M.A. (1970) Colorimetric method for determining hexachlorobutadiene in air and water (Russ.). In: Lyalikov, Y.S., ed., Methods of Pesticide Analysis, Kishinev, USSR, Academy of Sciences of the Moldavian SSR, pp. 57-59 [Chem. Abstr., 76, 32021t]

Li, R.T., Going, J.E. & Spigarelli, J.L. (1976) Sampling and Analysis of Selected Toxic Substances, Task IB-Hexachlorobutadiene, EPA-560/6-76-015, US Environmental Protection Agency, Report No. PB-253941, available from Springfield, VA, National Technical Information Service

Mann, J.B., Enos, H.F., Gonzalez, J. & Thompson, J.F. (1974) Development of sampling and analytical procedure for determining hexachlorobenzene and hexachloro-1,3-butadiene in air. Environ. Sci. Technol., 8, 584-585

McConnell, G., Ferguson, D.M. & Pearson, C.R. (1975) Chlorinated hydrocarbons and the environment. Endeavor, 34, 13-18

Pearson, C.R. & McConnell, G. (1975) Chlorinated C_1 and C_2 hydrocarbons in the marine environment. Proc. R. Soc. Lond. B., 189, 305-332

Podolenko, A.A. & Timofeeva, O.A. (1970) Spectrophotometric determination of hexachlorobutadiene in wine (Russ.). In: Lyalikov, Y.S., ed., Methods of Pesticide Analysis, Kishinev, USSR, Academy of Sciences of the Moldavian SSR, pp. 80-82 [Chem. Abstr., 76, 12780m]

Poteryaeva, G.E. (1966) The effect of hexachlorobutadien on offsprings of albino rats (Russ.). Gig. Sanit., 31, 33-36

Poteryaeva, G.E. (1972) Data for substantiating the maximum permissible
    concentration of hexachlorobutadiene in the air of industrial
    premises (Russ.). Gig. Sanit., 37, 32-36

Poteryaeva, G.E. (1973) Toxicity of hexachlorobutadiene during entry
    into the organism through the gastrointestinal tract (Russ.).
    Gig. Tr., 9, 98-100

Prager, B., Jacobson, P., Schmidt, P. & Stern, D., eds (1918)
    Beilsteins Handbuch der Organischen Chemie, 4th ed., Vol. 1,
    Syst. No. 12, Berlin, Springer, p. 250

Schwetz, B.A., Norris, J.M., Kociba, R.J., Keeler, P.A., Cornier, R.F. &
    Gehring, P.J. (1974) Reproduction study in Japanese quail fed
    hexachlorobutadiene for 90 days. Toxicol. appl. Pharmacol., 30,
    255-265

Schwetz, B.A., Smith, F.A., Humiston, C.G., Quast, J.F. & Kociba, R.J.
    (1977) Results of a reproduction study in rats fed diets containing
    hexachlorobutadiene. Toxicol. appl. Pharmacol., 42, 387-398

Shackelford, W.M. & Keith, L.H. (1976) Frequency of Organic Compounds
    Identified In Water, EPA-600/4-76-062, Athens, GA, US
    Environmental Protection Agency, p. 89

Shroit, I.G., Vasilos, A.F. & Gul'ko, A.G. (1972) Kidney lesions under
    experimental hexachlorobutadiene poisoning (Russ.). Aktual Vop.
    Gig. Epidemiol., 73-75 [Chem. Abstr., 81, 73128e]

Simonov, V.D., Popova, L.N. & Shamsutdinov, T.M. (1971) Spectrophotometric
    determination of perchlorinated hydrocarbons in water (Russ.).
    Dokl. Neftekhim. Sekts., Bashkir. Respub. Pravl., Vses. Khim.
    Obshchest., 6, 357-371 [Chem. Abstr., 78, 47526b]

Tardiff, R.G., Carlson, G.P. & Simmon, V. (1976) Halogenated organics
    in tap water: a toxicological evaluation. In: Jolley, R.L., ed.,
    The Environmental Impact of Water Chlorination, Springfield, VA,
    National Technical Information Service, pp. 213-227

Theiss, J.C., Stoner, G.D., Shimkin, M.B. & Weisburger, E.K. (1977)
    Test for carcinogenicity of organic contaminants of United States
    drinking waters by pulmonary tumor response in strain A mice.
    Cancer Res., 37, 2717-2720

US Environmental Protection Agency (1975a) Survey of Industrial Processing
    Data, Task I - Hexachlorobenzene and Hexachlorobutadiene Pollution
    from Chlorocarbon Processing, PB-243 641, Springfield, VA, National
    Technical Information Service, pp. 32,33,74,95,96,98,101

US Environmental Protection Agency (1975b) Preliminary Assessment of
    Suspected Carcinogens in Drinking Water, Washington DC, p. II-4

Vaintraub, F.P. (1970) Determination of hexachlorobutadiene [HCB], hexachlorocyclohexane [HCH], and DDT in wine and grape juice by thin-layer chromatography (Russ.). In: Lyalikov, Y.S., ed., Methods of Pesticide Analysis, Kishinev, USSR, Academy of Sciences of the Moldavian SSR, pp. 12-15 [Chem. Abstr., 76, 12781n]

Yip, G. (1976) Survey for hexachloro-1,3-butadiene in fish, eggs, milk and vegetables. J. Assoc. off. Anal. Chem., 59, 559-561

Yurawecz, M.P., Dreifuss, P.A. & Kamps, L.R. (1976) Determination of hexachloro-1,3-butadiene in spinach, eggs, fish, and milk by electron capture gas-liquid chromatography. J. Assoc. off. Anal. Chem., 59, 552-558

HEXACHLOROCYCLOHEXANE
(TECHNICAL HCH AND LINDANE)

These substances were considered by a previous Working Group, in October 1973 (IARC, 1974). Since that time new data have become available, and these have been incorporated into the monograph and taken into account in the present evaluation.

Two reviews on lindane are available (Mercier, 1975; Ulmann, 1972).

1. Chemical and Physical Data

1.1 Synonyms and trade names

Mixture of HCH isomers

Chem. Abstr. Services Reg. No.: 608-73-1

Chem. Abstr. Name: 1,2,3,4,5,6-Hexachlorocyclohexane

Synonyms: BHC; HCCH; hexachlor; hexachloran

Trade names: 666; Benzahex; Benzex; Dol; Dolmix; FBHC; Hexafor; Hexyclan; Kotol; Soprocide

α-isomer

Chem. Abstr. Services Reg. No.: 319-84-6

Chem. Abstr. Name: 1α,2α,3β,4α,5β,6β-Hexachlorocyclohexane

Synonyms: α-Benzene hexachloride; α-BHC; α-HCH; α-hexachloran; α-hexachlorane; α-hexachlorcyclohexane; α-1,2,3,4,5,6-hexachlorcyclohexane; α-hexachlorocyclohexane; α-1,2,3,4,5,6-hexachlorocyclohexane; α-lindane

β-isomer

Chem. Abstr. Services Reg. No.: 319-85-7

Chem. Abstr. Name: 1α,2β,3α,4β,5α,6β-Hexachlorocyclohexane

Synonyms: β-Benzene hexachloride; β-BHC; β-HCH; β-hexachlorobenzene; β-hexachlorocyclohexane; β-1,2,3,4,5,6-hexachlorocyclohexane; β-lindane

γ-isomer (lindane)

Chem. Abstr. Services Reg. No.:   58-89-9

Chem. Abstr. Name: 1α,2α,3β,4α,5α,6β-Hexachlorocyclohexane

Synonyms: γ-Benzene hexachloride;   BHC;   γ-BHC;   HCCH;   HCH;
γ-HCH;   γ-hexachlorobenzene;   γ-1,2,3,4,5,6-hexachlorocyclohexane;
γ-lindane

Trade names: 666;   Aalindan;   Aficide;   Agrocide;   Agrocide III;
Agrocide WP;   Ameisenmittel Merck;   Ameisentod;   Aparasin;   Aphtiria;
Aplidal;   Arbitex;   BBH;   Ben-Hex;   Bentox 10;   Bexol;   Celanex;
Chloresene;   Codechine;   DBH;   Detmol-Extrakt;   Devoran;   Dol Granule;
Drill tox-Spezial Aglukon;   ENT 7796;   Entomoxan;   Forlin;   Gamacid;
Gamaphex;   Gammalin;   Gammalin 20;   Gammaterr;   Gammexane;   Gexane;
Heclotox;   Hexa;   Hexachloran;   γ-Hexachloran;   Hexachlorane;
γ-Hexachlorane;   Hexatox;   Hexaverm;   Hexicide;   Hexyclan;   HGI;
Hortex;   Isotox;   Jacutin;   Kokotine;   Kwell;   Lendine;   Lentox;
Lidenal;   Lindafor;   Lindagam;   Lindatox;   Lindosep;   Lintox;
Lorexane;   Milbol 49;   Mszycol;   Neo-Scabicidol;   Nexen FB;   Nexit;
Nexit-Stark;   Nexol-E;   Nicochloran;   Novigam;   Omnitox;   Ovadziak;
Owadziak;   Pedraczak;   Pflanzol;   Quellada;   Sang-gamma;   Silvanol;
Spritz-Rapidin;   Spruehpflanzol;   Streunex;   TAP 85;   Tri-6;   Viton

δ-isomer

Chem. Abstr. Services Reg. No.:   319-86-8

Chem. Abstr. Name: 1α,2α,3α,4β,5α,6β-Hexachlorocyclohexane

Synonyms: δ-Benzene hexachloride;   δ-BHC;   δ-HCH;   δ-hexachlorocyclo-
hexane;   δ-1,2,3,4,5,6-hexachlorocyclohexane;   δ-(aeeeee)-1,2,3,4,5,6-
hexachlorocyclohexane;   δ-lindane

ε-isomer

Chem. Abstr. Services Reg. No. :   6108-10-7

Chem. Abstr. Name: 1α,2α,3α,4β,5β,6β-hexachlorocyclohexane

Synonyms: ε-Benzene hexachloride;   ε-BHC;   ε-HCH;   ε-hexachlorocyclo-
hexane;   ε-1,2,3,4,5,6-hexachlorocyclohexane;   ε-lindane

<u>ζ-isomer</u>

Chem. Abstr. Services Reg. No.:   6108-11-8

Chem. Abstr. Name: 1α,2α,3α,4α,5α,6α-Hexachlorocyclohexane

Synonyms: ζ-Hexachlorocyclohexane;   ζ-lindane

<u>η-isomer</u>

Chem. Abstr. Services Reg. No.:   6108-12-9

Chem. Abstr. Name: 1α,2α,3α,4α,5β,6β-Hexachlorocyclohexane

Synonyms: η-Hexachlorocyclohexane;   η-lindane

<u>θ-isomer</u>

Chem. Abstr. Services Reg. No.:   6108-13-0

Chem. Abstr. Name: 1α,2α,3α,4α,5α,6β-Hexachlorocyclohexane

Synonyms: θ-Hexachlorocyclohexane;   θ-lindane

1.2   <u>Structural and molecular formulae and molecular weight</u>

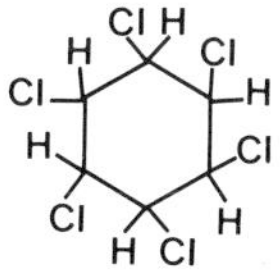

$C_6H_6Cl_6$ Mol. wt: 290.9

Isomers differ in the spatial positions of the chlorine atoms on the boat and chair forms.

1.3   <u>Chemical and physical properties of the mixture and of the pure substances</u>

Physical properties, except solubility, of the HCH isomers are given in Table 1.

(a)   <u>Solubility</u>:   The solubility of various HCH isomers in several organic solvents has been reported (Demozay & Marechal, 1972a).

(b)   <u>Stability</u>:   Fortified HCH is stable to light, air and heat (Hooker Chemical Corporation, 1969) (see section 1.4 for a definition of fortified HCH).   Lindane is stable to light under atmospheric conditions and is heat stable to 165.5°C (Hooker Chemical Corporation, 1973).

TABLE 1. PHYSICAL PROPERTIES OF HCH ISOMERS[a]

PROPERTY	MIXTURE (FORTIFIED)	α-ISOMER	β-ISOMER	γ-ISOMER (lindane)	δ-ISOMER	ε-ISOMER	ζ-ISOMER	η-ISOMER	θ-ISOMER
Description	Brownish-to-white crystals	Monoclinic prisms	Cubic crystals	White, monoclinic crystals	Crystals or fine platelets	Monoclinic needles or hexagonal, monoclinic crystals	-	-	-
Boiling-point (°C)	-	288	60 (0.58 mm)	323.4	60 (0.34 mm)	-	-	-	-
Melting-point (°C)	-	157.5-158	309.8-310.7	112.5-113	138.0-138.4	219.3	68-88	89.8-90.6	124-125
Density	-	1.87^{20}	1.89^{19}	1.85	-	-	-	-	-
Refractive index (n_D^{20})	-	1.60-1.626	1.630	1.60-1.635	1.576-1.674	1.00-1.635	-	-	-
Spectra[b]	-	ir	ir	ir, nmr	ir	-	-	-	-
Vapour pressure at 20°C (mm Hg)	-	0.02	0.005	0.03	0.02	-	-	-	-

[a] From Demozay & Marechal, 1972a; Grasselli & Ritchey, 1975; Hooker Chemical Corporation, 1969

[b] Spectral data tabulated by Grasselli & Ritchey, 1975 (ir – infra-red; nmr – nuclear magnetic resonance)

(c) Reactivity: Fortified HCH and lindane do not react with
     strong acids; they decompose in the presence of alkali at
     ambient temperatures, forming trichlorobenzenes (Hooker
     Chemical Corporation, 1969a, 1973).   Lindane decomposes in
     the presence of certain powdered metals such as iron, alu-
     minium and zinc (Demozay & Marechal, 1972a).

1.4 Technical products and impurities

Two forms of hexachlorocyclohexane are available commercially in the
US.   One, a mixture of isomers, is called HCH; the other, which consists
essentially of pure γ-isomer, is called lindane.

HCH

As produced initially by photochlorination of benzene, HCH contains
only 14-77% of the γ-isomer.   Technical grade HCH available commercially
in the US is 'fortified' HCH (FHCH) containing a varying mixture of at
least 5 isomers, with a minimum of 40% γ-isomer.   Typical isomer distribution is as follows (% by wt): γ, 40-45; δ, 20-22; α, 18-22;
β, 4; ε and inerts, 1; and heptachlorocyclohexane, 10 (Hooker Chemical
Corporation, 1969).

HCH is available in the US as dusts, wettable powders, oil solutions
and emulsifiable concentrates (Berg, 1978).

HCH available in Japan had a γ-isomer content of 12-15%.

Lindane

Commercial lindane available in the US contains a minimum of 99.9%
(by weight) of the γ-isomer.   The remaining 0.1% consists of other
unspecified isomers of HCH (Hooker Chemical Corporation, 1973).   It is
available in the US as emulsifiable concentrates, wettable powders, oil-
base sprays, dusts, aerosol sprays, granules and as a smoke generator
(Berg, 1978).

Lindane is available generally in Europe, with a purity of 99-99.5%.
Lindane available in Japan had a purity over 99% and a melting-point of
112-113°C.

2. Production, Use, Occurrence and Analysis

2.1 Production and use

(a) Production

HCH

HCH was first prepared by Faraday in 1825 by the addition of chlorine to benzene in sunlight (Hardie, 1964).   It is produced commercially in the US by the photochlorination of benzene, followed by fortification of the γ-isomer content by extraction (e.g., with methanol) and concentration of this isomer.

Commercial production of HCH in the US was first reported in 1945 (US Tariff Commission, 1946).   US production reached a maximum in 1951 when 16 companies produced 53 million kg containing 7 million kg of the γ-isomer (US Tariff Commission, 1952).   In 1963, the last year for which production data were reported, the number of US producers had dropped to 5 and total production of HCH amounted to 3.1 million kg, containing 0.8 million kg of the γ-isomer (US Tariff Commission, 1964). In 1976, only one US company reported production of an undisclosed amount (see preamble, p. 16) (US International Trade Commission, 1977a).

The following western European countries were reported to be producing HCH (technical grades) in 1973 (number of producing companies is given in parentheses):   Federal Republic of Germany (1), France (1) and Italy (2) (Economic Documentation Office, 1973).   One company in the UK may also be producing it.   France, the Federal Republic of Germany and Spain produce 30, 16 and 8.5 million kg/year, respectively.   HCH (technical grades) is also believed to be produced in the German Democratic Republic and to a lesser extend in Poland, Yugoslavia and Roumania.   Production of 18 million kg/year has been reported for the USSR.

Imports of this material by European countries in 1975 were as follows (thousands of kg):   Belgium and Luxembourg (42);   Federal Republic of Germany (580);   Italy (39);   The Netherlands (22);   and the UK (42).   Exports in 1975 were: Belgium and Luxembourg (30);   Federal Republic of Germany (2);   Italy (304);   The Netherlands (42) and the UK (5) (EUROSTAT, 1975).

HCH was first produced commercially in Japan in 1949;   however, it has not been produced there since 1971.   In 1974, exports amounted to an estimated 922 thousand kg (from inventory disposal), and none was imported.

Lindane

A review on lindane has been published (Blaquiere, 1972).

In 1944, the insecticidal properties of HCH were found to be due to the γ-isomer (lindane) (Hardie, 1964).   Lindane is extracted from HCH by the use of selected solvents, the most common of which is methanol.   The γ-isomer so obtained is treated with nitric acid to remove odour (Demozay & Marechal, 1972b).

Commercial production of lindane in the US was first reported in 1950 (US Tariff Commission, 1951).   The quantity produced in the US reached a maximum in the early 1950's and has declined since due to increased use of organophosphate insecticides.   One US company, the only one to have reported lindane production since 1956, is estimated to have produced 227 thousand kg in 1972 (US Environmental Protection Agency, 1976a).   US imports in 1976 through the principal US customs districts were 10,851 kg (US International Trade Commission, 1977b).

In Europe, 3.5, 1.7 and 1 million kg/year lindane are produced in France, the Federal Republic of Germany and Spain, respectively.   It is produced in the German Democratic Republic and to a lesser extent in Poland, Yugoslavia and Roumania.   In the USSR, 2 million kg lindane are produced annually.

Lindane was first produced commercially in Japan in 1949;   however, it has not been produced there since 1971, although one company produces minor quantities for industrial use.   In 1974, exports amounted to an estimated 153 thousand kg (from inventory disposal);   none was imported.

(b) Use

HCH

The only known use of HCH is as an insecticide.   It is registered for use in the US on a wide variety of fruits, vegetables, field crops, uncultivated land for general outdoor use and on breeding stock (US Environmental Protection Agency, 1970).

An estimated 450 thousand kg were used in the US in 1974, as follows: forests, 60%; livestock and poultry, 20%; and commercial, household and industrial establishments, 20%.

Tolerances in the US for residues of HCH in or on raw agricultural commodities are established at 1 mg/kg for a variety of 32 fruits and vegetables and at 0.01 mg/kg in or on pecan nuts (US Environmental Protection Agency, 1976b).

A notice of rebuttable presumption against registration and continued registration (RPAR) (see General Remarks on the Substances Considered, p. 31) of pesticide products containing HCH was issued by the US Environmental Protection Agency on 19 October, 1976 (US Environmental Protection Agency, 1976c) on the basis of carcinogenic effects.

The future use of HCH in the US depends largely on the outcome of these actions.

No data on its use in Europe were available.

HCH was used as an insecticide in Japan until 1971, when its use was discontinued.

Lindane

Lindane is used primarily as an insecticide (Demozay & Marechal, 1972c) and as a therapeutic agent in human and veterinary medicine.

It is registered in the US for insecticidal use on a wide variety of vegetable, fruit and field crops, as well as for use on animals, agricultural premises, general outdoor use and on uncultivated land (US Environmental Protection Agency, 1970).   An estimated 270 thousand kg lindane were used in the US for insecticidal purposes in 1974, with 67% on livestock and poultry and 33% on field crops.

Lindane is used in human medicine as a scabicide and pediculocide. Less than 1000 kg were used in the US for this purpose in 1971.   It is available for human use in preparations as a lotion (1%), cream (1%) and shampoo (1%) (Kastrup, 1976).

In Europe, it is used as an insecticide on various vegetables, fruits and crops and on animals and animal premises.   For specific uses in different countries, see Blaquière (1976a).

Domestic use of lindane in aerosol form has been prohibited in Sweden and Finland and restricted in Canada (Blaquière, 1976b).

Lindane was used as an insecticide in Japan until 1971 when its use was discontinued.

In November 1975, the Joint Meeting of the FAO Working Party of Experts on Pesticide Residues and the WHO Expert Committee on Pesticide Residues recommended maximum residue limits for 20 commodities ranging from 0.05 mg/kg on potatoes to 2 mg/kg on lettuce;   0.5 mg/kg was recommended for most fruit and vegetables (WHO, 1976).   Residue tolerances in the US range from 0.01 mg/kg for pecans to 7 mg/kg for the fat of meat, with most fruit and vegetables falling in the range of 1-3 mg/kg (US Environmental Protection Agency, 1976b).

A notice of rebuttable presumption against registration and continued registration (RPAR) (see General Remarks on the Substances Considered, p. 31) of pesticide products containing lindane was issued by the US Environmental Protection Agency on 17 February 1977 (US Environmental Protection Agency, 1977) on the basis of carcinogenic and delayed toxic effects and acute toxicity risk related to hazards in aquatic wildlife. The future use of lindane in the US depends largely on the outcome of these actions.

A maximum acceptable daily intake of lindane for humans was established at 0-0.01 mg/kg bw by the 1975 Joint Meeting of the FAO Working Party of Experts on Pesticide Residues and the WHO Expert Committee on Pesticide Residues (WHO, 1976). This level was re-established in 1977 (FAO/WHO, 1978).

The US Occupational Safety and Health Administration's standards for air contaminants require that an employee's exposure to lindane not exceed an 8-hr time-weighted average of 0.5 mg/m^3 in any 8-hr work shift of a 40-hr work week (US Occupational Safety & Health Administration, 1976).

The corresponding standard in the Federal Republic of Germany is 0.5 mg/m^3, and that in the German Democratic Republic, 0.2 mg/m^3; the ceiling concentration in the USSR is 0.05 mg/m^3 (Winell, 1975).

2.2 Occurrence

HCH and lindane are not known to occur as natural products.

(a) Air

The occurrence of residues of lindane in air has been reviewed by Sieper (1972).

In weekly air samples taken in the Mississippi Delta, maximum levels of lindane were 9.3 ng/m^3 and maximum levels of β-HCH were 49.4 ng/m^3 (Arthur et al., 1976). Lindane was also detected in the air of a plant producing hexachlorobenzene (Melnikova et al., 1975).

(b) Water and sediments

The presence of HCH and lindane in surface waters, drinking-water, and industrial and sewage effluents in the US and Europe has been reviewed and tabulated (Eurocop-Cost, 1976; Shackelford & Keith, 1976; Sieper, 1972).

The concentrations of α-HCH and lindane in rainwater in Tokyo were in the range of 45-830 ng/l and 29-398 ng/l, respectively (Masahiro & Takahisa, 1975).

HCH and lindane residues in ground-water used for drinking purposes were: (1) ≤ 15 ng/l lindane and 4 ng/l α-HCH in wells in Israel (Lahav & Kahanovitch, 1974); 10-340 ng/l lindane and 0-220 ng/l β-HCH in Czechoslovakia (Rosival & Szokolay, 1975); and < 10-319 ng/l lindane in 3 US rural areas (Achari *et al.*, 1975; Sandhu *et al.*, 1978). In a survey of finished US drinking-water, the highest reported level of HCH was 100 ng/l (US Environmental Protection Agency, 1975).

Levels of lindane in a US river during 1974 ranged from 1.25-2.9 ng/l (Brodtmann, 1976); lindane concentrations in two rivers in Canada ranged from 0.4-1.6 ng/l (Mamarbachi & St-Jean, 1976). HCH and lindane have been reported in rivers in the Federal Republic of Germany, at concentrations ranging from 5-2500 ng/l α-HCH and 5-7100 ng/l lindane (Herzel, 1972); at a river mouth in Italy, 9.5 ng/l lindane (Andryushchenko *et al.*, 1975); in Spain, 25 ng/l α-HCH and 47 ng/l lindane (Simal *et al.*, 1975); and in the UK, 15-55 ng/l lindane and 3-8 ng/l α-HCH (Musty & Nickless, 1976).

Lindane concentrations in a lake in Europe were 5 ng/l at the surface and 1.5-3 ng/l at a depth of 60 m (Maier & Wendlandt, 1976).

Rivers in Japan have been found to contain levels of HCH isomers ranging from traces to 860 ng/l (α-HCH), 10-30 ng/l (β-HCH), 5-410 ng/l (lindane) and 0-10 ng/l (δ-HCH) (Hirano & Katada, 1975; Kitayama *et al.*, 1976; Ochiai & Hanya, 1976; Saito & Kitayama, 1974); a maximum level of 10,000 ng/l total HCH has been found (Yamato *et al.*, 1975).

In a controlled study in a flooded limestone quarry, 41.1% of added lindane remained after 240 days: 40.6% in the water and 0.5% in the bottom sediments (Hamelink & Waybrant, 1973).

(c) Soil

A review on the degradation and persistence of lindane in soils has been published (Sieper, 1972).

In Japan after prohibition of the use of HCH on arable land, total HCH residues in soils declined from 7.9 mg/kg in 1970 to 0.4 µg/kg in 1973 in one area (Yamada & Sakamoto, 1975); in another area, lindane concentrations in soils declined from 0.06-1.12 mg/kg in 1970 to 0.013-0.848 mg/kg in 1972 (Saito & Kitayama, 1973).

Soil in southern Bohemia was reported to contain 1 µg/kg lindane (Hruska & Kocianova, 1975).

In a radioactive tracer study of lindane degradation in soils, approximately 89% and 86% of added lindane was recovered from moist and submerged organic soils, respectively, after 8 weeks, and 84% and 70% was recovered from moist and submerged mineral soils, respectively (Mathur & Saha, 1977).

(d)   Food and drink

A review has been published on lindane residues on vegetables in supervised trials (WHO, 1976).   The occurrence of lindane in foods has been reviewed (Sieper, 1972).

In a programme still in progress involving the monitoring of pesticide residues in food, the US Department of Health, Education, and Welfare monitored levels of lindane in foods during the period 1965-1974 and calculated the average daily intake.   For the period 1965-1970, the average daily intake of lindane was 3 µg/day;   in 1973, this dropped to 0.2223 µg/day, and it rose slightly in 1974 to 0.5856 µg/day (US Food & Drug Administration, 1975, 1977).

In total diet studies in Spain in 1971-1972, the estimated *per caput* intake of α-HCH was 11.52 µg/day;   that of lindane was 13.78 µg/day (Carrasco *et al.*, 1976).   In the German Democratic Republic, the estimated average daily intake of lindane of an adult male in 1971 was 10 µg, and that of nursery school children was 7 µg (Engst *et al.*, 1976a).   In Yugoslavia, the average daily intake of total HCH in 1970-1971 was 494 µg (Adamovic *et al.*, 1975).   A model daily diet for adult Japanese contained an average of 3.5 µg lindane (Ushio *et al.*, 1974).

In a 4-year study (1971-1974) in Japan, average levels of HCH in vegetables gradually decreased following prohibition of its use on arable land in 1970.   The proportion of isomers in total HCH residues was very different from that in the technical product: the β-isomer, in particular, was present in a much higher proportion in the residues than in the commercial product, due to its greater persistence (Suzuki *et al.*, 1976).

Apple and pear samples in Italy contained mean levels of 0.5 µg/kg α-HCH and 2.5 µg/kg lindane (Avancini & Stringari, 1974).

Honey and beeswax samples in the US contained α-HCH in ranges of 0.01-0.08 µg/kg and 0.21-3.5 µg/kg, respectively;   β-HCH in ranges of 0.03-0.3 µg/kg and 0.68-5.26 µg/kg;   and lindane in ranges of 0.01-0.38 µg/kg and 0.3-6 µg/kg (Estep *et al.*, 1977).

The lindane content of raw and processed vegetable oils in Iran was 29 µg/kg and 2 µg/kg, respectively (Hashemy-Tonkabony & Soleimani-Amiri, 1976).

Maximum residues of lindane in cultured fish and shellfish in Taiwan were 0.16 mg/kg (Jeng & Sun, 1974).

Lindane was present in 8/10 samples of cow's milk in Italy at concentrations ranging from 3-18 µg/l (Cerutti *et al.*, 1975).   Milk and milk products in the Federal Republic of Germany contained mean levels of 40 μg/l α-HCH and 72 μg/l lindane (Heeschen *et al.*, 1976). Samples of cow's milk in Roumania had concentrations of 124 μg/l and 255 μg/l lindane (Cocisiu *et al.*, 1975a). In Japan, after prohibition of use of HCH on arable land, lindane concentrations in cow's milk decreased from 244 μg/l in 1970 to 1 μg/l in 1973 (Yamada & Sakamoto, 1975).

Lindane concentrations in the fat of cattle given controlled feed for 112 days prior to slaughter (0.026 mg/kg) were higher than the original concentration in the feed (0.002 mg/kg) (Clark *et al.*, 1974).

In feeding experiments with broiler breeder hens, the ratio of the level of HCH in the animal fat to the level in the feed was 1.8 for α-HCH, 18 for β-HCH and 1.8 for lindane. The ratio of the level of HCH in eggs to the level in the feed was 0.10 for α-HCH, 1.5 for β-HCH and 0.13 for lindane on a whole egg basis (Kan & Tuinstra, 1976).

(e) Animals

The occurrence of lindane in animals has been reviewed (Sieper, 1972).

In Japan, crows were found to contain 8.2 mg/kg total HCH (Kaneshima *et al.*, 1976), and wild ducks contained 0-0.19 mg/kg total HCH (Ushio *et al.*, 1976). Levels of lindane in eggs of birds in France were 0.03-0.5 mg/kg (Mendola *et al.*, 1977). In the US, residues of HCH in starlings ranged from traces to 0.036 mg/kg in 1972 and from traces to 0.094 mg/kg in 1974 (Nickerson & Barbehenn, 1975; White, 1976).

Fat samples taken from 20 racoons in the US contained 0.17 mg/kg α-HCH (in one animal), 0.1-2.3 mg/kg β-HCH (in 15 animals) and 0.02-0.12 mg/kg lindane (in 5 animals) (Nalley *et al.*, 1975). Wild rabbits in Roumania had α-HCH and lindane in all tissues, with the highest concentration found in adipose tissue (Floru *et al.*, 1975).

Lindane was found in lake trout in the US at a mean concentration of 1.19 mg/kg (Parejko *et al.*, 1975). Molluscs in Spain contained maximum levels of 1.54 μg/kg α-HCH and 2.30 μg/kg lindane (Boado *et al.*, 1975). Fish in Iran contained residues of lindane ranging from 0-0.054 mg/kg (Hashemy-Tonkabony & Asadi Langaroodi, 1976); and fish in Lake Tanganyika contained 0.22-1.4 mg/kg lindane (Deelstra, 1974).

(f) Humans

The occurrence of lindane in humans has been reviewed (Sieper, 1972).

Milk samples taken from Italian women contained 0.06-0.52 mg/l β-HCH and 0.08-0.88 mg/l lindane (fat basis) (Cerutti *et al.*, 1976). Median values of HCH in mother's milk in The Netherlands were 0.01 mg/l α-HCH, 0.28 mg/l β-HCH and 0.02 mg/l lindane (fat basis) (Wegman & Greve, 1974). Milk fat from Austrian women contained mean concentrations of 0.2 mg/l

β-HCH and 0.048 mg/l lindane (Pesendorfer, 1975).   In Japan, mother's
milk contained 0.220 mg/l β-HCH in 1970; this declined to 0.013 mg/l
in 1973 after use of HCH had been prohibited (Yamada & Sakamoto, 1975).

In the US, β-HCH levels in the serum of new mothers in a rural area
ranged from 0-19 μg/l (mean, 1.9 μg/l) in blacks and 0-9 μg/l (mean,
3 μg/l) in whites; serum levels of β-HCH in the newborns ranged from
0-9 μg/l (means, 0.75 μg/l in black babies and 1 μg/l in white babies)
(D'Ercole *et al.*, 1976).   In a study of post-mortem human blood from
497 Virginia residents, 8.3% of samples contained lindane, in concentrations ranging from 1-17 μg/l, with a mean of 3.5 μg/l (Griffith & Blanke,
1975).

In Spain, lindane was detected in 94% of 199 samples of human serum
tested, with an average concentration of 0.066 mg/l (Santiago Laguna *et
al.*, 1975).

In 51 human fat samples analysed at autopsy in New Zealand in 1973,
measurable amounts of β-HCH were found in 37% and lindane in 22% (Solly
& Shanks, 1974).   HCH was present in 49/52 fat samples from autopsied
children in Argentina, at levels of 0.22 mg/kg α-HCH, 0.86 mg/kg β-HCH
and 0.09 mg/kg lindane (Astolfi *et al.*, 1973).

In a 1970 survey of pesticide residues in the adipose tissue of the
general population of the US, mean levels of α-HCH were 0.01 mg/kg, β-HCH
levels were 0.6 mg/kg, lindane levels were 0.01 mg/kg and δ-HCH levels
were 0.01 mg/kg (Kutz *et al.*, 1974).   Adipose tissue levels of β-HCH
in Spain averaged 2.55 mg/kg (Vioque & Sáez, 1976).   Lindane levels in
adipose tissue in Roumania averaged 4.76 mg/kg (Cocisiu *et al.*, 1975b).
In Japan, total HCH averaged 4.26 mg/kg in subjects less than 1 year old,
4.95 mg/kg in subjects from 1-19 years old, 8.45 mg/kg in subjects from
20-49 years old, and 7.46 mg/kg in subjects over 50 years of age (Yamada
et al., 1976).

The storage levels of total HCH isomers in adipose tissue in the
general populations of different countries varied from 0.02-1.43 mg/kg,
and the concentration in human blood was 0.003 mg/1 (Durham, 1969).
Sieper (1972) listed adipose tissue levels of lindane in the general
population: the lowest concentration was 0.015 mg/kg in the UK, and
the highest was 1.19 mg/kg in France.   In 241 human adipose tissue
samples from Japan, the mean concentration of α-HCH was 0.14 mg/kg,
that of β-HCH 1.28 mg/kg, and that of lindane 0.12 mg/kg (Curley *et al.*,
1973).   The total HCH concentration in human adipose tissue samples
taken in Budapest averaged 0.76 mg/kg (Soós *et al.*, 1972); and in
Australia, the value of total HCH varied from 0-2.6 mg/kg in 8/75 human
adipose tissue samples (Brady & Siyali, 1972).

(g) Occupational exposure

In Japan, β-HCH levels in human plasma were measured in 6 occupational groups. The lowest mean levels were found in female farmers (38 μg/1) and the highest mean levels in male workers in pesticide factories (94 μg/l) (Yamaguchi *et al.*, 1976).

2.3 Analysis

Methods used for the analysis of HCH and lindane in environmental samples are listed in Table 2.

The separation of 6 isomers of HCH by thin-layer chromatography alone (Thielemann, 1976) and in combination with gas chromatography (Szokolay *et al.*, 1975) has been investigated. The use of gel-permeation chromatography in an automated system has been proposed (Stalling, 1976).

3. Biological Data Relevant to the Evaluation
of Carcinogenic Risk to Humans

3.1 Carcinogenicity studies in animals[1]

(a) Oral administration

Mouse: Three groups of 20 male dd mice were fed diets containing either 6.6, 66 or 660 mg/kg diet technical HCH, comprising 66.5% α-isomer, 11.4% β-isomer, 15.2% lindane, 6.4% δ-isomer and 0.5% other isomers, for 24 weeks, at which time all animals were killed. Hepatomas were found in 20/20 animals fed 660 mg/kg diet technical HCH, but no such tumours were observed in mice receiving the lower doses. No liver tumours occurred in 14 male controls (Nagasaki *et al.*, 1971, 1972).

In a study reported while the experiment was still in progress, groups of 20 male ICR-JCL mice, aged 5 weeks, were fed 600 mg/kg diet technical HCH, pure α- or β-isomers or lindane or a mixture of δ- and ε-HCH. Further groups of 20 mice received 300 mg/kg diet lindane or a control diet. Gross examination of 10 animals of each group after 26 weeks showed the presence of liver nodules in those receiving 600 mg/kg diet technical HCH, α-HCH, lindane and the δ + ε mixture. Histologically benign liver tumours were observed in all treated groups, except in

---

[1]The Working Group was aware of studies in progress in mice in which α- and β-HCH are given in the diet, and of studies completed, but not published, in mice and rats given lindane in the diet (IARC, 1978).

TABLE 2. METHODS FOR THE ANALYSIS OF HEXACHLOROCYCLOHEXANE (TECHNICAL HCH AND LINDANE)

SAMPLE TYPE	ANALYTICAL METHOD			
	EXTRACTION/CLEAN-UP	DETECTION	LIMIT OF DETECTION	REFERENCE
Formulations	Dissolve (carbon disulphide)	IR	-	US Environmental Protection Agency (1976d) Horwitz (1975)
	Dissolve (chloroform), centrifuge, filter	IR	-	Goza (1972)
Powders (> 10% lindane)	Extract (nitromethane-hexane), filter, CC, evaporate solvent	Weigh residue	-	Horwitz (1975)
Air				
Workplace	Trap in iso-octane	GC/Electrolytic conductivity detection	50 $\mu g/m^3$	National Institute for Occupational Safety & Health (1977)
Atmosphere during field spraying	Trap on Chromosorb 102, extract (hexane-acetone) in Soxhlet	GC/ECD or thermionic detection	< 1 ng/m^3	Thomas & Seiber (1974)
Water	Filter, CC (reversed phase), elute (petroleum ether)	TLC	-	Musty & Nickless (1976)
Soil				
Sediments	Extract (acetone), double CC	TLC (revelation: silver nitrate/ultra-violet)	25 $\mu g/kg$	Taylor et al. (1975)
Sediments and sewage sludge	Centrifuge, extract solid (acetone), liquid/liquid partition, transfer into trimethylpentane, treat to remove sulphur, isolate in trimethylpentane	GC/ECD	1-10 $\mu g/kg$	Jensen et al. (1977)

TABLE 2. METHODS FOR THE ANALYSIS OF HEXACHLOROCYCLOHEXANE
(TECHNICAL HCH AND LINDANE) (continued)

SAMPLE TYPE	ANALYTICAL METHOD			
	EXTRACTION/CLEAN-UP	DETECTION	LIMIT OF DETECTION	REFERENCE
Food				
Vegetables and fruit (except citrus)	Extract (carbon tetrachloride), remove solvent, dechlorinate, nitrate, extract (ether), remove solvent, dissolve (methyl ethyl ketone), add potassium hydroxide	Spectrophotometry (565 nm)	-	Horwitz (1965)
Meat	Macerate with sulphuric acid, steam-distill with carbon tetrachloride, evaporate carbon tetrachloride phase, dissolve residue (acetone)	PC (revelation: fluorescein/ultra-violet)	20 µg/kg	Belonosov (1973)
Barley	Extract (petroleum ether), wash (acid), transfer to hexane	TLC (revelation: ultra-violet)	-	Tikhomirova *et al.* (1975)
Potatoes	Extract (petroleum ether-dichloromethane), CC	TLC	-	Piechocka (1975)
Fruit and vegetables	Extract (acetonitrile), liquid/liquid partition, CC	GC/Thermionic detection, TLC, PC	-	Horwitz (1975)
Eggs	Extract (acetonitrile), liquid/liquid partition, CC	GC/Thermionic detection	-	Finsterwalder (1976)
Biological				
Rat urine, faeces and tissues	Extract (hexane or acetone), liquid/liquid partition	TLC	-	Rao *et al.* (1975)
Rat serum	Extract (hexane) in vortex mixer, centrifuge, separate hexane layer	PC, GC/ECD	15 ng/l	Franken & Luyten (1976)
Bees	Homogenize with acetonitrile, liquid/liquid partition, CC	TLC (revelation: silver nitrate/ultra-violet)	0.1 µg (on the plate)	Stute & Kaufmann (1971)

Abbreviations: IR - infra-red spectrometry; CC - column chromatography; GC - gas chromatography; ECD - electron capture detection; PC - paper chromatography; TLC - thin-layer chromatography

those receiving 300 mg/kg diet lindane.   In animals administered diets
containing α-HCH and the δ + ε mixture, the histological appearance of
tumours was frequently malignant (Goto et al., 1972) [The Working
Group noted that this study was inadequately reported].

Twelve groups of 10-11 dd mice of each sex, aged 6 weeks, were
fed diets containing 100, 300 or 600 mg/kg diet of either α-, β- or
technical HCH or lindane for 32 weeks.   A control group of 21 male and
20 female mice were fed the basal diet.   At 26 weeks, 104 experimental
and 35 control mixe were still alive;   26 male and 27 female experimental animals were laparotomized at this time to observe the condition of
the liver.   All survivors were killed 5-6 weeks after the end of
exposure.   Proportions of mice found to have hepatomas at the end of
the study are shown in Table 3.

Table 3.   Proportions of mice fed various levels of HCH isomers that
developed hepatomas

HCH isomer	Sex	mg/kg diet		
		100	300	600
α-HCH	males	1/8	7/7	7/7
	females	0/8	2/3	6/8
β-HCH	males	0/9	0/8	0/8
	females	0/9	0/8	0/4
Lindane	males	0/10	0/9	3/4
	females	0/8	0/7	1/3
Technical HCH	males	0/10	4/4	4/4
	females	0/8	3/5	5/5

In mice receiving α-HCH and technical HCH, the average size of the
liver tumours was dose-related and ranged from 2 to 11 mm.   No liver
tumours were observed in 14 male and 15 female effective control mice
(Hanada et al., 1973)   [The Working Group noted the short duration of
the experiment and the small size of the experimental groups].

In a series of experiments in 8-week-old male dd mice, either
α-, β- or δ-HCH or lindane (99% pure by gas chromatography) was added
to the diet at concentrations of 100, 250 and 500 mg/kg diet.   Each
group included 20 mice, except for the group that received 250 mg/kg
diet α-HCH, which consisted of 38 mice.   Treatment lasted for 24 weeks,
at which time all survivors were killed.   Hepatocellular carcinomas
up to 2 cm in diameter were found in 10/38 mice that received 250 mg/kg
diet α-HCH and in 17/20 mice that received 500 mg/kg diet α-HCH;   in
the same groups, 30/38 and 20/20 mice, respectively, also had liver

nodular hyperplasia.   Nine additional groups of 26-30 mice were fed
diets containing 50, 100 or 250 mg/kg diet of either α- or β-HCH or
lindane for 24 weeks.   Hepatocellular carcinomas and/or nodular hyperplasia were found only in the group that received 250 mg/kg diet α-HCH
(23/30 with nodular hyperplasia and 8/30 with hepatocellular carcinoma)
(Ito *et al.*, 1973a) [The Working Group noted the short duration of the
experiment].

    In an experiment lasting 110 weeks, a group of 30 male and 30 female
CF1 mice were fed 200 mg/kg diet β-HCH (purity > 99%), and a group of 29
males and 29 females received 400 mg/kg diet lindane (purity, 99.5%).
A group of controls comprising 45 male and 44 female mice were fed a
standard diet.   Benign and malignant liver tumours were found in the
following numbers of animals receiving 0, 200 mg/kg β-HCH or 400 mg/kg
diet lindane: in males, 11 (24%), 22 (73%) and 27 (93%), respectively;
and in females, 10 (23%), 13 (43%) and 20 (69%), respectively.   Lung
metastases were found in 4 (13%) and 3 (10%) male animals receiving
β-HCH and lindane and in 9 (3%) females receiving lindane.   The incidence
of other tumours was not increased by exposure to either isomer (Thorpe
& Walker, 1973).

    The combined effect of the different HCH isomers was investigated
in another study lasting 24 weeks.   Groups of 8-week-old male dd mice
were given 250 mg/kg diet α-HCH only, or this concentration of the α-
isomer plus the same concentration of either β- or δ-HCH or lindane
(each isomer being > 99.0% pure).   Proportions of mice that developed
hepatocellular carcinomas with no metastases were 10/38 in animals given
only the α-isomer and 14/28, 12/28 and 7/28 in those receiving, respectively, α + β, α + lindane and α + δ;   75-93% of the animals also had
nodular hyperplasia.   These observations were considered to indicate
a lack of combined effects of the four HCH isomers.   Combined exposures
of groups of 29 mice to the β-isomer + lindane, to the β- + δ-isomers
and to lindane + the δ-isomer produced no hepatocellular carcinomas.
Only 1 nodular hyperplasia was seen among mice fed the β- + δ-HCH
mixture (Ito *et al.*, 1973b) [The Working Group noted the short duration
of the experiment].

    Twenty male DDY mice, aged 5-6 weeks, were fed a diet containing
500 mg/kg diet α-HCH for 24 weeks, at which time they were killed;
16 controls were fed the basal diet.   Average liver weight in treated
animals was 12.6% of body weight (*versus* 3.7% in controls);   6 treated
mice had well-differentiated hepatocellular carcinomas, and nodular
hyperplasia was found in all treated animals.   No liver lesions were
found in control mice.   In the same series of studies, groups including
13-29 mice of each sex, of the DDY, ICR, DBA/2, C57BL/6 and C3H/He
strains, were fed 500 mg/kg diet α-HCH for 24 weeks, at which time
they were killed;   controls were fed the basal diet.   Hepatocellular
carcinomas were observed in mice of the DDY strain (13/20 males and
5/20 females), the ICR strain (8/23 males and 6/29 females), the DBA/2

strain (1/16 males and 1/15 females) and the C3H/He strain (0/20 males
and 2/20 females), but not among 21 male and 18 female C57BL/6 mice.
Nodular hyperplasia was observed in mice of all strains, the incidence
being the lowest in C57BL/6 mice (4/21 males and 3/18 females) and the
highest in DDY mice (20/20 males and 16/20 females).   No hepatocellular
carcinomas or hyperplasia were found in control mice of any strain
(Nagasaki *et al.*, 1975).

Sixteen groups of 12-21 male DDY mice, 8 weeks old, were fed a
diet containing 500 mg/kg diet α-HCH (> 99.0% pure) for periods of 16,
20, 24 or 36 weeks and were killed at intervals 0-36 weeks later.   All
mice treated for 16 weeks were killed at the end of treatment, and 5/21
had liver tumours up to 1 cm in diameter.   Among mice treated for 20 weeks,
proportions with liver tumours were 14/20, 8/20, 5/20 and 2/19 in those
killed 0, 4, 8 and 12 weeks after the end of treatment, respectively.
Among mice treated for 24 weeks, proportions with liver tumours were
20/20, 18/19, 9/16, 7/17, 8/16, 12/15 and 14/14 among those killed 0,
4, 8, 12, 16, 24 and 32 weeks after the end of treatment.   Among mice
treated for 36 weeks, proportions with liver tumours were 14/14, 11/13,
12/12 and 13/13 in those killed 0, 12, 24 and 36 weeks after the end
of treatment.   No liver tumours were found among 18 control mice
observed for 72 weeks (Ito *et al.*, 1976).

Groups of 50 NMRI mice of each sex received diets containing 12.5,
25 or 50 mg/kg diet lindane (purity not specified), starting at 34 days
of age.   Untreated controls included 100 mice of each sex.   Treatment
lasted 80 weeks, at which time all survivors were killed;   a total of
79 control and treated mice died during the experiment, with no effects
related to treatment.   Liver tumours were found in 4 control males and
1 control female, in 2 males and 1 female fed 12.5 mg/kg diet and in 2
males fed 50 mg/kg diet;   all were liver-cell adenomas, except 1 malignant haemangioendothelioma in a male fed 12.5 mg/kg diet.   A total of
35 animals developed lymphocytic leukaemia or lymphosarcoma (17 controls
and 7, 4 and 7 mice fed 12.5, 25 and 50 mg/kg diet, respectively);   and
50 mice developed lung tumours (21 controls and 11, 8 and 10 mice fed
12.5, 25 and 50 mg/kg diet, respectively).   Other tumours included
8 reticulum-cell neoplasms (1 in controls), and 3 cutaneous or subcutaneous sarcomas (Weisse & Herbst, 1977)   [The Working Group noted the
relatively low dose administered, in comparison with other experiments
with lindane in mice].

Groups of 50 male and 50 female B6C3F1 hybrid mice, 5 weeks of age,
were fed diets containing 80 or 160 mg/kg diet lindane (100% pure)
for 80 weeks, and then observed for an additional 10-11 weeks.   Groups
of 50 mice of each sex were used as controls;   of these only 10 were
fully contemporary to the treated animals, whereas the other 40 overlapped the study with lindane by at least a year.   Survival rates were
similar for treated and control groups: at least 88% of the males and
80% of the females lived to the end of the study.   In males, hepato-

cellular carcinomas were found in 5/49 pooled controls (2/10 matched
controls), in 19/49 mice fed 80 mg/kg diet and in 9/46 mice fed 160 mg/
kg diet.   The corresponding proportions in females were 2/47 (0/10),
2/47 and 3/46.   In addition, 1 mouse of each sex in matched controls,
3 male and 1 female pooled controls, 2 females fed the low dose and 1
male fed the high dose had neoplastic nodules of the liver in the
absence of hepatocellular carcinoma.   Four hepatocellular carcinomas
in males given the low dose produced metastases.   Examination of data
on historical controls at this laboratory indicated that hepatocellular
carcinomas and neoplastic nodules of the liver occurred in 75/360 (20.8%)
male B6C3F1 mice.   In males, the first liver tumour was observed at
60 weeks in those given the low dose, at 77 weeks in controls and at
79 weeks in the high-dose group.   Tumours at other sites occurred
sporadically in all groups (National Cancer Institute, 1977) [The
Working Group noted the relatively low dose used and the small number
of controls contemporary to the experimental groups].

   Rat: Groups of 10 male and 10 female weanling Wistar rats were fed
for lifespan on diets containing 10, 50, 100 or 800 mg/kg diet technical
HCH;   10, 50, 100 or 800 mg/kg diet α-HCH;   10, 100 or 800 mg/kg diet
β-HCH;   5, 10, 50, 100, 400, 800 or 1600 mg/kg diet lindane as a solution
in corn oil;   or 10, 100 or 800 mg/kg diet powdered lindane.   The
technical HCH contained 64% α-, 10% β-, 9% δ- and 1.3% ε-isomers and
13% lindane;   the individual isomers were > 98% pure.   Average lifespan
was significantly reduced in all groups given the 800 mg/kg diet levels,
except for those given powdered lindane;   the mean age at death was 58
weeks in a group of 40 control animals and 33-70 weeks in experimental
groups (4 weeks in the group given 800 mg/kg diet β-HCH).   No increase
in tumour incidence was reported in treated animals;   however, organs were
examined microscopically in only 238 animals, with detailed sectioning of
86 animals (Fitzhugh et al., 1950) [The Working Group noted the early
mortality and the relatively small proportions of rats submitted to
pathological study].

   Male W rats, 5-8 weeks old, were fed diets containing either α-HCH
(500 or 1000 mg/kg diet for 24 or 48 weeks or 1000 or 1500 mg/kg diet
for 72 weeks), β-HCH (500 mg/kg diet for 24 or 48 weeks or 1000 mg/kg
diet for 24 weeks), lindane (500 mg/kg diet for 24 or 48 weeks) or
δ-HCH (500 or 1000 mg/kg diet for 24 or 48 weeks).   Each isomer was
more than 99% pure.   The original sizes of the groups and survival
rates were not reported.   Survivors (5-16 per group) were killed at
the end of the feeding period.   Hepatocellular carcinomas were found
in 3/13 and 1/16 rats fed 1500 and 1000 mg/kg diet α-HCH for 72 weeks.
No liver tumours were found in 31 rats fed 500 or 1000 mg/kg diet α-HCH
for 24 or 48 weeks, or in 59 rats fed the β- or δ-isomers or lindane at
concentrations of 500 or 1000 mg/kg diet for 24 or 48 weeks, or in 8
control rats observed for 72 weeks.   Liver nodular hyperplasia was
found in a total of 27/41 rats fed α-HCH at concentrations of 1000 or
1500 mg/kg diet for at least 48 weeks (Ito et al., 1975) [The Working

Group noted the relatively short duration of the study and the small
sizes of the control and experimental groups].

   Groups of 50 male and 50 female 5-week-old Osborne-Mendel rats
were fed diets containing lindane (100% pure) at two dose levels for
80 weeks and kept under observation for a further 29-30 weeks.   Preliminary experiments had indicated that a dietary concentration of
640 mg/kg diet caused a reversible early decrease in weight gain but
no deaths;   therefore, initial dietary concentrations of lindane were
set at 640 and 320 mg/kg diet.   Because of intercurrent deaths, however,
these concentrations were reduced to half after 2 and 38 weeks of treatment in females and males, respectively;   in females, a further reduction to one-fourth of the original dietary concentration was introduced
49 weeks after the beginning of treatment.   Time-weighted average
dietary concentrations were 236 and 472 mg/kg diet for males and 135
and 270 mg/kg diet for females.   Groups of 55 rats of each sex were
used as controls;   of these only 10 were fully contemporary to the
treated animals, whereas the other 45 overlapped the study with lindane
by at least a year.   Over 80% of rats lived for longer than 52 weeks.
Among male rats, 60%, 50% and 48% were still alive at the end of the
study in the control, low- and high-dose groups;   in females, only 40% of
the controls survived to the end of the study, while at least 60% of the
low- and high-dose groups survived.   Liver lesions were classified
according to Squire & Levitt (1975).   The proportions of animals that
developed neoplastic nodules in the liver and thyroid tumours are shown
in Table 4.   Tumours occurred sporadically at other sites, but their

Table 4.   Proportions of rats fed lindane with neoplastic liver nodules
and thyroid tumours

Tumour type	Sex	Group			
		Matched controls	Pooled controls	Low-dose	High-dose
Neoplastic liver nodules	males	0/10	0/49	3/45	2/45
	females	0/10	1/49	4/48	2/45
Thyroid follicular-cell adenomas or carcinomas	males	1/6	3/42	6/37	4/37
	females	0/8	0/48	2/44	1/42
Thyroid C-cell adenomas	males	1/6	2/42	3/37	1/37
	females	0/8	0/48	4/44^a	3/42

^{a} $p < 0.05$

incidence did not differ between control and treated animals (National
Cancer Institute, 1977)   [The Working Group noted the small number of
contemporary controls and the poor survival rates in all groups.   In

addition, there was no adequate evidence that the dose given to male rats corresponded to the maximum tolerated dose].

(b) Skin application

Mouse: In a study reported while still in progress, a group of 30 stock mice were given twice-weekly applications of a 0.5% solution of lindane in acetone to the skin for 15 months. Twenty-one mice were alive at the time of reporting (at least 15 months), and no skin tumours had occurred (Orr, 1948) [The Working Group noted the inadequacy of the report].

(c) Subcutaneous and/or intramuscular administration

Mouse: In an experiment reported while still in progress, no treatment-related tumours were observed in 12/20 stock mice still alive 10 months after s.c. implantation of a paraffin wax pellet containing 3% lindane (Orr, 1948) [The Working Group noted the inadequacy of the report].

(d) Intraperitoneal administration

Mouse: Three groups of 20 male A/St mice, 6-8 weeks of age, were given thrice weekly i.p. injectins of 8, 20 or 40 mg/kg bw lindane in tricaprylin for 8 weeks. All survivors were killed 24 weeks after the first injection. The number of lung tumours per mouse was not increased in comparison with that in controls injected with tricaprylin (Theiss *et al.*, 1977) [The Working Group noted the limitations of a negative result obtained with this test system; see General Remarks on the Substances Considered, p. 34].

(e) Carcinogenicity of metabolites

Mouse: Three metabolites of HCH, 1,2,4-trichlorobenzene, 2,3,5-trichlorophenol and 2,4,5-trichlorophenol, were administered at concentrations of 600 mg/kg diet to groups of 20 ICR-JCL male mice for 6 months, at which time 10 animals from each group were examined. No liver tumours were observed in these animals, in contrast to parallel experiments in which the same dose levels of HCH isomers (α, β, lindane or a δ + ε mixture) gave rise to benign and/or malignant liver tumours (Goto *et al.*, 1972) (See also monograph on 2,4,5- and 2,4,6-trichlorophenols, p. 349) [The Working Group noted the short duration of the experiment].

3.2 Other relevant biological data

A review on lindane is available (WHO, 1972).

(a) Experimental systems

Toxic effects

The oral LD_{50} of α-HCH is 1000 mg/kg bw in mice and 500-1700 mg/kg bw in rats; that of β-HCH is 1500 mg/kg bw in mice and 2000 mg/kg bw in rats; that of δ-HCH is 750-1000 mg/kg bw in rats; and that of a mixture of HCH isomers is 700 mg/kg bw in mice and 600-1250 mg/kg bw in rats (WHO, 1969).

The oral LD_{50} of lindane is 86 mg/kg bw in mice, 125-230 mg/kg bw in rats, 100-127 mg/kg bw in guinea-pigs and 60-200 mg/kg bw in rabbits (WHO, 1967). The LD_{50} of lindane by topical application in xylene to rats is 900-1000 mg/kg bw (Gaines, 1969).

Signs of acute lindane poisoning in rats include diarrhoea, hypo-thermia, epistaxis and convulsions; death is due to respiratory failure (Chen & Boyd, 1968).

Liver-cell hypertrophy was observed in rats and hamsters fed 500 mg/ kg diet α-HCH for 24 weeks (Nagasaki *et al.*, 1975).

Groups of 10 male and 10 female Wistar rats were administered diets containing 10-1600 mg/kg diet of α- or β-HCH isomers, lindane, technical HCH or powdered lindane for lifespan. Weight gain was reduced in females receiving 100 mg/kg diet β-HCH and in animals of both sexes receiving 800 mg/kg diet α-HCH or technical HCH. Mortality was increased significantly in all groups receiving 800 mg/kg diet of the test compounds, except in those receiving powdered lindane. Fatty dege-neration and focal necrosis of the liver were observed in the higher dose groups. Chronic nephritis with glomerular fibrosis and hyaline deposits was seen in rats fed 800 mg/kg diet α-HCH, powdered lindane or technical HCH (Fitzhugh *et al.*, 1950).

Embryotoxicity and teratogenicity

Daily doses of 0.5 mg/kg bw lindane given orally for 4 months to female rats produced disturbances of the oestrous cycle, inhibited the animals' capacity for conception and fertility, lowered the viability of embryos and delayed their physical development (Naishtein & Leibovich, 1971). Treatment of rats with 0.05 mg/kg bw did not produce such effects (Shtenberg & Mametkuliev, 1976).

No significant teratogenic effect was produced by administration of oral doses of 5, 10 or 20 mg/kg bw lindane on days 6-18 of gestation to rabbits or on days 6-15 of gestation to rats (Palmer *et al.*, 1978).

An increased incidence of stillborn pups was observed in litters of beagle bitches given 7.5 or 15 mg/kg bw/day lindane from day 5 throughout gestation (Earl *et al.*, 1973).

Injection of 2 mg/egg lindane did not decrease the hatchability of hens' eggs (Smith *et al.*, 1970). When Japanese quail eggs were sprayed with 0.15, 0.3 or 0.6% solutions of commercial lindane over 4 generations, reduced fertility, increased embryonic mortality and decreased egg hatchability, production and weight of eggs and chicks were observed (Lutz-Ostertag, 1974).

Absorption, distribution, excretion and metabolism

When single doses of ^{36}Cl-labelled α-HCH and lindane were given intraperitoneally to rats at levels of 200 mg/kg bw and 40 mg/kg bw, respectively, approximately 80% of the total radioactivity was excreted in the urine and 20% in the faeces (Koransky *et al.*, 1964). When labelled β-HCH was administered orally to female Sprague-Dawley rats, 80% was found to have been absorbed (Oshiba, 1972).

In rats fed 800 mg/kg diet α- and δ-HCH and lindane for 20 months, 3.5 mg/g α-isomer, 0.55 mg/g δ-isomer and 0.44 mg/g lindane were found in the adipose tissue; the levels in other tissues were lower by a factor of 5-10. β-HCH fed at 100 mg/kg diet for 20 months was stored to a greater extent, the concentration in adipose tissue being 1.9 mg/g; brain contained 130 μg/g and liver only 20 μg/g. Upon cessation of dietary exposure to HCH isomers, α- and δ-isomers and lindane disappeared from fat depots within 3 weeks, while the β-isomer persisted in the adipose tissue in small amounts after 14 weeks. The α-, β- and δ-isomers of HCH and lindane are stored in the adipose tissue of dogs; the α- and β-isomers are also stored to a lesser degree in the liver, kidneys and adrenals (Davidow & Frawley, 1951). Similar studies have been carried out by Kamada (1971), Koransky & Ullberg (1964), Oshiba (1972) and Oshiba & Kawakita (1972).

Pretreatment of rats with phenobarbital accelerated the rate of excretion of α-HCH and lindane (Koransky *et al.*, 1964).

In mice, urinary metabolites of a single i.p. injection of lindane accounted for 57% of the dose; these consisted mostly of glucuronide and sulphate conjugates of 2,4,6-trichlorophenol and 2,4-dichlorophenol. No mercapturic acid conjugates were detected (Kurihara & Nakajima, 1974).

When lindane was administered intraperitoneally to rats, 2,3,5- and 2,4,5-trichlorophenol were identified in their urine, either free or as conjugates with glucuronic and/or sulphuric acid (Grover & Sims, 1965). When weanling Sprague-Dawley rats were fed 400 mg/kg diet lindane, 3,4-dichlorophenol, 2,4,6-trichlorophenol, 2,3,4,5- and 2,3,4, 6-tetrachlorophenol and 2,3,4,5,6-pentachloro-2-cyclohexene-1-ol were identified in the urine (Chadwick & Freal, 1972). Pentachlorobenzene, 2,3,4,6- and 2,3,5,6-tetrachlorophenol and 2,4,6-trichlorophenol were excreted in the urine of rats given oral doses of lindane (Engst *et al.*, 1976b).

In vitro studies indicate that at least three mechanisms may lead to the formation of trichlorophenols: (1) as a major pathway, a direct hydroxylation of lindane and subsequent decomposition of the labile intermediate to yield 2,4,6-trichlorophenol; (2) dehydrochlorination to pentachlorocyclohexene or dehydrogenation to hexachlorocyclohexene, subsequent addition of oxygen and, following dehydrochlorination, formation of 2,4,5-trichlorophenol and 2,3,4,6-tetrachlorophenol (Freal & Chadwick, 1973); and (3) hydroxylation of the intermediate trichlorobenzene (Tanaka *et al.*, 1977). Pretreatment of rats with other organochlorine pesticides modified lindane metabolism (Chadwick *et al.*, 1977a,b; Freal & Chadwick, 1973).

In rats, 65% of an i.p. dose of ^{14}C-α-HCH was excreted in the urine and 16% in the faeces within 4 weeks. Conjugated 2,4,6-trichlorophenol was the major urinary metabolite; chlorothiophenols were also detected in the urine, and the proportion increased when animals were pretreated with α-HCH (Koransky *et al.*, 1975).

Mutagenicity and other related short-term tests

Lindane was not mutagenic in the host-mediated assay when *Salmonella typhimurium* (strain G46) and *Serratia marcescens* (strain a21) were used for reversion studies (Buselmaier *et al.*, 1972). HCH (a mixture of α- and β-isomers and lindane) was negative in the *rec* assay with *Bacillus subtilis* (Shirasu *et al.*, 1976). Exposure to lindane was not accompanied by an increase in respiration-deficient yeast mutants (Schubert, 1969). Reversion studies using *Saccharomyces cerevisiae* (strain XV185-14C) were also negative with α-HCH, both in the presence and absence of a mouse liver microsomal activation system (Shahin & von Borstel, 1977). No sex-linked recessive mutants were found in *Drosophila melanogaster* injected with a 0.001% solution of lindane (Benes & Sram, 1969).

Although it does not induce mutations, lindane is potent in inducing complete c-mitosis (colchicine-like effect; mitotic arrest at metaphase) in *Allium cepa* roots. The α-isomer, on the other hand, induced only partial c-mitosis, and the β-isomer was ineffective (Nybom & Knutsson, 1947). Induction of mitotic arrest, as well as polyploidy, by lindane have also been recorded in root tips of 8 varieties of common pulses, including *Pisum sativum* (Baquar & Khan, 1971; Sharma & Gosh, 1969). Commercially available powder and liquid insecticide preparations containing lindane (10 or 20%) and lindane crystals (100% pure) induced chromosome aberrations in *Allium cepa* roots (Sax & Sax, 1968).

In rats given 0.06% α-HCH in their diet for 3 weeks, there was a marked increase in mitotic rate in the liver parenchymal cells. Nearly one-third of the cells were tetraploid, and several cells had marker chromosomes. The cytogenetic changes observed were qualitatively similar to those seen in regenerating liver after partial hepatectomy (Hitachi *et al.*, 1975). Chromosome breaks and gaps were observed in

metaphase preparations of bone-marrow cells from rats injected with
0.01-10 mM/kg bw β-HCH solution (Shimazu *et al.*, 1976).

Lindane caused a slight increase in the frequencies of chromatid
gaps and breaks in Chinese hamster fibroblasts *in vitro* (Ishidate &
Odashima, 1977).

Concentrations of 5-10 µg/ml lindane inhibited cell division in
human peripheral blood lymphocytes *in vitro* and caused a concentration-
related increase in the frequency of chromatid breaks (Tzoneva-Maneva
et al., 1971).   In SV40-transformed human fibroblasts (VA-4), 1 or 1000
µM lindane failed to induce unscheduled DNA synthesis either in the
presence or absence of a rat liver microsomal activation system (Ahmed
et al., 1977).

(b)   Humans

The toxicity of lindane to humans has been reviewed; therapeutic
doses used in the treatment of scabies have been found to have neurotoxic and other effects (e.g., nausea, convulsions, cyanosis) (Solomon
et al., 1977).   Ingestion of large (unspecified) doses has led to muscle
and kidney necrosis and, in one case, to pancreatitis (Munk & Nantel,
1977).   Digestive tract inflammation, haemorrhage, coma and death have
been reported after lindane poisoning (Herbst & Bodenstein, 1972).

Cirrhosis and chronic hepatitis were observed in liver biopsies
from 8 workers heavily exposed to lindane, DDT or both for periods
ranging from 5-13 years (Schüttmann, 1968).

The occurrence of HCH isomers in human tissues is discussed in
section 2.2 (f).   Trace amounts of HCH have been detected in human milk
and blood (Curley & Kimbrough, 1969; D'Ercole *et al.*, 1976; Grasso
et al., 1973), and transplacental passage of HCH has been established
(Curley *et al.*, 1969; D'Ercole *et al.*, 1976; Grasso *et al.*, 1973).

In an 18-month-old infant fatally poisoned with lindane, about
350 mg/kg were found in the adipose tissue and 88 mg/kg in the liver
(Joslin *et al.*, 1958).   Following the accidental ingestion of lindane
by a 2½-year-old girl, 0.84 and 0.49 mg/l lindane were found in the
serum after 2 and 4 hrs, respectively.   Unchanged compound was found
in the faeces; and several urinary metabolites, 2,4-dichloro-, 2,4,6-
trichloro-, 2,3,5-trichloro-, 2,4,5-trichloro- and 2,3,4,6-tetrachloro-
phenols and 2,4-dichloromercapturic acid, were identified (Starr &
Clifford, 1972).

3.3 Case reports and epidemiological studies

Approximately 30 cases of aplastic anaemia associated with exposure
to HCH or lindane have been reported (Hans, 1976; Loge, 1965; West,
1967; Woodliff *et al.*, 1966).   At least 10 further cases were associated with exposure to HCH or lindane in combination with other
compounds, mainly DDT (Hans, 1976; Woodliff *et al.*, 1966).

Aplastic anaemia has also been reported in people exposed to HCH
or lindane in consumer products: 2 were exposed to lindane by frequent
treatment of dogs with products containing the compound, and at least
3 were exposed to lindane as a result of vaporization in their houses
(Hans, 1976; Loge, 1965; West, 1967; Woodliff *et al.*, 1966).

A case of acute myelomonocytic leukaemia, secondary to aplastic
anaemia, was associated with dermal exposure to a lindane/toxaphene
mixture (US Environmental Protection Agency, 1978).

The simultaneous development of acute paramyeloblastic leukaemia
in two cousins, both aged 20, exposed at the same time to lindane while
unloading sacks of insecticide, has also been reported (Jedlička *et al.*,
1958) [The Working Group noted that constitutional, hereditary,
familial and other common exposure factors may, or may not, have played
a role in the etiology of these two cases of leukaemia].

An increased incidence of lung cancer was reported between 1970
and 1975 in 285 workers who had applied various pesticides, including
HCH, in agricultural settings;   their ages ranged from 36-74 years
(Barthel, 1976) [The Working Group noted that since exposure may have
been to compounds other than HCH or in addition to HCH, no evaluation
of the carcinogenicity of HCH could be made on the basis of this study.
However, the increased incidence was too high to be accounted for by
smoking alone].

4. Summary of Data Reported and Evaluation

4.1 Experimental data

α-HCH was tested in several experiments in mice by oral administration: it produced benign and malignant liver tumours in animals of
both sexes;   a treatment of 16 weeks was sufficient to produce tumours.
Two feeding experiments in rats, one of which suggested a carcinogenic
effect on the liver, were considered to be inadequate.

β-HCH was tested in four experiments in mice by oral administration:
two were inadequate, and another was inadequately reported but suggested
hepatocarcinogenicity;   in the fourth study, β-HCH induced benign and
malignant liver tumours in animals of both sexes.   Two feeding experiments

in rats were considered to be inadequate.

Lindane was tested in six experiments in mice by oral administration: it produced benign and malignant liver tumours in animals of both
sexes in two experiments, one of which involved only small groups of
animals.   The results of a third experiment suggested hepatocarcinogenicity but were inadequately reported.   The results of a fourth experiment
also suggested hepatocarcinogenicity but were considered inadequate
because of the low number of control animals used.   The other experiments
were considered inadequate for an evaluation of carcinogenicity.   Lindane
was also tested in three feeding studies in rats: two were considered
inadequate; in the other a slight excess of thyroid tumours was observed
in females.   Lindane was tested inadequately in mice by skin application
and by subcutaneous and intraperitoneal administration.

Experimental data on the long-term effects of the δ- and ε-isomers
were considered to be inadequate.

Technical HCH was tested in three experiments in mice by oral administration, producing liver tumours.   A feeding experiment in rats was
considered to be inadequate.

Lindane is embryotoxic.   α- and β-HCH and lindane, when tested
individually and/or as a mixture, were not mutagenic in bacteria, yeast
or *Drosophila*.   Lindane induces chromosome aberrations, polyploidy and
mitotic arrest in a number of plant systems.   It also induced chromatid
breaks in human lymphocytes *in vitro*.

4.2 Human data

Several case reports indicate a relationship between exposure to HCH
or lindane and the occurrence of aplastic anaemia.   Two cases of acute
myeloid-type leukaemia in cousins exposed to lindane and one case of
acute myelomonocytic leukaemia, secondary to aplastic anaemia, that was
associated with dermal exposure to a lindane/toxaphene mixture have also
been reported.

The only epidemiological study related to possible carcinogenic
effects of HCH or lindane in humans involved exposure to many pesticides;
the Working Group was thus unable to draw any conclusion specific to
HCH or lindane.

The extensive production of HCH and lindane and their use in veterinary, agricultural and consumer products since the early 1950s indicate
that widespread human exposure occurs.   This is confirmed by many reports
of their occurrence in the general environment and by reports of their
presence in body fluids and tissues, both in the general population and
in exposed workers.

4.3 Evaluation

There is *sufficient evidence* that α-HCH, lindane and technical HCH are carcinogenic in mice; there is *limited evidence* that β-HCH is carcinogenic in mice.

5. References

Achari, R.G., Sandhu, S.S. & Warren, W.J. (1975) Chlorinated hydrocarbon residues in ground water. Bull. environ. Contam. Toxicol., 13, 94-96

Adamovic, V.M., Sokic, B., Petrovic, O., Pantovic, D. & Dragovic, R. (1975) Daily intake of some pesticides and total amount of arsenic in food by Belgrade residents (Croat). Hrana Ishrana, 16, 283-290 [Chem. Abstr., 84, 15779u]

Ahmed, F.E., Hart, R.W. & Lewis, N.J. (1977) Pesticide induced DNA damage and its repair in cultured human cells. Mutat. Res., 42, 161-174

Andryushchenko, V.V., Kulebakina, L.G. & Girenko, D.B. (1975) Organochlorine pesticides in the water and organisms of the Mediterranean Sea (Russ.). In: Polikarpov, G.G., ed., Radiochemo-Ecological Studies of the Mediterranean Sea, Kiev, Naukova Dumka, pp. 17-33 [Chem. Abstr., 85, 154824p]

Arthur, R.D., Cain, J.D. & Barrentine, B.F. (1976) Atmospheric levels of pesticides in the Mississippi delta. Bull. environ. Contam. Toxicol., 15, 129-134

Astolfi, E., Garcia Fernandez, J.C., DeJuarez, M.B. & Piacentino, H. (1973) Chlorinated pesticides found in the fat of children in the Argentine Republic. In: Deichmann, W.B., ed., Papers of the 8th Inter-America Conference on Toxicology and Occupational Medicine, Pesticides and the Environment: Continuing Controversy, New York, Stratton, pp. 233-243 [Chem. Abstr., 84, 145686x]

Avancini, D. & Stringari, G. (1974) Determination of chlorinated and phosphorated pesticide residues in fruit of Trentino-Alto Adige (Ital). Ind. Agrar., 12, 53-56 [Chem. Abstr., 83, 7316e]

Baquar, S.R. & Khan, N.R. (1971) Effect of γ-hexachlorocyclohexane (HCCH) on the mitotic cells of Pisum sativum L. Rev. Biol. (Lisbon), 7, 195-202

Barthel, E. (1976) High incidence of lung cancer in persons with chronic professional exposure to pesticides in agriculture (Germ.). Z. Erkrank. Atm.-Org., 146, 266-274

Belonosov, V.M. (1973) Use of paper chromatography to determine residual amounts of hexachloran in meat (Russ.). Tr. Uzb. Nauchno-Issled. Vet. Inst., 23, 62-65 [Chem. Abstr., 83, 191446w]

Benes, V. & Sram, R. (1969) Mutagenic activity of some pesticides in Drosophila melanogaster. Ind. Med., 38, 442-444

Berg, G.L., ed. (1978) Farm Chemicals Handbook, 1978, Willoughby, OH, Meister Publishing Co., pp. D35, D156

Blaquiere, C. (1972) H. Legal regulations pertaining to trade and use of lindane. In: Ulmann, E., ed., Lindane, Monograph of an Insecticide, Freiburg, K. Schillinger, pp. 263-335

Blaquiere, C. (1976a) H. Legal regulations pertaining to trade and use of lindane. In: Ulmann, E., ed., Lindane. II. Supplement 1976, Freiburg, K. Schillinger, pp. 74-122

Blaquiere, C. (1976b) Lindane - Legislation. In - European Symposium on Lindane, Lyon, 1976, Brussels, Centre International d'Etudes au Lindane, pp. 113-115

Boado, A., Simal, J., Charro, A. & Creus, J.M. (1975) Residues of poly-chlorinated biphenyl pesticides in the mollusks of Ria de Arosa (Span.). Anal. Bromatol., 27, 63-100

Brady, M.N. & Siyali, D.S. (1972) Hexachlorobenzene in human body fat. Med. J. Aust., 1, 158-161

Brodtmann, N.V., Jr (1976) Continuous analysis of chlorinated hydrocarbon pesticides in the lower Mississippi River. Bull. environ. Contam. Toxicol., 15, 33-39

Buselmaier, W., Röhrborn, G. & Propping, P. (1972) Mutagenicity investigations with pesticides in the host-mediated assay and the dominant lethal test in mice (Germ.). Biol. Zbl., 91, 311-325

Carrasco, J.M., Cunat, P., Martinez, M. & Primo, E. (1976) Pesticide residues in total diet samples, Spain - 1971-72. Pestic. Monit. J., 10, 18-23

Cerutti, G., Zappavigna, R., Gerosa, A. & Proverbio, A. (1975) Organo-chloride parasiticide residues in cow's and sheep's milk, yogurt, and cream (Ital.). Latte, 3, 547-552 [Chem. Abstr., 84, 103912n]

Cerutti, G., Gerosa, A., Zappavigna, R. & Pirovano, G. (1976) Residues of organochlorine pesticides in human milk (Ital.). Latte, 1, 317-321 [Chem. Abstr., 86, 134522f]

Chadwick, R.W. & Freal, J.J. (1972) The identification of five unreported lindane metabolites recovered from rat urine. Bull. environ. Contam. Toxicol., 7, 137-146

Chadwick, R.W., Chadwick, C.J., Freal, J.J. & Bryden, C.C. (1977a) Comparative enzyme induction and lindane metabolism in rats pre-treated with various organochlorine pesticides. Xenobiotica, 7, 235-246

Chadwick, R.W., Simmons, W.S., Bryden, C.C., Chuang, L.T., Key, L.M. & Chadwick, C.J. (1977b) Effect of dietary lipid and dimethyl sulfoxide on lindane metabolism. Toxicol. appl. Pharmacol., 39, 391-410

Chen, C.P. & Boyd, E.M. (1968) The acute oral toxicity of gamma benzene hexachloride (Abstract No. 377). Can. Fed. Biol. Soc., 11, 135

Clark, D.E., Smalley, H.E., Crookshank, H.R. & Farr, F.M. (1974) Chlorinated hydrocarbon insecticide residues in feed and carcasses of feedlot cattle, Texas - 1972. Pestic. Monit. J., 8, 180-183

Cocisiu, M., Nistor, C., Aizicovici, H., Pencescu, E., Alexandrescu, D., Mauca, M. & Iordachescu, D. (1975a) Residues of organochlorine insecticides DDT and HCH in total lunches and in samples of cow milk (Rom.). Rev. Ig., Bacteriol., Virusol., Parazitol., Epidemiol., Pneumoftiziol., Ig., 24, 83-86 [Chem. Abstr., 85, 158037g]

Cocisiu, M., Aizicovici, H. & Nistor, C. (1975b) Contamination of humans with DDT and HCH in some areas in our country [Roumania] (Rom.). Rev. Ig., Bacteriol., Virusol., Parazitol., Epidemiol., Pneumoftiziol., Ig., 24, 31-35 [Chem. Abstr., 85, 154801d]

Curley, A. & Kimbrough, R. (1969) Chlorinated hydrocarbon insecticides in plasma and milk of pregnant and lactating women. Arch. environ. Health, 18, 156-164

Curley, A., Copeland, M.F. & Kimbrough, R.D. (1969) Chlorinated hydrocarbon insecticides in organs of stillborn and blood of newborn babies. Arch. environ. Health, 19, 628-632

Curley, A., Burse, V.W., Jennings, R.W., Villanueva, E.C., Tomatis, L. & Akazaki, K. (1973) Chlorinated hydrocarbon pesticides and related compounds in adipose tissue from people of Japan. Nature (Lond.), 242, 338-340

Davidow, B. & Frawley, J.P. (1951) Tissue distribution, accumulation and elimination of the isomers of benzene hexachloride. Proc. Soc. exp. Biol. (NY), 76, 780-783

Deelstra, H. (1974) Secondary effects in the use of pesticides around Lake Tanganyika (Fr.). Trib. Cent. Belge Et. Doc. Eaux Air, 27, 93-96 [Chem. Abstr., 83, 54507c]

Demozay, D. & Marechal, G. (1972a) B. Physical and chemical properties. In: Ulmann, E., ed., Lindane, Monograph of an Insecticide, Freiburg, K. Schillinger, pp. 15-18

Demozay, D. & Marechal, G. (1972b) A. Introduction. In: Ulmann, E., ed., Lindane, Monograph of an Insecticide, Freiburg, K. Schillinger, p. 14

Demozay, D. & Marechal, G. (1972c) G. Applications of lindane. In: Ulmann, E., ed., Lindane, Monograph of an Insecticide, Freiburg, K. Schillinger, pp. 163-262

D'Ercole, A.J., Arthur, R.D., Cain, J.D. & Barrentine, B.F. (1976) Insecticide exposure of mothers and newborns in a rural agricultural area. Pediatrics, 57, 869-874

Durham, W.F. (1969) Body burden of pesticides in man. Ann. NY Acad. Sci., 160, 183-195

Earl, F.L., Miller, E. & Van Loon, E.J. (1973) Reproductive, teratogenic and neonatal effects of some pesticides and related compounds in beagle dogs and miniature swine. In: Deichmann, W.B., ed., Papers of the 8th Inter-America Conference on Toxicology and Occupational Medicine, Pesticides and the Environment: Continuing Controversy, Vol. 2, New York, Stratton, pp. 253-266

Economic Documentation Office (1973) Entoma Europe, 1973-1975, Hilversum, The Netherlands

Engst, R., Knoll, R., Morzek-Drux, A. & Hocke, R. (1976a) Chlorinated hydrocarbons in the daily diet (Ger.). Nahrung, 20, 359-368 [Chem. Abstr., 85, 121958g]

Engst, R., Macholz, R.M., Kujawa, M., Lewerenz, H.-J. & Plass, R. (1976b) The metabolism of lindane and its metabolites gamma-2,3,4,5,6-pentachlorocyclohexene, pentachlorobenzene, and pentachlorophenol in rats and the pathways of lindane metabolism. J. environ. Sci. Health, B11, 95-117

Estep, C.B., Menon, G.N., Williams, H.E. & Cole, A.C. (1977) Chlorinated hydrocarbon insecticide residues in Tennessee honey and beeswax. Bull. environ. Contam. Toxicol., 17, 168-174

Eurocop-Cost (1976) A Comprehensive List of Polluting Substances which have been Identified in Various Fresh Waters, Effluent Discharges, Aquatic Animals and Plants, and Bottom Sediments, 2nd ed., EUCO/MDU/73/76, XII/476/76, Luxembourg, Commission of the European Communities, pp. 26-28

EUROSTAT (1975) Analytical Tables of Foreign Trade, Vol. C, Chapters 28-38 (Products of the chemical and allied industries), Luxembourg, Statistical Office of the European Communities, pp. 48-49, 256-257

FAO/WHO (1978) Pesticide residues in food - 1977. FAO Plant Production and Protection Paper, 10th rev., pp. 39-40

Finsterwalder, C.E. (1976) Collaborative study of an extension of the Mills et al. method for the determination of pesticide residues in foods. J. Assoc. off. anal. Chem., 59, 169-171

Fitzhugh, O.G., Nelson, A.A. & Frawley, J.P. (1950) The chronic toxicities
    of technical benzene hexachloride and its alpha, beta and gamma
    isomers. J. Pharmacol. exp. Ther., 100, 59-66

Floru, S., Polizu, A. & Manolache, L. (1975) Organochlorine pesticide
    residues in the wild rabbit (Rom.). Stud. Cercet. Biol., 27, 353-355
    [Chem. Abstr., 85, 73128n]

Franken, J.J. & Luyten, B.J.M. (1976) Comparison of dieldrin, lindane,
    and DDT extractions from serum, and gas-liquid chromatography using
    glass capillary columns. J. Assoc. off. anal. Chem., 59, 1279-1285

Freal, J.J. & Chadwick, R.W. (1973) Metabolism of hexachlorocyclohexane
    to chlorophenols and effect of isomer pretreatment on lindane meta-
    bolism in rat. J. agric. Food Chem., 21, 424-427

Gaines, T.B. (1969) Acute toxicity of pesticides. Toxicol. appl. Pharmacol.
    11, 515-534

Goto, M., Hattori, M., Miyagawa, T. & Enomoto, M. (1972) Contribution
    to ecological chemistry. II. Hepatoma formation in mice after
    administration of HCH isomers in high doses (Germ.). Chemosphere,
    6, 279-282

Goza, S.W. (1972) Infrared analysis of pesticide formulations. J. Assoc.
    off. anal. Chem., 55, 913-917

Grasselli, J.G. & Ritchey, W.M., eds (1975) CRC Atlas of Spectral Data
    and Physical Constants for Organic Compounds, 2nd ed., Vol. III,
    Cleveland, OH, Chemical Rubber Co., pp. 111-112

Grasso, C., Bernardi, G. & Martinelli, F. (1973) Significance of the
    presence of chlorinated insecticides in the blood of newborn children
    and of their mothers (Ital.). Ig. Mod., 66, 362-371

Griffith, F.D., Jr & Blanke, R.V. (1975) Blood organochlorine pesticide
    levels in Virginia residents. Pestic. Monit. J., 8, 219-224

Grover, P.L. & Sims, P. (1965) The metabolism of γ-2,3,4,5,6-pentachloro-
    cyclohex-1-ene and γ-hexachlorocyclohexane in rats. Biochem. J., 96,
    521-525

Hamelink, J.L. & Waybrant, R.C. (1973) Factors Controlling the Dynamics
    of Non-Ionic Synthetic Organic Chemicals in Aquatic Environments,
    Technical Report No. 44, West Lafayette, IN, Purdue University,
    Water Resources Research Center, pp. 34-42

Hanada, M., Yutani, C. & Miyaji, T. (1973) Induction of hepatoma in
    mice by benzene hexachloride. Gann, 64, 511-513

Hans, R.J. (1976) Aplastic anemia associated with γ-benzene hexachloride. J. Am. med. Assoc., 236, 1009-1010

Hardie, D.W.F. (1964) Chlorocarbons and chlorohydrocarbons. Benzene hexachloride. In: Kirk, R.E. & Othmer, D.F., eds, Encyclopedia of Chemical Technology, 2nd ed., Vol. 5, New York, John Wiley & Sons, pp. 267-281, 374

Hashemy-Tonkabony, S.E. & Asadi Langaroodi, F. (1976) Detection and determination of chlorinated pesticide residues in Caspian Sea fish by gas-liquid chromatography. Environ. Res., 12, 275-280

Hashemy-Tonkabony, S.E. & Soleimani-Amiri, M.J. (1976) Detection and determination of chlorinated pesticide residues in raw and various stages of processed vegetable oil. J. Am. Oil Chem. Soc., 53, 752-753

Heeschen, W., Bluethgen, A. & Tolle, A. (1976) Residues of chlorinated hydrocarbons in milk and milk products - situation and evaluation (Ger.). Zbl. Bakteriol., Parasitenkd., Infektionskr., Hyg., Abt. 1: Orig., Reihe B,, 162, 188-197 [Chem. Abstr., 85, 107575y]

Herbst, M. & Bodenstein, G. (1972) C. Toxicology of lindane. In: Ulmann, E., ed., Lindane, Monograph of an Insecticide, Freiburg, K. Schillinger, pp. 23-113

Herzel, F. (1972) Organochlorine insecticides in surface waters in Germany - 1970 and 1971. Pestic. Monit. J., 6, 179-187

Hirano, C. & Katada, K. (1975) Residues of chlorinated hydrocarbon insecticides in some components of the Koso River in Kochi 5 years after the prohibition of their use (Jap.). Bochu-Kagaku, 40, 132-137 [Chem. Abstr., 84, 140556v]

Hitachi, M., Yamada, K. & Takayama, S. (1975) Cytologic changes induced in rat liver cells by short-term exposure to chemical substances. J. natl Cancer Inst., 54, 1245-1247

Hooker Chemical Corporation (1969) FBHC, Fortified Benzene Hexachloride, Bulletin No. 480, Industrial Chemicals Division, Niagara Falls, NY, pp. 1-4

Hooker Chemical Corporation (1973) Lindane HGI® (Hexachlorocyclohexane), Bulletin No. 475-A, Specialty Chemicals Division, Niagara Falls, NY, pp. 1-3

Horwitz, W., ed. (1965) Official Methods of Analysis of the Association of Official Agricultural Chemists, 10th ed., Washington DC, Association of Official Agricultural Chemists, pp. 386-390

Horwitz, W., ed. (1975) Official Methods of Analysis of the Association of Official Analytical Chemists, 12th ed., Washington DC, Association of Official Analytical Chemists, pp. 101-103, 518-528, 534

Hruska, J. & Kocianova, M. (1975) Contamination of the food chain by chlorinated insecticides in southern Bohemia (Czech.). Cesk. Hyg., 20, 421-428 [Chem. Abstr., 84, 100482m]

IARC (1974) IARC Monographs on the Evaluation of the Carcinogenic Risk of Chemicals to Man, 5, Some Organochlorine Pesticides, Lyon, pp. 47-74

IARC (1978) Information Bulletin on the Survey of Chemicals Being Tested for Carcinogenicity, No. 7, Lyon, pp. 127-128, 269

Ishidate, M., Jr & Odashima, S. (1977) Chromosome tests with 134 compounds on Chinese hamster cells in vitro - A screening for chemical carcinogens. Mutat. Res., 48, 337-354

Ito, N., Nagasaki, H. & Arai, M. (1973a) Interactions of liver tumorigenesi in mice treated with technical polychlorinated biphenyls (PCBs) and benzene hexachloride (BHC). In: Coulston, F., Korte, F. & Goto, M., eds, New Methods in Environmental Chemistry and Ecological Chemistry, Tokyo, International Academic Printing Company, pp. 141-147

Ito, N., Nagasaki, H., Arai, M., Sugihara, S. & Makiura, S. (1973b) Histologic and ultrastructural studies on the hepatocarcinogenicity of benzene hexachloride in mice. J. natl Cancer Inst., 51, 817-826

Ito, N., Nagasaki, H., Aoe, H., Sugihara, S., Miyata, Y., Arai, M. & Shirai, T. (1975) Development of hepatocellular carcinomas in rats treated with benzene hexachloride. J. natl Cancer Inst., 54, 801-805

Ito, N., Hananouchi, M., Sugihara, S., Shirai, T., Tsuda, H., Fukushima, S. & Nagasaki, H. (1976) Reversibility and irreversibility of liver tumors in mice induced by the α isomer of 1,2,3,4,5,6-hexachlorocyclohexane. Cancer Res., 36, 2227-2234

Jedlička, V., Heřmanská, Z., Šmída, I. & Kouba, A. (1958) Paramyeloblastic leukaemia appearing simultaneously in two blood cousins after simultaneous contact with gammexane (hexachlorcyclohexane). Acta med. scand., 161, 447-451

Jeng, S.S. & Sun, L.T. (1974) Organochlorine pesticide residues in cultured fishes of Taiwan. Bull. Inst. Zool., Acad. Sin., 13, 37-45 [Chem. Abstr., 83, 127136t]

Jensen, S., Renberg, L. & Reutergårdh, L. (1977) Residue analysis of sediment and sewage sludge for organochlorines in the presence of elemental sulfur. Anal. Chem., 49, 316-318

Joslin, E.F., Forney, R.L., Huntington, R.W., Jr & Hayes, W.J., Jr (1958) A fatal case of lindane poisoning. In: Proceedings of the National Association of Coroners, San Diego, California, 1958, pp. 53-57

Kamada, T. (1971) Hygienic studies on pesticide residues. I. Accumula-
    tion of BHC (α-, β-, γ- and δ-) isomers in rat bodies and excretion
    into urine following oral administration (Jap.). Nippon Eiseigaku
    Zasshi, 26, 358-364

Kan, C.A. & Tuinstra, L.G.M.T. (1976) Accumulation and excretion of
    certain organochlorine insecticides in broiler breeder hens.
    J. agric. Food Chem., 24, 775-778

Kaneshima, H., Kitayama, M., Yamada, M. & Ogawa, H. (1976) Environmental
    pollution and wild birds in Hokkaido. V. Chlorinated hydrocarbon
    pesticides and PCB residues in crows (Jap.). Hokkaidoritsu Eisei
    Kenkyusho Ho, 26, 70-72 [Chem. Abstr., 86, 145060e]

Kastrup, E.K., ed. (1976) Scabicides and/or pediculocides. Facts and
    Comparisons, St Louis, MO, Facts & Comparisons, Inc., p. 585

Kitayama, M., Kaneshima, H. & Ogawa, H. (1976) Prevention of poisoning
    by agricultural chemicals. XXII. Residues of agricultural chemicals
    in rivers of agricultural areas (Jap.). Hokkaidoritsu Eisei Kenkyusho
    Ho, 26, 63-66 [Chem. Abstr., 86, 145406x]

Koransky, W. & Ullberg, S. (1964) Distribution in the brain of ^{14}C-
    benzenehexachloride: autoradiographic study. Biochem. Pharmacol.,
    13, 1537-1538

Koransky, W., Portig, J., Vohland, H.W. & Klempau, I. (1964) Elimination of
    α- and γ-hexachlorocyclohexane and their influence on liver microsome
    enzymes (Germ.). Naunyn-Schmiedebergs Arch. exp. Path. Pharmakol., 247,
    49-60

Koransky, W., Münch, G., Noack, G., Portig, J., Sodomann, S. & Wirsching, M.
    (1975) Biodegradation of α-hexachlorocyclohexane. V. Characteri-
    zation of the major urinary metabolites. Naunyn-Schmiedeberg's Arch.
    exp. Path. Pharmacol., 288, 65-78

Kurihara, N. & Nakajima, M. (1974) Studies on BHC isomers and related
    compounds. VIII. Urinary metabolites produced from γ- and β-BHC in
    the mouse: chlorophenol conjugates. Pestic. Biochem. Physiol., 4,
    220-231

Kutz, F.W., Yobs, A.R., Johnson, W.G. & Wiersma, G.B. (1974) Pesticide
    residues in adipose tissue of the general population of the United
    States, FY 1970 survey. Bull. Soc. Pharmacol. Environ. Pathol., 2,
    4-10 [Chem. Abstr., 84, 13218m]

Lahav, N. & Kahanovitch, Y. (1974) Lindane residues in the southern coastal
    aquifer of Israel. Water Air Soil Pollut., 3, 253-259

Loge, J.P. (1965) Aplastic anemia following exposure to benzene hexachlo-
    ride (lindane). J. Am. med. Assoc., 193, 104-108

Lutz-Ostertag, Y. (1974) Study over several generations of the effects of
    lindane on fertility rate and embryo mortality, hatching, laying, and
    the weight of eggs and chicks (Fr.). Arch. Anat. Hist. Embr. norm.
    exp., 57, 269-282

Maier, D. & Wendlandt, E. (1976) Studies on the content of organochloride
    pesticides in Lake Constance, in the Ueberlinger area (Germ.).
    Z. Wasser-Abwasser-Forsch., 9, 53-55

Mamarbachi, G. & St-Jean, R. (1976) Pesticides and PCB in the Richelieu
    and Missisquoi rivers (Fr.). Eau Que., 9, 31, 33-35 [Chem. Abstr., 85,
    29559e]

Masahiro, O. & Takahisa, H. (1975) Alpha- and gamma-BHC in Tokyo rain-
    water (December 1968 to November 1969). Environ. Pollut., 9, 283-288

Mathur, S.P. & Saha, J.G. (1977) Degradation of lindane-^{14}C in a mineral
    soil and in an organic soil. Bull. environ. Contam. Toxicol., 17,
    424-430

Melnikova, L.V., Belyakov, A.A., Smirnova, V.G. & Kurenko, L.T. (1975)
    Sanitary-chemical method of determining noxious substances
    encountered in the production of sodium pentachlorophenolate (Russ.).
    Gig. Tr. Prof. Zabol., 7, 37-39

Mendola, J.T., Risebrough, R.W. & Blondel, J. (1977) Contamination of
    Camargue birds by residues of chlorinated organic compounds (Fr.).
    Environ. Pollut., 13, 21-31

Mercier, M. (1975) Preparatory Study for Establishing Criteria (Dose/
    Effect Relationships) for Humans on Organochlorine Compounds, i.e.
    Pesticides and their Metabolites, Doc. No. 1347/75e, Luxembourg,
    Commission of the European Communities, pp. 27, 67-77, 173-175, 217-218

Munk, Z.M. & Nantel, A. (1977) Acute lindane poisoning with development
    of muscle necrosis. Can. med. Assoc. J., 117, 1050-1054

Musty, P.R. & Nickless, G. (1976) Extractants for organochlorine insecti-
    cides and polychlorinated biphenyls from water. J. Chromatogr.,
    120, 369-378

Nagasaki, H., Tomii, S., Mega, T., Marugami, M. & Ito, N. (1971) Develop-
    ment of hepatomas in mice treated with bezene hexachloride. Gann,
    62, 431

Nagasaki, H., Tomii, S., Mega, T., Marugami, M. & Ito, N. (1972) Carcino-
    genicity of benzene hexachloride (BHC). In: Nakahara, W.,
    Takayama, S., Sugimura, T. & Odashima, S., eds, Topics in Chemical
    Carcinogenesis, Tokyo, University of Tokyo Press, pp. 343-353

Nagasaki, H., Kawabata, H., Miyata, Y., Inoue, K., Hirao, K., Aoe, H. &
    Ito, N. (1975) Effect of various factors on induction of liver
    tumors in animals by the α-isomer of benzene hexachloride. Gann,
    66, 185-191

Naishtein, S.Y. & Leibovich, D.L. (1971) Effect of small doses of DDT
    and lindane and their mixture on sexual function and embryogenesis
    in rats. Hyg. Sanit., 36, 190-195

Nalley, L., Hoff, G., Bigler, W. & Hull, W. (1975) Pesticide levels in
    the omental fat of Florida raccoons. Bull. environ. Contam. Toxicol.,
    13, 741-744

National Cancer Institute (1977) Bioassay of Lindane for Possible
    Carcinogenicity (Technical Report Series No. 14), Department of Health,
    Education, & Welfare Publication No. (NIH) 77-814

National Institute for Occupational Safety & Health (1977) NIOSH Manual of
    Analytical Methods, Part II, Standards Completion Program Validated
    Methods, 2nd ed., Vol. 3, Method S290, Department of Health, Education,
    & Welfare (NIOSH) Publ. No. 77-157-B, Washington DC, US Government
    Printing Office

Nickerson, P.R. & Barbehenn, K.R. (1975) Organochlorine residues in star-
    lings, 1972. Pestic. Monit. J., 8, 247-254

Nybom, N. & Knutsson, B. (1947) Investigations on c-mitosis in Allium
    cepa. I. The cytological effect of hexachlorocyclohexane. Hereditas,
    33, 220-234

Ochiai, M. & Hanya, T. (1976) Alpha- and gamma-BHC in Tamagawa River
    water, Japan (September 1968 to September 1969). Environ. Pollut.,
    11, 161-166

Orr, J.W. (1948) Absence of carcinogenic activity of benzene hexachloride
    ('gammexane'). Nature (Lond.), 162, 189

Oshiba, K. (1972) Experimental studies on the fate of β- and γ-BHC in vivo
    following daily administration (Jap.) Osaka Shiritsu Daigaku Igaku
    Zasshi, 21, 1-9 [Pestic. Abstr., 6, 73-0682]

Oshiba, K. & Kawakita, H. (1972) Interaction between toxicants and
    nutrition. III. Distribution and deposition of β-BHC in rat
    tissues (Jap.). Shokuhin Eiseigaku Zasshi, 13, 184-188 [Pestic.
    Abstr., 5, 72-1987]

Palmer, A.K., Bottomley, A.M., Worden, A.N., Frohberg, H. & Bauer, A. (1978)
    Effect of lindane on pregnancy in the rabbit and rat. Toxicology, 9,
    239-247

Parejko, R., Johnston, R. & Keller, R. (1975)   Chlorohydrocarbons in
    Lake Superior lake trout (*Salvelinus namacycush*).   Bull. environ.
    Contam. Toxicol., 14, 480-488

Pesendorfer, H. (1975)   Organochlorine pesticide (DDT etc.) and poly-
    chlorinated biphenyl (PCB) residues in human milk (from the area of
    Vienna and Lower Austria) (Ger.).   Wien. Klin. Wochenschr., 87,
    732-736

Piechocka, J. (1975)   Determination of active substances of Gamakarbatox
    in potatoes (Pol.).   Rocz. Panstw. Zakl. Hig., 26, 81-86   [Chem. Abstr.
    83, 41605h]

Rao, P.P., Jayaram, M., Visweswariah, K. & Majumder, S.K. (1975)   Deter-
    mination of residues of BHC components in different tissues of albino
    rats.   Bull. Grain Technol., 13, 18-22 [Chem. Abstr., 84, 130994x]

Rosival, L. & Szokolay, A. (1975)   Ecochemistry of BHC in Czechoslovakia.
    Pure appl. Chem., 42, 167-176

Saito, M. & Kitayama, M. (1973)   BHC and DDT residues in arable soil (Jap.).
    Hokkaidoritsu Eisei Kenkyusho Ho, 23, 116 [Chem. Abstr., 83, 159076q]

Saito, M. & Kitayama, M. (1974)   Prevention of poisoning by agricultural
    chemicals.   XIX.   Organochlorinated pesticide residues in water and
    soil (Jap.).   Hokkaidoritsu Eisei Kenkyusho Ho, 24, 126-127 [Chem.
    Abstr., 83, 54560q]

Sandhu, S.S., Warren, W.J. & Nelson, P. (1978)   Pesticidal residue in
    rural potable water.   J. Am. Water Works Assoc., 70, 41-45

Santiago Laguna, D., Alcaide Mejias, A., Garcia-Pantaleon Chamorro, A.
    & Infante Miranda, F. (1975)   Investigation of the organochloride
    pesticide residues in human serum (Span.).   Arch. Farmacol. Toxicol.,
    1, 173-184 [Chem. Abstr., 85, 57750d]

Sax, K. & Sax, H.J. (1968)   Possible mutagenic hazards of some food addi-
    tives, beverages and insecticides.   Jap. J. Genet., 43, 89-94

Schubert, A. (1969)   Investigations on the induction of respiration-deficient
    yeast mutants by chemical herbicides (Germ.).   Z. allg. Mikrobiol., 9,
    77-78

Schüttmann, W. (1968)   Chronic liver disease after occupational exposure
    to dichlorodiphenyltrichlorethane (DDT) and hexachlorocyclohexane (HCH)
    (Germ.).   Int. Arch. Gewerbepath. Gewerbehyg., 24, 193-210

Shackelford, W.M. & Keith, L.H. (1976) <u>Frequency of Organic Compounds Identified in Water</u>, EPA-600/4-76-062, Athens, GA, US Environmental Protection Agency, pp. 103-104, 151

Shahin, M.M. & von Borstel, R.C. (1977) Mutagenic and lethal effects of α-benzene hexachloride, dibutyl phthalate and trichloroethylene in *Saccharomyces cerevisiae*. <u>Mutat. Res.</u>, <u>48</u>, 173-180

Sharma, A.K. & Gosh, S. (1969) A comparative study of the effects of certain chemical agents on chromosomes. <u>Acta biol. acad. sci. hung.</u>, <u>20</u>, 11-21

Shimazu, H., Shiraishi, N., Akematsu, T., Ueda, N. & Sugiyama, T. (1976) Carcinogenicity screening tests on induction of chromosomal aberrations in rat bone marrow cells *in vivo* (Abstract no. 20). <u>Mutat. Res.</u>, <u>38</u>, 347

Shirasu, Y., Moriya, M., Kato, K., Furuhashi, A. & Kada, T. (1976) Mutagenicity screening of pesticides in the microbial system. <u>Mutat. Res.</u>, <u>40</u>, 19-30

Shtenberg, A.I. & Mametkuliev, C. (1976) The effect of gamma-isomer of hexachlorocyclohexane (HCCH) on the state of sexual glands in rats (Russ.). <u>Vop. Pitan.</u>, <u>4</u>, 62-67

Sieper, H. (1972) <u>D. Residues and Metabolism</u>. In: Ulmann, E., ed., <u>Lindane, Monograph of an Insecticide</u>, Freiburg, K. Schillinger, pp. 79-107

Simal, J., Charro, A., Creus, J.M. & Boado, A. (1975) Residues of polychlorinated biphenyls and pesticides in the water of Ria de Arosa (Span.). <u>Anal. Bromatol.</u>, <u>27</u>, 19-62

Smith, S.I., Weber, C.W. & Reid, B.L. (1970) The effect of injection of chlorinated hydrocarbon pesticides on hatchability of eggs. <u>Toxicol. appl. Pharmacol.</u>, <u>16</u>, 179-185

Solly, S.R.B. & Shanks, V. (1974) Polychlorinated biphenyls and organochlorine pesticides in human fat in New Zealand. <u>N.Z. J. Sci.</u>, <u>17</u>, 535-544

Solomon, L.M., Fahrner, L. & West, D.P. (1977) Gamma benzene hexachloride toxicity. A review. <u>Arch. Dermatol.</u>, <u>113</u>, 353-357

Soós, K., Cieleszky, V. & Tarján, R. (1972) The development of the level of chlorinated hydrocarbons in the adipose tissue of the population of Budapest in 1970 (Hung.). <u>Egészségtudomány</u>, <u>16</u>, 70-76

Squire, R.A. & Levitt, M.H. (1975) Report of a workshop on classification of specific hepatocellular lesions in rats. <u>Cancer Res.</u>, <u>35</u>, 3214-3223

Stalling, D.L. (1976) Application of analytical methods research to monitoring organic residues in fish. In: Proceedings of an International Conference on Environment Sensing Assessment, 1975, New York, Institute of Electrical & Electronic Engineers, pp. 1-4

Starr, H.G., Jr & Clifford, N.J. (1972) Acute lindane intoxication. A case study. Arch. environ. Health, 25, 374-375

Stute, K. & Kaufmann, I. (1971) Procedures for the determination of pesticides in poisoned bees (Ger.). Allg. Dtsch. Imkerztg., 5, 115-117 [Chem. Abstr., 83, 72801y]

Suzuki, M., Yamato, Y. & Watanabe, T. (1976) Organochlorine insecticide residues in vegetables of the Kitakyushu District, Japan - 1971-74. Pestic. Monit. J., 10, 35-40

Szokolay, A., Uhnák, J., Sackmauerová, M. & Maďarič, A. (1975) Analysis of HCB and BHC isomer residues in food. J. Chromatogr., 106, 401-404

Tanaka, K., Kurihara, N. & Nakajima, M. (1977) Pathways of chlorophenol formation in oxidative biodegradation of BHC. Agric. biol. Chem., 41, 723-725

Taylor, R., Bogacka, T. & Balcerska, M. (1975) Thin-layer chromatographic determination of chlorinated hydrocarbon insecticides in sediments (Pol.). Chem. Anal. (Warsaw), 20, 607-614 [Chem. Abstr., 83, 173898r]

Theiss, J.C., Stoner, G.D., Shimkin, M.B. & Weisburger, E.K. (1977) Test for carcinogenicity of organic contaminants of United States drinking waters by pulmonary tumor response in strain A mice. Cancer Res., 37, 2717-2720

Thielemann, H. (1976) Separation and identification of isomers of hexachlorocyclohexane on Kieselgel G layers (Ger.). Z. Chem., 16, 155-156 [Chem. Abstr., 85, 13495v]

Thomas, T.C. & Seiber, J.N. (1974) Chromosorb 102, an efficient medium for trapping pesticides from air. Bull. environ. Contam. Toxicol., 12, 17-25

Thorpe, E. & Walker, A.I.T. (1973) The toxicology of dieldrin (HEOD). II. Comparative long-term oral toxicity studies in mice with dieldrin, DDT, phenobarbitone, β-BHC and γ-BHC. Food Cosmet. Toxicol., 11, 433-442

Tikhomirova, G.P., Belen'kaya, S.L., Kalitvyanskaya, V.I. & Kostina, R.T. (1975) Determination of DDT and γ-hexachlorocyclohexane in raw material and waste products from the brewing industry (Russ.). Khim. Sel'sk. Khoz., 13, 303-304 [Chem. Abstr., 83, 41612h]

Tzoneva-Maneva, M.T., Kaloianova, F. & Georgieva, V. (1971) Influence of diazinon and lindan on the mitotic activity and the caryotype of human lymphocytes, cultivated *in vitro*. In: Proceedings of the XII International Congress of the Society of Blood Transfusion, Moscow, 1969, Bibl. Haemat., No. 38, part 1, Basel, Karger, pp. 344-347

Ulmann, E., ed. (1972) Lindane, Monograph of an Insecticide, Freiburg, K. Schillinger

US Environmental Protection Agency (1970) EPA Compendium of Registered Pesticides, Washington DC, US Government Printing Office, pp. III-B-6.1-III-B-6.6, III-L-2.1-III-L-2.12

US Environmental Protection Agency (1975) Preliminary Assessment of Suspected Carcinogens in Drinking Water, Report to Congress, Washington DC, p. II-4

US Environmental Protection Agency (1976a) Economic Analysis of Interim Final Effluent Guidelines for the Pesticides and Agricultural Chemicals Industry - Group II, EPA-230/1-76-065f, Washington DC, Office of Water Planning & Standards, p. 70

US Environmental Protection Agency (1976b) Protection of environment. US Code Fed. Regul., Title 40, parts 180.133, 180.140, pp. 319, 321

US Environmental Protection Agency (1976c) Rebuttable presumption against registration and continued registration of pesticide products containing benzene hexachloride (BHC). Fed. Regist., 41, 46024-46031

US Environmental Protection Agency (1976d) Manual of Chemical Methods for Pesticides and Devices, Office of Pesticide Programs, Washington DC, Association of Official Analytical Chemists

US Environmental Protection Agency (1977) Notice of rebuttable presumption against registration and continued registration of pesticide products containing lindane. Fed. Regist., 42, 9816-9822

US Environmental Protection Agency (1978) Summary of Reported Incidents Involving Toxaphene, Pesticide Incident Monitoring System, Report No. 113, Washington DC

US Food & Drug Administration (1975) Compliance Program Evaluation, Total Diet Studies: FY 1973 (7320.08), Bureau of Foods, Washington DC, US Government Printing Office, Table 5

US Food & Drug Administration (1977) Compliance Program Evaluation, FY 74 Total Diet Studies (7320.08), Bureau of Foods, Washington DC, US Government Printing Office, Table 6

Ushio, F., Fukano, S., Nishida, K., Kani, T. & Doguchi, M. (1974) Dietary intake of pesticides and PCB [polychlorinated biphenyl] residues and trace heavy metals (Jap.). Tokyo Toritsu Eisei Kenkyusho Kenkyu Nempo, 25, 307-312 [Chem. Abstr., 83, 91773g]

Ushio, F., Fukano, S., Doguchi, M. & Abe, M. (1976) Chlorinated hydrocarbons and pathological changes in the wild ducks suffering from mysterious disease (Jap.). Nippon Seitai Gakkaishi, 26, 13-18 [Chem. Abstr., 85, 73141m]

US International Trade Commission (1977a) Synthetic Organic Chemicals, US Production and Sales, 1976, USITC Publication 833, Washington DC, US Government Printing Office, p. 276

US International Trade Commission (1977b) Imports of Benzenoid Chemicals and Products, 1976, USITC Publication 828, Washington DC, US Government Printing Office, p. 102

US Occupational Safety & Health Administration (1976) Occupational safety and health standards, Subpart 2 - Toxic and hazardous substances, air contaminants. US Code Fed. Regul., Title 29, part 1910.1000, p. 31:8303

US Tariff Commission (1946) Synthetic Organic Chemicals, US Production and Sales, 1945, Report No. 157, Second Series, Washington DC, US Government Printing Office, p. 177

US Tariff Commission (1951) Synthetic Organic Chemicals, US Production and Sales, 1950, Report No. 173, Second Series, Washington DC, US Government Printing Office, p. 127

US Tariff Commission (1952) Synthetic Organic Chemicals, US Production and Sales, 1951, Report No. 175, Second Series, Washington DC, US Government Printing Office, pp. 54, 136

US Tariff Commission (1964) Synthetic Organic Chemicals, US Production and Sales, 1963, TC Publication 143, Washington DC, US Government Printing Office, pp. 52-53, 172

Vioque, A. & Sáez, J.M. (1976) Pollution of the Andalusian population by chlorine insecticide residues (Span.). Grasas Aceites, 27, 179-184

Wegman, R.C.C. & Greve, P.A. (1974) Levels of organochlorine pesticides and inorganic bromide in human milk. Meded. Fac. Landbouwwet., Rijksuniv, Gent., 39, 1301-1310

Weisse, I. & Herbst, M. (1977) Carcinogenicity study of lindane in the mouse. Toxicology, 7, 233-238

West, I. (1967) Lindane and hematologic reactions. Arch. environ. Health,
     15, 97-101

White, D.H. (1976) Nationwide residues of organochlorines in starlings,
     1974. Pestic. Monit. J., 10, 10-17

WHO (1967) 1966 Evaluations of some pesticide residues in food. WHO/Food
     Add./67.32, pp. 126-147

WHO (1969) 1968 Evaluations of some pesticide residues in food. WHO/Food
     Add./69.35, pp. 17-31

WHO (1972) 1971 Evaluations of some pesticide residues in food. WHO Pestic.
     Res. Ser., No. 1, pp. 333-345

WHO (1976) 1975 Evaluations of some pesticide residues in food. WHO Pestic.
     Res. Ser., No. 5, pp. 267-271, 396

Winell, M. (1975) An international comparison of hygienic standards for
     chemicals in the work environment. Ambio, 4, 34-36

Woodliff, H.J., Connor, P.M. & Scopa, J. (1966) Aplastic anaemia associated
     with insecticides. Med. J. Aust., 1, 628-629

Yamada, T. & Sakamoto, I. (1975) BHC residues in crops, soils, mother's
     milk, and cow's milk in Hiroshima Prefecture (Jap.). Hiroshima-ken
     Eisei Kenkyusho (To) Kogai Kenkyusho Kenkyu Hokoku, pp. 35-38
     [Chem. Abstr., 86, 110689q]

Yamada, T., Sugiyama, S., Noda, H., Mitsukuni, Y. & Yoshimura, M. (1976)
     Organochlorinated pesticides (BHC) in human organs and tissues (Jap.).
     Nippon Hoigaku Zasshi, 30, 416-426 [Chem. Abstr., 87, 79314h]

Yamaguchi, S., Kaku, S., Kuwahara, Y. & Yamada, A. (1976) Epidemiological
     findings and evaluation of the amount of organochlorine pesticides
     in human blood plasma in Japan. Arch. environ. Contam. Toxicol., 3,
     448-460

Yamato, Y., Suzuki, M. & Akiyama, T. (1975) Persistence of BHC in river
     water in the Kitakyushu district, Japan, 1970-1974. Bull. environ.
     Contam. Toxicol., 14, 380-384

HEXACHLOROPHENE

1. Chemical and Physical Data

1.1 Synonyms and trade names

Chem. Abstr. Services Reg. No.: 70-30-4

Chem. Abstr. Name: 2,2'-Methylenebis(3,4,6-trichlorophenol)

Synonyms: Bis(2-hydroxy-3,5,6-trichlorophenyl)methane; bis(3,5,6-trichloro-2-hydroxyphenyl)methane; 2,2'-dihydroxy-3,3',5,5',6,6'-hexachlorodiphenylmethane; 2,2'-dihydroxy-3,5,6,3',5',6'-hexachloro-diphenylmethane; 2,2',3,3',5,5'-hexachloro-6,6'-dihydroxydiphenyl-methane; hexachlorofen; hexachlorophane; hexachlorophen; hexophene; trichlorophene

Trade names: Acigena; Almederm; AT 7; AT-17; B32; Bilevon; Compound G-11; Cotofilm; Dermadex; Exofene; Fostril; G 11; G-11, Gamophen; Gamophene; G-Eleven; Germa-Medica; Hexabalm; Hexafen; Hexide; Hexosan; Isobac 20; Nabac; Neosept V; Phisodan; pHisoHex; Ritosept; Septisol; Septofen; Steral; Steraskin; Surgi-Cen; Surgi-Cin; Surofene; Tersaseptic; Turgex

1.2 Structural and molecular formulae and molecular weight

$C_{13}H_6O_2Cl_6$ Mol. wt: 406.9

1.3 Chemical and physical properties of the pure substance

(a) Description: White, free-flowing powder (Hawley, 1977)

(b) Melting-point: 166-167°C (Grasselli & Ritchey, 1975)

(c) Spectroscopy data: Infra-red and nuclear magnetic resonance spectral data have been tabulated (Grasselli & Ritchey, 1975).

(d) Solubility: Practically insoluble in water; soluble in
     ethanol, acetone, diethyl ether, chloroform, polypropylene
     glycol, polyethylene glycol, olive oil, cottonseed oil and
     dilute alkali (Windholz, 1976)

(e) Reactivity: Forms salts with alkali (Windholz, 1976)

1.4 Technical products and impurities

Hexachlorophene available in the US contains 98.0–100.5% of the
pure chemical, calculated on a dry basis. Hexachlorophene produced
from 2,4,5-trichlorophenol contains less than 15 µg/kg 2,3,7,8-tetra-
chlorodibenzo-*para*-dioxin (see IARC, 1977).

Hexachlorophene is available in the US as a detergent lotion
containing 3% active ingredient and as a liquid soap containing 0.25%
of the chemical (US Pharmacopeial Convention, Inc., 1975). The monosodium salt of hexachlorophene is available as a liquid soil fungicide
containing 20% of the salt.

2. Production, Use, Occurrence and Analysis

2.1 Production and use

(a) Production

The preparation of hexachlorophene was first reported in 1941, by
the reaction of 2,4,5-trichlorophenol with formaldehyde (Gump, 1941);
this is the method used currently for its production (Gump *et al.*, 1957).

Commercial production of this chemical in the US was first reported
in 1951 (US Tariff Commission, 1952). Only one company reported production of an undisclosed amount in 1976 (see preamble, p. 16) (US International Trade Commission, 1977).

It is produced in western Europe, but there has been no production
of hexachlorophene in Japan since 1972. Minor quantities of a product
containing 3% hexachlorophene are imported to Japan from the US.

(b) Use

The principal use of hexachlorophene has been in the manufacture
of germicidal soaps; it is also used as a topical anti-infective agent
for humans and as an anthelminthic in veterinary medicine (Windholz,
1976). The monosodium salt is used as a broad-spectrum soil fungicide
(Berg, 1978); it is also used widely as a disinfectant, particularly for
hospital equipment.

Hexachlorophene has been used extensively as a soap additive, particularly for deodorant soaps, because trace quantities are retained on the skin after washing with a soap or detergent containing it, imparting a bacteriostatic effect (Klarmann, 1963; Ryer, 1969).

On 27 September 1972, the US Food and Drug Administration (FDA) issued revised rules and regulations for the production, sale and use of drug and cosmetic products containing hexachlorophene.   Under this order, infant powders containing more than 0.75% of the chemical were recalled by the manufacturers.   All other products for infant use containing more than 0.75% hexachlorophene were made available only by prescription.   Nonprescription drugs and cosmetic products containing 0.75% or less of the chemical were not recalled, but future production and shipment were banned.   New labels for hexachlorophene-containing products were required to warn against its use on burned or denuded skin, or on any mucous membranes (Anon., 1972; US Food & Drug Administration, 1972).   Drug products formerly sold on a nonprescription (over-the-counter) basis are permitted to be sold as prescription drugs only after approval by the FDA of new drug applications proving safety and efficacy. These are approved only for surgical scrubbing and handwashing for controlled outbreaks of certain infections.   Of 20 such new drug applications filed in 1972, 7 were reported to be still under evaluation by the FDA in February 1978 (Anon., 1978a).   Hexachlorophene is permitted to be used as a preservative in drug and cosmetic products only at levels up to 0.1% (US Food & Drug Administration, 1972).

In April 1977, there were 54 registrants of 110 products containing hexachlorophene which are regulated by the US Environmental Protection Agency (1977); most are believed to be disinfectant products.

The sodium salt is used as a seed-treatment fungicide; an estimated 45 thousand kg of hexachlorophene were used for this purpose in 1975. In 1977, 3.2 thousand kg were used to treat cottonseed in California (California Department of Food & Agriculture, 1978).

A tolerance of 0.05 mg/kg is established for hexachlorophene in or on cottonseed, resulting from use of the monosodium salt.   The technical-grade hexachlorophene used in the formulation must not contain more than 0.1 mg/kg 2,3,7,8-tetrachlorodibenzo-*para*-dioxin (US Environmental Protection Agency, 1976).

No data on use patterns in Europe or Japan were available.

2.2 Occurrence

Hexachlorophene is not known to occur as a natural product.

(a) Water and sediments

Hexachlorophene has been found in two samples of finished drinking-water (Shackelford & Keith, 1976); in upstream and downstream water from 2 sewage treatment plants, at levels of 3.2-24 µg/l and 16.4-44.3 µg/l, respectively (Sims & Pfaender, 1975); in the influent and effluent water of 3 sewage plants at levels of 20-31 and 6-12 µg/l, respectively; and in a river, at levels of 0.01-0.1 µg/l (Buhler *et al.*, 1973).

Hexachlorophene has been detected in the sediment of a creek at levels of 9.3-377 µg/kg and in marine organisms, at levels of 333-27,800 µg/kg (Sims & Pfaender, 1975).

(b) Humans

Hexachlorophene has been detected in human milk at levels of 0-9 µg/l (West *et al.*, 1975).

In a study of the use of a 3% hexachlorophene solution as a body and hand soap, blood levels ranged from < 0.005-0.38 mg/l blood, compared with a mean baseline concentration in 30 control people of 0.02 mg/l blood. After prolonged use of a soap containing 0.75% hexachlorophene, levels ranged from 0.02-0.14 mg/l blood; and use of a mouthwash containing 0.5% hexachlorophene for 3 weeks produced levels of 0.02-0.12 mg/l blood. In a study of randomly selected hospital patients, hexachlorophene blood levels ranged from 0-0.12 mg/l, with a mean level of 0.03 mg/l (Butcher *et al.*, 1973).

Samples of adipose tissue obtained from the neck during routine surgery contained a mean concentration of 0.01 mg/kg tissue; abdominal fat obtained at autopsy contained 0.04 mg/kg tissue (Ulsamer *et al.*, 1973). In another study, hexachlorophene was detected at levels of 0-80 µg/kg adipose tissue (Shafik, 1973).

(c) Occupational exposure

In a controlled study of hospital operating-room personnel who scrubbed with hexachlorophene soaps or detergents, the mean hexachlorophene levels in the blood were 0.07 or 0.22 mg/l, respectively. Follow-up samples, taken 2-3 weeks after termination of hexachlorophene exposure, indicated a rapid return to the initial background level (Butcher *et al.*, 1973).

A 1974 National Occupational Hazard Survey estimated that exposure to hexachlorophene was primarily in hospitals, sanitariums, convalescent homes and rest homes (National Institute for Occupational Safety & Health, 1977).

2.3 Analysis

Schwedt (1973) has reviewed methods for extracting hexachlorophene from soaps, powders, creams and cosmetic sprays and its detection and determination at levels of 0.05-1.3% (with a precision of 0.01-0.05%) by thin-layer and gas chromatography and ultra-violet spectrometry.

Methods used for the analysis of hexachlorophene in environmental samples are listed in Table 1.

Collaborative studies have been carried out with the method of the Association of Official Analytical Chemists (Sheppard & Wilson, 1975; Wilson, 1974). Tentative methods using high-performance liquid chromatography of hexachlorophene or its derivatives have been described (Carr, 1974; Porcaro & Shubiak, 1972); and thin-layer chromatography can also be used to determine hexachlorophene in formulations (Amin & Jakobs, 1977).

3. Biological Data Relevant to the Evaluation
of Carcinogenic Risk to Humans

3.1 Carcinogenicity studies in animals[1]

(a) Oral administration

Rat: Groups of 24 male and 24 female Fischer 344 rats, 52 days old, were fed diets containing 0, 17, 50 or 150 mg/kg diet hexachlorophene (98% minimum purity) for 105-106 weeks. Of male rats, 79% of the high-dose group, 88% of the mid-dose group, 67% of the low-dose group and 88% of controls were still alive at the end of the study. In females, the respective percentages were 75%, 79%, 50% and 63%. No increased incidence of tumours was observed compared with that in controls (National Cancer Institute, 1978).

---

[1]The Working Group was aware of a study in progress in rats to assess the carcinogenicity of hexachlorophene by oral administration (IARC, 1978).

TABLE 1. METHODS FOR THE ANALYSIS OF HEXACHLOROPHENE

SAMPLE TYPE	ANALYTICAL METHOD			
	EXTRACTION/CLEAN-UP	DETECTION	LIMIT OF DETECTION	REFERENCE
Water				
Urban drainage	Extract (ether), dry, concentrate, take up into benzene, acetylate	GC/ECD		Sims & Pfaender (1975)
Sediments	Dry, extract (ether) in Soxhlet, acetylate	GC/ECD		Sims & Pfaender (1975)
Food				
Peanuts and soya beans	Homogenize, extract (ether), centrifuge, recover ether, concentrate, add benzene-hexane, CC, methylate	GC/ECD	1 µg/kg	Van Auken & Hulse (1977); Van Auken et al. (1977)
Biological				
Blood	Extract (ether-absolute ethanol), add water, evaporate to dryness, acetylate, evaporate, take up into benzene	GC/ECD		Ulsamer (1972)
Organs	Homogenize (water), extract (chloroform-methanol), liquid/liquid partition, methylate	GC/ECD		Ulsamer (1972)
Human adipose tissue	Grind, extract (hexane), add caustic soda, mix, discard hexane layer, re-extract (hexane), discard, acidify, extract (ether), ethylate, transfer to hexane	GC/ECD	10 µg/kg	Shafik (1973)
Blood	Add citrate buffer pH5, extract (ether), concentrate to 1 ml, methylate, evaporate to dryness, take up into hexane, wash hexane with acid, dry hexane phase	GC/ECD		Ferry & McQueen (1973)

TABLE 1. METHODS FOR THE ANALYSIS OF HEXACHLOROPHENE (continued)

SAMPLE TYPE	ANALYTICAL METHOD			REFERENCE
	EXTRACTION/CLEAN-UP	DETECTION	LIMIT OF DETECTION	
Miscellaneous				
Cosmetics	Reflux sample (ethanol-hydrochloric acid), cool, add water, extract (chloroform), wash extracts (water), concentrate, CC	Spectrophotometry		Horwitz (1975)
Cosmetics	Mix with ethanol, filtrate	TLC (many revelations)		Wilson (1975)

Abbreviations: CC – column chromatography; GC/ECD – gas chromatography/electron capture detection; TLC – thin-layer chromatography

(b) Skin application

Mouse: Hexachlorophene was applied to the dorsal skin of groups
of 50 random-bred female Swiss mice twice a week for life, starting at
8 weeks of age, in doses of 0.02 ml of concentrations of 50, 25 and 5%
in acetone, corresponding to 10, 5 and 1 mg hexachlorophene per application. A further group of 50 mice was used as controls [It was not
specified whether they were untreated or given the solvent]. The
treatment caused skin ulceration, necrosis and inflammation, as well
as neurological symptoms. About 25% of treated animals at all dose
levels died within 40 weeks of treatment, *versus* 5% of controls; 60
weeks after the start of treatment, 50-65% of treated animals had died,
compared with 10% of controls. In the treated groups, tumours developed
in 10/50 (15 tumours), 14/50 (17 tumours) and 15/50 (19 tumours) animals,
respectively; 20/50 controls developed a total of 29 tumours. Among
treated animals, only one benign skin papilloma developed. Lymphomas,
lung adenomas, liver haemangiomas and other tumours occurred sporadically
with similar frequencies in treated and experimental groups (Stenbäck,
1975) [The Working Group noted that lifespan was greatly reduced in all
experimental groups].

3.2 Other relevant biological data

The toxicity of hexachlorophene in both experimental animals and
humans has been reviewed recently (Kimbrough, 1976).

(a) Experimental systems

Toxic effects

The oral LD_{50} of hexachlorophene in male rats is 66 mg/kg bw, in
females 56 mg/kg bw and in weanling rats 120 mg/kg bw (Gaines *et al.*,
1973); in suckling rats (10-days old), it is 9 mg/kg bw (Nieminen *et
al.*, 1973)

When rats were maintained on diets containing 400 mg/kg diet
hexachlorophene, or given large dermal or oral doses, they exhibited
neurotoxic symptoms which were characterized initially by a weakness
in the hind legs; this has also been reported in mice, dogs, rabbits
and monkeys (Kimbrough, 1974, 1976). The effect is at least partly
reversible if the hexachlorophene-containing diet is replaced (Nakaue
et al., 1973; de Jesus & Pleasure, 1973). Hexachlorophene induces a
lesion in the white matter of brain and sciatic nerves, called *status
spongiosus*, characterized by oedema and intramyelinic vacuolization at
the interperiod line (Gaines *et al.*, 1973; Kimbrough & Gaines, 1971;
Pleasure *et al.*, 1974).

Hexachlorophene inhibits rat liver mitochondrial oxidative phosphorylation (Caldwell *et al.*, 1972).

Topical exposure of neonatal rats to 3% hexachlorophene solution caused reduced fertility in 7-month-old males, due to inability to ejaculate (Geller *et al.*, 1978).

Embryotoxicity and teratogenicity

Placental transfer of hexachlorophene has been demonstrated in rats (Kennedy *et al.*, 1977).

Administration of 500 mg/kg diet or 20-30 mg/kg bw/day by gavage to rats caused some malformations (angulated ribs, cleft palate, micro- and anophthalmia) and reduction in litter size (Gaines *et al.*, 1973; Kennedy *et al.*, 1975a, 1976; Oakley & Shepard, 1972). These dosages approached those that resulted in maternal death. A 45% suspension of hexachlorophene applied into the vagina of pregnant rats caused maternal toxicity and malformations in some offspring (hydrocephaly, micro- and anophthalmia, wavy ribs, urogenital defects) (Kimmel *et al.*, 1974). In rabbits, an oral dose of 6 mg/kg bw/day caused a low frequency of rib malformations (Kennedy *et al.*, 1975a). S.c. injection of 12.5 or 25 mg/kg bw/day hexachlorophene to mice on days 3-8, 7-12 or 11-17 of gestation caused foetal resorptions but no malformations (Majumdar *et al.*, 1975).

A dose of 100 mg/kg diet hexachlorophene caused reduced survival in the Fl generation offspring of rats (Gaines *et al.*, 1973). In another study, doses of up to 50 mg/kg diet failed to produce any effects in 3 generations of rats (Kennedy *et al.*, 1975b). Hexachlorophene did not interfere with reproduction in hamsters (Alleva, 1973).

Absorption, distribution, excretion and metabolism

Hexachlorophene can be absorbed through the skin in rats (Nakaue & Buhler, 1976), especially when applied to skin lesions (Carroll *et al.*, 1967).

Hexachlorophene administered orally to rats was recovered (80-90%) unchanged in the faeces within 10 days (Bjondahl & Isomaa, 1976); however, after i.p. administration, extensive biliary excretion (31-47% of the dose within 24 hrs) and enterohepatic circulation occurred (Edelson & McMullen, 1976; Gandolfi & Buhler, 1974). The principal metabolite in bile was the monoglucuronide. Much of the unchanged hexachlorophene in the faeces is probably a result of intestinal bacterial hydrolysis of the conjugate: when the bile duct was ligated, 55% of the dose was excreted as the monoglucuronide in the urine (Gandolfi & Buhler, 1974). It does not accumulate extensively in the brain at doses which induce lesions (Ulsamer *et al.*, 1975).

Hexachlorophene is excreted in the milk of rats (Kennedy *et al.*, 1977).

Mutagenicity and other related short-term tests

Hexachlorophene did not induce reverse mutations in *Salmonella typhimurium* G46 in a host-mediated assay using male albino rats that received 100 or 200 mg/kg diet for 90 days (Arnold *et al.*, 1975). Dominant lethal tests with male mice treated with single i.p. injections of 2.5 or 5.0 mg/kg bw hexachlorophene were negative (Kennedy *et al.*, 1975c).

In human peripheral blood lymphocytes treated with hexachlorophene *in vitro* at concentrations ranging from 1–200 mg/l and with treatment times extending from 6–21 hrs, there was no evidence of increased chromosome aberrations; however, mitosis was suppressed with concentrations as low as 40 mg/l applied for 6 hrs, and this effect was found to be both concentration- and treatment time-dependent (Vig, 1972).

(b) Humans

Poisoning by hexachlorophene, for example, by its liberal application to patients with burns or to infants, leads to circulatory failure, body temperature fluctuations and central nervous symptoms, including headache, twitching, convulsions and death (Kimbrough, 1976). Some infants treated with high doses of hexachlorophene have died; premature infants and newborns appear to be most susceptible. The spongiform brain changes seen in animals were also observed in infants who died from overexposure to hexachlorophene (Powell *et al.*, 1973).

In newborn infants exposed to soap containing hexachlorophene, its half-life ranged from 6–44 hrs; the time of peak blood concentrations following a bath ranged from 6–10 hrs. One infant has a blood concentration of 4.3 µg/ml and developed symptoms comparable with hexachlorophene-induced toxicity (Tyrala *et al.*, 1977).

Halling (1977, 1979) reported severe malformations in children of hospital personnel who had been exposed to hexachlorophene soap during pregnancy as compared with children of a group of unexposed personnel: 4 severe and 6 slight malformations were observed in 82 babies born to the exposed group *versus* 1 slight malformation in 46 babies born to mothers not exposed to hexachlorophene. The occurrence of chlorinated, so-called 'predioxins' in the soap was discussed. In a more recent report, 25 severe malformations, such as eye and central nervous system defects, were reported among 460 live births to these women, compared with no severe malformations seen in a control group of 233 live births from unexposed mothers. Minor malformations were also more frequent in the hexachlorophene exposed group (Anon., 1978b; Hay, 1978).

3.3 Case reports and epidemiological studies

No data were available to the Working Group.

4. Summary of Data Reported and Evaluation

4.1 Experimental data[1]

Hexachlorophene was tested in one experiment in rats by oral administration; it had no carcinogenic effect.   It was inadequately tested in one experiment in mice by skin application.

Hexachlorophene is embryotoxic and produces some teratogenic effects.   It was not mutagenic in *Salmonella typhimurium* and was negative in a dominant lethal assay in male mice.   Cytogenetic tests with cultured human lymphocytes were also negative.

4.2 Human data

No case reports or epidemiological studies were available to the Working Group.

Malformations have been reported in children born to mothers repeatedly exposed to hexachlorophene.

The extensive production and use, particularly in germicidal soap, of hexachlorophene over the past several decades indicate that widespread human exposure occurs in both the general and the working environment.   This is confirmed by its presence in human body fluids. Episodes of intoxication have also been reported..

4.3 Evaluation

The available data do not allow an evaluation of the carcinogenicity of hexachlorophene to be made.

---

[1]Subsequent to the meeting of the Working Group, the Secretariat became aware of completed studies on the carcinogenicity of hexachlorophene in which no carcinogenic effects were observed in mice or rats following its oral administration or in mice following exposure prenatally or *via* the mother's milk or following its s.c. injection to newborn mice (Rudali & Assa, 1978).

5. References

Alleva, F.R. (1973) Failure of neonatal injection of hexachlorophene to affect reproduction in hamsters. Toxicology, 1, 357-360

Amin, M. & Jakobs, U. (1977) Thin-layer chromatography of active compounds from ointments and suppositories followed by direct quantitative analysis by remission (Germ.). J. Chromatogr., 131, 391-398

Anon. (1972) FDA limits availability of hexachlorophene. J. Am. med. Assoc., 222, 421

Anon. (1978a) Antiseptics and germicides. The Food & Drug Letter, 17 February, p. 5

Anon. (1978b) Study links birth defects to hexachlorophene. FDA Consumer, July-August, p. 16

Arnold, D.W., Kennedy, G.L., Jr & Keplinger, M.L. (1975) Mutagenic evaluation of hexachlorophene (Abstract no. 158). Toxicol. appl. Pharmacol., 33, 185

Berg, G.L., ed. (1978) Farm Chemicals Handbook 1978, Willoughby, OH, Meister, pp. D139, D147

Bjondahl, K. & Isomaa, B. (1976) The distribution and excretion of hexachlorophene in rats of different ages. Food Cosmet. Toxicol., 14, 179-182

Buhler, D.R., Rasmusson, M.E. & Nakaue, H.S. (1973) Occurrence of hexachlorophene and pentachlorophenol in sewage and water. Environ. Sci. Technol., 7, 929-934

Butcher, H.R., Ballinger, W.F., Gravens, D.L., Dewar, N.E., Ledlie, E.F. & Barthel, W.F. (1973) Hexachlorophene concentrations in the blood of operating room personnel. Arch. Surg., 107, 70-74

Caldwell, R.S., Nakaue, H.S. & Buhler, D.R. (1972) Biochemical lesion in rat liver mitochondria induced by hexachlorophene. Biochem. Pharmacol., 21, 2425-2441

California Department of Food and Agriculture (1978) Pesticide Use Report Annual 1977, Sacramento, p. 90

Carr, C.D. (1974) Use of a new variable wavelength detector in high performance liquid chromatography. Anal. Chem., 46, 743-749

Carroll, F.E., Jr, Salak, W.W., Howard, J.M. & Pairent, F.W. (1967)
    Absorption of antimicrobial agents across experimental wounds.
    Surg. Gynecol. Obstet., 125, 974-978

Edelson, J. & McMullen, J.P. (1976) Hexachlorophene metabolism in rats:
    the hepatic route. Arch. int. Pharmacodyn., 220, 140-147

Ferry, D.G. & McQueen, E.G. (1973) Hexachlorophene analysis in blood
    by electron capture gas chromatography. J. Chromatogr., 76,
    233-235

Gaines, T.B., Kimbrough, R.D. & Linder, R.E. (1973) The oral and dermal
    toxicity of hexachlorophene in rats. Toxicol. appl. Pharmacol., 25,
    332-343

Gandolfi, A.J. & Buhler, D.R. (1974) Biliary metabolites and enterohepatic
    circulation of hexachlorophene in the rat. Xenobiotica, 4, 693-704

Gellert, R.J., Wallace, C.A., Wiesmeier, E.M. & Shuman, R.M. (1978)
    Topical exposure of neonates to hexachlorophene: long-standing
    effects on mating behaviour and prostatic development in rats.
    Toxicol. appl. Pharmacol., 43, 339-349

Grasselli, J.G. & Ritchey, W.M., eds (1975) CRC Atlas of Spectral Data
    and Physical Constants for Organic Compounds, 2nd ed., Vol III,
    Cleveland, OH, Chemical Rubber Co., p. 589

Gump, W.S. (1941) 2,2'-Dihydroxy-3,5,6,3',5',6'-hexachlorodiphenylmethane.
    US Patent 2,250,480, 29 July, to Burton T. Bush, Inc. [Chem. Abstr.
    35, 7120 (2)]

Gump, W.S., Luthy, M. & Krebs, H.G. (1957) Bis(3,5,6-trichloro-2-hydroxy-
    phenyl)methane. US Patent 2,812,365, 5 November, to Givaudan Corp.
    [Chem. Abstr., 52, 5473d]

Halling, H. (1977) Suspected link between exposure to hexachlorophene
    and birth of malformed infants (Swed.) Läkartidningen, 74, 542-546

Halling, H. (1979) New report on suspected link between exposure to
    hexachlorophene and congenital malformations. Lancet (in press)

Hawley, G.G., ed. (1977) The Condensed Chemical Dictionary, 9th ed.,
    New York, Van Nostrand-Reinhold, p. 437

Hay, A. (1978) Halogenated hydrocarbon effects. Nature (Lond.), 274,
    533-534

Horwitz, W., ed. (1975) Official Methods of Analysis of the Association
    of Official Analytical Chemists, 12th ed., Washington DC, Association
    of Offical Analytical Chemists, pp. 649-650

IARC (1977)   IARC Monographs on the Evaluation of the Carcinogenic Risk
      Of Chemicals to Man, Vol. 15, Some Fumigants, the Herbicides 2,4-D
      and 2,4,5-T, Chlorinated Dibenzodioxins and Miscellaneous Industrial
      Chemicals, Lyon, p. 49

IARC (1978)   Information Bulletin on the Survey of Chemicals Being Tested
      for Carcinogenicity, No. 7, Lyon, p. 250

de Jesus, P.V., Jr & Pleasure, D.E. (1973) Hexachlorophene neuropathy.
      Arch. Neurol., 29, 180-182

Kennedy, G.L., Jr, Smith, S.H., Keplinger, M.L. & Calandra, J.C. (1975a)
      Evaluation of the teratological potential of hexachlorophene in
      rabbits and rats. Teratology, 12, 83-88

Kennedy, G.L., Jr, Smith, S.H., Keplinger, M.L. & Calandra, J.C. (1975b)
      Effect of hexachlorophene on reproduction in rats. J. agric. Food
      Chem., 23, 866-868

Kennedy, G.L., Jr, Arnold, D.W., Keplinger, M.L. & Calandra, J.C. (1975c)
      Investigation of hexachlorophene for dominant lethal effects in the
      mouse. Toxicology, 5, 159-162

Kennedy, G.L., Jr, Smith, S.H., Plank, J.B., Keplinger, M.L. & Calandra, J.
      (1976) Reproductive and peri- and postnatal studies with hexachloro-
      phene. Food Cosmet. Toxicol., 14, 421-423

Kennedy, G.L., Jr, Dressler, I.A., Keplinger, M.L. & Calandra, J.C. (1977)
      Placental and milk transfer of hexachlorophene in the rat. Toxicol.
      appl. Pharmacol., 40, 571-576

Kimbrough, R.D. (1974) The toxicity of polychlorinated polycyclic compound
      and related chemicals. CRC Crit. Rev. Toxicol., 2, 445-498

Kimbrough, R.D. (1976) Hexachlorophene: toxicity and use as an antibacter
      agent. Essays Toxicol., 7, 99-120

Kimbrough, R.D. & Gaines, T.B. (1971) Hexachlorophene effects on the rat
      brain. Study of high doses by light and electron microscopy.
      Arch. environ. Health, 23, 114-118

Kimmel, C.A., Moore, W., Jr, Hysell, D.L. & Stara, J.F. (1974) Teratogenic
      of hexachlorophene in rats. Comparison of uptake following various
      routes of administration. Arch. environ. Health, 28, 43-48

Klarmann, E.G. (1963) Antiseptics and disinfectants. In: Kirk, R.E. &
      Othmer, D.F., eds, Encyclopedia of Chemical Technology, 2nd ed., Vol.
      New York, John Wiley & Sons, pp. 630-637

Majumdar, S.K., Franco, R.A., Filippone, E.J. & Sobel, J.H. (1975) Teratologic evaluation of hexachlorophene in mice. Proc. Pennsylvania Acad. Sci., 49, 110-112

Nakaue, H.S. & Buhler, D.R. (1976) Percutaneous absorption of hexachlorophene in the rat. Toxicol. appl. Pharmacol., 35, 381-391

Nakaue, H.S., Dost, F.N. & Buhler, D.R. (1973) Studies on the toxicity of hexachlorophene in the rat. Toxicol. appl. Pharmacol., 24, 239-249

National Cancer Institute (1978) Bioassay of Hexachlorophene for Possible Carcinogenicity (Tech. Rep. Ser. No. 40), DHEW Publication No. (NIH) 78-840, Washington DC, US Government Printing Office

National Institute for Occupational Safety & Health (1977) National Occupational Hazard Survey, Vol. III, Survey Analysis and Supplemental Tables, DHEW Publication No. (NIOSH) 76, Draft, Cincinnati, OH, US Department of Health, Education, & Welfare, pp. 5583-5587

Nieminen, L., Bjondahl, K. & Mättönen, M. (1973) Effect of hexachlorophene on the rat brain during ontogenesis. Food Cosmet. Toxicol., 11, 635-639

Oakley, G.P. & Shepard, T.H. (1972) Possible teratogenicity of hexachlorophene in rats (Abstract). Teratology, 5, 264

Pleasure, D., Towfighi, J., Silberberg, D. & Parris, J. (1974) The pathogenesis of hexachlorophene neuropathy: *in vivo* and *in vitro* studies. Neurology, 24, 1068-1075

Porcaro, P.J. & Shubiak, P. (1972) Detection of nanogram quantities of hexachlorophene by ultraviolet liquid chromatography. Anal. Chem., 44, 1865-1867

Powell, H., Swarner, O., Gluck, L. & Lampert, P. (1973) Hexachlorophene myelinopathy in premature infants. J. Pediatr., 82, 976-981

Rudali, G. & Assa, R. (1978) Lifespan carcinogenicity studies with hexachlorophene in mice and rats. Cancer Lett., 5, 325-332

Ryer, F.V. (1969) Soap. Speciality soaps. In: Kirk, R.E. & Othmer, D.F., eds, Encyclopedia of Chemical Technology, 2nd ed., Vol. 18, New York, John Wiley & Sons, p. 429

Schwedt, G. (1973) Identification and determination of hexachlorophene in cosmetics (Germ.) Dtsch. Lebensm.-Rundsch., 69, 221-223 [Chem. Abstr., 79, 45624d]

Shackelford, W.M. & Keith, L.H. (1976) Frequency of Organic Compounds Identified in Water, EPA-600/4-76-062, Athens, GA, US Environmental Protection Agency, p. 142

Shafik, T.M. (1973) The determination of pentachlorophenol and hexachloro-
    phene in human adipose tissue. Bull. environ. Contam. Toxicol., 10,
    57-63

Sheppard, E.P. & Wilson, C.H. (1975) Preservatives in cosmetics: partition
    chromatography and ultraviolet spectrophotometry. J. Assoc. off. anal.
    Chem., 58, 937-940

Sims, J.L. & Pfaender, F.K. (1975) Distribution and biomagnification of
    hexachlorophene in urban drainage areas. Bull. environ. Contam.
    Toxicol., 14, 214-220

Stenbäck, F. (1975) Hexachlorophene in mice. Effects after long-term
    percutaneous applications. Arch. environ. Health, 30, 32-35

Tyrala, E.E., Hillman, L.S., Hillman, R.D. & Doolson, W.E. (1977)
    Clinical pharmacology of hexachlorophene in newborn infants.
    J. Pediatr., 91, 481-486

Ulsamer, A.G. (1972) The determination of hexachlorophene in mammalian
    tissues by gas-liquid chromatography. J. Assoc. off. anal. Chem.,
    55, 1294-1299

Ulsamer, A.G., Marzulli, F.N. & Coen, R.W. (1973) Hexachlorophene
    concentrations in blood associated with the use of products containing
    hexachlorophene. Food Cosmet. Toxicol., 11, 625-633

Ulsamer, A.G., Yoder, P.D., Kimbrough, R.D. & Marzulli, F.N. (1975)
    Effects of hexachlorophene on developing rats: toxicity, tissue
    concentrations and biochemistry. Food Cosmet. Toxicol., 13, 69-80

US Environmental Protection Agency (1976) Hexachlorophene; tolerance
    for residues. US Code Fed. Regul., Title 40, part 180.302,
    p. 353

US Environmental Protection Agency (1977) Product Label File Active
    Ingredients, 04/04/77, Washington DC, US Government Printing Office,
    p. 122

US Food & Drug Administration (1972) Hexachlorophene as a component in
    drug and cosmetic products for human use. Fed. Regist., 37,
    20160-20164

US International Trade Commission (1977) Synthetic Organic Chemicals, US
    Production and Sales, 1976, USITC Publication 833, Washington DC,
    US Government Printing Office, p. 306

US Pharmacopeial Convention, Inc. (1975) The US Pharmacopeia, 19th rev.,
    Rockville, MD, pp. 230-231

US Tariff Commission (1952) Synthetic Organic Chemicals, US Production
     and Sales, 1951, Report No. 175, Second Series, Washington DC,
     US Government Printing Office, p. 138

Van Auken, O.W. & Hulse, M. (1977) Extraction and gas-liquid chromatographic
     determination of hexachlorophene from several plant tissues. J. Assoc.
     off. anal. Chem., 60, 1081-1086

Van Auken, O.W., Hulse, M. & Durocher, C.L. (1977) Extraction, gas-liquid
     chromatographic detection, and quantitation of hexachlorophene
     residues from plant tissues high in lipid content. J. Assoc. off
     anal. Chem., 60, 1087-1092

Vig, B.K. (1972) No chromosome aberrations induced in cultured human
     leukocytes by hexachlorophene. EMS Newslett., 6, 5-6

West, R.W., Wilson, D.J. & Schaffner, W. (1975) Hexachlorophene
     concentrations in human milk. Bull. environ. Contam. Toxicol., 13,
     167-169

Wilson, C.H. (1974) Hexachlorophene in cosmetics by partition chromatography
     and ultraviolet spectrophotometry. J. Assoc. off. anal. Chem., 57,
     563-564

Wilson, C.H. (1975) Identification of preservatives in cosmetic products
     by thin-layer chromatography. J. Soc. Cosmet. Chem., 26, 75-81

Windholz, M., ed. (1976) The Merck Index, 9th ed., Rahway, NJ, Merck &
     Co., pp. 612-613

METHOXYCHLOR

This substance was considered by a previous IARC Working Group, in October 1973 (IARC, 1974). Since that time new data have become available, and these have been incorporated into the monograph and taken into account in the present evaluation.

A recent review on methoxychlor is available (Mercier, 1977).

1. Chemical and Physical Data

1.1 Synonyms and trade names

Chem. Abstr. Services Reg. No.: 72-43-5

Chem. Abstr. Name: 1,1'-(2,2,2-Trichloroethylidene)bis(4-methoxy-benzene)

Synonyms: 1,1-Bis(*para*-methoxyphenyl)-2,2,2-trichloroethane; 2,2-bis(*para*-methoxyphenyl)-1,1,1-trichloroethane; 2,2-di-*para*-anisyl-1,1,1-trichloroethane; *para,para'*-dimethoxydiphenyl-trichloroethane; dimethoxy-DDT; dimethoxy-DT; di(*para*-methoxy-phenyl)trichloromethyl methane; DMDT; *para,para'*-DMDT; *para,para'*-methoxychlor; methoxy-DDT; 1,1,1-trichloro-2,2-bis(*para*-methoxyphenyl)ethane; 1,1,1-trichloro-2,2-di(4-methoxyphenyl)-ethane

Trade names: Maralate; Marlate; Metox

1.2 Structural and molecular formulae and molecular weight

$C_{10}H_{15}Cl_3O_2$ Mol. wt: 345.7

1.3 Chemical and physical properties of the pure substance

From Spencer (1973), unless otherwise specified

(a) Description: Colourless crystals

(b) Melting-point: 89°C

(c) Spectroscopy data: λ_{max} 275, 270, 238 and 230 nm (E_1^1 = 183, 241, 458 and 575) in benzene; infra-red and nuclear magnetic resonance spectral data have also been tabulated (Grasselli & Ritchey, 1975).

(d) Solubility: Insoluble in water (0.1 mg/1 at 25°C); moderately soluble in ethanol and petroleum oils; readily soluble in aromatic solvents

(e) Stability: Resistant to oxidation

(f) Reactivity: More stable than DDT to dehydrochlorination in alcoholic alkali; susceptible to catalytic dehydrochlorination by heavy metal catalysts

1.4 Technical products and impurities

Methoxychlor is available commercially in the US as a technical grade containing 88% of the pure chemical and 12% of isomers and other reaction products. 3,6,11,14-Tetramethoxydibenzo(g,p)chrysene is one of the impurities present in commercial samples (Grant et al., 1976).

In the US, formulations of methoxychlor for various uses include wettable powders, emulsifiable concentrates, oil solutions, aerosols and dusts (Berg, 1978).

2. Production, Use, Occurrence and Analysis

2.1 Production and use

(a) Production

Methoxychlor was first synthesized in 1893, by the reaction of chloral hydrate with anisole in the presence of acetic acid and sulphuric acid (Prager et al., 1918). It is produced commercially by the condensation of anisole with chloral in the presence of sulphuric acid (Windholz, 1976).

Commercial production of methoxychlor in the US was first reported in 1946 (US Tariff Commission, 1948).   In 1975, 3 companies in the US produced a total of 2.5 million kg (US International Trade Commission, 1977a);   2 companies produced an undisclosed amount in 1976 (see pre-amble, p. 16) (US International Trade Commission, 1977b).

No data on its production in Europe or Japan were available.

(b) Use

The only known use for methoxychlor is as an insecticide.   It is approved in the US for use on 78 agricultural crops (including several types of seed), with restrictions on the use of treated seeds.   Metho-xychlor is also approved for use as an insecticide on beef cattle, dairy cattle, goats, sheep and swine and for spray treatment of barns, grain bins, mushroom houses and other agricultural premises (US Environmental Protection Agency, 1972a).

In 1974, 1.5 million kg methoxychlor were used in the US, as follows: home and garden applications, 30%; livestock and poultry, 15%; alfalfa, 10%; soya beans, 10%; forests, 10%; ornamental shrubs, 10%; deciduous fruits and nuts, 5%; and vegetables, 5%.

Domestic use of methoxychlor as a substitute for DDT is increasing and is estimated to be 4.5 million kg a year in the US (Safe Drinking Water Committee, 1977).

Residue tolerances on raw agricultural commodities range from 0 in milk and 2 mg/kg on stored grains treated after harvest to 100 mg/kg on alfalfa (US Environmental Protection Agency, 1972b).

The US Occupational Safety and Health Administration's health standards for exposure to air contaminants require that an employee's exposure to methoxychlor not exceed an 8-hr time-weighted average of 15 mg/m^3 in the working atmosphere in any 8-hr work shift of a 40-hr work week (US Occupational Safety & Health Administration, 1977).

In March 1965, the Joint Meeting of the FAO Working Party of Experts on Pesticide Residues and the WHO Expert Committee on Pesticide Residues established a temporary acceptable daily intake for man of 0-0.1 mg/kg bw (WHO, 1975); this was confirmed in 1977 (FAO/WHO, 1978).

No data on its use in Europe or Japan were available.

2.2 Occurrence

Methoxychlor is not known to occur as a natural product.

(a) Water and sediments

The half-life of methoxychlor in water is about 46 days. No residues of methoxychlor were detected in 500 samples of finished drinking-water from the Mississippi and Missouri Rivers or in 101 water samples from Hawaii. No methoxychlor was found during a survey of the drinking-water in New Orleans (Safe Drinking Water Committee, 1977).

Methoxychlor has been detected in: (1) several rivers, at levels of 2.9-89.1 µg/l; (2) one lake, at levels of up to 0.1 g/l (surface) and of 0.13-175 mg/l (sediment); (3) the effluent water from a biological sewage treatment plant, at levels of up to 106 µg/l (Eurocop-Cost, 1976); (4) 2 samples of ground-water (Shackelford & Keith, 1976); (5) the inlet waters of Lake Utah, in concentrations of 0-5.2 µg/l (Bradshaw *et al.*, 1972); (6) rural drinking-water supplies, at levels of 0-312 ng/l (Sandhu *et al.*, 1978); (7) municipal water in 5 locations (Luczak *et al.*, 1972, 1973); and (8) shallow, underground waters in some rural regions (Uminska *et al.*, 1973).

In studies of water and sediment pollution, methoxychlor has been detected in surface water and in drainage ditch and streambed sediments in a farming area, at levels of 0-43 µg/l (Burns *et al.*, 1975); it has been found in tributary streams and in tributary and ravine sediments of Lake Michigan, at levels of 2.9-89.1 ng/l and 0.19-175 µg/l, respectively (Schacht, 1974).

(b) Soil

Of 1729 cropland soil samples tested in the US National Soils Monitoring Program, only one contained methoxychlor, at a level of 0.28 mg/kg (Wiersma *et al.*, 1972). It was detected in the surface soils of 31 apple orchards, at levels in the range of 0-4 µg/kg (Frank *et al.*, 1976).

(c) Food and drink

In a continuing programme involving the monitoring of pesticide residues in food, levels of methoxychlor in foods were measured during the period 1965-1974 and an average daily intake of methoxychlor was calculated. For the period 1965-1970, the average daily intake was 0.5 µg/day; this level dropped to 0.1134 µg/day in 1973 and rose to 0.7974 µg/day (US Food & Drug Administration, 1975, 1977).

Methoxychlor has also been detected in: (1) samples of liver pâté, at maximum concentrations of 0.27 mg/kg (De Battistis & Lucisano, 1973);

(2) fruit and vegetables (Polizu & Serban, 1973);   (3) milk products,
at maximum concentrations of 0.089 mg/l (Laskowski & Bierska, 1976);
(4) meat and milk (Knoeppler, 1976);   (5) cherries, at residue levels
of more than 4 mg/kg (Haefner, 1976); and (6) lard, after storage for
17 months (Dzilinski & Raslawski, 1974).

Levels of pesticides (including methoxychlor) in specific crops in
Finland have been tabulated by Siltanen & Rosenberg (1976).

(d) Animals

Methoxychlor has been detected in: (1) fat samples from racoons,
at levels of 0.16-36.82 mg/kg (Bigler *et al.*, 1975; Nalley *et al.*,
1975); (2) 61 frogs (Jaskoski & Kinders, 1974); (3) goldeye fish
muscle tissue, at levels of < 0.01-1.5 mg/kg (Fredeen *et al.*, 1975);
(4) 2 lake fish, at levels of 56 and 62 µg/kg (Bradshaw *et al.*, 1972);
and (5) the edible portions of 5 species of lake fish, at levels of
0-0.1 mg/kg (wet-weight basis) (Schacht, 1974).

(e) Occupational exposure

Methoxychlor has been detected in the blood of agricultural workers
(Kontek *et al.*, 1976).

(f) Other

Methoxychlor has been detected in the following poultry feeds:
soya bean meal (2-53 µg/kg); corn meal (91-151 µg/kg); alfalfa meal
(7-1947 µg/kg); fish meal (15-232 µg/kg); and fats (91-151 µg/kg)
(Waldron & Naber, 1974).   Extensive tables have been published on the
levels of pesticides, including methoxychlor, in over 9000 samples of
animal feed (Maletto & Mussa, 1975).

Sixty days after spray application of 2.24 kg/ha methoxychlor, the
residue level on pine branches was 4.63 mg/kg (Sundaram, 1977).   Residues
were also detected on four Dutch elm trees at levels of 50-955 mg/kg
(Sundaram, 1976).

Methoxychlor has been detected in raw tobacco (Thurm, 1974) and in
finished tobacco products (Thurm & Fensterer, 1972).

2.3 Analysis

Methods used for the analysis of methoxychlor in environmental
samples are listed in Table 1.

Other methods for the separation of various pesticides include
gel-permeation chromatography (Johnson *et al.*, 1976); reverse-phase
liquid chromatography, with a detection limit of 10 ng/sample (Seiber,

TABLE 1. METHODS FOR THE ANALYSIS OF METHOXYCHLOR

SAMPLE TYPE	ANALYTICAL METHOD			
	EXTRACTION/CLEAN-UP	DETECTION	LIMIT OF DETECTION	REFERENCE
Formulations				
Powders	Extract (carbon disulphide)	IR; GC/FID		US Environmental Protection Agency (1976)
Powders	Extract (toluene), treat with sodium biphenyl	Titration (Vohlard)		Pease (1975)
	Extract (toluene)	TLC (revelation: silver nitrate-ultra-violet)		
Water	Extract (benzene), TLC, elute from plate	Polarography		Maultz (1975)
	Extract (hexane)	GC/ECD	1 µg/kg	Solomon & Lockhart (1977)
Sediments	Extract (acetone), double CC	TLC (revelation: silver nitrate-ultra-violet)	25 µg/kg	Taylor et al. (1975)
Food & drink				
Fruit	Extract (benzene), evaporate, dissolve in petroleum ether, liquid/liquid partition, remove solvent, treat with potassium hydroxide, extract (petroleum ether), wash (ethanol), remove solvent, treat with sulphuric acid	Spectrophotometry (550 nm)		Horwitz (1965)
Fruit, vegetables, silage, dairy products	Extract (acetonitrile or aqueous acetonitrile), liquid/liquid partition, CC	GC/ECD, TLC & PC (revelation: silver nitrate-ultra-violet)	0.005 µg on TLC plate	Horwitz (1975)

TABLE 1. METHODS FOR THE ANALYSIS OF METHOXYCHLOR (continued)

SAMPLE TYPE	ANALYTICAL METHOD			
	EXTRACTION/CLEAN-UP	DETECTION	LIMIT OF DETECTION	REFERENCE
Fish	Extract (hexane), defat by freezing, CC	GC/ECD	10 µg/kg	Solomon & Lockhard (1977)
Raw sugar & sugar products	Extract (petroleum ether-acetone), CC	GC/ECD	0.15 mg/kg	Kubacki & Kasprowicz (1972)
Margarine & butter	Extract (petroleum ether), liquid/liquid partition, CC	GC/ECD		Kubacki et al. (1974)
Beer and hops	Beer: extract (petroleum ether-acetone); hops: extract (petroleum ether), CC of appropriate extract	GC/ECD	25.8 pg/sample	Lipowska et al. (1972)
Apples, potatoes and dry feed	Extract (naphtha ether), steam distill, CC	GC/ECD		Lewandowski et al. (1975)
Fruit	Extract (chloroform), remove solvent, redissolve (petroleum ether), liquid/liquid partition, CC	TLC (revelation: silver nitrate-ultra-violet)	0.4 mg/kg	Cwiertniewska (1973)
Animal fat	Homogenize (anhydrous sodium sulphate), extract (petroleum ether), CC	TLC (revelation: silver nitrate-ultra-violet)		Batista (1974)

Abbreviations: IR - infra-red spectrometry; GC/FID - gas chromatography/flame ionization detection; TLC - thin-layer chromatography; CC - column chromatography; ECD - electron capture detection; PC - paper chromatography

1974); gas chromatography on 9 different columns (Thompson *et al.*, 1975); and a rapid thin-layer chromatographic method (Ludwick *et al.*, 1977). Clean-up procedures prior to thin-layer chromatography of various food extracts have been described by Pordab & Maik (1972a,b).

Gas chromatography has been used to determine methoxychlor in formulations (Sundaram, 1975) and in the tissues of chickens fed 7 chlorinated hydrocarbon insecticides at low levels (Onley *et al.*, 1975).

3. Biological Data Relevant to the Evaluation
of Carcinogenic Risk to Humans

3.1 Carcinogenicity studies in animals

(a) Oral administration

Mouse: Groups of 50 male and 50 female 5-7-week-old B6C3F1 hybrid mice were fed technical-grade methoxychlor (95% minimum purity) in the diet.   Initially, high-dose animals received 2800 mg/kg diet for males and 1500 mg/kg diet for females, and low-dose animals received 1400 mg/kg diet for males and 750 mg/kg diet for females.   After 1 week these doses were increased to 3500 mg/kg diet and 2000 mg/kg diet for high-dose groups and 1750 and 1000 mg/kg diet for low-dose groups; animals were maintained on these diets for 77 weeks, followed by 14-15 weeks on methoxychlor-free diets.   The measured, time-weighted, average doses were 1746 (low dose) and 3491 (high dose) mg/kg diet for males and 997 (low dose) and 1994 (high dose) mg/kg diet for females.   Groups of 20 male and 20 female mice served as matched controls and were maintained on methoxychlor-free diets for 92 weeks.   Survival was reduced in male animals: 69% of the high-dose, 58% of the low-dose and 45% of control animals survived to 81 weeks.   In females, survival to 92 weeks was 98% of high-dose, 90% of low-dose and 85% of control animals.   In necropsied male mice, the numbers of tumour-bearing animals were 3/12 controls compared with 5/44 in the low-dose group and 9/47 in the high-dose group.   In necropsied female mice, the respective numbers of tumour-bearing animals were 3/20 controls, 6/46 in the low-dose group and 3/50 in the high-dose group. Only 60-70% of the males and 28-32% of the females were examined histo-pathologically.   Statistical analysis of the results revealed no obvious increase in the yield of benign and malignant neoplasms which could be ascribed to treatment with methoxychlor.   There were no significant differences between test and control groups in the age at which tumours occurred (National Cancer Institute, 1978).

Rat: In a study by Nelson & Fitzhugh reported and reviewed by Lehman (1952, 1965) and by Deichmann *et al.* (1967), 6 groups of 24 Osborne-Mendel rats were fed diets containing 10-2000 mg/kg diet metho-xychlor for 2 years, at which time 52% of the animals were still alive.

One rat fed 500 mg/kg diet and 5 rats fed 2000 mg/kg diet were found to have liver nodules, 4 of which were diagnosed as liver-cell adenomas. All but one liver-tumour-bearing animal survived for 2 years [The Working Group noted that the inaccessibility of the original data precluded any evaluation of this experiment].

Four groups of 25 male and 25 female rats (strain unspecified), about 4 weeks of age, were fed diets containing 0, 25, 200 or 1600 mg/kg diet methoxychlor for 2 years. No tumours were found in 13 controls which survived until the end of the experiment. One neurofibroma and 1 lung tumour were found in 13 survivors administered 25 mg/kg diet; 1 mammary tumour was found in 10 survivors administered 200 mg/kg diet; and 1 mammary tumour, 1 ovarian cystadenoma, 1 tumour of the abdominal wall, 1 adenocarcinoma of the pancreas and 1 epidermoid carcinoma were found in 16 survivors administered 1600 mg/kg diet (Hodge et al., 1952) [The increased number of tumours in animals fed 1600 mg/kg diet was considered by the authors to be coincidental; all of these tumours, with the exception of the adenocarcinoma of the pancreas, occur commonly in rats of that colony].

Two groups of 30 male and 30 female Osborne-Mendel rats were administered diets containing 0 or 80 mg/kg diet methoxychlor for 2 years. Malignant tumours were found in 5 treated females and in 9 control rats; benign tumours were present in 8 treated and in 6 control rats. The distribution of tumours by site and type was similar in the two groups (Radomski et al., 1965) [The Working Group noted the low dose used].

In a 27-month study, 30 male and 30 female Osborne-Mendel rats, about 4 weeks old, were administered 1000 mg/kg diet methoxychlor. At 18 months, 54/60 treated rats were still alive, compared with 48/60 controls. The incidence and distribution of benign and malignant tumours (mainly mammary and subcutaneous) were similar in treated (10 benign, 1 malignant) and control (14 benign, 1 malignant) groups (Deichmann et al., 1967).

Groups of 50 male and 50 female 5-7-week-old Osborne-Mendel rats were fed diets containing technical-grade methoxychlor of 95% minimum purity. High-dose animals received 720 mg/kg diet for 29 weeks in males and 1500 mg/kg diet for 55 weeks in females; the dose was increased to 1000 mg/kg diet for a further 29 weeks in males. For the remaining 16-17 weeks of treatment, males were fed 1000 mg/kg diet and females 1500 mg/kg diet for 4 weeks, followed by 1 week without treatment, and then the cycle was repeated. Low-dose animals received 360 mg/kg diet for 29 weeks and 500 mg/kg diet for 49 weeks for males and 750 mg/kg diet for 78 weeks for females. Low- and high-dose groups were maintained for a further 33-34 weeks on a methoxychlor-free diet. Time-weighted average doses were 448 and 750 mg/kg diet for males and females of the low-dose group and 845 and 1385 mg/kg diet for males and

females of the high-dose group.   Groups of 20 animals of each sex were
used as matched controls.   At 100 weeks, 86% of high-dose males and 94%
of high-dose females, 74% of low-dose males and 94% of low-dose females
and 85% of male and 90% of female controls were still alive.   Histopathology of all organ systems was performed on 82% or more of the
animals entered into the study.   The numbers of tumour-bearing animals
(benign and malignant neoplasms) were, <u>males</u>: controls, 11/20; low
dose, 23/44; high dose, 21/41; <u>females</u>: controls, 12/20; low dose,
30/47; high dose, 30/49.   Haemangiosarcomas of the spleen in male rats
were the only tumours that showed an increased incidence (1/20 controls,
6/44 in low dose, 2/42 in high dose).   S.c. and abdominal haemangiosarcomas were observed in 3 low-dose males; although their incidence
was not significantly increased, these tumours occur rarely in untreated
Osborne-Mendel rats (National Cancer Institute, 1978).

(b) Skin application

<u>Mouse</u>: Two groups of 50 male and 50 female 2-4-month old C3H/Anf
mice were painted weekly with either 0.1 or 10 mg/animal methoxychlor
in 0.2 ml acetone (total dose, 0.1-10.4 mg/animal at the low level and
10-980 mg/animal at the high level).   The mean survival time ranged
from 342 days in females given the low dose to 450 days in the other
groups.   No skin tumours were observed (Hodge *et al.*, 1966) [The
Working Group noted the low dose used].

(c) Subcutaneous and/or intramuscular administration

<u>Mouse</u>: A group of 50 male and 50 female 2-4-month-old C3H/Anf
mice were given single s.c. injections of 10 mg/animal methoxychlor in
0.02 ml trioctanoin.   The mean survival times were 372 days in males
and 419 days in females.   No s.c. tumours were observed; histological
observation was confined to 24 mice (Hodge *et al.*, 1966) [The Working
Group noted that a negative result obtained with a single s.c. injection is not an adequate basis for discounting carcinogenicity].

3.2 Other relevant biological data

(a) Experimental systems

Toxic effects

The oral LD_{50} in rats is 5000-7000 mg/kg bw (Hodge *et al.*, 1950),
in mice, 2900 mg/kg bw and in monkeys, > 2500 mg/kg bw (Coulston &
Serrone, 1969).

Dermal application of 2-3 ml of a 30% solution in dimethyl phthalate
to rabbits on 5 days a week for 13 weeks produced paralysis of the fore-
limbs, some fatty degeneration of the liver and lesions of the central
nervous system (Haag *et al.*, 1950).

Dogs and pigs were fed 1000, 2000 or 4000 mg/kg diet methoxychlor for 2 years; and rats and monkeys were given 400, 1000 and 2500 mg/kg bw/day by gavage in 1% gum tragacanth for 3 and 6 months, respectively. In dogs, the 2 higher dose levels produced nervousness, apprehension, excess salivation, tremors and convulsions; in rats and monkeys, damage to the liver and small intestine was observed. Nephritis and mammary hyperplasia were observed in the pigs at autopsy (Stein, 1968).

Near-lethal doses of methoxychlor increased liver:body-weight ratios in rats (Davison & Cox, 1976). Methoxychlor or a metabolite has an oestrogenic effect (Nelson et al., 1976, 1977; Welch et al., 1969).

Atrophy of the testes was observed in rats given 1% methoxychlor in their diet (Hodge et al., 1950). In rats given 100 or 200 mg/kg bw/day, arrested spermatogenesis was noticed after 70 consecutive days of treatment; and corpora lutea failed to develop in female rats treated with similar dosages for 14 days before and continuously after mating (Bal & Mungkornkarn, 1977).

Embryotoxicity and teratogenicity

It was reported in an abstract that methoxychlor did not affect the development of the chick embryo (Marlia, 1964). It was toxic to sea urchins and led to abnormal embryos (Bresch & Arendt, 1977).

Administration of 1000 mg/kg diet methoxychlor to pregnant rats caused early vaginal openings in their offspring; and both male and female offspring had reduced fertility when they attained maturity (Harris et al., 1974).

Oral administration of technical-grade and formulations of methoxychlor to pregnant rats reduced maternal body weight gain during gestation at all doses, ranging from 50-400 mg/kg bw. Both methoxychlor samples were foetotoxic at 200 and 400 mg/kg bw and produced a dose-related increase in the incidence of wavy ribs at 100, 200 and 400 mg/kg bw (Khera et al., 1978). No abortions were produced in pregnant cows given 10 mg/kg bw/day methoxychlor (Macklin & Ribelin, 1971).

Absorption, distribution, excretion and metabolism

In mice, 98% of labelled methoxychlor given orally was eliminated within 24 hrs. The main metabolic pathway was O-dealkylation to 2-(para-hydroxyphenyl)-2-(para-methoxyphenyl)-1,1,1-trichloroethane, 2,2-bis(para-hydroxyphenyl)-1,1,1-trichloroethane and its ethylene, and 4,4'-dihydroxybenzophenone which were extreted mainly as conjugates (Kapoor et al., 1970).

[^{14}C-1-phenyl]-Methoxychlor in oil emulsion given intravenously to rats at a dose of 1 mg in 0.5 ml emulsion was metabolized rapidly by the liver to unidentified hydrophilic products, which were excreted mainly in the faeces, by secretion from the liver into the bile, and to a lesser extent in the urine.   Very little reabsorption occurred from the gastrointestinal tract (Weikel, 1957).

Weanling rats fed 500 mg/kg diet methoxychlor for 4-18 weeks stored 14-36 mg/kg in fat.   Equilibrium was reached within 4 weeks, and methoxychlor disappeared from the fatty tissue within 2 weeks after end of exposure.   Rats fed 100 mg/kg stored 1-7 mg/kg.   No methoxychlor was stored in animals given 25 mg/kg diet, and no sex differences in storage were observed (Kunze *et al.*, 1950).

Cluett *et al.* (1960) found residues in milk shortly after cows were sprayed with aqueous suspensions of methoxychlor.   A maximum level of 0.1 mg/l was found 1 day after treatment, and detectable levels persisted for 1 week.

Mutagenicity and other related short-term tests

Technical-grade and purified methoxychlor were not mutagenic in plate tests with *Salmonella typhimurium* TA1535, TA1537, TA1538, TA98 and TA100, even with metabolic activation (Grant *et al.*, 1976; Poole *et al.*, 1977); however, 3,6,11,14-tetramethoxydibenzo(*g,p*)chrysene, one of the impurities present in commercial samples of methoxychlor, was mutagenic in strain TA98 in the presence of a liver microsomal activation system from phenobarbital-treated rats at concentrations of 100 and 200 µg/plate (Grant *et al.*, 1976).   Negative results were obtained with *Escherichia coli* WP2 and *Saccharomyces cerevisiae* D3 (Poole *et al.*, 1977).

It was reported in an abstract that Phosan-plus (a mixture of methoxychlor and two organophosphates, dimethoate and malathion) did not induce reverse mutations in *Schizosaccharomyces pombe* (strain *ade 7-C8*) either in the presence or absence of a liver microsomal activation system (Degraeve *et al.*, 1977).

Male mice that received a single i.p. injection of 30 mg/kg bw Phosan-plus showed no significant increase in chromosomal damage in their bone-marrow cells (polychromatic erythrocyte micronuclei, chromosome breakage) during the first 3 days after injection.   In testis preparations from mice injected similarly, made at intervals ranging from 12 hrs to 44 days, a slight increase in chromosome breakage was detectable in spermatogonia after 24 and 48 hrs.   However, there was no increase in sperm abnormalities 40 and 44 days after injection, and spermatocyte metaphases revealed no significant cytological damage. Dominant lethal tests were also negative (Degraeve *et al.*, 1977).

Injection of a 0.1% solution of methoxychlor did not induce sex-linked recessive lethals in male *Drosophila melanogaster* (Benes & Sram, 1969).

(<u>b</u>) <u>Humans</u>

The estimated fatal oral dose for humans is 450 g/subject (approximately 6 g/kg bw). An oral dose of 350 mg/subject/day (100 mg/kg diet) for 2 years produced no toxic symptoms, whereas 500 mg/kg diet (1750 mg/subject/day) produced unspecified tissue changes (American Conference of Governmental Industrial Hygienists, 1974).

3.3 <u>Case reports and epidemiological studies</u>

No data were available to the Working Group.

4. <u>Summary of Data Reported and Evaluation</u>[1]

4.1 <u>Experimental data</u>

Methoxychlor was tested in one experiment in mice and in several experiments in rats by oral administration. The study in mice gave negative results. In at least four experiments in rats, dietary concentrations of 1000 mg/kg or more were used. A suggestion that it was hepatocarcinogenic, made in an earlier study that was inadequately reported, was not confirmed in three more recent experiments. Methoxychlor was inadequately tested in mice by repeated skin application and by subcutaneous injection of single doses.

Methoxychlor was not mutagenic in bacteria, yeast or *Drosophila melanogaster*. Cytogenic and dominant lethal tests in mice were also negative.

Methoxychlor is foetotoxic.

---

[1]Subsequent to the meeting of the Working Group, the Secretariat became aware of a paper by Reuber (1979a), reporting the results of a study carried out in 1969 in which oral administration of methoxychlor induced testicular carcinomas in 27/51 male Balb/c mice, compared with 8/71 controls, but in none of the C3H mice tested. A further paper by Reuber (1979b) reported the results of a study carried out in 1951 in which oral administration of methoxychlor to Osborne-Mendel rats induced liver carcinomas.

4.2 Human data

No case reports or epidemiological studies were available to the Working Group.

The extensive production and the widespread use of methoxychlor over the past several decades, together with the persistent nature of the compound, indicate that widespread human exposure occurs. This is confirmed by many reports of its occurrence in the general environment and by its presence in human blood.

4.3 Evaluation

The available data did not provide evidence that methoxychlor is carcinogenic in experimental animals.

5. References

American Conference of Government Hygienists (1974)   Documentation of
    the Threshold Limit Values for Substances in Air, Cincinnati, OH,
    p. 152

Bal, H.S. & Mungkornkarn, P. (1977)   Chronic toxicity effects of
    methoxychlor on the reproductive system of the rat (Abstract).
    In: Abstracts of the International Congress on Toxicology, Toronto,
    Canada, 1977, p. 4

Batista, M.T.P.M. (1974)   Qualitative analysis of DDT and related
    compounds in animal fat (Port.).   Bol. Fac. Farm., Univ. Coimbra,
    Ed. Didact.: Not. Farm., 40, 5, 7 [Chem. Abstr., 83, 191415k]

Benes, V. & Sram, R. (1969)   Mutagenic activity of some pesticides in
    Drosophila melanogaster.   Ind. Med., 38, 50-52

Berg, G.L., ed. (1978)   Farm Chemicals Handbook 1978, Willoughby, OH,
    Meister, p. D 171

Bigler, W.J., Jenkins, J.H., Cumbie, P.M., Hoff, G.L. & Prather, E.D.
    (1975)   Wildlife and environmental health: racoons as indicators
    of zoonoses and pollutants in southeastern United States.   J. Am.
    vet. Med. Assoc., 167, 592-597

Bradshaw, J.S., Loveridge, E.L., Rippee, K.P., Peterson, J.L., White, D.A.,
    Barton, J.R. & Fuhriman, D.K. (1972)   Seasonal variations in residues
    of chlorinated hydrocarbon pesticides in the water of the Utah Lake
    drainage system - 1970 and 1971.   Pestic. Monit. J., 6, 166-170

Bresch, H. & Arendt, U. (1977)   Influence of different organochlorine
    pesticides on the development of the sea urchin embryo.   Environ. Res.,
    13, 121-128

Burns, B.G., Peach, M.E. & Stiles, D.A. (1975)   Organochlorine pesticide
    residues in a farming area, Nova Scotia - 1972-73.   Pestic. Monit. J.,
    9, 34-38

Cluett, M.L., Lowen, W.K., Pease, H.L. & Woodhouse, C.A. (1960)   Determination
    of methoxychlor and/or metabolites in milk following topical
    application to dairy cows.   J. agric. Food Chem., 8, 277-281

Coulston, F. & Serrone, D.M. (1969)   The comparative approach to the role
    of nonhuman primates in evaluation of drug toxicity in man: a
    review.   Ann. N.Y. Acad. Sci., 62, 681-704

Cwiertniewska, E. (1973)   Residues of captan and methoxychlor in certain
    fruits (Pol.).   Rocz. Panstw. Zakl. Hig., 24, 309-314 [Chem. Abstr.,
    80, 46573u]

Davison, K.L. & Cox, J.H. (1976) Methoxychlor effects on hepatic storage of vitamin A in rats. Bull. environ. Contam. Toxicol., 16, 145-148

De Battistis, P. & Lucisano, A. (1973) Organochlorinated insecticides in liver pate (Ital.). Acta med. vet., 19, 157-161 [Chem. Abstr., 81, 103340n]

Degraeve, N., Moutschen, J., Moutschen-Dahmen, M., Gilot-Delhalle, J., Houbrechts, N. & Colizzi, A. (1977) Cytogenetic and genetic effects of Phosan-plus (Abstact no. 20). Mutat. Res., 46, 204

Deichmann, W.B., Keplinger, M., Sala, F. & Glass, E. (1967) Synergism among oral carcinogens. IV. The simultaneous feeding of four tumorigens to rats. Toxicol. appl. Pharmacol., 11, 88-103

Dzilinski, E. & Raslawski, Z. (1974) Speed of disappearing of γ-HCH, methoxychlor, and DDT and its metabolites in lard (Pol.). Med. Wet., 30, 97-99 [Chem. Abstr., 81, 103343r]

Eurocop-Cost (1976) A Comprehensive List of Polluting Substances which have been Identified in Various Fresh Waters, Effluent Discharges, Aquatic Animals and Plants, and Bottom Sediments, 2nd ed., EUCO/MDU/73/76, XII/476/76, Luxembourg, Commission of the European Communities, p. 49

FAO/WHO (1978) Pesticide residues in food - 1977. FAO Plant Production and Protection Paper, 10 Rev., pp. 41-42

Frank, R., Braun, H.E., Ishida, K. & Suda, P. (1976) Persistant organic and inorganic pesticide residues in orchard soils and vineyards of Southern Ontario. Can. J. Soil Sci., 56, 463-484

Fredeen, F.J.H., Saha, J.G. & Balba, M.H. (1975) Residues of methoxychlor and other chlorinated hydrocarbons in water, sand, and selected fauna following injections of methoxychlor black fly larvicide into the Saskatchewan River, 1972. Pestic. Monit. J., 8, 241-246

Grant, E.L., Mitchell, R.H., West, P.R., Mazuch, L. & Ashwood-Smith, M.J. (1976) Mutagenicity and putative carcinogenicity tests of several polycyclic aromatic compounds associated with impurities of the insecticide methoxychlor. Mutat. Res., 40, 225-228

Grasselli, J.G. & Ritchey, W.M., eds (1975) CRC Atlas of Spectral Data and Physical Constants for Organic Compounds, 2nd ed., Vol. III, Cleveland, OH, Chemical Rubber Co., p. 241

Haag, H.B., Finnegan, J.K., Larson, P.S., Riese, W. & Dreyfuss, M.L. (1950) Comparative chronic toxicity for warm-blooded animals of 2,2-bis-(p- chlorophenyl)-1,1,1-trichloroethane (DDT) and 2,2-bis-(p-methoxyphenyl)-1,1,1-trichloroethane (DMDT, methoxychlor). Arch. int. Pharmacodyn., 83, 491-504

Haefner, M. (1976) Residues of methoxychlor on cherries – application of methoxychlor using a helicopter (Germ.). Gesunde Pflanz., 28, 249–259 [Chem. Abstr., 86, 104552y]

Harris, S.J., Cecil, H.C. & Bitman, J. (1974) Effect of several dietary levels of technical methoxychlor on reproduction in rats. J. agric. Food Chem., 22, 969–973

Hodge, H.C., Maynard, E.A., Thomas, J.F., Blanchet, H.J., Jr, Wilt, W.G., Jr & Mason, K.E. (1950) Short-term oral toxicity tests of methoxychlor [2,2 di-(p-methoxy phenyl)-1,1,1-trichloroethane] in rats and dogs. J. Pharmacol. exp. Ther., 99, 140–148

Hodge, H.C., Maynard, E.A., & Blanchet, H.J., Jr (1952) Chronic oral toxicity tests of methoxychlor (2,2-di-(p-methoxyphenyl)-1,1,1-trichloroethane) in rats and dogs. J. Pharmacol. exp. Ther., 104, 60–66

Hodge, H.C., Maynard, E.A., Downs, W.L., Ashton, J.K. & Salerno, L.L. (1966) Tests on mice for evaluating carcinogenicity. Toxicol. appl. Pharmacol., 9, 583–596

Horwitz, W., ed. (1965) Official Methods of Analysis of the Association of Official Agricultural Chemists, 10th ed., Washington DC, Association of Official Agricultural Chemists, p. 399

Horwitz, W., ed. (1975) Offical Methods of Analysis of the Association of Official Analytical Chemists, 12th ed., Washington DC, Association of Official Analytical Chemists, pp. 518–533, 547

IARC (1974) IARC Monographs on the Evaluation of Carcinogenic Risk of Chemicals to Man, 5, Some Organochlorine Pesticides, Lyon, pp. 193–202

Jaskoski, B.J. & Kinders, R.J. (1974) DDT and methoxychlor in a frog population in Cook County. Trans. Illinois State Acad. Sci., 67, 341–344 [Chem. Abstr., 83, 38484n]

Johnson, L.D., Waltz, R.H., Ussary, J.P. & Kaiser, F.E. (1976) Automated gel permeation chromatographic cleanup of animal and plant extracts for pesticide residue determination. J. Assoc. off. anal. Chem., 59, 174–187

Kapoor, I.P., Metcalf, R.L., Nystrom, R.F. & Sangha, G.K. (1970) Comparative metabolism of methoxychlor, methiochlor, and DDT in mouse, insects, and in a model ecosystem. J. agric. Food Chem., 18, 1145–1152

Khera, K.S., Whalen, C. & Trivett, G. (1978) Teratogenicity studies on linuron, malathion, and methoxychlor in rats. Toxicol. appl. Pharmacol., 45, 435–444

Knoeppler, H.O. (1976) Pesticide residues in food of animal origin
    (Germ.). Fleischwirtschaft, 56, 1643-1646 [Chem. Abstr., 86, 41939g]

Kontek, M., Glogowski, K. & Paradowski, S. (1976) Chlorinated hydrocarbons
    in the blood of agricultural workers with occupational exposure to
    pesticides (Pol.). Pol. Tyg. Lek., 31, 265-267

Kubacki, S.J. & Kasprowicz, W. (1972) Determination of organochlorine
    pesticide residues in sugar raw materials and sugar products by gas
    chromatography (Pol.). Pr. Inst. Lab. Badaw. Przem. Spozyw., 22,
    295-306 [Chem. Abstr., 79, 3929b]

Kubacki, S., Bednarek-Karbul, W., Kasprowicz, W. & Danielewska, B.
    (1974) Estimation of chloroorganic pesticide residues in margarine
    and butter by gas-liquid chromatography (Pol.). Rocz. Inst. Przem.
    Mlecz., 16, 15-25 [Chem. Abstr., 82, 71662w]

Kunze, F.M., Laug, E.Q. & Prickett, C.S. (1950) The storage of
    methoxychlor in the fat of the rat. Proc. Soc. exp. Biol. (NY),
    75, 415-416

Laskowski, K. & Bierska, J. (1976) Residues of chlorinated organic
    pesticides in milk products in Poland during 1968-1974 (Germ.).
    Tagungsber., Akad. Landwirtschaftswiss. D.D.R., 144, 91-94
    [Chem. Abstr., 85, 190888w]

Lehman, A.J. (1952) Chemicals in foods: a report to the Association of
    Food and Drug Officials on current developments. II. Pesticides.
    V. Pathology. Bull. Assoc. Food Drug Off. US, 16,
    126-132

Lehman, A.J. (1965) Summaries of Pesticide Toxicity, Food & Drug
    Administration, US Department of Health, Education, & Welfare,
    Washington DC, US Government Printing Office, pp. 29-31

Lewandowski, A., Dorozalska, A. & Schroeder, G. (1975) Purification of
    organochlorine pesticides from plant materials in gaseous phase
    (Pol.). Chem. Anal. (Warsaw), 20, 829-834 [Chem. Abstr., 84,
    57440g]

Lipowska, T., Kubacki, S.J. & Goszcz, H. (1972) Rapid method for one-
    stage purification of beer and hops for the determination of
    organochlorine pesticide content by gas chromatography (Pol.).
    Pr. Inst. Lab. Badaw. Przem. Spozyw., 22, 307-316 [Chem. Abstr.,
    79, 3767x]

Luczak, J., Chrostowska, K., Kazmierczyk, J., Kraus, W. & Traczyk, J.
    (1972) Occurrence of persistent pesticides in the municipal water
    in Rzeszow, Katowice, and Opote Provinces (Pol.) Rocz. Panstw.
    Zakl. Hig., 23, 513-520 [Chem. Abstr., 78, 88437s]

Luczak, J., Brudny, E., Chmielewska, Z., Traczyk, J., Jurkiewicz, J., Krzeczkowska, I., Siudak, F. & Lewtak, M. (1973) Persistent pesticides in waters used for community purposes in the cities of Krakow and Warsaw and in the provinces of Gdansk, Olsztyn, and Lodz (Pol.). Rocz. Panstw. Zakl. Hig., 24, 101-107 [Chem. Abstr., 79, 23264j]

Ludwick, A.G., Lau, A.N.K. & Ludwick, L.M. (1977) Simple sensitive technique for detecting organochlorine pesticides on thin layer chromatograms. J. Assoc. off. anal. Chem., 60, 1077-1080

Macklin, A.W. & Ribelin, W.E. (1971) The relation of pesticides to abortion in dairy cattle. J. Am. vet. med. Assoc., 159, 1743-1748

Maletto, S. & Mussa, P.P. (1975) Quantity and frequency of pesticides in forage and fodder used in Italy. Folio Vet. Lat., 5, 549-586 [Chem. Abstr., 85, 92305j]

Marliac, J.-P. (1964) Toxicity and teratogenic effects of 12 pesticides in the chick embryo (Abstract no. 26). Fed. Proc., 23, 105

Maultz, S. (1975) Polarographic modification of determination of DDT, methoxychlor, and γ-HCH in water by thin-layer chromatography (Pol.). Gaz, Woda Tech. Sanit., 49, 83-85 [Chem. Abstr., 83, 173694w]

Mercier, M. (1977) Preparatory Study for Establishing Criteria (Exposure, Effect Relationships) for Humans on Organochlorine Compounds, i.e. Pesticides, 2nd Series, Doc. V/F/2500/1/76e, Luxembourg, Commission of the European Communities, pp. 18-24

Nalley, L., Hoff, G., Bigler, W. & Hull, W. (1975) Pesticide levels in the omental fat of Florida raccoons. Bull. environ. Contam. Toxicol., 13, 741-744

National Cancer Institute (1978) Bioassay of Methoxychlor for Possible Carcinogenicity (Technical Report Series No. 35), DHEW Publication No. (NIH) 78-835, Washington DC, US Department of Health, Education, & Welfare

Nelson, J.A., Struck, P.F. & James, R. (1976) Estrogenically-active forms of o,p'-DDT and methoxychlor (Abstract no. 730). Pharmacologist, 18, 247

Nelson, J.A., Struck, R.F. & James, R. (1977) Role of metabolism in the estrogenic activities of methoxychlor and o,p'-DDT (Abstract). J. Toxicol. environ. Health, 3, 366-367

Onley, J.H., Giuffrida, L., Watts, R.R., Ives, N.F. & Storherr, R.W. (1975) Residues in broiler chick tissues from low level feedings of seven chlorinated hydrocarbon insecticides. J. Assoc. off. anal. Chem., 58, 785-792

Pease, H.L. (1975) Collaborative study of a method for the analysis of
    dry methoxychlor formulations. J. Assoc. off. anal. Chem., 58, 40-43

Polizu, A. & Serban, V. (1973) Dynamics of methylchlor and DDT residues
    in fruits and vegetables (Rom.). An. Inst. Cercet. Prot. Plant.,
    Acad. Stŭnte Agric. Silvice, 10, 473-478 [Chem. Abstr., 83, 7329m]

Poole, D.C., Simmon, V.F. & Newell, G.W. (1977) In vitro mutagenic
    activity of fourteen pesticides (Abstract no. 155). Toxicol. appl.
    Pharmacol., 41, 196

Pordab, Z. & Maik, L. (1972a) Thin-layer chromatographic determination
    of residues of DDT and its metabolites (DDE, DDD), lindane, and
    DMDT in meat for baby foods production and in baby foods (Pol.).
    Biul. Inst. Orchr. Rosl., 54, 521-533 [Chem. Abstr., 81, 62208e]

Pordab, Z. & Maik, L. (1972b) Thin-layer chromatographic determination
    of residues of DDT and its metabolites (DDE,DDD), lindane, and DMDT
    in vegetable raw materials for baby food production (Pol.). Biul.
    Inst. Ochr. Rosl., 54, 535-551 [Chem. Abstr., 81, 62237p]

Prager, B., Jacobson, P., Schmidt, P. & Stern, D. (1918) Beilsteins
    Handbuch der Organischen Chemie, 4th ed., Vol. 6, Syst. No. 563,
    Berlin, Springer, p. 1007

Radomski, J.L., Deichmann, W.B., MacDonald, W.E. & Glass, E.M. (1965)
    Synergism among oral carcinogens. I. Results of the simultaneous
    feeding of four tumorigens to rats. Toxicol. appl. Pharmacol.,
    7, 652-656

Reuber, M.D. (1979a) Interstitial cell carcinomas of the testis in Balb/C
    male mice ingesting methoxychlor. J. Cancer Res. clin. Oncol., 93, 173-
    180

Reuber, M.D. (1979b) Carcinomas of the liver in Osborne-Mendel rats
    ingesting methoxychlor. Life Sci., 24, 1367-1372

Safe Drinking Water Committee (1977) Drinking Water and Health,
    Washington DC, National Academy of Sciences, pp. 579, 581

Sandhu, S.S, Warren, W.J. & Nelson, P. (1978) Pesticidal residue in rural
    potable water. J. Am. Water Works Assoc., 70, 41-45

Schacht, R.A. (1974) Pesticides in the Illinois Waters of Lake Michigan,
    EPA 660/3-74-002, Washington DC, US Government Printing Office, p. 10

Seiber, J.N. (1974) Reversed-phase liquid chromatography of some
    pesticides and related compounds. Solubility-retention relationships.
    J. Chromatogr., 94, 151-157

Shackelford, W.M. & Keith, L.H. (1976) Frequency of Organic Compounds
    Identified in Water, EPA-600/4-76-062, Athens, GA, US
    Environmental Protection Agency, p. 169

Siltanen, H. & Rosenberg, C. (1976) Investigations on Pesticide Residues
    1975. Publications of the State Institute of Agricultural Chemistry,
    11, Helsinki, Finland

Solomon, J. & Lockhart, W.L. (1977) Rapid preparation of micro sample
    and gas-liquid chromatographic determination of methoxychlor
    residues in animal tissues and water. J. Assoc. off. anal. Chem.,
    60, 690-695

Spencer, E.Y. (1973) Chemicals Used in Crop Protection, 6th ed, Research
    Branch, Agriculture Canada, Publication 1093, London, Ontario,
    University of Western Ontario, pp. 337-338

Stein, A.A. (1968) Comparative methoxychlor toxicity in dogs, swine,
    rats, monkeys and man. Ind. med. Surg., 37, 540-541

Sundaram, K.M.S. (1975) Gas chromatographic analysis of methoxychlor
    formulations and spray mixtures. Information Report CC-X, CC-X-94,
    Ottawa, Chemical Control Research Institute [Chem. Abstr., 84, 17493j]

Sundaram, K.M.S. (1976) Persistence and fate of methoxychlor used for
    elm bark beetle control in the urban environment of the national
    capitol area. Information Report CC-X, CC-X-118, Ottawa, Chemical
    Control Research Institute [Chem. Abstr., 85, 105325t]

Sundaram, K.M.S. (1977) A study on the comparative deposit levels and
    persistence of two methoxychlor formulations used in white pine
    weevil control. Information Report CC-X, CC-X-142, Ottawa, Chemical
    Control Research Institute [Chem. Abstr., 87, 178663c]

Taylor, R., Bogacka, T. & Balcerska, M. (1975) Thin-layer chromatographic
    determination of chlorinated hydrocarbon insecticides in sediments
    (Pol.) Chem. Anal. (Warsaw), 20, 607-614 [Chem. Abstr., 83, 173898r]

Thompson, J.F., Mann, J.B., Apodaca, A.O. & Kantor, E.J. (1975) Relative
    retention ratios of ninety-five pesticides and metabolites on nine
    gas-liquid chromatographic columns over a temperature range of 170
    to 204°C in two detection modes. J. Assoc. off. anal. Chem., 58,
    1037-1050

Thurm, V. (1974) Pesticide residues on tobacco products. II. Insecticide
    content of raw tobaccos (Germ.). Nahrung, 18, 445-449 [Chem. Abstr.,
    82, 11945f]

Thurm, V. & Fensterer, C. (1972) Pesticide residues on tobacco products.
    I. Content of chlorinated hydrocarbons in tobacco products (Germ.).
    Nahrung, 16, 353-358 [Chem. Abstr., 78, 108414n]

Uminska, R., Bujalska, U., Rotter, A. & Sochan, M. (1973) Evaluation
    of the contamination of shallow, underground waters with chlorinated
    hydrocarbon pesticides in some rural regions of the Lublin District
    (Pol.). Bromatol. Chem. Toksykol., 6, 75-82 [Chem. Abstr., 80,
    112374h]

US Environmental Protection Agency (1972a) EPA Compendium of Registered
    Pesticides, Washington DC, US Government Printing Office, pp. III-M-10.1
    - III-M-10.9

US Environmental Protection Agency (1972b) Methoxychlor; tolerances for
    residues. US Code Fed. Regul., Title 40, subpart 180.120,
    pp. 417-418

US Environmental Protection Agency (1976) Manual of Chemical Methods for
    Pesticides and Devices, Methoxychlor EPA-1, EPA-2, Washington DC,
    Association of Official Analytical Chemists

US Food & Drug Administration (1975) Compliance Program Evaluation,
    Total Diet Studies: FY 1973 (7320.08), Washington DC, US Government
    Printing Office, Table 5

US Food and Drug Administration (1977) Compliance Program Evaluation,
    FY 74 Total Diet Studies (7320.08), Washington DC, US Government
    Printing Office, Table 6

US International Trade Commission (1977a) Synthetic Organic Chemicals,
    US Production and Sales, 1975, USITC Publication 804, Washington DC,
    US Government Printing Office, p. 186

US International Trade Commission (1977b) Synthetic Organic Chemicals,
    US Production and Sales, 1976, USITC Publication 833, Washington DC,
    US Printing Office, p. 276

US Occupational Safety & Health Administration (1977) Air contaminants.
    US Code Fed. Regul., Title 29, part 1910.1000, p. 27

US Tariff Commission (1948) Synthetic Organic Chemicals, US Production
    and Sales, 1946, Report no. 159, Second Series, Washington DC,
    US Government Printing Office, p. 133

Waldron, A.C. & Naber, E.C. (1974) Importance of feed as an unavoidable
    source of pesticide contamination in poultry meat and eggs. I.
    Residues in feedstuffs. Poult. Sci., 53, 1359-1371

Weikel, J.H., Jr (1957) The metabolism of methoxychlor [1,1,1 tri-
     chloro-2-2-bis-(p-methoxyphenyl)ethane]. I. The role of the liver
     and biliary excretion in the rat. Arch. int. Pharmacodyn., 110,
     423–432

Welch, R.M., Levin, W. & Conney, A.H. (1969) Estrogenic action of DDT
     and its analogs. Toxicol. appl. Pharmacol., 14, 358–367

WHO (1975) Pesticide residues in food. World Health Organ. tech. Rep.
     Ser., No. 574, pp. 578, 579, 583

Wiersma, G.B., Tai, H. & Sand, P.F. (1972) Pesticide residue levels in
     soils, FY 1969 – National Soils Monitoring Program. Pestic. Monit. J.,
     6, 194–228

Windholz, M., ed. (1976) The Merck Index, 9th ed., Rahway, NJ, Merck
     & Co, pp. 783–784

MIREX

This substance was considered by a previous IARC Working Group, in October 1973 (IARC, 1974). Since that time new data have become available, and these have been incorporated into the monograph and taken into account in the present evaluation.

A review on mirex is available (French *et al.*, 1977).

1. Chemical and Physical Data

1.1 Synonyms and trade names

Chem. Abstr. Services Reg. No.: 2385-85-5

Chem. Abstr. Name: 1,1a,2,2,3,3a,4,5,5,5a,5b,6-Dodecachlorooctahydro-1,3,4-metheno-1*H*-cyclobuta(*cd*)pentalene

Synonyms: Dodecachlorooctahydro-1,3,4-methano-2*H*-cyclobuta(*cd*)-pentalene; dodecachloropentacyclo$(3.3.2.0^{2,6}.0^{3,9}.0^{5,10})$ decane; ENT 25,719; hexachlorocyclopentadiene dimer; 1,2,3,4,5,5-hexa-chloro-1,3-cyclopentadiene dimer; perchlorodihomocubane; perchloro-pentacyclodecane; perchloropentacyclo$(5.2.1.0^{2,6}.0^{3,9}.0^{5,8})$decane

Trade names: CG-1283; Dechlorane; Dechlorane 515; Dechlorane 4070; Dechlorane Plus; Dechlorane Plus 515; Ferriamicide; HRS 1276

1.2 Structural and molecular formulae and molecular weight

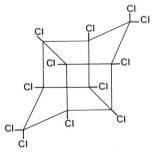

$C_{10}Cl_{12}$ Mol. wt: 545.5

1.3 Chemical and physical properties of the pure substance

From Spencer (1973), unless otherwise specified

(<u>a</u>) <u>Description</u>: White crystals

(<u>b</u>) <u>Melting-point</u>: 485°C

(<u>c</u>) <u>Solubility</u>: Insoluble in water; soluble in dioxane (15.3%), xylene (14.3%), benzene (12.2%), carbon tetrachloride (7.2%) and methyl ethyl ketone (5.6%) (Windholz, 1976)

(<u>d</u>) <u>Volatility</u>: Vapour pressure is 3×10^{-7} mm at 25°C (Hooker Chemical Corporation, 1968).

(<u>e</u>) <u>Stability</u>: Very stable at normal temperatures. Decomposes above 500°C to give hexachlorobenzene; hexachloropentadiene was found in small amounts in the thermal residue; the products identified from the vapour phase were carbon monoxide, carbon dioxide, hydrogen chloride, chlorine, carbon tetra-chloride and phosgene (Holloman *et al.*, 1975). Degrades in soil to give chlordecone (see monograph, p. 67) (Carlson *et al.*, 1976). Its photodecomposition gives mainly photomirex (8-monohydromirex) (Hallett *et al.*, 1978).

(<u>f</u>) <u>Reactivity</u>: Unaffected by sulphuric, nitric and hydrochloric acids

1.4 Technical products and impurities

A technical grade of mirex was formerly available in the US as a white crystalline solid in two average particle size ranges, 5-10 and 40-70 microns (Hooker Chemical Corporation, 1968). The term 'mirex' is also used in reference to a bait comprising corncob grits, soya bean oil and mirex (US Environmental Protection Agency, 1976a).

Insect bait formulations for aerial application, containing 0.3-0.5% mirex, and fire ant formulations containing 0.075-0.3% mirex have been used in the US (US Environmental Protection Agency, 1976a). Another formulation under consideration for limited interim use in the use is called 'Ferriamicide' and contains an amine and a metal salt, thus rendering the mirex unstable (Anon., 1977a).

Chlordecone has been found to be present in technical mirex at levels of up to 2.58 mg/kg and in mirex bait at levels of up to 0.25 mg/kg (US Environmental Protection Agency, 1976a).

2. Production, Use, Occurrence and Analysis

2.1 Production and use

(a) Production

Mirex was first synthesized in the mid-1940's but was not offered for sale in commercial quantities in the US until 1958. It is made by the dimerization of hexachlorocyclopentadiene in the presence of aluminium chloride.

Only one company in the world is known to have manufactured technical-grade mirex, and that US company ceased production in 1967. Another company manufactured the insecticidal bait containing mirex, but discontinued this in 1975, when production of the bait was taken over by the state of Mississippi (Holden, 1976) until the supply of the chemical was exhausted. On the basis of reports of quantities used for fire ant control in the US (Anon., 1977b), it is estimated that at least 225 thousand kg of the chemical were produced in the US before production was stopped in 1967.

Mirex has been imported to the US from Brazil (Cookson, 1979).

(b) Use

The only known current use for mirex is as an insecticide, and by far the major application to date is believed to have been in the control of fire ants in the southern US, although it is reportedly also used against leaf cutters in South America, against harvester termites in South Africa, against Western harvester ants in the US, against the mealybug of pineapple in Hawaii, and has been investigated for use against yellow jacket wasps in the US (US Environmental Protection Agency, 1976a; Vaughn, 1971).

Under the name 'Dechlorane', mirex was marketed in the US in the period 1959-1972 as a stable, fire-retardant additive for use in thermoplastic, thermosetting and elastomeric resin systems. It was also reported to be useful in paper, paint, rubber, electrical, adhesive and textile applications (Hooker Chemical Corporation, 1968).

Mirex was introduced in the southern US in 1962 when the US Department of Agriculture initiated a 12-year programme to eradicate the fire ant. In the period 1962-1976, about 132 million acres (53.4 million hectares) in 10 states were treated with about 226 thousand kg

of mirex, initially at a rate of 4.2 g/ha, which was later reduced to
1.16 g/ha (Anon., 1977b).   This programme was decelerated from 1971 when
the US Environmental Protection Agency (EPA) issued a cancellation order
for mirex.   The order was appealed, and in 1972, following hearings,
the EPA reinstated all mirex registrations and issued new guidelines
calling for a modified spraying programme aimed at control, rather than
eradication, of the ants.   Hearings were reconvened in 1973, during
which new evidence became available from the US National Cancer Institute
(Holden, 1976).   On 20 October 1976, a plan was announced by the EPA
for phasing out the use of mirex for control of the fire ant in the
southern US and suspension of the then pending hearings.   The plan,
developed by the state of Mississippi and the EPA, led to cessation of
aerial application of the more concentrated forms of bait by the end of
1976 and of the dilute formulation by the end of 1977.   Selective ground
application of the dilute formulation was to be permitted through June
1978, at which time the use of the product was to be banned in the US,
with the exception of continued use in Hawaii on pineapple until stocks
on hand are exhausted (Holden, 1976; US Environmental Protection Agency,
1976a).

In December 1977, the state of Mississippi filed a request with the
EPA for a specific exemption from the requirements of the law regulating
the use of pesticides for a formulation of mirex called Ferriamicide,
claiming the existence of emergency conditions.   Approval was requested
for aerial, ground and mound application of this formulation (Anon.,
1977a).   The requested exemption was granted in March 1978, but with
the following limitations: application by ground equipment only; use
to begin after 30 June 1978 and to end 1 July 1979; mound-to-mound
application only on agricultural land and non-crop land other than parks
and cemeteries; and not more than 5.3 thousand kg of mirex (2.7 million
kg of bait) to be applied.   Eight other states will be allowed to use
Ferriamicide under the conditions granted to Mississippi (Anon., 1978a,
b,c).   The granting of this exemption by the EPA was challenged by the
Environmental Defense Fund in a suit filed on 30 March 1978 (Anon.,
1978d).

Tolerances for residues of mirex in food products in the US are as
follows: 0.1 mg/kg in fat of meat from cattle, goats, hogs, horses,
poultry and sheep, and in eggs and milk fat; and 0.01 mg/kg in or on
all other raw agricultural commodities (US Environmental Protection
Agency, 1976b).

No data on its use in Europe or Japan were available.

2.2 Occurrence

Mirex is not known to occur as a natural product.   Its occurrence
in the environment has been reviewed (Waters, 1976).

(a) Water

Mirex has been found in one sample of ground-water in the US
(Shackelford & Keith, 1976).   It has also been determined in rural
drinking-water, at levels of 0-437 ng/1 (Sandhu et al., 1978).

(b) Soil

Mirex has been detected in: (1) pineapple field soils, at levels
of 10-18 µg/kg, 9 months after its application (Bevenue et al., 1975);
(2) soil, at levels of 190-500 µg/kg, 12 years after application of
1 mg/kg; and (3) mud, at a level of 0.2 mg/kg, 5 years after the crash
of an airplane carrying mirex bait; chlordecone was also found as a
degradation product (Carlson et al., 1976).

(c) Food and drink

A survey of items in the human food chain showed that detectable
residues of mirex were still present 1 year after a single aerial
application of mirex bait, at levels of 1.7 g/acre (4.2 g/ha).   The
levels observed in various species were: (1) quail, 36 µg/kg; (2)
bluegill fish, 18 µg/kg; (3) domestic chickens, 14 µg/kg; and (4)
chicken eggs, 1 µg/kg.   No mirex residues were detected in beef fat
or milk after 1 year (Collins et al., 1974).   Mirex has been detected
at levels of 5-24 µg/kg in 9/77 composite samples of seafood, including
oysters, crabs, shrimp, fish and fish products (Markin et al., 1974a).

Milk from cows grazed on pastures treated repeatedly with mirex
contained residues of up to 0.3 µg/1 (Hawthorne et al., 1974).

Residues of mirex were detected at levels of 0.01-1.71 mg/kg in
soya bean, garden bean, sorghum and wheat seedlings when these were
grown in prepared substrates containing 0.3-3.5 mg/kg mirex (de la
Cruz & Rajanna, 1975).

(d) Animals

Mirex residues have been detected in pineapple-growing areas in:
(1) birds, at levels of 0-10,400 µg/kg; (2) rodents, at levels of
5-9410 µg/kg; and (3) mongooses, at levels of 30-11,760 µg/kg
(Bevenue et al., 1975).

Mirex residues have been detected in various wildlife samples
including: (1) adipose tissue of deer, at levels of up to 0.3 mg/kg;
(2) liver (up to 7.5 mg/kg) and fat (up to 104 mg/kg) from fish and
birds; (3) brain tissue of birds, at levels of up to 1.8 mg/kg; (4)
heart and muscle tissue of birds, at levels of up to 1.9 mg/kg; (5)
insects, at levels of up to 1.2 mg/kg; and (6) earthworms, at levels of
0.03-0.076 mg/kg (Baetcke et al., 1972).

One year after a single aerial application of 0.6 g mirex/ha, residues were detected in 61 vertebrates, including: (1) mammals, at levels of 0.01-0.054 mg/kg; (2) birds, at levels of 0.012-3.6 mg/kg; (3) reptiles, at levels of 0-0.2 mg/kg; and (4) amphibians, at levels of 0.008-0.074 mg/kg (Collins *et al.*, 1974). Seven months after a single aerial application of 0.85 g/acre (2.1 g/ha) mirex bait, residues were also detected in rodents (rats, mice, shrews) at levels of 0.01-1.9 mg/kg (Wolfe & Norment, 1973).

Mirex has been identified in seal fat (Ten Noever de Brauw *et al.*, 1973); it has been detected in beef fat at levels of 0.001-0.125 mg/kg, with an average of 0.025 mg/kg (Ford *et al.*, 1973).

As part of the US National Pesticides Monitoring Program, mirex was detected at levels of 0.01-1.66 mg/kg in starlings from 10/12 sites (Oberheu, 1972). Residues of mirex have been detected in the eggs of the following birds: (1) double-crested cormorants, at levels of 0.058-0.113 mg/kg (wet weight) (Zitko, 1976); (2) herring gulls, at levels of 0.028 mg/kg (wet weight) (Zitko, 1976); and (3) estuarine birds, at levels of 0-2.9 mg/kg (wet weight) (Ohlendorf *et al.*, 1974).

Continuous exposure to low levels of mirex in feed (0.001-0.03 mg/kg) and in the soil of pens (0.03-0.25 mg/kg) resulted in residues at levels of 0.072-1.09 mg/kg in the abdominal fat of chicken within 8 weeks (Putnam *et al.*, 1974). In a similar study, eggs of laying hens fed 0.01-1.06 mg/kg diet mirex showed residue levels of < 0.01-0.07 mg/kg within a week and levels of 0.01-2.03 mg/kg for the next 39 weeks. Residues in the tissues of hens fed 0.01 mg/kg and 1.06 mg/kg for 39 weeks were 0.01-0.3 mg/kg and 0.3-25 mg/kg, respectively (Woodham *et al.*, 1975).

The milk of cattle fed 0.01 and 1 mg/kg diet mirex for 3 weeks showed residue levels of < 0.01-0.02 mg/l and 0.01-0.08 mg/l, respectively. Mirex was detected in the omental fat of these cows at levels of 0.06 and 1.87 mg/kg, respectively, and at levels of 0.08-2.52 mg/kg in the tissues of calves that received the milk (Bond *et al.*, 1975).

Mirex residues have been detected in: (1) aquatic animals, at levels of 3-7 µg/kg (Bevenue *et al.*, 1975); (2) crab and fish, at levels of < 0.01-0.12 mg/kg (Borthwick *et al.*, 1974); (3) fish in streams, at levels of 0.01-1.02 mg/kg (Wolfe & Norment, 1973); (4) two lake fish, at levels of 0.02-0.05 mg/kg (Kaiser, 1974); (5) edible red crawfish, at levels of 0-0.07 mg/kg (Markin *et al.*, 1972); (6) terrestrial and aquatic invertebrates 1 year after application of 2.5 kg/ha mirex bait, at levels of 0-0.092 mg/kg (Markin *et al.*, 1974b); (7) fish and invertebrates, at levels of 0-1.02 mg/kg (Wolfe & Norment, 1973); and (8) catfish and aquatic organisms 16 months after application, at levels of 0.02-0.44 mg/kg (Collins *et al.*, 1973).

(e) Humans

Human exposure to mirex has been reviewed (US Environmental Protection Agency, 1976a).

Mirex has been detected in adipose tissue from 6 human subjects at
levels of 0.16-5.94 mg/kg (Kutz et al., 1974).   Average residues of
mirex in the fat of residents of states where mirex is applied were 1.32
mg/kg fat (US Environmental Protection Agency, 1976a).

Traces of mirex have been detected in some human milk samples at
0.1-0.6 µg/kg (wet-weight basis) and 2.3-21.5 µg/kg (fat basis) (Mes
et al., 1978).

2.3 Analysis

Methods used for the analysis of mirex in environmental samples are
listed in Table 1.

Collaborative studies have been carried out to evaluate mirex in
natural samples (Krause, 1973).

Other analytical methods to isolate and identify mirex include
gel-permeation chromatography (Johnson et al., 1976) and gas chromato-
graphy/Coulson electrolytic conductivity detection (Su & Price, 1973).
Mirex can be analysed among polychlorobiphenyls by gas chromatography/
electron capture detection after photodegradation of the polychlorobiphenyls (Lewis et al., 1976).

3. Biological Data Relevant to the Evaluation
of Carcinogenic Risk to Humans

3.1 Carcinogenicity studies in animals[1]

(a) Oral administration

Mouse: Groups of 18 male and 18 female (C57BL/6xC3H/Anf)F1 mice
and 18 male and 18 female (C57BL/6xAKR)F1 mice received mirex (98% pure)
according to the following schedule: 10 mg/kg bw in 0.5% gelatin at 7
days of age by stomach tube and the same amount (not adjusted for

---

[1]The Working Group was aware of a study in progress to assess the
carcinogenicity in mice and rats administered mirex in the diet (IARC,
1978).

TABLE 1. METHODS FOR THE ANALYSIS OF MIREX

SAMPLE TYPE	ANALYTICAL METHOD			
	EXTRACTION/CLEAN-UP	DETECTION	LIMIT OF DETECTION	REFERENCE
Air	Trap on polyurethane foam, extract (hexane-ether) in Soxhlet, wash	GC/ECD	0.1 ng/m³	Lewis et al. (1977)
Water				
Rural potable	Extract (hexane), CC	GC/ECD	10 ng/l	Sandhu et al. (1978)
Soil				
Soil, sediments	Extract (petroleum ether or acetone-petroleum ether) in Soxhlet, CC	GC/ECD	3-6 µg/kg	Bevenue et al. (1975)
Food				
Fruit and vegetables	Extract (acetonitrile or aqueous acetonitrile), liquid/liquid partition, CC	GC/ECD, TLC, PC		Horwitz (1975)
Fatty products and fish	Mix with Florisil, extract (acetonitrile), liquid/liquid partition, CC	GC/ECD		Bong (1975, 1977)
Catfish	Grind with anhydrous sodium sulphate, extract (hexane), CC	GC/ECD	10 µg/kg	Collins et al. (1973)
Biological				
Wildlife	Grind with anhydrous sodium sulphate, extract (hexane-isopropanol), wash (water), CC	GC/ECD	1 µg/kg	Collins et al. (1974)
Wildlife	Mix with Florisil, extract (5% water in acetonitrile), liquid/liquid partition, CC, chlorinate	GC/FID/ECD/CD, GC/MS		Hallett et al. (1976)

Abbreviations: GC/ECD - gas chromatography/electron capture detection; CC - column chromatography; TLC - thin-layer chromatography; PC - paper chromatography; FID - flame-ionization detection; CD - conductivity detection; MS - mass spectrometry

increasing body weight) daily up to 4 weeks of age; subsequently, the mice were fed 26 mg/kg diet mirex.   The dose was the maximum tolerated dose for infant and young mice [but not necessarily that for adults]. The experiment was terminated at 70 weeks of age, when all animals had died.   Tumour incidences were compared with those in 79-90 necropsied mice of each sex and strain, which had either been untreated or had received gelatine only.   Hepatomas were found in 6/18 male and 8/16 female necropsied mice of the first strain (compared with 8/79 and 0/87 in the corresponding controls) and in 5/15 male and 10/16 female mice of the second strain (compared with 5/90 and 1/82 in the corresponding controls) [For each of the two sexes of the two strains, $P < 0.05$] (Innes *et al.*, 1969; National Technical Information Service, 1968).

Rat: In a preliminary report of a study by the National Cancer Institute, groups of 26 CD rats of each sex, 6 weeks old, were fed 50 or 100 mg/kg diet mirex (99% pure) for 18 months, except during the first 10 weeks of treatment, when dietary concentrations were 40 and 80 mg/kg diet, respectively.   The dietary concentration of 100 mg/kg had been identified from previous short-term experiments as the maximum tolerated dose.   Twenty untreated rats of each sex were used as controls. All survivors were killed 24 months after treatment began; a dose-related effect on survival was noticed after the first year of treatment: at the end of the study 65% of the female and 55% of the male controls were still alive, but survival rates were poorer in the treated group.   Liver changes were classified according to Squire & Levitt (1975).   Neoplastic liver nodules up to 5 cm in diameter were observed in 2 males and 4 females given the lowest dose and in 7 males ($P < 0.05$) and 4 females given the highest dose.   Of the 17 rats with neoplastic nodules, 1 male at the lowest dose and 4 males and 1 female at the highest dose also had well-differentiated liver-cell carcinomas.   No metastases were observed (all lobes of the lung were examined routinely in histological sections).   No neoplastic liver nodules were found among controls.   Liver megalocytosis was observed in a total of 48 treated rats *versus* 0 in controls.   Tumours of the breast and endocrine system were distributed uniformly among control and treated animals. Eight other tumours were found in treated animals: 1 lipoma and 1 squamous-cell carcinoma of the ear-duct in males given the lowest dose; 2 fibromas, 1 fibrosarcoma and 1 squamous-cell carcinoma of the ear-duct in males given the highest dose; 2 fibrosarcomas in females given the highest dose.   No such tumours were observed in controls (Ulland *et al.*, 1977).

(b) Subcutaneous and/or intramuscular administration

Mouse: Groups of 18 male and 18 female (C57BL/6xC3H/Anf)F1 mice and 18 male and 18 female (C57BL/6xAKR)F1 mice were given single s.c. injections of 1000 mg/kg bw mirex (98% pure) in 0.5% gelatin on the 28th day of life and were observed until they were about 78 weeks of age, at which time 16, 17, 17 and 15 mice were still alive.   A group of negative controls comprised untreated animals and animals treated with gelatine, corn oil or dimethylsulphoxide.   Proportions

of necropsied mice that developed reticulum-cell sarcomas were 6/18,
0/17, 1/17 and 3/18 in the four groups, respectively; 2/16 gelatin-
treated control males and 8/141 negative control males of the first
strain developed these tumours [P > 0.05 and P < 0.01, respectively].
The corresponding proportions of mice with hepatomas were 2/18, 0/17,
4/17 and 1/18; 1/18 gelatin-treated control males and 1/161 negative
control males of the second strain developed such tumours [P > 0.05 and
P < 0.01, respectively]. The total incidences in the two strains (males
plus females) of reticulum-cell sarcomas was significantly greater than
that in controls (6/35 *versus* 9/295, and 4/35 *versus* 5/318) (National
Technical Information Service, 1968) [The Working Group noted that the
statistical significance of the results disappears when only matched
controls are considered].

3.2 Other relevant biological data

(a) Experimental systems

Toxic effects

The oral LD_{50} of mirex in corn oil in male rats is 740 mg/kg bw and
in females, 600 mg/kg bw (Gaines, 1969). Acute hepatotoxic effects in
rats after oral administration of mirex included hepatocyte enlargement,
glycogen depletion, focal surface necrosis and periportal liposis
(Kendall, 1974). Oral administration of 1 and 10 mg/kg bw to rats for
14 days enlarged the liver and led to fatty infiltration in the centrilobular region (Villeneuve *et al.*, 1977).

I.p. injections of mirex increased liver mixed-function oxidase
activity in mice, rats and monkeys (Baker *et al.*, 1972; Byard *et al.*,
1975; Davison *et al.*, 1976; Fulfs *et al.*, 1977). In rats, it increased
microsomal protein and cytochrome P450 but did not affect hydroxylation
of aniline or demethylation of aminopyrine (Davison *et al.*, 1976).

When chickens were fed 5-160 mg/kg diet mirex for 12 and 16 weeks,
and Japanese quail 5-80 mg/kg diet for 12 weeks, no effect was seen on
the concentration of protein or cytochrome P450 in hepatic microsomes,
nor on aniline hydroxylase or aminopyrine-*N*-demethylase levels. However,
structural changes were apparent in the livers of chickens fed mirex at
10 mg/kg diet and above, including regions of necrosis, non-specific
cellular aberrations and alterations of sinusoids and bile canaliculi
(Davison *et al.*, 1976).

Embryotoxicity and teratogenicity

Reduced litter size was noted in 2 strains of mice fed a dietary concentration of 5 mg/kg diet mirex before and after mating (Ware & Good, 1967). Progeny from female rats fed a diet containing 25 mg/kg diet mirex before and after mating had a reduced survival rate and a high incidence of cataracts, while progeny from females maintained on a level of 5 mg/kg diet appeared to be normal (Gaines & Kimbrough, 1970).

Rats were given daily oral doses of 1.5, 3, 6 and 12.5 mg/kg bw mirex on days 6-15 of gestation; the highest dose caused maternal toxicity, pregnancy failure, decreased foetal survival, reduced foetal weight and an increased incidence of visceral anomalies. Maternal toxicity and an increased incidence of foetal visceral anomalies were also observed with 6 mg/kg bw. Lower doses produced minimal or no adverse effects (Khera *et al.*, 1976).

No perceptible reproductive effects were observed in bobwhite quail fed 40 mg/kg diet mirex or in mallard ducks fed 1 or 10 mg/kg diet (Heath & Spann, 1973).

Absorption, distribution, excretion and metabolism

In rats, more than 50% of an oral dose of 6 mg/kg bw ^{14}C-mirex was excreted unchanged in the faeces within 48 hrs; thereafter, excretion dropped rapidly. Less than 1% unchanged mirex was found in the urine after 7 days, and tissues contained about 34%. No metabolites were found (Mehendale *et al.*, 1972).

Rats given single oral doses of 0.2 mg/kg bw ^{14}C-mirex excreted 15% in the faeces within 2 days and 3% over the subsequent 5 days; only traces were found in the urine. About 1 µg/g was found in adipose tissue throughout the 28 days of the experiment. Other tissue concentrations were lower and declined within the first 7 days after dosing (Gibson *et al.*, 1972).

In a reproduction study in rats, mirex crossed the placental barrier and was also secreted in their milk (Gaines & Kimbrough, 1970).

[14]C-Mirex administered at concentrations of 30 mg/kg diet was stored unchanged in the fat of quail and rats at levels up to 5500 mg/ kg and was not appreciably metabolized or excreted, even when mirex was removed from the diet (Ivie *et al.*, 1974). Similar observations were made in *Macaca mulatta* monkeys; a minor metabolite, accounting for less than 3% of the faecal radioactivity, was identified as a 9- or 10-monohydro derivative. The highest concentration of ^{14}C was found in fat, followed by adrenal gland, peripheral nerve, thyroid gland and skin (Stein & Pittman, 1977; Wiener *et al.*, 1976).

Mutagenicity and other related short-term tests

Male Wistar rats that received daily doses of 1.5, 3 and 6 mg/kg bw
mirex by stomach tube for 10 consecutive days were mated sequentially
with untreated females (1 male × 2 females) every 5 days over a period
of 70 days (a total of 14 mating periods).   The pregnant females were
dissected 13-15 days after separation from the males to assess the
incidence of dominant lethality.   In none of the mating periods was
there any significant difference (relative to controls) in the proportion of fertile matings, embryos/pregnancy or deciduomas/pregnancy,
except for a decrease in the incidence of pregnancies in the group
receiving 6 mg/kg bw in the first trial (Khera *et al.*, 1976).

(b) Humans

Levels of mirex in human tissues are discussed in section 2.2 (e).

3.3 Case reports and epidemiological studies

No data were available to the Working Group.

4.   Summary of Data Reported and Evaluation

4.1 Experimental data

Mirex has been tested in one experiment in two strains of mice and
in one experiment in rats by oral administration.   It has also been
tested in two strains of mice by subcutaneous injection of single doses.
In the studies using oral administration, it produced benign and malignant liver tumours in mice and rats of both sexes.   An excess of liver
tumours was also found in males of one of the two strains of mice following a single subcutaneous injection;   this experiment also suggested
that it produced reticulum-cell sarcomas in males of both strains.

Mirex is foetotoxic and produces **teratogenic effects**.   It was
negative in a dominant lethal assay in mice.

4.2 Human data

No case reports or epidemiological studies were available to the
Working Group.

The extensive production and the widespread use of mirex since the
late 1950s, together with the persistent nature of the compound, indicate
that widespread human exposure has occurred.   This is confirmed by many
reports of its occurrence in the general environment and by its presence
in human fat.

4.3 Evaluation

There is *sufficient evidence* that mirex is carcinogenic in mice
and rats.   In the absence of adequate data in humans, it is reasonable, for practical purposes, to regard mirex as if it presented a
carcinogenic risk to humans.

5. References

Anon. (1977a) Section 18 exemption requested for Ferriamicide to control fire ants. Pestic. Tox. Chem. News, 6, 13-14

Anon. (1977b) Mississippi set to sell mirex insecticide bait for spray application. Chemical Marketing Reporter, 7 March, p. 4

Anon. (1978a) EPA outlines Ferriamicide testing plans; notes registration possibility. Pestic. Tox. Chem. News, 6, 13-14

Anon. (1978b) Maximum formulated Ferriamicide product expected to be 7 million pounds. Pestic. Tox. Chem. News, 6, 16-17

Anon. (1978c) EDF 'extremely unhappy' with EPA decision on Ferriamicide Section 18. Pestic. Tox. Chem. News., 6, 24-26

Anon. (1978d) EDF asks court to set aside Ferriamicide Section 18 exemption granted by EPA. Pestic. Tox. Chem. News, 6, 14-15

Baetcke, K.P., Cain, J.D. & Poe, W.E. (1972) Mirex and DDT residues in wildlife and miscellaneous samples in Mississippi - 1970. Pestic. Monit. J., 6, 14-22

Baker, R.C., Coons, L.B., Mailman, R.B. & Hodgson, E. (1972) Induction of hepatic mixed function oxidases by the insecticide, mirex. Environ. Res., 5, 418-424

Bevenue, A., Ogata, J.N., Tengan, L.S. & Hylin, H.W. (1975) Mirex residues in wildlife and soils, Hawaiian pineapple-growing areas - 1972-74. Pestic. Monit. J., 9, 141-149

Bond, C.A., Woodham, D.W., Ahrens, E.H. & Medley, J.G. (1975) The cumulation and disappearance of mirex residues. II. In milk and tissues of cows fed two concentrations of the insecticide in their diet. Bull. environ. Contam. Toxicol., 14, 25-31

Bong, R.L. (1975) Determination of hexachlorobenzene and mirex in fatty products. J. Assoc. off. Anal. Chem., 58, 557-561

Bong, R.L. (1977) Collaborative study of the recovery of hexachloro-benzene and mirex in butterfat and fish. J. Assoc. off. Anal. Chem., 60, 229-232

Borthwick, P.W., Cook, G.H. & Patrick, J.M., Jr (1974) Mirex residues in selected estuaries of South Carolina - June 1972. Pestic. Monit. J., 7, 144-145

Byard, J.L., Koepke, U.C., Abraham, R., Golberg, L. & Coulston, F. (1975) Biochemical changes in the liver of mice fed mirex. Toxikol. appl. Pharmacol., 33, 70-77

Carlson, D.A., Konyha, K.D., Wheeler, W.B., Marshall, G.P. & Zaylskie, R.G. (1976) Mirex in the environment: its degradation to kepone and related compounds. Science, 194, 939-941

Collins, H.L., Davis, J.R. & Markin, G.P. (1973) Residues of mirex in channel catfish and other aquatic organisms. Bull. environ. Contam. Toxicol., 10, 73-77

Collins, H.L., Markin, G.P. & Davis, J. (1974) Residue accumulation in selected vertebrates following a single aerial application of mirex bait, Louisiana - 1971-72. Pestic. Monit. J., 8, 125-130

Cookson, C. (1979) Environmentalists fight use of 'untested' pesticide. The EPA has been accused of playing politics over Mississippi's fire ant 'emergency'. Nature (Lond.), 278, 2

de la Cruz, A.A. & Rajanna, B. (1975) Mirex incorporation in the environment: uptake and distribution in crop seedlings. Bull. environ. Contam. Toxicol., 14, 38-42

Davison, K.L., Mollenhauer, H.H., Younger, R.L. & Cox, J.H. (1976) Mirex-induced hepatic changes in chickens, Japanese quail, and rats. Arch. environ. Contam. Toxicol., 4, 469-482

Ford, J.H., Hawthorne, J.C. & Markin, G.P. (1973) Residues of mirex and certain other chlorinated hydrocarbon insecticides in beef-fat - 1971. Pestic. Monit. J., 7, 87-94

French, I.W. et al. (1977) Mirex (Environmental Health Criteria Document 77-EHD-12), Ottawa, Canada, Information Directorate, Department of National Health & Welfare

Fulfs, J., Abraham, R., Drobeck, B., Pittman, K. & Coulston, F. (1977) Species differences in the hepatic response to mirex: ultrastructural and histochemical studies. Ecotoxicol. environ. Safety, 1, 327-342

Gaines, T.B. (1969) Acute toxicity of pesticides. Toxicol. appl. Pharmacol., 14, 515-534

Gaines, T.B. & Kimbrough, R.D. (1970) Oral toxicity of mirex in adult and suckling rats with notes on the ultrastructure of liver changes. Arch. environ. Health, 21, 7-14

Gibson, J.R., Ivie, G.W. & Dorough, H.W. (1972) Fate of mirex and its major photodecomposition product in rats. J. agric. Food Chem., 20, 1246-1248

Hallett, D.J., Norstrom, R.J., Onuska, F.I., Comba, M.E. & Sampson, R. (1976) Mass spectral confirmation and analysis by the Hall detector of mirex and photomirex in herring gulls from Lake Ontario. J. agric. Food Chem., 25, 1189-1193

Hallett, D.J., Khera, K.S., Stoltz, D.R., Chu, I., Villeneuve, D.C. &
    Trivett, G. (1978) Photomirex: synthesis and assessment of acute
    toxicity, tissue distribution, and mutagenicity. J. agric. Food
    Chem., 26, 388-391

Hawthorne, J.C., Ford, J.H., Loftis, C.D. & Markin, G.P. (1974)
    Mirex in milk from southeastern United States. Bull. environ.
    Contam. Toxicol., 11, 238-240

Heath, R.G. & Spann, J.W. (1973) Reproduction and related residues in
    birds fed mirex. In: Deichmann, W.B., ed., Papers of the 8th
    Inter-America Conference on Toxicology and Occupational Medicine,
    Pesticides and the Environment: Continuing Controversy, Vol. 2,
    New York, Stratton, pp. 421-435

Holden, C. (1976) Mirex: persistent pesticide on its way out. Science,
    194, 301-303

Holloman, M.E., Layton, B.R., Kennedy, M.V. & Swanson, C.R. (1975)
    Identification of the major thermal degradation products of the
    insecticide mirex. J. agric. Food Chem., 23, 1011-1012

Hooker Chemical Corporation (1968) Dechlorane® (Perchloropentacyclode-
    cane), Hooker Industrial Chemicals for Basic Industries, Houston,
    TX, p. 5

Horwitz, W., ed. (1975) Official Methods of Analysis of the Association
    of Official Analytical Chemists, 12th ed., Washington DC,
    Association of Official Analytical Chemists, pp. 518-528

IARC (1974) IARC Monographs on the Evaluation of Carcinogenic Risk
    of Chemicals to Man, 5, Some Organochlorine Pesticides, Lyon,
    pp. 203-210

IARC (1978) Information Bulletin on the Survey of Chemicals Being
    Tested for Carcinogenicity, No. 7, Lyon, p. 226

Innes, J.R.M., Ulland, B.M., Valerio, M.G., Petrucelli, L., Fishbein, L.,
    Hart, E.R., Pallotta, A.J., Bates, R.R., Falk, H.L., Gart, J.J.,
    Klein, M., Mitchell, I. & Peters, J. (1969) Bioassay of pesticides
    and industrial chemicals for tumorigenicity in mice: a preliminary
    note. J. natl Cancer Inst., 42, 1101-1114

Ivie, G.W., Gibson, J.R., Bryant, H.E., Begin, J.J., Barnett, J.R. &
    Dorough, H.W. (1974) Accumulation, distribution, and excretion
    of mirex-^{14}C in animals exposed for long periods to the insecticide
    in the diet. J. agric. Food Chem., 22, 646-653

Johnson, L.D., Waltz, R.H., Ussary, J.P. & Kaiser, F.E. (1976)
    Automated gel permeation chromatographic cleanup of animal and
    plant extracts for pesticide residue determination. J. Assoc. off.
    anal Chem., 59, 174-187

Kaiser, K.L.E. (1974) Mirex: an unrecognized contaminant of fishes from Lake Ontario. Science, 185, 523-525

Kendall, M.W. (1974) Acute hepatoxic effects of mirex in the rat. Bull. environ. Contam. Toxicol., 12, 617-621

Khera, K.S., Villeneuve, D.C., Terry, G., Panopio, L., Nash, L. & Trivett, G. (1976) Mirex: a teratogenicity, dominant lethal and tissue distribution study in rats. Food Cosmet. Toxicol., 14, 25-29

Krause, R.T. (1973) Determination of several chlorinated pesticides by the AOAC multiresidue method with additional quantitation of perthane after dehydrochlorination: collaborative study. J. Assoc. off. anal. Chem., 56, 721-727

Kutz, F.W., Yobs, A.R., Johnson, W.G. & Wiersma, G.B. (1974) Mirex residues in human adipose tissue. Environ. Entomol., 3, 882-884

Lewis, R.G., Hanisch, R.C., MacLeod, K.E. & Sovocool, G.W. (1976) Photochemical confirmation of mirex in the presence of polychlorinated biphenyls. J. agric. Food Chem., 24, 1030-1035

Lewis, R.G., Brown, A.R. & Jackson, M.D. (1977) Evaluation of polyurethane foam for sampling of pesticides, polychlorinated biphenyls and polychlorinated naphthalenes in ambient air. Anal. Chem., 49, 1668-1672

Markin, G.P., Ford, J.H. & Hawthorne, J.C. (1972) Mirex residues in wild populations of the edible red crawfish (Procambarus clarki). Bull. environ. Contam. Toxicol., 8, 369-374

Markin, G.P. Hawthorne, J.C., Collins, H.L. & Ford, J.H. (1974a) Levels of mirex and some other organochlorine residues in seafood from Atlantic and Gulf coastal states. Pestic. Monit. J., 7, 139-143

Markin, G.P., Collins, H.L. & Davis, J. (1974b) Residues of the insecticide mirex in terrestrial and aquatic invertebrates following a single aerial application of mirex bait, Louisiana - 1971-72. Pestic. Monit. J., 8, 131-134

Mehendale, H.M., Fishbein, L., Fields, M. & Matthews, H.B. (1972) Fate of mirex-^{14}C in the rat and plants. Bull environ. Contam. Toxicol., 8, 200-207

Mes, J., Davies. D.J. & Miles, W. (1978) Traces of mirex in some Canadian human milk samples. Bull. environ. Contam. Toxicol., 19, 564-570

National Technical Information Service (1968) Evaluation of Carcinogenic, Teratogenic and Mutagenic Activities of Selected Pesticides and Industrial Chemicals, Vol. 1, Carcinogenic Study, Washington DC, US Department of Commerce

Oberheu, J.C. (1972) The occurrence of mirex in starlings collected in seven southeastern states - 1970. Pestic. Monit. J., 6, 41-42

Ohlendorf, H.M., Klaas, E.E. & Kaiser, T.E. (1974) Environmental pollution in relation to estuarine birds. In: Khan, M.A.Q. & Bederka, J.P., eds, Proceedings of a Symposium. Survival in Toxic Environments, Houston, TX, 1973, New York, Academic Press, pp. 53-81

Putnam, E.M., Brewer, R.N. & Cottier, G.J. (1974) Low level pesticide contamination of soil and feed and its effect on broiler tissue residue. Poult. Sci., 53, 1695-1698

Sandhu, S.S., Warren, W.J. & Nelson, P. (1978) Pesticidal residue in rural potable water. J. Am. Water Works Assoc., 70, 41-45

Shackelford, W.M. & Keith, L.H. (1976) Frequency of Organic Compounds Identified in Water, EPA-600/4-76-062, Athens, GA, US Environmental Protection Agency, p. 170

Spencer, E.Y. (1973) Guide to the Chemicals Used in Crop Protection, Research Branch, Agriculture Canada, Publication 1093, 6th ed., London, Ontario, University of Western Ontario, p. 359

Squire, R.A. & Levitt, M.H. (1975) Report of a workshop on classification of specific hepatocellular lesions in rats. Cancer Res., 35, 3214-3223

Stein, V.B. & Pittman, K.A. (1977) Identification of a mirex metabolite from monkeys. Bull. environ. Contam. Toxicol., 18, 425-427

Su, G.C.C. & Price, H.A. (1973) Element specific gas chromatographic analyses of organochlorine pesticides in the presence of PCB's by selective cancellation of interfering peaks. J. agric. Food Chem., 21, 1099-1102

Ten Noever de Brauw, M.C., Van Ingen, C. & Koeman, J.H. (1973) Mirex in seals. Sci. total Environ., 2, 196-198

Ulland, B.M., Page, N.P., Squire, R.A., Weisburger, E.K. & Cypher, R.L. (1977) A carcinogenicity assay of mirex in Charles River CD rats. J. natl Cancer Inst., 58, 133-140

US Environmental Protection Agency (1976a) Administrator's decision to accept plan of Mississippi Authority and order suspending hearing for the pesticide chemical mirex. Fed. Regist., 41, 56694-56704

US Environmental Protection Agency (1976b) Dodecachlorooctahydro-1,3,4-
    metheno-2*H*-cyclobuta(*cd*)pentalene; tolerances for residues.
    US Code Fed. Regul., Title 40, part 180.251, p. 343

Vaughn, W.L. (1971) Mirex: next on 'EEK-ology ban wagon'?
    Farm Chemicals, April, pp. 46,48

Villeneuve, D.C., Yagminas, A.P., Marino, I.A., Chu, I. & Reynolds, L.M.
    (1977) Effects of food deprivation in rats previously exposed
    to mirex. Bull. environ. Contam. Toxicol., 18, 278-284

Ware, G.W. & Good, E.E. (1967) Effects of insecticides on reproduction
    in the laboratory mouse. II. Mirex, telodrin, and DDT. Toxicol.
    appl. Pharmacol., 10, 54-61

Waters, E.M. (1976) Mirex. I. An Overview. II. An Abstracted
    Literature Collection, 1947-1976, Toxicology Information Program,
    National Library of Medicine, ORNL/TIRC-76/4, Oak Ridge, TN, Oak
    Ridge National Laboratory

Wiener, M., Pittman, K.A. & Stein, V. (1976) Mirex kinetics in the
    rhesus monkey. I. Disposition and excretion. Drug Metab. Disp.,
    4, 281-287

Windholz, M., ed. (1976) The Merck Index, 9th ed., Rahway, NJ,
    Merck & Co., p. 807

Wolfe, J.L. & Norment, B.R. (1973) Accumulation of mirex residues
    in selected organisms after an aerial treatment, Mississippi -
    1971-72. Pestic. Mont. J., 7, 112-116

Woodham, D.W., Bond, C.A., Ahrens, E.G. & Medley, J.G. (1975) The
    cumulation and disappearance of mirex residues. III. In eggs
    and tissues of hens fed two concentrations of the insecticide in
    their diet. Bull. environ. Contam. Toxicol., 14, 98-104

Zitko, V. (1976) Levels of chlorinated hydrocarbons in eggs of double-
    crested cormorants from 1971 to 1975. Bull. environ. Contam.
    Toxicol., 16, 399-405

PENTACHLOROPHENOL

A review on pentachlorophenol is available (Mercier, 1977).

1. Chemical and Physical Data

1.1 Synonyms and trade names

Chem. Abstr. Services Reg. No.: 87-86-5

Chem. Abstr. Name: Pentachlorophenol

Synonyms: Chlorophen; PCP; penchlorol; penta; pentachloro-
fenol; pentachlorofenolo; pentachlorophenate; pentachlorphenol;
2,3,4,5,6-pentachlorophenol; pentanol

Trade names: Chem-Tol; Cryptogil ol; Dowcide 7; Dowicide 7;
Dowicide G; Durotox; EP 30; Fungifen; Grundier Arbezol;
Lauxtol; Lauxtol A; Liroprem; Pentacon; Penta-Kil; Pentasol;
Penwar; Peratox; Permacide; Permagard; Permasan; Permatox;
Permite; Santobrite; Santophen; Santophen 20; Sinituho; Termi-
i-Trol; Thompson's Wood Fix; Weedone

1.2 Structural and molecular formulae and molecular weight

C_6HCl_5O Mol. wt: 266.3

1.3 Chemical and physical properties of the pure substance

From Grasselli & Ritchey (1975), unless otherwise specified

(a) Description: White crystals

(b) Boiling-point: 309-310°C (decomposition) at 754 mm

(c) <u>Melting-point</u>:   174°C

(d) <u>Spectroscopy data</u>: λ_{max} 280 nm (E_1^1 = 34), 273 nm (E_1^1 = 39),
224 nm (E_1^1 = 309) in methanol; infra-red and ultra-violet
spectra have been tabulated (Gore *et al.*, 1971).

(e) <u>Solubility</u>: Slightly soluble in water (8 mg/100 ml) and
cold petroleum ether; soluble in benzene, ethanol, diethyl
ether (Windholz, 1976), and paraffinic petroleum oils
(Mercier, 1977)

(f) <u>Stability</u>: Stable; prolonged heating above 200°C produces
traces of octachlorodibenzo-*para*-dioxin (Langer *et al.*, 1973).

(g) <u>Reactivity</u>: Forms salts with alkaline metals (Windholz, 1976);
sodium pentachlorophenate is converted exothermically to
octachlorodibenzo-*para*-dioxin at 360°C (Langer *et al.*, 1973);
heating of the sodium salt to 280°C produced 0.9 mg/kg octa-
and 0.3 mg/kg hepta-chlorodibenzo-*para*-dioxins, together with
0.02-0.03 mg/kg hexa-, penta- and tetra-chlorodibenzo-*para*-
dioxins (Rappe *et al.*, 1978).

1.4 <u>Technical products and impurities</u>

Pentachlorophenol is available commercially in the US in prill,
flake or block form (von Rumker *et al.*, 1975). The typical composition
of commercial pentachlorophenol is as follows: pentachlorophenol, 88.4%;
tetrachlorophenol, 4.4%; trichlorophenol, < 0.1%; and higher chlorinated
phenoxyphenols, 6.2%. The non-phenolic components fall into two chemical classes: polychlorinated dibenzo-*para*-dioxins and polychlorinated
dibenzofurans. Commercial pentachlorophenol typically contains the
following chlorinated dioxins: 2,3,7,8-tetrachlorodibenzo-*para*-dioxin,
< 0.05 mg/kg; hexachlorodibenzo-*para*-dioxin, 4 mg/kg; heptachlorodi-
benzo-*para*-dioxin, 125 mg/kg; and octachlorodibenzo-*para*-dioxin, 2500 mg/
kg. The typical dibenzofuran content of commercial pentachlorophenol is
as follows: hexachlorodibenzofuran, 30 mg/kg; heptachlorodibenzofuran,
80 mg/kg; and octachlorodibenzofuran, 80 mg/kg (Schwetz *et al.*, 1974).
Hexachlorobenzene is also found, at levels of 400 mg/kg, in commercial
pentachlorophenol (Schwetz *et al.*, 1978). One producer offers a
commercial product in which the dioxin content is minimized; this
product has the following composition: pentachlorophenol, 88%; 2,3,4,-
6-tetrachlorophenol, 12%; octachlorodibenzo-*para*-dioxin, 30 mg/kg max;
and hexachlorodibenzo-*para*-dioxins, 1 mg/kg max (von Rumker *et al.*, 1975).

In Japan, the technical-grade chemical contained a minimum of 95%
pentachlorophenol.

Pentachlorophenol is available as its sodium salt as a 5% emulsifiable concentrate or as 3-40% solutions in oil or grease, and in formulations with other chlorophenols, methylene bisthiocyanate and copper
naphthenate (von Rumker *et al.*, 1975; US Environmental Protection
Agency, 1975).

2. Production, Use, Occurrence and Analysis

A review is available (Gebefügi & Parlar, 1978).

2.1 Production and use

(a) Production

Pentachlorophenol was first prepared by Merz & Weith in 1872, by
chlorination of a mixture of phenol and antimony trichloride at elevated
temperatures (Prager *et al.*, 1923).   The process for commercial production of pentachlorophenol is similar, involving the chlorination of
phenol at progressively higher temperatures, using anhydrous aluminium
chloride (von Rumker *et al.*, 1975) or ferric chloride as a catalyst in
the final stages of chlorination.   One commercial process is reported
to involve a mixture of phenol and *ortho*-, 2,6-di- and 2,4,6-trichloro-
phenols as starting material.   Pentachlorophenol has also been manufactured by the hydrolysis of hexachlorobenzene (Doedens, 1964).

In Japan, pentachlorophenol has been produced by chlorination of
2,4-dichlorophenol, derived from 1,2,4-trichlorobenzene.

Although use of pentachlorophenol as a wood preservative started
in the late 1930's (Doedens, 1964), commercial production in the US
was first reported only in 1950, by 2 companies (US Tariff Commission,
1951).   US production of pentachlorophenol in the decade 1967-1976 was
in the range of 20-23 million kg, with production in 1976 at the lower
extreme of that range, at just under 20 million kg (US International
Trade Commission, 1977).   US imports of pentachlorophenol were last
reported in 1974 when 56 thousand kg were imported through the principal
customs districts (US International Trade Commission, 1976).

No data on its production in Europe were available.

In Japan, pentachlorophenol was first produced commercially in 1960.
Production reached a level of 14.5 million kg in 1966 and decreased to
3.3 million kg in 1971, when production was discontinued.

(b) Use

The use pattern for the 23.4 million kg pentachlorophenol used in the US in 1974 was as follows: wood preservation, 84%; synthesis of sodium pentachlorophenate, 12%; and miscellaneous uses, 4%.

Pentachlorophenol is used to protect wood (primarily construction lumber, but also poles and posts) from attack by fungal rots and decay and to prevent stain. It may be used in combination with other chlorophenols, 2,4-dinitrophenol, sodium fluoride, dichromate salts, sodium arsenate or arsenious oxide (US Environmental Protection Agency, 1973).

It is also used as a herbicide and defoliant. About 700 thousand kg are used in the US in home and garden applications (von Rumker *et al.*, 1975), primarily for preservation of various wooden articles and structures.

Sodium pentachlorophenate, produced from pentachlorophenol, is used as a wood preservative, as a fungicide in water-based latex paints, as a herbicide and as a slimicide.

The fungicidal and herbicidal uses of pentachlorophenol, including those cited above, are regulated by the US Environmental Protection Agency. It is registered in the US as a preharvest desiccant on alfalfa, clovers, lespedeza and vetch, but only when these crops are grown for the production of seed. Treated areas may not be grazed, and the treated forage or threshings may not be fed to livestock (US Environmental Protection Agency, 1970).

Other registered fungicidal uses of pentachlorophenol include treatment of beans to prevent seedling disease and a variety of miscellaneous agricultural uses involving preservation of wood, leather, burlap, twine and rope from attack by various fungi. Registered homeowner uses include maintenance of boats, trailers, station wagons, siding, fences, outdoor furniture and similar articles. There are a large number of registered industrial uses, such as in construction of boats and buildings, mould control in petroleum drilling and production, and treatment of cable coverings, canvas belting, nets, construction lumber and poles. Other industrial uses include incorporation in paints, pulp stock, in pulp and paper, cooling tower water, hardboard and particle board (US Environmental Protection Agency, 1975).

In France, pentachlorophenol is used as a fungicide, bactericide, algicide and anti-termite. In Japan, essentially all of the pentachlorophenol produced was used as a herbicide, with minor use as a fungicide.

Pentachlorophenol is being reviewed by the US Environmental Protection Agency for possible issuance of a notice of a rebuttable presumption

against renewal of registration (RPAR) (See General Remarks on Substances Considered, p. 31) on the basis of reproductive effects in
experimental animals (Anon., 1978).

The US Occupational Safety and Health Administration's health
standards for exposure to air contaminants require that an employee's
exposure to pentachlorophenol not exceed an 8-hr time-weighted average
of 0.5 mg/m^3 in the working atmosphere in any 8-hr work shift of a
40-hr work week (US Occupational Safety & Health Administration, 1977).
The corresponding standard in the Federal Republic of Germany, the
German Democratic Republic and Sweden is also 0.5 mg/m^3; and the
acceptable ceiling concentration of pentachlorophenol in the USSR is
0.1 mg/m^3 (Winell, 1975).

2.2 Occurrence

It has been suggested, but not proven, that pentachlorophenol is
a natural product, possibly a product of fungus metabolism (Arsenault,
1976).   The occurrence of pentachlorophenol in the environment has
been reviewed (Arsenault, 1976; Howard & Durkin, 1973).

(a) Air

Pentachlorophenol has been detected in the atmosphere of two
towns, at levels of 0.25-0.93 and 5.7-7.8 ng/m^3 air (Cautreels *et al.*,
1977).

(b) Water

Pentachlorophenol has been detected in: (1) river water and
effluent water from a chlorinated biological sewage treatment plant
(Eurocop-Cost, 1976); (2) the effluent waters from various manufacturing
and processing plants (Shackelford & Keith, 1976); and (3) well-water
(Nomura, 1974).

It has also been detected in: (1) the sewage influent and effluent
water of 3 cities, at levels of 1-5 µg/l; (2) a river, at levels of
0.1-0.7 µg/l (Buhler *et al.*, 1973); (3) rain-, snow- and lake-water,
at levels of 2-284, 14 and 10 ng/l, respectively (Bevenue *et al.*, 1972);
and (4) creek-water containing industrial discharges, at levels of
0.1-10 mg/l (Fountaine *et al.*, 1976).

(c) Soil

After treatment of greenhouse soil with pentachlorophenol at levels
of 15 and 45 kg/ha, residues in the soil were 20.4 and 69.1 mg/kg,
respectively.   Lettuce grown on this soil contained residues of 0.73
and 1.56 mg/kg, respectively.   In a second experiment, the greenhouse
soil was treated with 15 and 30 kg pentachlorophenol/ha, and residues

of 0.46 and 0.87 mg/kg, respectively, were detected in the lettuce
(Casanova & Dubroca, 1973).

(d) Food

In a continuing programme involving the monitoring of pesticide
residues in food, levels of pentachlorophenol in foods were measured
for the period 1965-1970, and an average daily intake of pentachlorophenol was calculated.   For the period 1965-1970, the average daily
intake was 1.67 µg/day; this level dropped to 0.725 µg/day in 1973 and
rose to 0.76 µg/day in 1974 (US Food & Drug Administration, 1975,
1977).

(e) Animals

Pentachlorophenol has been detected in: (1) fish, white shark
liver, bird eggs and fish food, at levels of < 0.5-4, 10.8, 0.36-0.51
and 2.23 µg/kg (wet weight), respectively (Zitko et al., 1974); (2)
birds, snails, frogs and fish, at levels of 0.04-0.49, 36.8, 8.1 and
0.37-59.4 mg/kg (mean wet weight), respectively (Vermeer et al., 1974);
(3) fish extracts (Tokunaga, 1971); and (4) fish, at levels of 0.35-
26 mg/kg (Renberg, 1974).

In the state of Michigan, herds of dairy cattle were contaminated
with pentachlorophenol used to treat the wood of barns where they were
housed and from feed bins treated with pentachlorophenol; the
contaminating pentachlorophenol was said to contain 1-1000 mg/kg
dioxin.   Pentachlorophenol levels in 18 cows ranged from 58-1136 µg/kg
(Anon., 1977a).   Pentachlorophenol has been found in the blood of 8 such
herds (Anon., 1977b).   One sample of milk was found to contain 0.09 mg/
kg (Anon., 1977c).

(f) Humans

Pentachlorophenol has been detected in human blood plasma at levels
of 15.69-15.86 µg/1 in haemodialysed patients and of 15.0 µg/1 in the
persons used as controls (Pearson et al., 1976).   It has also been
detected in the urine, seminal fluid (20-70 µg/kg) and fingernails of
non-occupationally exposed individuals (Dougherty & Piotrowska, 1976a).

Pentachlorophenol was found in 85% of 416-418 samples of urine
collected from the general population during the Health and Nutritional
Examination Survey.   The maximum level was 193 µg/1, and the mean
level 6.3 µg/1 (Kutz et al., 1978).

(g) Occupational exposure

The 1974 National Occupational Hazard Survey indicated that the
workers primarily exposed to pentachlorophenol are those in the gas and

electric service industries;   the potential exposure of hospital workers was also noted (National Institute for Occupational Safety & Health, 1977).

Air and urine samples taken at 25 factories using pentachlorophenol as a wood preservative showed that the average worker's exposure to penta-chlorophenol in air was 0.013 mg/m^3, with a maximum range of 0.004-1.000 mg/m^3, and the level in urine ranged from 0.12-9.68 mg/l (Arsenault, 1976).

When worker exposure to pentachlorophenol at a wood-treatment plant was measured over a 5-month period, serum and urine levels of penta-chlorophenol were 348.4-3963 μg/l and 41.3-760 μg/l, respectively. Pentachlorophenol residues in the workplace air were in the range of 5.1-15275.1 ng/m^3 (Wyllie *et al.*, 1975).   It has also been detected in the workplace air of a sodium pentachlorophenate production plant (Melnikova *et al.*, 1975).

(h) Other

Pentachlorophenol has been detected in 9/65 commercial samples of paints used on children's toys, at levels of 100-2700 mg/kg (van Langeveld, 1975);   and in wood-shaving litter from chicken houses, at levels of 0.6-83 mg/kg (fresh) and 0-4.1 mg/kg (after 8 weeks) (Parr *et al.*, 1974).

2.3 Analysis

Methods used for the analysis of pentachlorophenol in environmental samples are listed in Table 1 (Howard & Durkin, 1973).

Other proposed methods include high-pressure liquid chromatography (Ayres & Gopalan, 1976;   US Environmental Protection Agency, 1976) and thin-layer chromatography (Dietz *et al.*, 1976).   Background levels of trace impurities in analytical reagents can introduce error in gas chromatography/electron capture determinations of 1.0 ng/kg to 1.0 μg/kg levels (Bevenue & Ogata, 1971).

3. Biological Data Relevant to the Evaluation

of Carcinogenic Risk to Humans

3.1 Carcinogenicity studies in animals

(a) Oral administration

Mouse: Groups of 18 male and 18 female (C57BL/6xC3H/Anf)Fl mice and 18 male and 18 female (C57BL/6xAKR)Fl mice received pentachlorophenol

TABLE 1. METHODS FOR THE ANALYSIS OF PENTACHLOROPHENOL

SAMPLE TYPE	ANALYTICAL METHOD			
	EXTRACTION/CLEAN-UP	DETECTION	LIMIT OF DETECTION	REFERENCE
Formulations	Ignite with lime, neutralize	Volhard titration		Adams et al. (1974)
Air	Trap in potassium hydroxide, extract (hexane), methylate, CC	GC/ECD	20 µg/kg	Hoben et al. (1976a)
Water				
Natural and waste	Extract (benzene), re-extract (potassium carbonate), acetylate, extract (hexane)	GC/ECD	10 ng/l	Chau & Coburn (1974)
Domestic waste	Acidify, extract (dichloromethane), liquid/liquid partition, methylate	GC/FID GC/MS	0.2 µg/l	Garrison et al. (1976)
Natural	Adsorb on ion exchanger, remove water, extract (benzene), methylate	GC/ECD	1 ng/l	Renberg (1974)
River and waste	Make alkaline, wash (chloroform), acidify, extract (chloroform), re-extract (sodium hydroxide), acidify	UV, IR		Fountaine et al. (1976)
Soil				
Sediment and sewage	Centrifuge, extract solid (acetone), liquid/liquid partition, transfer into trimethyl pentane, treat to remove sulphur, isolate in trimethyl pentane, methylate or acetylate	GC/ECD	1-10 µg/kg	Jensen et al. (1977)
Soil	Centrifuge slurry with alkali, adsorb on ion exchanger, extract (benzene), methylate	GC/ECD	0.1-1 µg/kg	Renberg (1974)

TABLE 1. METHODS FOR THE ANALYSIS OF PENTACHLOROPHENOL (continued)

SAMPLE TYPE	ANALYTICAL METHOD			
	EXTRACTION/CLEAN-UP	DETECTION	LIMIT OF DETECTION	REFERENCE
Food and drink				
Milk	Extract (benzene), re-extract from benzene (potassium carbonate solution), form pentachlorophenol acetate, extract (hexane)	GC/ECD	5 µg/kg	Erney (1978)
Beef fat and milk chocolate	Macerate, extract (hot caustic soda), cool, extract (hexane-2-propanol), reduce bulk, CC	MS (negative chemical ionization)	5 µg/kg	Dougherty & Piotrowska (1976a,b)
Biological				
Tissue	Digest (potassium hydroxide), acidify, steam distill, extract distillate (toluene), ethylate	GC/ECD	1 µg/kg for fat, 0.1 µg/kg for muscle	Gee et al. (1974)
Tissue	Acidify, extract (hexane) in mixer, centrifuge, methylate, CC	GC/ECD	20 µg/kg	Hoben et al. (1976a)
Tissue	Homogenize with hexane-acetone, liquid/liquid partition, adsorb on ion exchanger, extract (benzene), methylate	GC/ECD	0.1 µg/kg	Renberg (1974)
Human adipose tissue	Extract (hexane) in mixer, make alkaline, re-extract (hexane), acidify residue, extract (ether), ethylate, CC	GC/ECD	5 µg/kg	Shafik (1973)
Plasma	Acidify, extract (benzene), centrifuge, ethylate, CC	GC/ECD	20 µg/l	Hoben et al. (1976a)
Blood and urine	Acidify, extract (benzene), centrifuge, methylate	GC/ECD	10 µg/l	Rivers (1972)
Rat urine	Acidify, reflux, make alkaline, extract (ether), ethylate, transfer to hexane, CC	GC/ECD	10 µg/l	Shafik et al. (1973)
Human urine	Make alkaline, extract (hexane), make acid, extract (hexane), methylate	GC/ECD	2.2 µg/l	US Food & Drug Administration (1970)

TABLE 1. METHODS FOR THE ANALYSIS OF PENTACHLOROPHENOL (continued)

SAMPLE TYPE	EXTRACTION/CLEAN-UP	DETECTION	LIMIT OF DETECTION	REFERENCE
ANALYTICAL METHOD				
Biological				
Human urine	Hydrolyse (acid), extract (hexane-2-propanol), concentrate to 100 μl	MS (negative chemical ionization)	4-40 ng/l	Dougherty & Piotrowska (1976a)
Urine	Acidify, extract (hexane), centrifuge, ethylate, CC	GC/ECD	20 μg/l	Hoben et al. (1976a)
Seminal fluid	Hydrolyse (acid), extract (hexane-ether), concentrate to 100 μl	MS (negative chemical ionization)	1-10 μg/l	Dougherty & Piotrowska (1976a)
Miscellaneous				
Wood	Ignite with lime, neutralize	Volhard titration		Adams et al. (1974)
Wood	Extract (chloroform)	TLC (revelation: silver nitrate)	60 ng (on unwashed plates) 25 μg (on plates pre-washed with acetone)	Henshaw et al. (1975)
Wood shavings	Digest (potassium hydroxide), acidify, steam distill, extract (toluene), ethylate	GC/ECD	10 μg/kg	Gee et al. (1974)

Abbreviations: CC - column chromatography; GC/ECD - gas chromatography/electron capture detection; MS - mass spectrometry; FID - flame-ionization detection; UV - ultra-violet spectrometry; IR - infra-red spectrometry

as the commercial product Dowcide-7 (impurities unspecified) according
to the following schedule: 46.4 mg/kg bw in 0.5% gelatin at 7 days of
age by stomach tube and the same amount (not adjusted for increasing
body weight) daily up to 4 weeks of age;   subsequently, the mice were
fed 130 mg/kg diet until they reached 78 weeks of age, at which time
16, 18, 17 and 16 mice were still alive in the four groups, respectively.
The dose was the maximum tolerated dose for infant and young mice [but
not necessarily that for adults].   Tumours developed in 3/18, 4/18,
3/17 and 2/18 male and female necropsied mice;   these incidences were
not significantly greater than in 79-90 necropsied mice of each sex
and strain, which had either been untreated or had received gelatin
only (Innes *et al.*, 1969;   National Technical Information Service,
1968).

Rat: Six groups of 27 male and 27 female weanling Sprague-Dawley
(Spartan substrain) rats were given laboratory chow diet containing
pentachlorophenol (sample XD-9108.002:   pentachlorophenol, 90.4%;
tetrachlorophenol, 10.4%;   trichlorophenol, < 0.1%;   hepta- and octa-
chlorodibenzo-*para*-dioxins, about 21 mg/kg;   hexa- and heptachlorodibenzofurans, about 5.2 mg/kg;   and hexachlorobenzene, 400 mg/kg) to
provide dose levels of 0, 1, 3, 10 or 30 mg pentachlorophenol/kg bw/
day.   The pentachlorophenol was dissolved in anisole, and the concentrations were adjusted on a monthly basis to maintain the designated
dose levels on a mg/kg bw/day according to the food consumption and
body weight of the rats.   Groups of 27 male and 27 female control rats
received laboratory chow containing anisole only.   Female rats were
maintained on test diets for 24 months, but the male rats were taken
off the test diets after 22 months because of high mortality among both
control and experimental animals.   The mean body weight of male rats
was not significantly altered by ingestion of diets containing pentachlorophenol;   among the female rats, the mean body weight of those
receiving the highest dose level was significantly less than that of
the control group;   in the other groups body weight was comparable with
that of the control groups.   The total and individual tumour incidences
by sites, the times of appearance of tumours and the average numbers of
tumours per animal (predominantly benign neoplasms) were not significantly different from those observed in control rats.   The numbers of rats
with tumours/those examined were, in <u>males</u>:   11/27 (controls), 13/26
(1 mg/kg), 13/27 (3 mg/kg), 12/27 (10 mg/kg), 11/27 (30 mg/kg);   in
<u>females</u>:   27/27 (controls), 26/27 (1 mg/kg), 25/27 (at all other doses)
(Schwetz *et al.*, 1978).

(b)   Subcutaneous and/or intramuscular administration

Mouse: Groups of 18 male and 18 female (C57BL/6xC3H/Anf)F1 mice
and 18 male and 18 female (C57BL/6xAKR)F1 mice were given single s.c.
injections of 46.4 mg/kg bw commercial pentachlorophenol (Dowcide-7;
impurities unspecified) in corn oil at 28 days of age and were observed
up to 78 weeks of age, at which time 14, 18, 18 and 16 mice in the four

groups, respectively, were still alive.   Negative control groups consisted
of animals that were either untreated or received gelatin, corn oil or
dimethylsulphoxide and comprised 141 males and 154 females of the first
strain and 161 males and 157 females of the second strain.   The incidence
of hepatomas (4/17) in males of the first strain was significantly increased
[$P < 0.05$] over that in controls (9/141) (National Technical Information
Service, 1968).

3.2 Other relevant biological data

Commercially produced pentachlorophenol contains significant
amounts of chlorinated dibenzo-*para*-dioxins and polychlorinated dibenzofurans (see section 1.4).   These contaminants may not be important in
relation to the acute toxicity of pentachlorophenol but may be associated
with those toxic or other biological effects that are seen after long-
term exposure (Baader & Bauer, 1951; Goldstein *et al.*, 1977).

(a) Experimental systems

Toxic effects

The oral LD_{50} in rats is 146-174 mg/kg bw, that by skin application
320-330 mg/kg bw (Gaines, 1969), and that by inhalation of aerosol
11.7 mg/kg bw (Hoben *et al.*, 1976b).

The acutely toxic state is characterized by accelerated respira-
tion, elevated body temperature, tachycardia, progressive neuromuscular
weakness and death due to cardiac failure.   Rigor mortis is instantane-
ous (Deichmann *et al.*, 1942).

A commercial sample of pentachlorophenol produced positive responses
in the chick oedema test and in the rabbit ear acnegenic test.   Rats
fed doses of 3, 10 and 30 mg/kg bw/day for 90 days showed haemolytic
changes, increased liver and kidney weights and hepatic alterations
(Johnson *et al.*, 1973).

With a pentachlorophenol formulation that had 'markedly reduced
levels of impurities', mild toxicity was observed in rats that received
30 mg/kg bw for 2 years.   'No effect' levels were reported to be 3 mg/
kg bw/day for females and 10 mg/kg bw/day for males (Schwetz *et al.*,
1978).

In an 8-month feeding study with female rats, analytical grade
pentachlorophenol was compared with a technical grade.   The latter
produced hepatic porphyria and increased aryl hydrocarbon hydroxylase
activity and glucuronyl transferase activity when given at 100 mg/kg

diet.   Pure pentachlorophenol had no significant effect on aryl hydrocarbon hydroxylase activity, but it increased glucuronyl transferase
when given at 500 mg/kg diet (Goldstein et al., 1977).   The authors
attributed these effects to the chlorinated dibenzo-para-dioxins present
in the commercial product.

Weinbach (1954) demonstrated that pentachlorophenol uncouples
oxidative phosphorylation in mitochondria.   It also disturbs electron
transport from flavins to cytochromes in microsomes, suggesting microsomal detoxification malfunction (Arrhenius et al., 1977a,b).

Embryotoxicity and teratogenicity

Purified and commercial grades of pentachlorophenol were given
orally to rats at doses ranging from 5-50 mg/kg bw/day at various intervals during days 6-15 of pregnancy.   Signs of embryotoxicity and
foetotoxicity, such as resorptions, subcutaneous oedema, dilated ureters
and anomalies of the skull, ribs, vertebrae and sternebrae, were observed
at an incidence which increased with dose.   Early organogenesis was the
most sensitive period.   The no-effect dose level of the commercial
grade was 5 mg/kg bw/day; purified pentachlorophenol given at the same
dose level caused a statistically significant increase in the incidence
of delayed ossification of the skull bones but had no other effect on
embryonal or foetal development (Schwetz et al., 1974).   Ingestion of
3 mg/kg bw/day of a commercially available purified grade of pentachlorophenol had no effect on reproduction, neonatal growth, survival or development (Schwetz et al., 1978).

A dose of 60 mg/kg bw pentachlorophenol (purity > 99%) was given to
Charles River CD rats as a single oral dose at various times during days
8-13 of gestation.   The incidence of resorptions was not significantly
greater than that in controls.   Although malformations were observed,
the number was minimal, and the authors suggested that the effect could
have been due to toxic effects of the compound on the mothers (Larsen
et al., 1975).

In Syrian golden hamsters, foetal deaths and resorptions were
reported in 3/6 test groups after oral administration of doses varying
from 1.25-20.0 mg/kg bw/day pentachlorophenol from days 5-10 of gestation (Hinkle, 1973).

Absorption, distribution, excretion and metabolism

In mice, pentachlorophenol is excreted primarily in the urine, and
the rest in the faeces (Jakobson & Yllner, 1971).   Urinary excretion
in mice and rats is principally as free pentachlorophenol or tetrachlorohydroquinone, although glucuronide conjugates of both pentachlorophenol
and tetrachlorohydroquinone have been identified in rats (Ahlborg et al.,
1974, 1978).   The metabolite tetrachlorohydroquinone was not found in
the urine of Macaca mulatta monkeys (Braun & Sauerhoff, 1976).

In rats, dechlorination of pentachlorophenol is mediated by micro-somal enzymes that can be induced by phenobarbital (Ahlborg *et al.*, 1978) or by tetrachlorodibenzo-*para*-dioxin (Ahlborg & Thunberg, 1978).

Enterohepatic circulation of pentachlorophenol occurs in monkeys and mice (Braun & Sauerhoff, 1976; Jakobsen & Yllner, 1971). In rats, it is found mainly in plasma protein; liver and kidney have the highest tissue concentrations (Braun *et al.*, 1977). The plasma half-lives of a 10 mg/kg bw dose were about 15 hrs in rats and 78 hrs in *Macaca mulatta* monkeys. There is no pharmacokinetic evidence that pentachloro-phenol *per se* would have cumulative toxic effects (Braun & Sauerhoff, 1976; Braun *et al.*, 1977).

Mutagenicity and other related short-term tests

In feeding experiments with *Drosophila melanogaster*, 7 mM penta-chlorophenol failed to induce sex-linked recessive lethals in meiotic and postmeiotic stages of male germ cells (Vogel & Chandler, 1974).

In lateral roots of *Vicia faba* seedlings treated with 43.5-174 mg/1 pentachlorophenol, there was an increase in the frequency of abnormal cell divisions (e.g., stickiness and lagging of chromosomes and chromosome fragmentation); these abnormalities were more frequent during meta-phase than in later stages and, in general, increased with increasing concentration (Amer & Ali, 1969).

(b) Humans

Toxic effects and fatalities due to occupational and accidental exposures to pentachlorophenol have been reviewed by Mercier (1977). Nine sawmill workers died after exposure to impregnated wood (Menon, 1958); 2 deaths were reported among 20 infants intoxicated in a hospital in which there was misuse of a laundry product containing 22.9% sodium pentachlorophenol, 4% 3,4,4-trichlorocarbanilide and sodium salts of other chlorophenols and inert materials (Mercier, 1977; Robson *et al.*, 1969).

One case of fatal aplastic anaemia was associated with exposure to pentachlorophenol and tetrachlorophenol (Roberts, 1963).

Extended periods of exposure to pentachlorophenol have resulted in persistent chloracne and disorders of the nervous system and liver (Baader & Bauer, 1951; Vinogradova *et al.*, 1973).

Average serum and urine levels of pentachlorophenol were about 30% and 50% higher in 6 exposed workers than in 4 control workers (Wyllie *et al.*, 1975). The urine of workers exposed to pentachloro-phenol contained unchanged compound and tetrachlorohydroquinone (Ahlborg *et al.*, 1974). For the occurrence of pentachlorophenol in serum and urine, see section 2.2 (e).

In lymphocyte cultures of 6 workers exposed to pentachlorophenol at a factory, the incidence of chromosome aberrations (breaks and gaps) was not significantly different from that in 4 'control' workers (Wyllie *et al.*, 1975).

3.3 Case reports and epidemiological studies

No data were available to the Working Group.

4. Summary of Data Reported and Evaluation

4.1 Experimental data

Pentachlorophenol was tested in one experiment in two strains of mice and in one experiment in rats by oral administration at dose levels sufficiently high to cause mild toxicity: no carcinogenic effect was seen in either species. Pentachlorophenol was also tested in one experiment in mice of two strains by subcutaneous injection of single doses; it produced hepatomas in males of one strain.

Pentachlorophenol did not induce sex-linked recessive lethals in *Drosophila melanogaster*.

4.2 Human data

No case reports or epidemiological studies were available to the Working Group.

The extensive production of pentachlorophenol and its use for wood preservation and, to a lesser extent, in homes and gardens, together with the persistent nature of the compound, indicate that widespread human exposure occurs. This is confirmed by many reports of its occurrence in the general environment and its presence in body fluids, both in the general population and in exposed workers. Several episodes of occupational intoxication have been reported.

4.3 Evaluation

The available data do not permit an evaluation of the carcinogenicity of pentachlorophenol to be made.

5. References

Adams, W.J., Arsenault, R.D., Behr, E.A., Burdell, C.A., Cantrell,
    W.R., Han, S.S., Hartford, W.H., Hudson, C.D., Hudson, M.S.,
    Keefe, D.E., Kulp, D.A., Leutritz, J., Jr, Lindsay, D.R.,
    Mathur, V.N.P., Suggitt, J.W. & Wetzel, W.H. (1974) Report of
    Committee P-5, methods for chemical analysis of preservatives.
    Proc. Am. Wood-Preserv. Assoc., 70, 259-264

Ahlborg, U.G. & Thunberg, T. (1978) Effects of 2,3,7,8-tetrachloro-
    dibenzo-p-dioxin in the in vivo and in vitro dechlorination
    of pentachlorophenol. Arch. Toxicol., 40, 55-61

Ahlborg, U.G., Lindgren, J.-E. & Mercier, M. (1974) Metabolism of
    pentachlorophenol. Arch. Toxicol., 32, 271-281

Ahlborg, U.G., Larsson, K. & Thunberg, T. (1978) Metabolism of
    pentachlorophenol in vivo and in vitro. Arch. Toxicol., 40, 45-53

Amer, S.M. & Ali, E.M. (1969) Cytological effects of pesticides. IV.
    Mitotic effects of some phenols. Cytologia, 34, 533-540

Anon. (1977a) PCP pesticides suspended in Michigan; dioxin found in
    cow livers. Pestic. Tox. Chem. News, 16 March, pp. 30-32

Anon. (1977b) FDA, Dow sample milk from Michigan herds for PCP, dioxin
    residues. Food Chem. News, 21 March, p. 36

Anon. (1977c) FDA finds 6 of 7 milk samples clean of PCP, dioxin. Food
    Chem. News, 28 March, p. 54

Anon. (1978) OSPR updates and expands RPAR actions summary to add post
    RPAR status. Pestic. Tox. Chem. News, 1 February, p. 22

Arrhenius, E., Renberg, L. & Johansson, L. (1977a) Subcellular
    distribution, a factor in risk evaluation of pentachlorophenol.
    Chem.-biol. Interact., 18, 23-34

Arrhenius, E., Renberg, L., Johansson, L. & Zetterqvist, M.-A. (1977b)
    Disturbance of microsomal detoxication mechanisms in liver by
    chlorophenol pesticides. Chem.-biol. Interact., 18, 35-46

Arsenault, R.D. (1976) Pentachlorophenol and contained chlorinated
    dibenzodioxins in the environment. A study of environmental fate,
    stability, and significance when used in wood preservation.
    Proc. Am. Wood-Preserv. Assoc., 72, 122-148

Ayres, D.C. & Gopalan, R. (1976) HPLC analysis of chlorophenolic
    pollutants and of their oxidation products. In: Dixon, P.F.,
    Gray, C.H. & Lim, C.K., eds, Proceedings of a Symposium on High
    Pressure Liquid Chromatography in Clinical Chemistry, London,
    Academic Press, pp. 195-199

Baader, E.W. & Bauer, H.J. (1951) Industrial intoxication due to
    pentachlorophenol. Ind. Med. Surg., 20, 286-290

Bevenue, A. & Ogata, J.N. (1971) A contributive error from analytical
    reagents in the analysis of chlorophenoxy acids and pentachlorophenol
    by electron capture gas chromatography. J. Chromatogr., 61, 147-148

Bevenue, A., Ogata, J.N. & Hylin, J.W. (1972) Organochlorine pesticides
    in rainwater, Oahu, Hawaii, 1971-1972. Bull. environ. Contam.
    Toxicol., 8, 238-241

Braun, W.H. & Sauerhoff, M.W. (1976) The pharmacokinetic profile of
    pentachlorophenol in monkeys. Toxicol. appl. Pharmacol., 38,
    525-533

Braun, W.H., Young, J.D., Blau, G.E. & Gehring, P.J. (1977) The
    pharmacokinetics and metabolism of pentachlorophenol in rats.
    Toxicol. appl. Pharmacol., 41, 395-406

Buhler, D.R., Rasmusson, M.E. & Nakaue, H.S. (1973) Occurrence of
    hexachlorophene and pentachlorophenol in sewage and water. Environ.
    Sci. Technol., 7, 929-934

Casanova, M. & Dubroca, J. (1973) Residues of pentachloronitrobenzene
    and its hexachlorobenzene impurity in soils and lettuce (Fr.). C.R.
    Seances Acad. Agr. Fr., 58, 990-998 [Chem. Abstr., 79, 1062q]

Cautreels, W., Van Cauwenberghe, K. & Guzman, L.A. (1977) Comparison
    between the organic fraction of suspended matter at a background and
    an urban station. Sci. total Environ., 8, 79-88

Chau, A.S.Y. & Coburn, J.A. (1974) Determination of pentachlorophenol in
    natural and waste waters. J. Assoc. off. anal. Chem., 57, 389-393

Deichmann, W., Machle, W., Kitzmiller, K.V. & Thomas, G. (1942) Acute
    and chronic effects of pentachlorophenol and sodium pentachlorophenate
    upon experimental animals. J. Pharmacol. exp. Ther., 76, 104-117

Dietz, F., Traud, J., Koppe, P. & Rübelt, C. (1976) Systems for the
    identification of phenolic compounds by thin-layer chromatography
    (Germ.). Chromatographia, 9, 380-396

Doedens, J.D. (1964) Chlorophenols. In: Kirk, R.E. & Othmer, D.F., eds,
    Encyclopedia of Chemical Technology, 2nd ed., Vol. 5, New York,
    John Wiley & Sons, pp. 336-337

Dougherty, R.C. & Piotrowska, K. (1976a) Screening by negative chemical
    ionization mass spectrometry for environmental contamination with
    toxic residues: application to human urines. Proc. natl Acad.
    Sci. (Wash.), 73, 1777-1781

Dougherty, R.C. & Piotrowska, K. (1976b) Multiresidue screening by
    negative chemical ionization mass spectrometry of organic poly-
    chlorides. J. Assoc. off. anal. Chem., 59, 1023-1027

Erney, D.R. (1978) Gas-liquid chromatographic determination of
    pentachlorophenol in milk. J. Assoc. off. anal. Chem., 61, 214-216

Eurocop-Cost (1976) A Comprehensive List of Polluting Substances Which
    Have Been Identified in Various Fresh Waters, Effluent Discharges,
    Aquatic Animals and Plants, and Bottom Sediments, 2nd ed., EUCO/
    MDU/73/76, XII/476/76, Luxembourg, Commission of the European
    Communities, p. 52

Fountaine, J.E., Joshipura, P.B. & Keliher, P.N. (1976) Some observa-
    tions regarding pentachlorophenol levels in Haverford Township,
    Pennsylvania. Water Res., 10, 185-188

Gaines, T.B. (1969) Acute toxicity of pesticides. Toxicol. appl. Pharmacol
    14, 515-534

Garrison, A.W., Pope, J.D. & Allen, F.R. (1976) GC/MS analysis of
    organic compounds in domestic wastewaters. In: Keith, L.H., ed.,
    Identification and Analysis of Organic Pollutants in Water,
    Ann Arbor, MI, Ann Arbor Sci., pp. 517-556

Gebefügi, I. & Parlar, H. (1978) Estimation of the Risk of Pentachloropheno
    in the Environment (Germ.), GSF-Bericht Ö 414, Munich, Gesellschaft
    für Strahlen und Umweltforchung, mbH

Gee, M.G., Land, D.G & Robinson, D. (1974) Simultaneous analysis of
    2,3,4,6-tetrachloroanisole, pentachloroanisole and the corresponding
    chlorophenols in biological tissue. J. Sci. Food Agric., 25,
    829-834

Goldstein, J.A., Friesen, M., Linder, R.E., Hickman, P., Hass, J.R. &
    Bergman, H. (1977) Effects of pentachlorophenol on hepatic drug-
    metabolizing enzymes and porphyria related to contamination with
    chlorinated dibenzo-p-dioxins and dibenzofurans. Biochem.
    Pharmacol., 26, 1549-1557

Gore, R.C., Hannah, R.W., Pattacini, S.C. & Porro, T.J. (1971) Infra-
    red and ultraviolet spectra of seventy-six pesticides. J. Assoc.
    off. anal. Chem., 54, 1040-1043, 1068-1069, 1082

Grasselli, J.G. & Ritchey, W.M., eds (1975) CRC Atlas of Spectral Data
    and Physical Constants for Organic Compounds, 2nd ed., Vol. IV,
    Cleveland, OH, Chemical Rubber Co., p. 93

Henshaw, B.G., Morgan, J.W.W. & Williams, N. (1975)   The detection of organic
    solvent preservatives in wood by thin-layer chromatography.
    J. Chromatogr., 110, 37-41

Hinkle, D.K. (1973) Fetotoxic effects of pentachlorophenol in the
    golden Syrian hamster (Abstract no. 42). Toxicol. appl. Pharmacol.,
    25, 455

Hoben, H.J., Ching, S.A., Casarett, L.J. & Young, R.A. (1976a) A study
    of the inhalation of pentachlorophenol by rats. I. A method for
    the determination of pentachlorophenol in rat plasma, urine and
    tissue and in aerosol samples. Bull. environ. Contam. Toxicol., 15,
    78-85

Hoben, H.J., Ching, S.A. & Casarett, L.J. (1976b) A study of inhalation
    of pentachlorophenol by rats. III. Inhalation toxicity study.
    Bull. environ. Contam. Toxicol., 15, 463-465

Howard, P.H. & Durkin, P.R. (1973) Preliminary Environmental Hazard
    Assessment of Chlorinated Naphthalenes, Silicones, Fluorocarbons,
    Benzenepolycarboxylates, and Chlorophenols, EPA-560/2-74-001,
    US Environmental Protection Agency, Report No. PB238074, available
    from Springfield, VA, National Technical Information Service, pp. 204-
    205, 214, 217-221, 256-263

Innes, J.R.M., Ulland, B.M., Valerio, M.G., Petrucelli, L., Fishbein, L.,
    Hart, E.R., Pallotta, A.J., Bates, R.R., Falk, H.L., Gart, J.J.,
    Klein, M., Mitchell, I. & Peters, J. (1969) Bioassay of pesticides
    and industrial chemicals for tumorigenicity in mice. A preliminary
    note. J. natl Cancer Inst., 42, 1101-1114

Jakobson, I. & Yllner, S. (1971) Metabolism of ^{14}C-pentachlorophenol
    in the mouse. Acta pharmacol. toxicol., 29, 513-524

Jensen, S., Renberg, L. & Reutergårdh, L. (1977) Residue analysis of
    sediment and sewage sludge for organochlorines in the presence
    of elemental sulfur. Anal. Chem., 49, 316-318

Johnson, R.L., Gehring, P.J., Kociba, R.J. & Schwetz, B.A. (1973)
    Chlorinated dibenzodioxins and pentachlorophenol. Environ. Health
    Perspect., 5, 171-175

Kutz, F.W., Murphy, R.S. & Strassman, S.C. (1978) Survey of pesticide
    residues and their metabolites in urine from the general population.
    In: Ranga Rao, K., ed., Pentachlorophenol, New York, Plenum,
    pp. 363-369

Langer, H.G., Brady, T.P., Dalton, L.A., Shannon, T.W. & Briggs, P.R.
    (1973) Thermal chemistry of chlorinated phenols. In: Blair,
    E.H., ed., Chlorodioxins - Origin and Fate (Advances in Chemistry
    Series, No. 120), Washington DC, American Chemical Society,
    pp. 26-32

van Langeveld, H.E.A.M. (1975) Determination of pentachlorophenol in toy paints. J. Assoc. off. anal. Chem., 58, 19-22

Larsen, R.V., Born, G.S., Kessler, W.V., Shaw, S.M. & Van Sickle, D.C. (1975) Placental transfer and teratology of pentachlorophenol in rats. Environ. Lett., 10, 121-128

Melnikova, L.V., Belyakov, A.A., Smirnova, V.G. & Kurenko, L.T. (1975) Sanitary-chemical method of determining noxious substances encountered in the production of sodium pentachlorophenolate (Russ.). Gig. Tr. Prof. Zabol., 7, 37-39

Menon, J.A. (1958) Topical hazards associated with the use of pentachlorophenol. Br. med. J., ii, 1156-1158

Mercier, M. (1977) Preparatory Study for Establishing Criteria (Exposure/Effect Relationships) for Humans on Organochlorine Compounds, i.e. Pesticides, 2nd Series, Doc. No. V/F/2500/1/76e, Luxembourg, Commission of the European Communities, pp. 26-50

National Institute for Occupational Safety & Health (1977) National Occupatic Hazard Survey, Vol. III, Survey Analyses and Supplemental Tables, December, Draft, Cincinnati, OH, pp. 8,285-8,288

National Technical Information Service (1968) Evaluation of Carcinogenic, Teratogenic and Mutagenic Activities of Selected Pesticides and Industrial Chemicals, Vol. 1, Carcinogenic Study, Washington DC, US Department of Commerce

Nomura, N. (1974) Polluting materials in the wells in the O district, Toyama City (Jap.). Toyama Daigaku Kyoikugakubu Kiyo, 22, 115-118 [Chem. Abstr., 83, 48033d]

Parr, L.J., Gee, M.G., Land, D.G., Robinson, D. & Curtis, R.F. (1974) Chlorophenols from wood preservatives in broiler house litter. J. Sci. Food Agric., 25, 835-841

Pearson, J.E., Schultz, C.D., Rivers, J.E. & Gonzalez, F.M. (1976) Pesticide levels of patients on chronic hemodialysis. Bull. environ. Contam. Toxicol., 16, 556-558

Prager, B., Jacobson, P., Schmidt, P. & Stern, D., eds (1923) Beilsteins Handbuch der Organische Chemie, 4th ed., Vol. 6, Syst. No. 522, Berlin, Springer, p. 194

Rappe, C., Marklund, S., Buser, H.R. & Bosshardt, H.-P. (1978) Formation of polychlorinated dibenzo-p-dioxins (PCDDs) and dibenzofurans (PPFs) by burning or heating chlorophenates. Chemosphere, 3, 269-281

Renberg, L. (1974) Ion exchange technique for the determination of chlorinated phenols and phenoxy acids in organic tissue, soil, and water. Anal. Chem., 46, 459-461

Rivers, J.B. (1972) Gas chromatographic determination of pentachlorophenol in human blood and urine. Bull. environ. Contam. Toxicol., 8, 294-296

Roberts, H.J. (1963) Aplastic anemia due to pentachlorophenol and tetra-chlorophenol. South. med. J., 56, 632-635

Robson, A.M., Kissane, J.M., Elvick, N.H. & Pundavela, L. (1969) Pentachlorophenol poisoning in a nursery for newborn infants. I. Clinical features and treatment. J. Pediat., 75, 309-316

von Rumker, R., Lawless, E.W. & Meiners, A.F. (1975) Production, Distribution, Use and Environmental Impact Potential of Selected Pesticides, EPA 540/1-74-001, Washington DC, US Environmental Protection Agency, pp. 308-319

Schwetz, B.A., Keeler, P.A. & Gehring, P.J. (1974) The effect of purified and commercial grade pentachlorophenol on rat embryonal and fetal development. Toxicol. appl. Pharmacol., 28, 151-161

Schwetz, B.A., Quast, J.F., Keeler, P.A., Humiston, C.G. & Kociba, R.J. (1978) Results of two-year toxicity and reproduction studies on pentachlorophenol in rats. In: Ranga Rao, K., ed., Pentachlorophenol, New York, Plenum, pp. 301-309

Shackelford, W.M. & Keith, L.H. (1976) Frequency of Organic Compounds Identified in Water, EPA-600/4-76-062, Athens, GA, US Environmental Protection Agency, pp. 190-191

Shafik, T.M. (1973) The determination of pentachlorophenol and hexachlorophene in human adipose tissue. Bull. environ. Contam. Toxicol., 10, 57-63

Shafik, T.M., Sullivan, H.C. & Enos, H.R. (1973) Multiresidue procedure for halo- and nitrophenols. Measurement of exposure to biodegradable pesticides yielding these compounds as metabolites. J. agric. Food Chem., 21, 295-298

Tokunaga, S. (1971) Identification of poisonous substances in dead fish. II. Detection and determination of pentachlorophenol from fish extract (Jap.) Kagaku Keisatsu Kenkyusho Hokoku, 24, 138-146 [Chem. Abstr., 77, 18157f]

US Environmental Protection Agency (1970) EPA Compendium of Registered Pesticides, Vol. I, Herbicides and Plant Regulators, Washington DC, US Government Printing Office, p. I-P-3

US Environmental Protection Agency (1973) EPA Compendium of Registered
    Pesticides, Vol. II, Fungicides and Nematicides, Washington DC,
    US Government Printing Office, pp. S-59-001 - S-59-00.03

US Environmental Protection Agency (1975) EPA Compendium of Registered
    Pesticides, Vol. II, Fungicides and Nematicides, Washington DC,
    US Government Printing Office, p. I-P-3

US Environmental Protection Agency (1976) Manual of Chemical
    Methods for Pesticides and Devices, Office of Pesticide Programs,
    Washington DC, Association of Official Analytical Chemists, pp. EPA-
    5:1 - EPA-5:3

US Food & Drug Administration (1970) Pesticide Analytical Manual, Vol. III,
    Methods which Detect Pesticide Residues in Human and Environmental
    Media, Rockville, MD, pp. 1-6

US Food & Drug Administration (1975) Compliance Program Evaluation.
    Total Diet Studies: FY 1973 (7320.08), Bureau of Foods, Washington DC,
    US Government Printing Office, Table 5

US Food & Drug Administration (1977) Compliance Program Evaluation.
    Total Diet Studies: FY 74 (7320.08), Bureau of Foods, Washington DC,
    US Government Printing Office, Table 6

US International Trade Commission (1976) Imports of Benzenoid Chemicals
    and Products, 1974, USITC Publication 762, Washington DC, US
    Government Printing Office, p. 97

US International Trade Commission (1977) Synthetic Organic Chemicals,
    US Production and Sales, 1976, USITC Publication 833, Washington
    DC, US Government Printing Office, p. 269

US Occupational Safety & Health Administration (1977) Air contaminants.
    US Code Fed. Regul., Title 29, part 1910.1000, p. 27

US Tariff Commission (1951) Synthetic Organic Chemicals, US Production
    and Sales, 1950, Report No. 173, Second Series, Washington DC,
    US Government Printing Office, p. 128

Vermeer, K., Risebrough, R.W., Spaans, A.L. & Reynolds, L.M. (1974)
    Pesticide effects on fishes and birds in rice fields of Surinam,
    South America. Environ. Pollut., 7, 217-236

Vinogradova, V.K., Kalyaganov, P.I., Sudonina, L.T. & Elizarov, G.P.
    (1973) Hygienic characteristics of working conditions and health
    status of workers engaged in the production of sodium pentachloro-
    phenolate (Russ.). Gig. Tr. Prof. Zabol., 8, 11-13

Vogel, E. & Chandler, J.L.R. (1974) Mutagenicity testing of cyclamate
    and some pestcides in *Drosophila melanogaster*. Experientia, 30,
    621-623

Weinbach, E.C. (1954) The effect of pentachlorophenol on oxidative
    phosphorylation. J. biol. Chem., 210, 545-550

Windholz, M., ed. (1976) The Merck Index, 9th ed., Rahway, NJ, Merck
    & Co., p. 921

Winell, M. (1975) An international comparison of hygienic standards
    for chemicals in the work environment. Ambio, 4, 34-36

Wyllie, J.A., Gabica, J., Benson, W.W. & Yoder, J. (1975) Exposure
    and contamination of the air and employees of a pentachlorophenol
    plant, Idaho - 1972. Pestic. Monit. J., 9, 150-153

Zitko, V., Hutzinger, O. & Choi, P.M.K. (1974) Determination of
    pentachlorophenol and chlorobiphenyl in biological samples.
    Bull. environ. Contam. Toxicol., 12, 649-653

TOXAPHENE (POLYCHLORINATED CAMPHENES)

A literature compilation (Mashburn, 1978) and one review on
toxaphene (French & Assoc. Ltd, 1977) are available.

1. Chemical and Physical Data

1.1 Synonyms and trade names

Chem. Abstr. Services Reg. No.: 8001-35-2

Chem. Abstr. Name: Toxaphene

Synonyms: Camphechlor; camphochlor; chlorinated camphene;
chlorocamphene; kamfochlor; octachlorocamphene; polychlor-
camphene; polychlorocamphene; toxafeen; toxaphen

Trade names: Agricide Maggot Killer; Alltex; Alltox; Camphofene
Huileux; Chem-Phene; Clor Chem T-590; Compound 3956; Crestoxo;
Cristoxo-90; ENT 9,735; Estonox; Fasco-Terpene; Geniphene; Gy-
Phene; Hercules 3956; Hercules Toxaphene; M 5055; Melipax;
Motox; Penphene; Phenacide; Phenatox; Strobane-T; Synthetic
3956; Toxadust; Toxakil; Toxon 63; Toxyphen; Vertac 90%

1.2 Structural and molecular formulae and molecular weight

Empirical formula: $C_{10}H_{10}Cl_8$ Mol. wt: 414 (average)

1.3 Chemical and physical properties of the substance

From Hawley (1977), unless otherwise specified

(a) Description: Amber, waxy solid

(b) Melting range: 65-90°C

(c) Solubility: Soluble in common organic solvents; practically
     insoluble in water (Windholz, 1976)

(d) Stability: Dehydrochlorinates in the presence of alkali,
     prolonged exposure to sunlight and at temperatures of about
     155°C (Windholz, 1976)

(e) Reactivity: Noncorrosive in absence of moisture (Spencer,
     1973)

1.4 Technical products and impurities

The exact composition of toxaphene is unknown.   Technical toxaphene
consists predominantly of polychlorinated camphenes with 4-12 chlorine
atoms per molecule, and contains 67-69% chlorine (Parlar *et al.*, 1977).
In one study, toxaphene was found to contain at least 177 components
(Holmsted *et al.*, 1974).

Toxaphene is available in the US in the following formulations:
a wettable powder (40% active), emulsifiable concentrates of various
strengths, dusts (10% and 20%), granules (10% and 20%), baits (1% in
bran), an oil solution (90%), an emulsion containing 2 parts toxaphene
and 1 part DDT, and a dust containing 14% toxaphene and 7% DDT.

2. Production, Use, Occurrence and Analysis

2.1 Production and use

(a) Production

It is believed that toxaphene was first introduced in 1948.   It
was prepared by chlorination of camphene in 1953 (Buntin, 1953).   Toxaphene is currently produced commercially in the US by chlorination of
camphene until a chlorine content of 67-69% is obtained (Spencer, 1973).

Commercial production of toxaphene in the US was first reported in
1947 (US Tariff Commission, 1948).   In 1976, 3 US companies produced a
total of 19 million kg (US International Trade Commission, 1977), which
represented a decline of 29% from the 1975 production level of 27 million
kg (US International Trade Commission, 1976).   No data were available
on US imports and exports.

Toxaphene is not known to be produced commercially in western
Europe or Japan; all toxaphene used in western Europe is imported from
the US.

(b) Use

Toxaphene is used as an insecticide for the control of grasshoppers, army-worms, cutworms and all major cotton pests.   It is also recommended for the control of livestock pests such as flies, lice, ticks, scab mites and mange (Berg, 1978).   An estimated 20 million kg toxaphene were used in the US in 1974, as follows: cotton, 85%; livestock and poultry, 7%; other field crops, 5%; soya beans, 3%; and sorghum, less than 1%.

No data on its use in Europe were available; it is not known to have been used in Japan.

Tolerances for residues of toxaphene in or on raw agricultural commodities in the US have been established at 0.1-7 mg/kg for a variety of about 50 fruit, vegetable and meat products (US Environmental Protection Agency, 1976a).   The ambient water criterion for toxaphene in US navigable waters is 5 ng/l (US Environmental Protection Agency, 1977a).

A notice of rebuttable presumption against registration and continued registration (RPAR) (see General Remarks on Substances Considered, p. 31) of pesticide products containing toxaphene was issued by the US Environmental Protection Agency on 25 May, 1977 on the basis of possible mutagenic, endocrine, enzymatic and reproductive effects and population reductions in avian species (US Environmental Protection Agency, 1977b). The future insecticidal use of toxaphene will depend largely on the outcome of this action.

The US Occupational Safety and Health Administration's health standards for air contaminants require that an employee's exposure to toxaphene not exceed an 8-hr time-weighted average of 0.5 mg/m^3 in any 8-hr work shift of a 40-hr work week (US Occupational Safety & Health Administration, 1977).

2.2 Occurrence

Toxaphene is not known to occur as a natural product.   Reviews on its occurrence and environmental fate have been published (Sheets et al., 1972; US Environmental Protection Agency, 1976b).

(a) Air

Atmospheric levels of toxaphene measured during 1973-1974 ranged from < 0.02-3.3 ng/m^3 at a tower on the south shore of Bermuda to < 0.04-1.6 ng/m^3 from the bow of a ship in the western North Atlantic; 1.7-5.2 ng/m^3 were found in the spring of 1975 at Sapelo Island, Georgia (Bidleman & Olney, 1975).

Weekly air samples were taken in a primary cotton-growing area during 1972-1974.   Average monthly atmospheric levels of toxaphene were found to range from 0-1540 ng/m^3, with maximum levels occurring during the late summer months and minimum levels in winter (Arthur *et al.*, 1976).

(b) Water

Toxaphene has been found in 2 US rivers (Shackelford & Keith, 1976), in land run-off water from crop spraying, and in river-water, lakes, aquatic plants, fish and sediments (Eurocop-Cost, 1976). It was detected in 5/8 samples of rainwater, at levels ranging from 44-280 ng/l (Munson, 1976).

(c) Soil and sediments

Toxaphene levels in soil samples from 3 locations in 8 cities during the summer and autumn of 1969 were 0.11, 12 and 15-53 mg/kg (Wiersma *et al.*, 1972); those in 14 US cities during the summer and autumn of 1970 were 7.7-33.4 mg/kg in 3/28 samples from one location and 16.1 mg/kg in 1/27 samples from another (Carey *et al.*, 1976).

Sediment samples, collected at varying depths by 10 cm increments up to 80 cm, were taken 0.2, 0.8 and 1.4 miles from the outfall of a toxaphene plant. Toxaphene levels ranged from 5.27 mg/kg (in a 70-80 cm sediment sample from the site farthest from the plant) to 1,858 mg/kg (in a surface-10 cm sample from the site closest to the toxaphene plant) (Durant & Reimold, 1972).

Forty-five percent of toxaphene applied to sandy loam soil in 1951 remained 20 years later (Nash *et al.*, 1973).

(d) Animals

Toxaphene was found in 96% of samples of 50 catfish taken from commercial ponds in spring 1970, at an average concentration of 1.98 mg/kg (Hawthorne *et al.*, 1974).

Samples of meat were collected from bobwhite quail, rabbits and white-tailed deer found in or near toxaphene-treated soya bean fields during the summer and autumn of 1960 and 1969. Toxaphene was found in 5/20 quail, in amounts ranging from 10.3-88.9 mg/kg; in 2/31 rabbits, at levels of 1.2 and 12.35 mg/kg; and in 3/22 deer, at levels of 1.7-8.7 mg/kg (Causey *et al.*, 1972).

Toxaphene was detected in all 21 brown pelican eggs collected during 1973 in a small breeding colony, at levels ranging from 0.12-0.58 mg/kg (Blus *et al.*, 1975). It was also detected in 3/50 bats (Reidinger, 1976).

(e) Occupational exposure

Toxaphene levels in the air of manufacturing plants in the USSR were found to exceed by 5-6 times the permissible level of 0.2 mg/m^3. By the end of the work shift, concentrations on uncovered parts of the skin of employees were 30-1000 mg/m^2; covered skin areas had toxaphene concentrations of up to 40 mg/m^2 (Ashirova, 1971).

(f) Other

Toxaphene levels in samples of cigarettes, cigars, smoking tobacco, chewing tobacco and snuff purchased at a retail market over the period 1971-1973 were found to decrease: in cigarettes, the average concentration decreased from 3.3 to 1.4 mg/kg (Domanski et al., 1974).

Residues of toxaphene in 6 brands of cigars purchased in 5 cities ranged from < 0.5-3.42 mg/kg (Domanski & Guthrie, 1974).

Toxaphene levels in auction-market flue-cured, Burley and fire- and air-cured tobacco were sampled in 1970 and 1972. In 1972, 90% of the flue-cured samples contained toxaphene, at mean concentrations of 0.51-1.93 mg/kg; whereas in 1970 less than 30% contained toxaphene. In 1972, 50% of the Burley tobacco samples had toxaphene concentrations greater than 0.5 mg/kg, whereas in 1970, only 18% of the samples were found to contain toxaphene. Fire- and air-cured tobaccos contained mean levels of 0.19-1.69 mg/kg toxaphene in 1972 (Domanski et al., 1975). Toxaphene residues in individual samples of flue-cured tobacco ranged from < 0.3-7.7 mg/kg (Domanski & Sheets, 1976).

Toxaphene residue levels in sugarbeet pulp samples collected from 57 processing plants in 16 states in the autumn of 1970 ranged from 0-0.34 mg/kg (Yang et al., 1976).

2.3 Analysis

After fractionation using silica-gel column chromatography, combined gas chromatography/chemical ionization/mass spectrometry was used to establish that commercial toxaphene is a complex mixture of at least 177 polychlorinated 10-carbon derivatives (Holmsted et al., 1974). Infra-red and mass spectrometry and hydrogen and carbon-13 nuclear magnetic resonance spectral analysis have been used to characterize its composition (Parlar et al., 1977).

The Association of Official Analytical Chemists' method to deter- mine the contamination of other pesticide formulations by chlorinated pesticides (Horwitz, 1975) has been studied collaboratively, and a dis- cussion of the method and the problems encountered has been published (Bontoyan & Jung, 1972). The recovery procedures of this method have also been discussed in detail in the Pesticide Analytical Manual,

published by the US Food and Drug Administration.   More than 80% of
toxaphene was found to be recovered by this procedure (US Food & Drug
Administration, 1975).

Pesticide residues, including toxaphene, have been recovered quanti-
tatively from flour, fruit, vegetables and tobacco by steam distillation
followed by continuous extraction of the distillate with toluene (Stijve
& Cardinale, 1973).

Methods used for the analysis of toxaphene in environmental samples
are listed in Table 1.

Reverse-phase partition thin-layer chromatography has also been
used to separate toxaphene from other chlorinated hydrocarbons, with
detection of levels of 2.5 µg/sample (Ismail & Bonner, 1974).   Thin-layer
chromatography has been used to determine toxaphene in soil, beetroots
and potatoes (Kosmatyi & Gritsaenko, 1970) and in prepared samples
(Geike, 1971; Thielemann, 1973).

The Pesticide Analytical Manual cites two colorimetric methods to
determine toxaphene: (1) in all types of environmental samples, by
fusion with diphenylamine in the presence of zinc chloride, with a limit
of detection of 2 mg/kg in fats and 0.1 mg/kg in crops; and (2) by extraction in ethanol, boiling with dilute nitric acid, treatment with sodium
hydroxide and pyridine, and measurement at 410 and 440 nm (US Food & Drug
Administration, 1975).

Toxaphene has been determined colorimetrically in water by treatment
with pyridine, alkali and ethyl cyanoacetate and measurement of the resulting complex at 550 nm, with a limit of detection of 15 µg/l (Hempel *et
al.*, 1971).

3.   Biological Data Relevant to the Evaluation
of Carcinogenic Risk to Humans

3.1 Carcinogenicity studies in animals

Oral administration

Mouse: Groups of 50 male and 50 female 5-week-old B6C3F1 mice were
fed technical-grade toxaphene in the diet.   Initially, high-dose
animals received 320 mg/kg diet for 19 weeks followed by 160 mg/kg diet
for a further 61 weeks; low-dose animals received 160 mg/kg diet for
19 weeks and 80 mg/kg diet for a further 61 weeks.   A toxaphene-free
diet was then fed for 10-11 weeks.   A group of 10 male and 10 female mice
served as matched controls and received untreated diet for 90-91 weeks.
The time-weighted average doses were 99 mg/kg diet (low dose) and 198 mg/kg

TABLE 1. METHODS FOR THE ANALYSIS OF TOXAPHENE

SAMPLE TYPE	ANALYTICAL METHOD		LIMIT OF DETECTION	REFERENCE
	EXTRACTION/CLEAN-UP	DETECTION		
Formulations				
Formulations contaminated with 0.05-0.1% toxaphene	Extract (acetone), centrifuge	TLC (revelation: silver nitrate-ultra-violet		Horwitz (1975)
Air				
Workplace	Trap on cellulose membrane, extract (petroleum ether)	GC/ECD	0.225-1.155 mg/m^3	National Institute for Occupational Safety & Health (1977)
Water				
Fish-tank	Extract (acetone-petroleum ether) in a special syphon system, wash resulting water-acetone layer (petroleum ether), bulk petroleum ether fractions, CC	GC/ECD, GC/MS	10 µg/l	Stalling & Huckins (1976)
Soil				
	Extract (hexane-acetone-methanol) in Soxhlet or on a column, or extract by shaking (hexane-acetone-ammonium chloride solution)	GC/ECD		Nash et al. (1973)
	Moisten (water), extract (hexane-isopropanol), wash (water)	GC/ECD	0.05-0.1 mg/kg	Carey et al. (1976)
	Extract (hexane-isopropanol), filter, wash (water)	GC/flame photometric detection	50 µg/kg	Wiersma et al. (1972)

TABLE 1. METHODS FOR THE ANALYSIS OF TOXAPHENE (continued)

SAMPLE TYPE	EXTRACTION/CLEAN-UP	DETECTION	LIMIT OF DETECTION	REFERENCE
ANALYTICAL METHOD				
Food				
Molasses	Dilute (water), extract (hexane-isopropanol)	GC/ECD	0.03 mg/kg	Yang et al. (1976)
Fish	Extract (hexane-isopropanol) in blender, filter, wash (water), liquid/liquid partition, CC	GC/ECD	0.01 mg/kg	Hawthorne et al. (1974)
Fruits and vegetables	Extract (acetone) in blender, filter, extract (petroleum ether-dichloromethane), wash aqueous phase (dichloromethane), bulk solvent extracts, evaporate to small bulk, add acetone, reduce volume and repeat, CC	GC/ECD		Luke et al. (1975)
Fish	Freeze, grind in blender with dry ice, place in freezer overnight to allow dry ice to sublime, mix with anhydrous sodium sulphate, extract (ether-petroleum ether) in a column, add cyclohexane, reduce volume, multiple CC (an additional wash with sodium hydroxide may be required)	GC/ECD GC/MS	30 µg/kg	Stalling & Huckins (1976)
Biological				
Tissues	Macerate, add anhydrous sodium sulphate, extract (acetone), add water, extract (chloroform), wash (potassium hydroxide-water)	TLC (revelation: 14 reagents compared)	1 µg (on the plate)	Tewari & Sharma (1977)
Stomach washings and urine	Extract (hexane)	TLC (revelation: 14 reagents compared)		Tewari & Sharma (1977)
Blood	Add dilute sulphuric acid and sodium tungstate solution, filter extract (hexane)	TLC (revelation: 14 reagents compared)		Tewari & Sharma (1977)

Abbreviations: TLC - thin-layer chromatography; GC/ECD - gas chromatography/electron capture detection; CC - column chromatography; MS - mass spectrometry

diet (high dose).   Further control data were obtained from 50 male and
50 female pooled controls from other experiments.   There was a dose-
related decrease in survival of male mice and a decrease in the survival of high-dose females: in male mice, 46/50 (92%) of the high-dose
group, 49/50 (98%) of the low-dose group and all 10 animals of the
matched control group lived beyond week 52 of the study; in females,
46/50 (92%) of the high-dose group, 46/50 (92%) of the low-dose group
and 9/10 (90%) of the matched control group lived beyond week 52 of
the study; at 90 weeks, 21/50 (42%) high-dose males and 37/50 (74%)
high-dose females were still alive.   An increased incidence of hepatocellular carcinomas was found in treated mice: in <u>males</u>: matched
controls, 0/10; pooled controls, 4/48 (8%); low dose, 34/49 (69%);
high dose, 45/46 (98%); in <u>females</u>: matched controls, 0/9; pooled
controls, 0/48; low dose, 5/49 (10%); high dose, 34/49 (69%).   In
addition, neoplastic nodules of the liver occurred in 2/10 matched
control males, 6/49 low-dose males, 0/9 matched control females, 13/49
low-dose females and 6/49 high-dose females (National Cancer Institute,
1979).

  <u>Rat</u>: Groups of 50 male and 50 female 5-week-old Osborne-Mendel
rats were fed diets containing technical-grade toxaphene.   High-dose
male rats received 2560 mg/kg diet for 2 weeks, 1280 mg/kg diet for
53 weeks, 640 mg/kg diet for a further 25 weeks, followed by a toxaphene-
free diet for 28 weeks.   High-dose females received 1280 mg/kg diet for
55 weeks, 640 mg/kg diet for 25 weeks, followed by a toxaphene-free diet
for 30 weeks.   Low-dose males received 1280 mg/kg diet for 2 weeks,
640 mg/kg diet for 53 weeks, 320 mg/kg diet for 25 weeks, followed by
a toxaphene-free diet for 28 weeks.   Low-dose females received 640 mg/kg
diet for 55 weeks, 320 mg/kg diet for 25 weeks, followed by a toxaphene-
free diet for 30 weeks.   Time-weighted average doses were 556 and 540
mg/kg diet for low-dose males and females, and 1112 and 1080 mg/kg diet
for high-dose males and females, respectively.   Groups of 10 male and
10 female rats that served as matched controls were given a toxaphene-
free diet for 108-109 weeks; 55 untreated male and 55 untreated female
rats from other experiments served as pooled controls.   In male rats,
45/50 (90%) of the high-dose group, 47/50 (94%) of the low-dose group
and all 10 rats of the matched control group were still alive at week
52 of the study; in females, 48/50 (96%) of the high-dose group, 46/50
(92%) of the low-dose group and all 10 rats of the matched control
group were still alive at week 52.   In male rats, the combined incidence of follicular-cell carcinomas and adenomas of the thyroid was
increased to a statistically significant extent in the high-dose group,
compared with pooled controls ($P = 0.008$) (1/7 in matched controls,
2/44 in pooled controls, 7/41 in low-dose and 9/35 in high-dose animals).
In females, the incidences of follicular-cell adenomas of the thyroid
were 0/6 in matched controls, 1/46 in pooled controls, 1/43 in low-dose
animals and 7/42 in high-dose animals ($P = 0.021$ compared with pooled
controls).   The incidence of adenomas, chromophobe adenomas or carcinomas of the pituitary in high-dose females was 23/39, compared with

17/51 in pooled controls (P = 0.013) (National Cancer Institute, 1979).

3.2 Other relevant biological data

A review on toxaphene is available (Pollock & Kilgore, 1978).

(a) Experimental systems

Toxic effects

In Sherman rats, the oral LD_{50} of technical-grade toxaphene is 90 mg/kg bw in males and 80 mg/kg bw in females (Gaines, 1960). In male Wistar rats fed a 3.5% casein diet, the oral LD_{50} of technical-grade toxaphene is 80 mg/kg bw; in those fed a 26% casein diet, 293 mg/kg bw; and in those fed standard laboratory chow, 220 mg/kg bw (Boyd & Taylor, 1971). In fasted dogs, the oral LD_{50} of toxaphene is 25 mg/kg bw (Lackey, 1949). In male mice, the i.p. LD_{50} of technical-grade toxaphene is 42 mg/kg bw. Two toxic fractions gave i.p. LD_{50} values of 3.1 and 6.6 mg/kg bw (Khalifa et al., 1974); the first was identified as a mixture of 2,2,5-endo,6-exo,8,8,9,10-octachlorobornane and 2,2,5-endo,6-exo, 8,9,9,10-octachlorobornane (Turner et al., 1975) and the second as 2,2,5-endo-6-exo,8,9,10-heptachlorobornane (Casida et al., 1974).

In Sherman rats, the dermal LD_{50} of technical-grade toxaphene is 1075 mg/kg bw in males and 780 mg/kg bw in females (Gaines, 1960).

The LC_{50} in mice for inhalation of an oil-based mist of toxaphene was 20 mg/m^3 air over a 2-hr exposure (Conley, 1952).

Signs of acute toxaphene poisoning are clonic-tonic convulsions, salivation, vomiting and hyperreflexia; death has been attributed to respiratory failure (Boyd & Taylor, 1971; Conley, 1952; Lackey, 1949). In rats, renal tubular damage and fatty degeneration of the liver with necrosis are observed (Boyd & Taylor, 1971).

Feeding of 5, 50 and 100 mg/kg diet toxaphene to chickens for 31 weeks produced sternal deformation, resembling osteomalacia, and nephrosis of the kidney. Occasional keel deformation, involving the cartilaginous tissue as well as an apparent increase in the growth of cartilage, was found in birds fed 0.5 mg/kg diet toxaphene (Bush et al., 1977).

In some Sherman rats fed 50 and 200 mg/kg diet toxaphene for 2-9 months, centrilobular hypertrophy of liver cells was observed (Ortega et al., 1957); however, no effects on liver-cell histology were observed by Clapp et al. (1971) in rats fed up to 189 mg/kg diet toxaphene for 12 weeks.

Alterations to serum alkaline phosphatase activity, indicating liver damage, have been observed in rats fed toxaphene (Gertig & Nowaczyk, 1975; Grebenyuk, 1970); it induces various hepatic microsomal enzymes, such as O- and N-demethylases (Kinoshita et al., 1966) and androgen hydroxylase (Peakall, 1976); it also stimulates oestrone metabolism in rats (Welch et al., 1971). Phenobarbital sleeping times were reduced in rats given toxaphene orally by gavage (Schwabe & Wendling, 1967).

Administration of 5, 50 or 500 mg/kg diet toxaphene to quail for up to 4 months produced hypertrophy of the thyroid, with increased uptake of ^{131}I and adrenal hypertrophy (Hurst et al., 1974).

Embryotoxicity and teratogenicity

Administration of 25 mg/kg diet toxaphene to mice through 5 generations produced no embryotoxicity or teratogenicity (Keplinger et al., 1968). In a 3-generation reproduction study, Sprague-Dawley rats received either 25 or 100 mg/kg diet toxaphene; no effects on litter size, pup survival, weanling body weights or reproductive capacity were observed (Kennedy et al., 1973).

Toxaphene was administered by oral intubation to CD-1 mice and CD rats during the period of embryonic organogenesis (days 7-16 of gestation) at dose levels of 0, 15, 25 and 35 mg/kg bw/day. The highest dose produced marked maternal mortality in rats and mice and an increase in the incidence of encephaloceles among offspring of mice. Foetal mortality was slightly increased in mice at all three dose levels. Small decreases in foetal body weight and in the number of sternal and caudal ossification centres were seen in rats, mostly in those receiving the 25 mg/kg bw dose (Chernoff & Carver, 1976).

Injection of 1.5 mg/egg toxaphene had no effect on hatchability rates of the eggs of chickens (Smith et al., 1970). In a similar study, no embryotoxicity was observed in chicken embryos hatched from eggs previously injected with 400 or 500 mg/kg toxaphene in acetone; although when it was dissolved in corn oil embryotoxicity was seen with 300-400 mg/kg (Dunachie & Fletcher, 1969).

Absorption, excretion, distribution and metabolism

In mice and rats, toxaphene is absorbed through the skin and gastro-intestinal tract, at a rate depending upon the vehicle used for its administration. Of a single oral dose of 20 mg/kg bw technical-grade ^{36}Cl-toxaphene administered in 0.5 ml peanut oil/acacia gum to rats, about 52% was excreted within 9 days: 15% in the urine, mainly as $^{36}Cl^-$ ion, and 37% in the faeces (Crowder & Dindal, 1974).

Three percent of an oral dose of ^{14}C-toxaphene was excreted unchanged in the faeces of rats. More than 5% of the administered dose was excreted in the urine and faeces as completely dechlorinated metabolites and 27% as partially dechlorinated metabolites; 2% of the activity was found in expired air, probably as $^{14}CO_2$. Less than 1 μg toxaphene or metabolites was found in each of fat, liver, kidney, blood, bone, brain, heart, lung, muscle, spleen and testis 14 days after a 19 mg/kg bw dose of ^{14}C-toxaphene. Following administration of ^{36}Cl-toxaphene, 50% of the activity was excreted as ^{36}Cl-ion in the urine (Ohsawa et al., 1975).

Administration of 2.5-20 mg/kg diet toxaphene to cows resulted in a dose-related increase in the excretion of toxaphene in the milk (0.043-0.179 mg/l) (Zweig et al., 1963).

Mutagenicity and other related short-term tests

Toxaphene is mutagenic in the Salmonella typhimurium test without requiring liver homogenate for activity (Hooper et al., 1979).

Toxaphene did not induce dominant lethal mutations in ICR/Ha Swiss mice. When males were injected intraperitoneally with 36 and 180 mg/kg bw and bred with untreated females during 8 weeks, the frequency of early foetal deaths and preimplantation losses was within control limits. Negative results were also obtained in animals treated orally for 5 successive days with 40 or 80 mg/kg bw (Epstein et al., 1972).

(b) Humans

The acute lethal dose for humans has been estimated to be between 2-7 g/person (Conley, 1952).

A 9-month-old child poisoned with a 2:1 mixture of toxaphene:DDT died after convulsions and respiratory arrest. The ratio of toxaphene: DDT in the brain and liver was 10:1 and in the kidneys 3:1 (Haun & Cueto, 1967). Four other cases of acute poisoning in children, 3 of which were fatal, have been reported (McGee et al., 1952).

Allergic bronchopneumonia was observed in two workers using toxaphene sprays (Warraki, 1963).

Eight women working in an area which had been sprayed with 2 kg/ha toxaphene by aircraft had a higher incidence of chromosome aberrations (acentric fragments and chromatid exchanges), as observed in lymphocyte cultures, compared with an unspecified number of control individuals: 13.1% versus 1.6% (Samosh, 1974).

No significant levels of toxaphene were found in skin fat and attached subcutaneous tissue taken from 68 newborns in 13 cities in the US (Zavon et al., 1969).

3.3 Case reports and epidemiological studies

Two cases of acute aplastic anaemia associated with dermal exposure to toxaphene:lindane mixtures have been reported. One of these
cases terminated in death due to acute myelomonocytic leukaemia
(US Environmental Protection Agency, 1978).

An increased incidence of lung cancer (10 observed *versus* 0.54
expected) was reported among 285 workers who applied various pesticides in agricultural settings. Some of these workers were exposed
to toxaphene (Barthel, 1976) [The Working Group noted that since they
may have been exposed to compounds other than toxaphene or in addition
to toxaphene, no evaluation specific for toxaphene could be made on
the basis of this study; see also monograph on hexachlorocyclohexane
(technical HCH and lindane), p. 195].

In a survey of 199 employees who worked or had worked with toxaphene
between 1949 and 1977, with exposures ranging from 6 months to 26 years
(mean, 5.23 years), 20 employees died, 1 with cancer of the colon;
none of these deaths appeared to be related to exposure to toxaphene
(Anon., 1977; Ottoboni, 1977; US Environmental Protection Agency,
1977c).

4. Summary of Data Reported and Evaluation

4.1 Experimental data

Toxaphene (polychlorinated camphenes) was tested in one experiment
in mice and in one in rats by oral administration: a dose-related
increase in the incidence of hepatocellular carcinomas was observed in
male and female mice, and an increased incidence of thyroid tumours was
observed in male and female rats.

Toxaphene is mutagenic in *Salmonella typhimurium*; it did not
induce dominant lethals in mice.

4.2 Human data

No epidemiological studies relating specifically to the carcinogenicity of toxaphene were available to the Working Group.

Two cases of acute aplastic anaemia associated with dermal exposure to toxaphene:lindane mixtures have been reported, one terminating
in death due to acute myelomonocytic leukaemia. The only epidemiological study that related to possible carcinogenic effects of toxaphene
in humans has weaknesses which prevented the Working Group from drawing
any conclusion specific to toxaphene.

An increased frequency of chromosomal aberrations has been observed in the lymphocytes of workers exposed to toxaphene.

The extensive production and the widespread use of toxaphene, together with the persistent nature of the compound, indicate that human exposure occurs.   This is confirmed by many reports of its occurrence in the general environment.

4.3 Evaluation

There is *sufficient evidence* that toxaphene is carcinogenic in mice and rats.   In the absence of adequate data in humans, it is reasonable, for practical purposes, to regard toxaphene as if it presented a carcinogenic risk to humans.

5. References

Anon. (1977) EPA criticized for pesticide ban process. Chem. Eng.
    News, 26 September, p.22

Arthur, R.D., Cain, J.D. & Barrentine, B.F. (1976) Atmospheric levels
    of pesticides in the Mississippi delta. Bull. environ. Contam.
    Toxicol., 15, 129-134

Ashirova, S.A. (1971) Work hygiene and effectiveness of health measures
    in the manufacture of chlorinated terpenes (Russ.). Nauch. Tr.
    Leningrad. Gos. Inst. Usoversh. Vrachei, 98, 26-30 [Chem. Abstr., 79,
    13949n]

Barthel, E. (1976) High incidence of lung cancer in persons with chronic
    professional exposure to pesticides in agriculture (Germ.). Z.
    Erkrank. Arm. -Org., 146, 266-274

Berg, G.L., ed. (1978) Farm Chemicals Handbook 1978, Willoughby, OH,
    Meister Publishing Co., p. D 265

Bidleman, T.F. & Olney, C.E. (1975) Long range transport of toxaphene
    insecticide in the atmosphere of the western North Atlantic.
    Nature (Lond.), 257, 475-477

Blus, L.J., Joanen, T., Belisle, A.A. & Prouty, R.M. (1975) The brown
    pelican and certain environmental pollutants in Louisiana. Bull.
    environ. Contam. Toxicol., 13, 646-655

Bontoyan, W.R. & Jung, P.D. (1972) Thin layer chromatographic detection
    of chlorinated hydrocarbons as cross-contaminants in pesticide
    formulations. J. Assoc. off. anal. Chem., 55, 851-856

Boyd, E.M. & Taylor, F.I. (1971) Toxaphene toxicity in protein-deficient
    rats. Toxicol. appl. Pharmacol., 18, 158-167

Buntin, G.A. (1953) Chlorinated camphor and fenchone as insecticides.
    US Patent 2,657,164, 27 October, to Hercules Powder Co. [Chem. Abstr.
    48, 2977d]

Bush, P.B., Kiker, J.T., Page, R.K., Booth, N.H. & Fletcher, O.J. (1977)
    Effects of graded levels of toxaphene on poultry residue accumulation,
    egg production, shell quality, and hatchability in white Leghorns.
    J. agric. Food Chem., 25, 928-932

Carey, A.E., Wiersma, G.B. & Tai, H. (1976) Pesticide residues in urban
    soils from 14 United States cities, 1970. Pestic. Monit. J., 10,
    54-60

Casida, J.E., Holmstead, R.L., Khalifa, S., Knox, J.R., Ohsawa, T., Palmer, K.J. & Wong, R.Y. (1974) Toxaphene insecticide: a complex biodegradable mixture. Science, 183, 520-521

Causey, K., McIntyre, S.C., Jr & Richburg, R.W. (1972) Organochlorine insecticide residues in quail, rabbits, and deer from selected Alabama soybean fields. J. agric. Food Chem., 20, 1205-1209

Chernoff, N. & Carver, B.D. (1976) Fetal toxicity of toxaphene in rats and mice. Bull. environ. Contam. Toxicol., 15, 660-664

Clapp, K.L., Nelson, D.M., Bell, J.T. & Rousek, E.J. (1971) Effect of toxaphene on the hepatic cells of rats. In: Proceedings of Annual Meeting, Western Section, American Society of Animal Science, Vol. 22, Fresno, CA, Fresno State College, pp. 313-323 [Chem. Abstr., 76, 701y]

Conley, B.E. (1952) Pharmacologic properties of toxaphene, a chlorinated hydrocarbon insecticide. J. Am. med. Assoc., 149, 1135-1137

Crowder, L.A. & Dindal, E.F. (1974) Fate of ^{36}Cl-toxaphene in rats. Bull. environ. Contam. Toxicol., 12, 320-327

Domanski, J.J. & Guthrie, F.E. (1974) Pesticide residues in 1972 cigars. Bull. environ, Contam. Toxicol., 11, 312-314

Domanski, J.J. & Sheets, T.J. (1976) Environmental contamination of flue-cured tobacco with chlorinated hydrocarbon insecticides. Beitr. Tabakforsch., 8, 330-333

Domanski, J.J., Haire, P.L. & Sheets, T.J. (1974) Insecticide residues on 1973 US tobacco products. Tobacco Sci., 18, 108-109

Domanski, J.J., Haire, P.L. & Sheets, T.J. (1975) Insecticide residues on 1972 US auction-market tobacco. Beitr. Tabakforsch., 8, 39-43

Dunachie, J.F. & Fletcher, W.W. (1969) An investigation of the toxicity of insecticides to birds' eggs using the egg-injection technique. Ann. appl. Biol., 64, 409-423

Durant, C.J. & Reimold, R.J. (1972) Effects of estuarine dredging of toxaphene-contaminated sediments in Terry Creek, Brunswick, Ga. - 1971. Pestic. Monit. J., 6, 94-96

Epstein, S.S., Arnold, E., Andrea, J., Bass, W. & Bishop, Y. (1972) Detection of chemical mutagens by the dominant lethal assay in the mouse. Toxicol. appl. Pharmacol., 23, 288-325

Eurocop-Cost (1976) A Comprehensive List of Polluting Substances which Have Been Identified in Various Fresh Waters, Effluent Discharges, Aquatic Animals and Plants, and Bottom Sediments, 2nd ed., EUCO/MDU/ 73/76, XII/476/76, Luxembourg, Commission of the European Communities, 55

French, I.W. & Associates Limited (1977) Toxaphene, 77-EHD-11, Ottawa, Canada, Department of National Health & Welfare

Gaines, T.B. (1960) The acute toxicity of pesticides to rats. Toxicol. appl. Pharmacol., 2, 88-99

Geike, F. (1971) Thin-layer chromatographic-enzymatic identification and the mode of action of chlorinated hydrocarbon insecticides. III. Identification by inhibition of phosphatase (Germ.). J. Chromatogr., 61, 279-283

Gertig, H. & Nowaczyk, W. (1975) The influence of carathane and toxaphene on the activity of some enzymes in rat's tissues in the studies in vivo. Pol. J. Pharmacol. Pharm., 27, 357-364

Grebenyuk, S.S. (1970) Effect of polychlorocamphene on liver functions (Russ.). Gig. Primen. Toksikol. Pestits. Klin. Otravlenii, 8, 166-169 [Chem. Abstr., 77, 122758p]

Haun, E.C. & Cueto, C., Jr (1967) Fatal toxaphene poisoning in a 9-month-old infant. Am. J. Dis. Child., 113, 616-618

Hawley, G.G., ed. (1977) The Condensed Chemical Dictionary, 9th ed., New York, Van Nostrand-Reinhold, p. 871

Hawthorne, J.C., Ford, J.H. & Markin, G.P. (1974) Residues of mirex and other chlorinated pesticides in commercially raised catfish. Bull. environ. Contam. Toxicol., 11, 258-264

Hempel, D., Liebmann, R. & Hellwig, A. (1971) New colorimetric determination of toxaphene in water (Germ.). Fortrschr. Wasserchem. Ihrer Grenzgeb., 13, 181-188 [Chem. Abstr., 76, 109003y]

Holmstead, R.L., Khalifa, S. & Casida, J.E. (1974) Toxaphene composition analyzed by combined gas chromatography-chemical ionization mass spectrometry. J. agric. Food Chem., 22, 939-944

Hooper, N.K., Ames, B.N., Saleh, M.A. & Casida, J.E. (1979) Toxaphene, a complex mixture of polychloroterpenes and a major insecticide, is mutagenic. Science, 205, 591-593

Horwitz, W., ed. (1975) Official Methods of Analysis of the Association of Official Analytical Chemists, 12th ed., Washington DC, Association of Official Analytical Chemists, pp. 81-82, 518-528

Hurst, J.G., Newcomer, W.S. & Morrison, J.A. (1974) Some effects of DDT, toxaphene and polychlorinated biphenyl on thyroid function in bobwhite quail. Poult. Sci., 53, 125-133

Ismail, R.J. & Bonner, F.L. (1974) New, improved thin layer chromatography
for polychlorinated biphenyls, toxaphene and chlordane components.
J. Assoc, off. anal. Chem., 57, 1026-1032

Kennedy, G.L., Jr, Frawley, J.P. & Calandra, J.C. (1973) Multigeneration
reproductive effects of three pesticides in rats. Toxicol. appl.
Pharmacol., 25, 589-596

Keplinger, M.L., Deichmann, W.B. & Sala, F. (1968) Effects of combinations
of pesticides on reproduction in mice. Ind. med. Surg., 37, 525

Khalifa, S., Mon, T.R., Engel, J.L. & Casida, J.E. (1974) Isolation of
2,2,5-*endo*,6-*exo*,8,9,10-heptachlorobornane and an octachloro
toxicant from technical toxaphene. J. agric. Food Chem., 22,
653-657

Kinoshita, F.K., Frawley, J.P. & DuBois, K.P. (1966) Quantitative
measurement of induction of hepatic microsomal enzymes by various
dietary levels of DDT and toxaphene in rats. Toxicol. appl.
Pharmacol., 9, 505-513

Kosmatyi, E.S. & Gritsaenko, N.N. (1970) Determination of polychlorocamphene in soil by thin-layer chromatography without purification (Ukr.).
Zashch. Rast. (Kiev), 11, 101-103 [Chem. Abstr., 77, 30114x]

Lackey, R.W. (1949) Observations on the acute and chronic toxicity of
toxaphene in the dog. J. ind. Hyg. Toxicol., 31, 117-120

Luke, M.A., Froberg, J.E. & Masumoto, H.T. (1975) Extraction and clean-
up of organochlorine, organophosphate, organonitrogen, and hydrocarbon pesticides in produce for determination by gas-liquid
chromatography. J. Assoc. off. anal. Chem., 58, 1020-1026

Mashburn, S.A. (1978) Health and Environmental Effects of Toxaphene –
A Literature Compilation, 1962-1978, ORNL/TIRC-78/5, Oak Ridge, TN,
Oak Ridge National Laboratory

McGee, L.C., Reed, H.L. & Fleming, J.P. (1952) Accidental poisoning by
toxaphene. Review of toxicology and case reports. J. Am. med.
Assoc., 149, 1124-1126

Munson, R.O. (1976) A note on toxaphene in environmental samples from
the Chesapeake Bay region. Bull. environ. Contam. Toxicol., 16,
491-494

Nash, R.G., Harris, W.G., Ensor, P.D. & Woolson, E.A. (1973) Comparative
extraction of chlorinated hydrocarbon insecticides from soils 20
years after treatment. J. Assoc. off. anal. Chem., 56, 728-732

National Cancer Institute (1979) Bioassay of Toxaphene for Possible Carcinogenicity, DHEW Publ. No. (NIH) 79-837, Carcinogenesis Testing Program, Division of Cancer Cause & Prevention, Bethesda, MD

National Institute for Occupational Safety & Health (1977) NIOSH Manual of Analytical Methods, 2nd ed., Vol. II, Method No. S67, DHEW (NIOSH), Publ. No. 77-157-B, Washington DC, US Government Printing Office, pp. S67-1-S67-7

Ohsawa, T., Knox, J.R., Khalifa, S. & Casida, J.E. (1975) Metabolic dechlorination of toxaphene in rats. J. agric. Food Chem., 23, 98-106

Ortega, O., Hayes, W.J., Jr & Durham, W.F. (1957) Pathologic changes in the liver of rats after feeding low levels of various insecticides. Arch. Pathol., 64, 614-622

Ottoboni, A. (1977) Rebuttal to the Philosophy and Methodology Employed by EPA in its RPAR Program and to the Presumption that the Current Uses of Toxaphene Constitute a Chronic Risk to Humans, September, Berkeley, CA, Department of Health, State of California, Health & Welfare Agency, pp. 23-24

Parlar, H., Nitz, S., Gab, S. & Korte, F. (1977) A contribution to the structure of the toxaphene components. Spectroscopic studies on chlorinated bornane derivatives. J. agric. Food Chem., 25, 68-72

Peakall, D.B. (1976) Effects of toxaphene on hepatic enzyme induction and circulating steroid levels in the rat. Environ. Health Perspect., 13, 117-120

Pollock, G.A. & Kilgore, W.W. (1978) Toxaphene. Residue Rev., 69, 87-140

Reidinger, R.F., Jr (1976) Organochlorine residues in adults of six south-western bat species. J. Wildl. Manage., 40, 677-680 [Chem. Abstr., 86, 51271x]

Samosh, L.V. (1974) Chromosome aberrations and character of satellite associations after accidental exposure of the human body to poly-chlorocamphene. Tsitol. Genet., 8, 24-27

Schwabe, U. & Wendling, I. (1967) Stimulation of drug metabolism by low doses of DDT and other chlorinated hydrocarbon insecticides Germ.). Arzneimittel-Forsch., 17, 614-618

Shackelford, W.M. & Keith, L.H. (1976) Frequency of Organic Compounds Identified in Water, EPA-600/4-76-062, Athens, GA, US Environmental Protection Agency, p. 226

Sheets, T.J., Bradley, J.R., Jr & Jackson, M.D. (1972) Contamination
    of Surface and Ground Water with Pesticides Applied to Cotton,
    Report 60, Raleigh, NC, University of North Carolina Water Resources
    Research Institute. Available from Springfield, VA, National
    Technical Information Service, No. PB 210148

Smith, S.I., Weber, C.W. & Reid, B.L. (1970) The effect of injection
    of chlorinated hydrocarbon pesticides on hatchability of eggs.
    Toxicol. appl. Pharmacol., 16, 179-185

Spencer, E.Y. (1973) Guide to the Chemicals Used in Crop Protection,
    Publication 1093, Research Branch, Agriculture Canada, 6th ed., London,
    Ontario, University of Western Ontario, p. 506

Stalling, D.L. & Huckins, J.N. (1976) Analysis and GC-MS Characterization
    of Toxaphene in Fish and Water, EPA-600/3-76-076, Duluth, MN, US
    Environmental Protection Agency. Available from Springfield, VA,
    National Technical Information Service, No. PB-257773

Stijve, T. & Cardinale, E. (1973) Determination of chlorinated pesticide
    residues by entrainment distillation with water. Mitt. Gab.
    Lebensmittelunters. Hyg., 64, 415-426 [Chem Abstr., 80, 131711g]

Tewari, S.N. & Sharma, I.C. (1977) Isolation and determination of
    chlorinated organic pesticides by thin-layer chromatography and the
    application to toxicological analysis. J. Chromatogr., 131, 275-284

Thielemann, H. (1973) Thin-layer chromatographic separation and semi-
    quantitative determination of toxaphene and lindane (γ-hexachloro-
    cyclohexane) on activated Silufol foils (Germ.). Fresenius' Z. Anal.
    Chem., 264, 32 [Chem. Abstr., 78, 155331t]

Turner, W.V., Khalifa, S. & Casida, J.E. (1975) Toxaphene toxicant A.
    Mixture of 2,2,5-endo,6-exo,8,8,9,10-octachlorobornane and 2,2,5-
    endo,6-exo,8,8,9,10-octachlorobornane. J. agric. Food Chem., 23,
    991-994

US Environmental Protection Agency (1976a) Protection of environment.
    US Code Fed. Regul., Title 40, part 180.138, pp. 320-321

US Environmental Protection Agency (1976b) Criteria Document for
    Toxaphene, EPA-440/9-76-014, Washington DC, Office of Water Planning
    and Standards. Available from Springfield, VA, National Technical
    Information Service, No. PB-253677

US Environmental Protection Agency (1977a) Standards for aldrin/dieldrin,
    DDT (DDD,DDE), endrin and toxaphene; final decision. Fed. Regist.,
    42, 2588-2617

US Environmental Protection Agency (1977b) Rebuttable presumption against registration and continued registration of pesticide products containing toxaphene. Fed., Regist., 42, 26860-26862

US Environmental Protection Agency (1977c) Assessment of Toxaphene in Agriculture, USDA/State Assessment Team on Toxaphene, 9 September, Washington DC

US Environmental Protection Agency (1978) Summary of Reported Incidents Involving Toxaphene, Report No. 113, Washington DC, Pesticide Incident Monitoring System

US Food & Drug Administration (1975) Pesticide Analytical Manual, Vol. I, Methods Which Detect Multiple Residues, Rockville, MD, Table 201-A

US International Trade Commission (1976) Synthetic Organic Chemicals, US Production and Sales, 1975, USITC Publication 804, Washington DC, US Government Printing Office, p. 181

US International Trade Commission (1977) Synthetic Organic Chemicals, US Production and Sales, 1976, USITC Publication 833, Washington DC, US Government Printing Office, pp. 269, 276

US Occupational Safety & Health Administration (1977) Air contaminants, US Code Fed. Regul., Title 29, part 1910.1000, pp. 59-60

US Tariff Commission (1948) Synthetic Organic Chemicals, US Production and Sales, 1947, Report No. 162, Second Series, Washington DC, US Government Printing Office, p. 138

Warraki, S. (1963) Respiratory hazards of chlorinated camphene. Arch. environ. Health, 7, 253-256

Welch, R.M., Levin, W., Kuntzman, R., Jacobson, M. & Conney, A.H. (1971) Effect of halogenated hydrocarbon insecticides on the metabolism and uterotropic action of estrogens in rats and mice. Toxicol. appl. Pharmacol., 19, 234-246

Wiersma, G.B., Tai, H. & Sand, P.F. (1972) Pesticide residues in soil from eight cities - 1969. Pestic. Monit. J., 6, 126-129

Windholz, M., ed. (1976) The Merck Index, 9th ed., Rahway, NJ, Merck & Co., pp. 1228-1229

Yang, H.S.C., Wiersma, G.B. & Mitchell, W.G. (1976) Organochlorine pesticide residues in sugarbeet pulps and molasses from 16 states, 1971. Pestic. Monit. J., 10, 41-43

Zavon, M.R., Tye, R. & Latorre, L. (1969) Chlorinated hydrocarbon
    content of the neonate. Ann. N.Y. Acad. Sci., 160, 196-200

Zweig, G., Pye, E.L., Sitlani, R. & Peoples, S.A. (1963) Residues in
    milk from dairy cows fed low levels of toxaphene in their daily
    ration. J. agric. Food Chem., 11, 70-72

2,4,5- AND 2,4,6-TRICHLOROPHENOLS

1. Chemical and Physical Data

1.1 Synonyms and trade names

2,4,5-Trichlorophenol

Chem. Abstr. Services Reg. No.: 95-95-4

Chem. Abstr. Name: 2,4,5-Trichlorophenol

Trade names: Collunosol; Dowicide 2; Dowicide B; Nurelle;
Preventol I

2,4,6-Trichlorophenol

Chem. Abstr. Services Reg. No.: 88-06-2

Chem. Abstr. Name: 2,4,6-Trichlorophenol

Synonym: Trichlorfenol

Trade names: Dowicide 2S; Omal; Phenachlor

1.2 Structural and molecular formulae and molecular weights

2,4,5-Trichlorophenol

$C_6H_3Cl_3O$ Mol. wt: 197.5

2,4,6-Trichlorophenol

$C_6H_3Cl_3O$ Mol. wt: 197.5

1.3 Chemical and physical properties of the pure substances

2,4,5-Trichlorophenol

From Windholz (1976), unless otherwise specified

(<u>a</u>) <u>Description</u>: Grey flakes (Hawley, 1977)

(<u>b</u>) <u>Boiling-point</u>: 248°C (746 mm); 253°C (760 mm)

(<u>c</u>) <u>Melting-point</u>: 67°C

(<u>d</u>) <u>Spectroscopy data</u>: λ_{max} 299 nm (E_1^1 = 140); 292 nm (E_1^1 = 145) in methanol; infra-red, nuclear magnetic resonance and mass spectral data have been tabulated (Grasselli & Ritchey, 1975).

(<u>e</u>) <u>Solubility</u>: g/100 g solvent at 25°C: acetone, 615; benzene, 163; carbon tetrachloride, 51; diethyl ether, 525; denatured ethanol, 525; methanol, 615; liquid petrolatum (at 50°C), 56; soya bean oil, 79; toluene, 122; water, < 0.2

(<u>f</u>) <u>Volatility</u>: Vapour pressure is 1 mm at 72°C (Perry & Chilton, 1973).

(<u>g</u>) <u>Stability</u>: Stable up to its melting-point

(<u>h</u>) <u>Reactivity</u>: Can be converted to sodium salt by reaction with sodium carbonate; the hydroxyl group forms ethers, esters and salts with metals and amines; aromatic portion undergoes substitution reactions such as nitration, alkylation, acetylation and halogenation; chlorine atoms can be hydrolysed to produce polyhydroxyl benzenes, by reaction with bases at elevated temperatures and pressures; oxidative decomposition occurs with strong oxidizing agents (Howard & Durkin, 1973).

2,3,7,8-Tetrachlorodibenzo-*para*-dioxin may be formed as a by-product during the synthesis of 2,4,5-trichlorophenol by the hydrolysis of 1,2,4,5-tetrachlorobenzene using methanol and sodium hydroxide at elevated pressure or ethylene glycol and sodium hydroxide at atmospheric pressure. In the latter case, if the reaction temperature exceeds the normal 180°C process temperature, 2,3,7,8-tetrachlorodibenzo-*para*-dioxin is formed by the condensation of two molecules of sodium 2,4,5-trichlorophenate under the influence of the exothermic decomposition of sodium-2-hydroxyethanol (Milnes, 1971). For additional information see IARC monograph on chlorinated dibenzo-*para*-dioxins (IARC, 1977a).

2,4,6-Trichlorophenol

From Windholz (1976), unless otherwise specified

(<u>a</u>) Description: Yellow flakes (Hawley, 1977)

(<u>b</u>) Boiling-point: 246°C

(<u>c</u>) Melting-point: 69°C

(<u>d</u>) Spectroscopy data: λ_{max} 296 nm (E_1^1 = 129); 289 nm (E_1^1 = 125) in methanol; infra-red, nuclear magnetic resonance and mass spectral data have been tabulated (Grasselli & Ritchey, 1975).

(<u>e</u>) Solubility: g/100 g solvent at 25°C: acetone, 525; benzene, 113; carbon tetrachloride, 37; diacetone alcohol, 335; diethyl ether, 354; denatured ethanol, 400; methanol, 525; pine oil, 163; Stoddard solvent, 16; toluene, 100; turpentine, 37; water, < 0.1

(<u>f</u>) Volatility: Vapour pressure is 1 mm at 76.5°C (Perry & Chilton, 1973).

(<u>g</u>) Stability: Stable up to its melting-point. Heating of the phenate to 280°C produced < 0.1 mg/kg octa- and heptachlorinated dibenzo-*para*-dioxins and < 0.02-0.03 mg/kg hexa-, penta- and tetrachlorinated dibenzo-*para*-dioxins (Rappe *et al.*, 1978).

(<u>h</u>) Reactivity: Can be converted to sodium salt by reaction with sodium carbonate; the hydroxyl group forms ethers, esters and salts with metals and amines; the aromatic portion undergoes substitution reactions such as nitration, alkylation, acetyl-

ation and halogenation; chlorine atoms can be hydrolysed to

produce polyhydroyl benzenes, by reaction with bases at

elevated temperatures and pressures; oxidative decomposition

occurs with strong oxidizing agents (Howard & Durkin, 1973).

1.4 Technical products and impurities

2,4,5-Trichlorophenol is available in the US as a 95% technical
grade product.   Formulations available in the US are concentrated
aqueous and non-aqueous solutions, concentrated solids and emulsifiable
concentrates.   A liquid formulation contains 45.9% 2,4,5-trichloro-
phenol as the sodium salt.

2,4,6-Trichlorophenol available in Japan has a purity of 97%.
It is available in the US in aqueous formulations.

2,3,7,8-Tetrachlorodibenzo-*para*-dioxin was found in 3/6 samples of
2,4,5-trichlorophenol (or its sodium salt) in the range of 0.07-6.2 mg/kg.
2,7-Dichloro-, 1,3,6,8-tetrachloro- and pentachlorodibenzo-*para*-dioxins
were found in concentrations of 0.72, 0.30 and 1.5 mg/kg, respectively
(Firestone *et al.*, 1972).

1,3,6,8-Tetrachlorodibenzo-*para*-dioxin and 2,3,7-trichlorodibenzo-
para-dioxin were found in a sample of 2,4,6-trichlorophenol at levels of
49 and 93 mg/kg, respectively.   In the same study, tri-, tetra- and
pentachlorodimethoxy-dibenzofurans were present in 3/6 samples of 2,4,5-
trichlorophenol or its sodium salt;   and tetra-, penta- and hexachloro-
dibenzofurans were found in one sample of 2,4,6-trichlorophenol
(Firestone *et al.*, 1972).

In a Swedish sample of 2,4,6-trichlorophenol, 1.5 mg/kg 2,3,7,8-
tetrachlorodibenzofuran was found, as well as 17.5, 36 and 4.8 mg/kg
penta-, hexa- and heptachlorodibenzofurans;   less than 3 mg/kg polychlorinated dibenzo-*para*-dioxins were found (Rappe *et al.*, 1979).

2. Production, Use, Occurrence and Analysis

2.1 Production and use

(a) Production

2,4,5-Trichlorophenol

2,4,5-Trichlorophenol was first prepared in 1920 by heating 1,2,4,5-
tetrachlorobenzene with sodium methoxide (Richter, 1944).   It was

manufactured in the US by the hydrolysis of 1,2,4,5-tetrachlorobenzene
with methanolic sodium hydroxide at 160°C (Doedens, 1964).

Commercial production of 2,4,5-trichlorophenol in the US was first
reported in 1950 (US Tariff Commission, 1951).   In 1976, one US
company reported production of an undisclosed amount (see preamble,
p. 16) (US International Trade Commission, 1977a); 87.2 thousand kg
were imported through the principal US customs districts in that year
(US International Trade Commission, 1977b).

Annual production of 2,4,5-trichlorophenol in Austria is estimated
to be 1-10 million kg.   It was previously produced in Italy (see IARC,
1977a).

Japanese production of 2,4,5-trichlorophenol was stopped in 1971.
Imports since that year have amounted to approximately 10-15 thousand
kg annually.

2,4,6-Trichlorophenol

2,4,6-Trichlorophenol was prepared by Laurent in 1836 by chlorination of phenol (Prager *et al.*, 1923), and this method is currently
used in the US (Doedens, 1964).   In Japan, it is produced as a coproduct of *ortho*- or *para*-chlorophenol manufacture by the chlorination
of phenol.

Commercial production of 2,4,6-trichlorophenol in the US was first
reported in 1950 (US Tariff Commission, 1951).   In 1974, the last year
in which production was reported, one company reported production of an
undisclosed amount (see preamble, p. 16) (US International Trade
Commission, 1975).   In 1976, 1000 kg were imported through the
principal US customs districts (US International Trade Commission,
1977b).

No data on its production in Europe were available.

2,4,6-Trichlorophenol has been produced commercially in Japan
since 1965.   In 1977, one company produced an estimated 120 thousand
kg.   None was imported or exported.

(b)   Use

2,4,5-Trichlorophenol

The major use for 2,4,5-trichlorophenol is as an intermediate in
the manufacture of the herbicide 2,4,5-trichlorophenoxyacetic acid
(2,4,5-T) (see IARC, 1977b) and its esters (Doedens, 1964).   It is also
used in the manufacture of 3 other chemicals used as pesticides: Silvex
[2-(2,4,5-trichlorophenoxy)propionic acid], Ronnel (*O,O*-dimethyl-*O*-2,4,5-

trichlorophenyl phosphorothioate) and sodium 2,4,5-trichlorophenate
(Sittig, 1977).   Minor uses of 2,4,5-trichlorophenol itself are as
a fungicide and in the manufacture of hexachlorophene (see monograph,
p. 241).

The systemic herbicide 2,4,5-T is used to control woody and herbace-
ous weeds by air or ground spray applications (Hilton et al., 1974).
In 1975, an estimated 2 million kg were used for commercial and industrial (non-crop) weed control, and 1 million kg were used on pasture
and rangeland.   For additional information on 2,4,5-T, see IARC (1977b).

The herbicide Silvex is used to control woody plants, particularly
oak and maple; it is also used for weed control in water and turf
(Spencer, 1973).   In 1975, an estimated 454 thousand kg were used for
industrial and commercial weed control, 227 thousand kg for aquatic weed
control and 227 thousand kg on pasture and rangeland.

The systemic insecticide Ronnel is used primarily on livestock
(Spencer, 1973).   In 1974, an estimated 318 thousand kg were used on
livestock and poultry and 182 thousand kg for commercial, household
and industrial establishment uses.

Sodium 2,4,5-trichlorophenate is registered for use as a fungicide
by the US Environmental Protection Agency for pulp and paper mill wet-
end systems (US Environmental Protection Agency, 1973) and is approved
by the US Food and Drug Administration for use as a preservative in
defoaming agents and as a slimicide in the manufacture of paper and
paperboard intended for contact with food (US Food & Drug Administration,
1977).

2,4,5-Trichlorophenol is registered for use in the US as a fungicide
in polyvinyl acetate emulsions used in adhesives (see IARC, 1979) and as
a rubber additive (US Environmental Protection Agency, 1973).

A notice of rebuttable presumption against renewal of registration
(RPAR) (see General Remarks on Substances Considered, p. 31) has been
issued for 2,4,5-trichlorophenol and its salts, because of carcinogenic and foetotoxic effects and possible effects of chlorinated dibenzo-
para-dioxins (US Environmental Protection Agency, 1978).

No data on its use in Europe were available.

2,4,5-Trichlorophenol is used in Japan primarily for antiseptic
applications in industrial use.

2,4,6-Trichlorophenol

2,4,6-Trichlorophenol has been used as a wood preservative, glue
preservative, insecticide ingredient, bactericide and an antimildew

treatment for textiles (Doedens, 1964).   It can also be used to prepare
the following fungicides (although they are not believed to be produced
commercially from 2,4,6-trichlorophenol):   chloranil (2,3,5,6-tetra-
chloro-1,4-benzoquinone), pentachlorophenol and 2,3,4,6-tetrachloro-
phenol (Doedens, 1964; Sittig, 1977).

No data on its use in Europe were available.

In Japan, 2,4,6-trichlorophenol is used primarily as a wood
preservative.

2.2 Occurrence

2,4,5- and 2,4,6-Trichlorophenol are not known to occur as natural
products.   2,4,5-Trichlorophenol is a major contaminant of 2,4,5-T,
Silvex and Ronnel (IARC, 1977b; Sittig, 1977).

(a) Water

Trichlorophenol (unspecified isomers) has been found in 1 river-
water sample, 4 finished drinking-water samples, 4 chemical plant
effluent water samples and 2 sewage treatment plant effluent samples in
the US (Shackelford & Keith, 1976).

Trichlorophenol (unspecified isomers) has been detected in river-
water, landfill leachate (at a level of 40 µg/l), tap-water (at levels
of 2 and 4 ng/l), and in chlorinated, biologically-treated effluent
from a sewage plant (Eurocop-Cost, 1976).

2,4,5-Trichlorophenol was detected at unspecified concentrations
in drinking-water in 1975 (Deinzer et al., 1975).

(b) Animals

2,4,6-Trichlorophenol was found at levels of 16-45 mg/kg in body
fat of rainbow trout after experimental exposure to sulphate pulp
bleachery effluents diluted 40 times with brackish water (Landner et al.,
1977).

(c) Food

Following treatment of corn and pea seedlings with γ-pentachloro-
cyclohex-1-ene, a metabolic product of lindane in plants, the plant roots
were homogenized and extracted with hexane.   The extract of corn seedlings
were found to contain 2,4,5-trichlorophenol and the pea seedling extract
both 2,4,5- and 2,4,6-trichlorophenol (Mostafa & Maza, 1973).

(d) Occupational exposure

A 1974 National Occupational Hazard Survey estimated that workers primarily exposed to 2,4,5-trichlorophenol were those in the crude petroleum and natural gas and telephone and telegraph industries. Worker exposure to 2,4,6-trichlorophenol was primarily in hospitals, where it is used as a bactericide, and in the leather tanning and finishing industry (National Institute for Occupational Safety & Health, 1977).

2.3 Analysis

Analytical techniques used to determine chlorophenols, including 2,4,5- and 2,4,6-trichlorophenols, in trace amounts in environmental samples have been reviewed (Howard & Durkin, 1973).

Methods used for the analysis of 2,4,5- and 2,4,6-trichlorophenols in environmental samples are listed in Table 1.

A method employing reverse osmosis to concentrate 2,4,6-trichloro-phenol and other organic contaminants from a 1600-litre sample of tap-water has been described (Deinzer *et al.*, 1975). Ultra-violet spectro-metry at 312 nm has been evaluated as a method for the determination of 2,4,6-trichlorophenol in water samples in the range of 0-20 mg/l (Shibata *et al.*, 1976).

3. Biological Data Relevant to the Evaluation
of Carcinogenic Risk to Humans

3.1 Carcinogenicity studies in animals[1]

(a) Oral administration

Mouse: Groups of 18 male and 18 female (C57BL/6xC3H/Anf)F1 mice and 18 male and 18 female (C57BL/6xAKR)F1 mice received commercial 2,4,6-trichlorophenol (Omal; Dowicide 2S; impurities unspecified) according to the following schedule: 100 mg/kg bw in 0.5% gelatin at 7 days of age by stomach tube and the same amount (not adjusted for increasing body weight) daily up to 4 weeks of age; subsequently, the mice were fed 260 mg/kg diet until they reached 78 weeks of age, at which time 10, 16, 16 and 17 mice were still alive in the 4 groups, respectively. The dose was the maximum tolerated dose for infant

---

[1]The Working Group was aware of studies in progress in which rats and mice are administered 2,4,6-trichlorophenol by oral administration (IARC, 1978).

TABLE 1. METHODS FOR THE ANALYSIS OF 2,4,5- AND 2,4,6-TRICHLOROPHENOLS

| SAMPLE TYPE | EXTRACTION/CLEAN-UP | ANALYTICAL METHOD | | REFERENCE |
		DETECTION	LIMIT OF DETECTION	
Water	Adsorb on ion exchanger, remove water, extract (benzene), methylate	GC/ECD	1 ng/l	Renberg (1974)
Soil				
Sediment and sewage sludge	Centrifuge, extract solid (acetone), liquid/liquid partition, transfer into trimethyl pentane, treat to remove sulphur, isolate in tri-methylpentane, methylate or acetyl-ate	GC/ECD	1-10 µg/kg	Jensen et al. (1977)
Soil	Centrifuge slurry with alkali, adsorb on ion exchanger, extract (benzene), methylate	GC/ECD	0.1 µg/kg	Renberg (1974)
Food				
Milk and cream	Hydrolyse (acid), extract (ether), CC	GC/ECD or micro-coulometry	50 µg/l	Bjerke et al. (1972)
Biological				
Muscle, fat, liver and kidney	Distill from acid into alkali, acidify distillate, extract (dichloromethane), remove solvent, dissolve (hexane), silylate	GC/ECD	50 µg/kg	Clark et al. (1975)
	Digest (caustic potash), then proceed as above	GC/ECD	50 µg/kg	Clark et al. (1975)
Rat urine	Hydrolyse (acid), extract (ether), ethylate, CC	GC/ECD	10 µg/l	Shafik et al. (1973)
Tissue	Homogenize (hexane-acetone), liquid/liquid partition, adsorb on ion exchanger, extract (benzene), methylate	GC/ECD	0.1 µg/kg	Renberg (1974)

TABLE 1. METHODS FOR THE ANALYSIS OF 2,4,5- AND 2,4,6-TRICHLOROPHENOLS (continued)

SAMPLE TYPE	ANALYTICAL METHOD			
	EXTRACTION/CLEAN-UP	DETECTION	LIMIT OF DETECTION	REFERENCE
Miscellaneous				
Broiler house litter	Extract (pentane), re-extract (sodium hydroxide), acidify, extract (pentane), methylate	GC/ECD GC/FID GC/MS		Land *et al.* (1975)
Bleach liquors from paper manufacture	Extract (ether), wash extract (sodium hydrogen carbonate), re-extract (sodium hydroxide), acidify, extract (ether), transfer to isooctane-ethanol, purify by HPLC, ethylate	GC/FID GC/ECD GC/MS	pg range	Lindström & Nordin (1976)

Abbreviations: CC - column chromatography; GC/ECD - gas chromatography/electron capture detection; FID - flame-ionization detection; MS - mass spectrometry; HPLC - high-pressure liquid chromatography

and young mice [but not necessarily that for adults].   The total numbers
of tumour-bearing animals were 9/18, 7/18, 3/17 and 2/17 in treated males
and females of the 2 strains, compared with 22/79, 8/87, 16/90 and 7/82
in pooled controls.   Statistically significant increases [$P < 0.05$] in
the incidences of hepatomas (5/36) and reticulum-cell sarcomas (6/36)
were observed in mice of the first strain when the numbers of tumours
in males and females were combined (Innes *et al.*, 1969; National
Technical Information Service, 1968) [The Working Group noted, however,
that the statistical significance of the results disappears when the
incidences in males and females are considered separately, or when
matched controls are considered].

(b) Subcutaneous and/or intramuscular administration

Mouse: Groups of 18 male and 18 female (C57BL/6xC3H/Anf)Fl mice
and 18 male and 18 female (C57BL/6xAKR)Fl mice were given single s.c.
injections of 464 mg/kg bw commercial 2,4,6-trichlorophenol (Omal;
Dowicide 2S; impurities unspecified) in corn oil at 28 days of age.
Similar groups received 1000 mg/kg bw commercial 2,4,5-trichlorophenol
(Collunosol; Dowicide 2; impurities unspecified) in corn oil.
Animals were observed until about 78 weeks of age, when all mice treated
with 2,4,6-trichlorophenol and 16, 11, 18 and 18 mice treated with 2,4,5-
trichlorophenol were still alive in the 8 groups, respectively.   A
negative control group consisted of animals that were either untreated
or received gelatin, corn oil or dimethylsulphoxide and comprised 141
males and 154 females of the first strain and 161 males and 157 females
of the second strain.   Tumour incidences were not increased in the
treated mice [$P > 0.05$] (National Technical Information Service, 1968)
[The Working Group noted that a negative result obtained with a single
s.c. injection is not an adequate basis for discounting carcinogenicity].

(c) Other experimental systems

Promotion: A single application of 75 µg dimethylbenz[*a*]anthracene
(DMBA) (25 µl of a 0.3% solution in acetone) was painted on the dorsal
skin of 20 female Sutter mice, 2-3 months old, followed by application
of one drop (approximately 25 µl) of commercial 2,4,5-trichlorophenol
(producer and impurities unspecified) dissolved in reagent-grade
acetone (21% solution), twice a week for 16 weeks, at which time the
experiment was terminated.   No mice were treated with 2,4,5-trichloro-
phenol alone.   At termination of the experiment, skin papillomas were
observed in 8/19 surviving mice.   No skin tumours were found in 18
surviving controls of the same strain and sex treated with acetone alone;
1/21 surviving male mice (strain unspecified) treated with 75 µg DMBA
alone developed a papilloma (Boutwell & Bosch, 1959) [The Working Group
noted the inadequacy of the experimental design].

3.2 Other relevant biological data

(a) Experimental systems

Toxic effects

Trichlorophenols may contain 2,3,7,8-tetrachlorodibenzo-*para*-dioxin (TCDD), which is formed during its synthesis (IARC, 1977a).

The acute i.p. LD_{50}s in rats for the 2,4,5- and 2,4,6-trichlorophenols are 355 and 276 mg/kg bw, respectively (Farquharson *et al.*, 1958).   The acute oral LD_{50} in rats of 2,4,5-trichlorophenol administered by gavage is about 3 g/kg bw (McCollister *et al.*, 1961).

In a 98-day feeding study in rats, 0.3 g and 1 g/kg bw/day doses of 2,4,5-trichlorophenol retarded weight gain and caused diuresis, mild centrilobular changes in the liver, moderate degenerative changes in the convoluted tubules of the kidneys and early proliferative changes in kidney interstitial tissue.   Slight proliferation of bile ducts and early portal cirrhosis were also observed.   The severity of effects was dose-related.   No significant effects were observed with doses of 100 mg/kg bw/day (0.1% in diet) or less (McCollister *et al.*, 1961).

2,4,6-Trichlorophenol produces symptoms of central nervous depression. The toxicity of 2,4,5-trichlorophenol was characterized by an ascending hypotonia leading to prostration, flaccid paralysis, dyspnoea and death. Rapid development of rigor mortis, sometimes evident before death, is a characteristic finding, analogous to that seen with pentachlorophenol (Farquharson *et al.*, 1958).   It has been suggested that the mechanism of action of 2,4,6-trichlorophenol is interference with mitochondrial oxidative phosphorylation and inhibition of cytochrome P450-dependent mixed-function oxidases (Arrhenius *et al.*, 1977).

No data on the embryotoxicity or teratogenicity of trichlorophenols were available to the Working Group.

Absorption, distribution, excretion and metabolism

The 2,4,5-trichlorophenol-derived herbicides, 2,4,5-T and Silvex, were fed at dose levels of 0, 300, 1000 and 2000 mg/kg aiet to adult cattle and sheep for 28 days;   tissues were sampled 1 day and 1 week after the last dose was given.   No residues of 2,4,5-trichlorophenol were found in the fat of sheep receiving 2000 mg/kg diet 2,4,5-T (0.05 mg/kg detection limit);   average residue levels in liver were over 6 times the average in kidney: 6.1 *versus* 0.90 and 4.4 *versus* 0.81 mg/kg in tissues taken 1 day and 7 days after treatment, respectively.   Muscle and fat of sheep and cattle fed Silvex contained no detectable levels of 2,4,5-trichlorophenol residues;   levels were slightly higher in liver than in

kidney: 0.06-0.63 mg/kg in liver and < 0.05-0.17 mg/kg in kidney
(Clark *et al.*, 1975).

Cows were fed rations containing 2,4,5-T and Silvex at 6 levels
(10-1000 mg/kg diet) for 2 or 3 weeks; milk and cream samples were
collected at various intervals during the feeding of the chemicals and
during the 7 days following withdrawal of the highest level.   No
residue of 2,4,5-trichlorophenol greater than 0.05 mg/kg was found in
milk or cream from those fed the 10-30 mg/kg diet levels; with 1000 mg/
kg diet, average residues were 0.23 mg/kg 2,4,5-trichlorophenol in milk
and 0.19 mg/kg in cream.   No residues of 2,4,5-trichlorophenol were
found in any of the samples of milk or cream from cows fed Silvex
(Bjerke *et al.*, 1972).

<u>Mutagenicity and other related short-term tests</u>

Repeated spraying of flower buds of *Vicia faba* with an aqueous
solution of 2,4,5-trichlorophenol increased the frequency of abnormalities in pollen mother cells, including stickiness and lagging of
chromosomes during cell division and chromosome fragments (Amer & Ali,
1974).

(<u>b</u>)   <u>Humans</u>

Adverse health effects have been seen in workers exposed to
chlorophenols contaminated with TCDD or to products synthesized from
trichlorophenol (IARC, 1977c; Jirasek *et al.*, 1974; Schulz, 1957).
These effects, probably due to TCDD, include persistent chloracne,
liver dysfunction, neuromuscular weakness, porphyria and psychological
changes.

The general population was exposed to 2,4,5-trichlorophenol and
its contaminants (in particular, TCDD) in Seveso, Italy, due to an
accident in a 2,4,5-trichlorophenol plant (see IARC, 1977c).

3.3   <u>Case reports and epidemiological studies</u>

No data were available to the Working Group.

4. Summary of Data Reported and Evaluation[1]

4.1 Experimental data

2,4,6-Trichlorophenol was tested in one experiment in two strains of mice by oral administration, and 2,4,5- and 2,4,6-trichlorophenols were tested in one experiment by subcutaneous injection in two strains of mice. 2,4,5-Trichlorophenol was also tested in one experiment for its promoting activity in female mice. All three experiments were considered to be inadequate.

4.2 Human data

No case reports or epidemiological studies were available to the Working Group.

The extensive production and the widespread use of trichloro-phenols over the past several decades in agriculture indicate that exposure of workers and of the general population occurs.

4.3 Evaluation

The available data do not permit an evaluation of the carcino-genicity of 2,4,5- and 2,4,6-trichlorophenols to be made.

---

[1] Subsequent to the meeting of the Working Group, the Secretariat became aware of carcinogenicity studies in B6C3F1 mice and Fischer rats given 2,4,6-trichlorophenol (96-97% pure) orally. Groups of 50 male mice were administered 5000 and 10,000 mg/kg diet 2,4,6-trichlorophenol for 105 weeks; and groups of 50 female mice were given 10,000 and 20,000 mg/kg diet for 38 weeks, then 2500 and 5000 mg/kg diet for 67 weeks. Survival was 80% or more in all groups. Hepatocellular carcinomas or adenomas occurred in both male and female mice; their incidence was statistically higher in low-dose males (32/49) and high-dose males (39/47) (controls, 4/20) and in high-dose females (24/48) (low-dose, 12/50; controls, 1/20). Groups of 50 rats of each sex were given 5000 or 10,000 mg/kg diet 2,4,6-trichlorophenol for 106-107 weeks. Survival to the end of the experiment was 68% or more in all groups. In male rats, the increased incidences of lymphomas and leukaemias were statis-tically significant in low-dose (25/50) and high-dose (29/50) groups (controls, 4/20). The incidence of leukaemia in female rats was not significantly greater than in controls (National Cancer Institute, 1979).

5. References

Amer, S.M. & Ali, E.M. (1974) Cytological effects of pesticides. V. Effects of some herbicides on *Vicia faba*. Cytologia, 39, 633-643

Arrhenius, E., Renberg, L., Johansson, L. & Zetterqvist, M.A. (1977) Disturbance of microsomal detoxication mechanisms in liver by chlorophenol pesticides. Chem.-biol. Interact., 18, 35-46

Bjerke, E.L., Herman, J.L., Miller, P.W. & Wetters, J.H. (1972) Residue study of phenoxy herbicides in milk and cream. J. agric. Food Chem., 20, 963-967

Boutwell, R.K. & Bosch, D.K. (1959) The tumor-promoting action of phenol and related compounds for mouse skin. Cancer Res., 19, 413-424

Clark, D.E., Palmer, J.S., Radeleff, R.D., Crookshank, H.R. & Farr, F.M. (1975) Residues of chlorophenoxy acid herbicides and their phenolic metabolites in tissues of sheep and cattle. J. agric. Food Chem., 23, 573-578

Deinzer, M., Melton, R. & Mitchell, D. (1975) Trace organic contaminants in drinking water; their concentration by reverse osmosis. Water Res., 9, 799-805

Doedens, J.D. (1964) Chlorophenols. In: Kirk, R.E. & Othmer, D.F., eds, Encyclopedia of Chemical Technology, 2nd ed., Vol. 5, New York, John Wiley & Sons, pp. 333-335

Eurocop-Cost (1976) A Comprehensive List of Polluting Substances Which Have Been Identified in Various Fresh Waters, Effluent Discharges, Aquatic Animals, and Plants, and Bottom Sediments, 2nd ed., EUCO/ MDU/73/76, XII/476/76, Luxembourg, Commission of the European Communities, p. 58

Farquharson, M.E., Gage, J.C. & Northover, J. (1958) The biological action of chlorophenols. Br. J. Pharmacol., 13, 20-24

Firestone, D., Ress, J., Brown, N.L., Barron, R.P. & Damico, J.N. (1972) Determination of polychloridobenzo-*para*-dioxins and related compounds in commercial chlorophenols. J. Assoc. off. anal. Chem., 55, 85-92

Grasselli, J.G. & Ritchey, W.M., eds (1975) CRC Atlas of Spectral Data and Physical Constants for Organic Compounds, 2nd ed., Vol. IV, Cleveland, OH, Chemical Rubber Co., p. 95

Hawley, G.G., ed. (1977) The Condensed Chemical Dictionary, 9th ed., New York, Van Nostrand-Reinhold, p. 879

Hilton, J.L., Bovey, R.W., Hull, H.M., Mullison, W.R. & Talbert, R.E.
    (1974) Herbicide Handbook of the Weed Science Society of America,
    3rd ed., Champaign, IL, Weed Science Society of America,
    pp. 375-378

Howard, P.H. & Durkin, P.R. (1973) Preliminary Environmental Hazard Assess-
    ment of Chlorinated Naphthalenes, Silicones, Fluorocarbons, Benzenepoly-
    carboxylates, and Chlorophenols, EP-560/2-74-001, Washington DC,
    US Environmental Protection Agency, pp. 220-222, 256-263

IARC (1977a) IARC Monographs on the Evaluation of the Carcinogenic
    Risk of Chemicals to Man, 15, Some Fumigants, the Herbicides
    2,4,-D and 2,4,5-T, Chlorinated Dibenzodioxins and Miscellaneous
    Industrial Chemicals, Lyon, pp. 41-102

IARC (1977b) IARC Monographs on the Evaluation of the Carcinogenic
    Risk of Chemicals to Man, 15, Some Fumigants, the Herbicides
    2,4-D and 2,4,5-T, Chlorinated Dibenzodioxins, and Miscellaneous
    Industrial Chemicals, Lyon, pp. 273-299

IARC (1977c) Long Term Hazards of Polychlorinated Dibenzodioxins and
    Polychlorinated Dibenzofurans, Internal Technical Report 78/001, Lyon

IARC (1978) Information Bulletin on the Survey of Chemicals Being
    Tested for Carcinogenicity, No. 7, Lyon, p. 228

IARC (1979) IARC Monographs on the Evaluation of the Carcinogenic
    Risk of Chemicals to Humans, 19, Some Monomers, Plastics and
    Synthetic Elastomers, and Acrolein, Lyon, pp. 346-351

Innes, J.R.M., Ulland, B.M., Valerio, M.G., Petrucelli, L., Fishbein, L.,
    Hart, E.R., Pallotta, A.J., Bates, R.R., Falk, H.L., Gart, J.J.,
    Klein, M., Mitchell, I. & Peters, J. (1969) Bioassay of pesticides
    and industrial chemicals for tumorigenicity in mice. A preliminary
    note. J. natl Cancer Inst., 42, 1101-1114

Jensen, S., Renberg, L. & Reutergårdh, L. (1977) Residue analysis of
    sediment and sewage sludge for organochlorines in the presence of
    elemental sulfur. Anal. Chem., 49, 316-318

Jirásek, L., Kalenský, J., Kubeck, K., Pazderová, J. & Lukáš, E. (1974)
    Acne chlorina, porphyria cutanea tarda and other manifestations of
    general intoxication during the manufacture of herbicides. II.
    Cs. Dermatol., 49, 145-157

Land, D.G., Gee, M.G., Gee, J.M. & Spinks, C.A. (1975) 2,4,6-Trichloroanisol
    in broiler house litter: a further cause of musty taint in chickens.
    J. Sci. Food Agric., 26, 1585-1591

Landner, L., Lindström, K., Karlsson, M., Nordin, J. & Sörensen, L.
    (1977) Bioaccumulation in fish of chlorinated phenols from kraft
    pulp mill bleachery effluents. Bull. environ. Contam. Toxicol.
    18, 663-673

Lindström, K. & Nordin, J. (1976) Gas chromatography-mass spectrometry
    of chlorophenols in spent bleach liquors. J. Chromatogr., 128, 13-26

McCollister, D.D., Lockwood, D.T. & Rowe, V.K. (1961) Toxicologic
    information on 2,4,5-trichlorophenol. Toxicol. appl. Pharmacol., 3,
    63-70

Milnes, M.H. (1971) Formation of 2,3,7,8-tetrachlorodibenzodioxin by
    thermal decomposition of sodium 2,4,5-trichlorophenate. Nature
    (Lond.), 232, 395-396

Mostafa, I.Y. & Moza, P.N. (1973) Degradation of gamma-pentachloro-
    cyclohex-1-ene (γ-PCCH) in corn and pea seedlings. Egypt. J.
    Chem. (Special Issue Tourky), 235-242

National Cancer Institute (1979) Bioassay of 2,4,6-Trichlorophenol for
    Possible Carcinogenicity (Tech. Rep. Series No. 155) DHEW Publications
    No. (NIH) 79-1711, Washington DC, US Department of Health, Education, &
    Welfare

National Institute for Occupational Safety & Health (1977)
    National Occupational Hazard Survey, Vol. III, Survey Analyses and
    Supplemental Tables, Cincinnati, OH, US Department of Health,
    Education, & Welfare, pp. 11,619-11,620

National Technical Information Service (1968) Evaluation of Carcinogenic,
    Teratogenic and Mutagenic Activities of Selected Pesticides and
    Industrial Chemicals, Vol. 1, Carcinogenic Study, Washington DC, US
    Department of Commerce

Perry, R.H. & Chilton, C.H., eds (1973) Chemical Engineers' Handbook,
    5th ed., New York, McGraw-Hill, p. 3-60

Prager, B., Jacobson, P., Schmidt, P. & Stern, D., eds (1923)
    Beilsteins Handbuch der Organischen Chemie, 4th ed., Vol. 6,
    Syst. no. 522, Berlin, Springer, p. 190

Rappe, C., Marklund, S., Buser, H.R. & Bosshardt, H.-P. (1978)
    Formation of polychlorinated dibenzo-para-dioxins (PCDDs) and
    dibenzofurans (PCDFs) by burning or heating chlorophenates.
    Chemosphere, 7, 269-281

Rappe, C., Garå, A. & Buser, H.R. (1979) Identification of polychlorinated
    dibenzofurans (PCDFs) in commercial chlorophenol formulations.
    Chemosphere (in press)

Renberg, L. (1974) Ion exchange technique for the determination of
    chlorinated phenols and phenoxy acids in organic tissue, soil, and
    water. Anal. Chem., 46, 359-461

Richter, F., ed. (1944) Beilsteins Handbuch der Organischen Chemie,
    4th ed., Vol. 6, 2nd Suppl., Syst. no. 522, Berlin, Springer,
    p. 180

Schulz, K.H. (1957) Clinical and experimental examinations of etiology
    of chloracne (Germ.). Arch. Klin. Exp. Dermatol., 206, 589-596

Shackelford, W.M. & Keith, L.H. (1976) Frequency of Organic Compounds
    Identified in Water, EPA-600/4-76-062, Athens, GA, US
    Environmental Protection Agency, pp. 191-192

Shafik, T.M., Sullivan, H.C. & Enos, H.R. (1973) Multiresidue procedure
    for halo- and nitrophenols. Measurement of exposure to biodegradable
    pesticides yielding these compounds as metabolites. J. agric. Food
    Chem., 21, 295-298

Shibata, S., Furukawa, M. & Nakashima, R. (1976) Dual-wavelength spectro-
    photometry. VI. Determination of phenol in industrial waste and the
    determination of 2,4-dichlorophenol and 2,4,6-trichlorophenol in
    mixtures by first derivative spectra. Anal. chem. acta, 81, 206-210

Sittig, M. (1977) Pesticides Process Encyclopedia, Park Ridge, NJ,
    Noyes Data Corporation, pp. 94-95, 415-416, 423, 429-430, 439, 441

Spencer, E.Y. (1973) Guide to the Chemicals Used in Crop Protection,
    Publication 1093, 6th ed., Research Branch, Agriculture Canada,
    London, Ontario, University of Western Ontario, pp. 447, 458

US Environmental Protection Agency (1973) EPA Compendium of Registered
    Pesticides, Vol. II, Fungicides and Nematicides, Washington DC,
    US Government Printing Office, pp. A-05-00.01, S-62-00.03, T-13-00.01,
    T-87-95.01

US Environmental Protection Agency (1978) Rebuttable presumption against
    registration and continued registration of pesticide products
    containing 2,4,5-trichlorophenol and its salts. Fed. Regist., 43,
    34026-34053

US Food & Drug Administration (1977) Food and drugs. US Code Fed. Regul.,
    Title 21, parts 176.200, 176.300, pp. 490-491

US International Trade Commission (1975) Synthetic Organic Chemicals,
    US Production and Sales, 1974, USITC Publication 776, Washington
    DC, US Government Printing Office, p. 187

US International Trade Commission (1977a) Synthetic Organic Chemicals,
    US Production and Sales, 1976, USITC Publication 833, Washington
    DC, US Government Printing Office, pp. 269, 272 & 275

US International Trade Commission (1977b) Imports of Benzenoid Chemicals
    and Products, 1976, USITC Publication 828, Washington DC, US
    Government Printing Office, p. 103

US Tariff Commission (1951) Synthetic Organic Chemicals, US Production
    and Sales, 1950, Report No. 173, Second Series, Washington DC,
    US Government Printing Office, p. 130

Windholz, M., ed. (1976) The Merck Index, 9th ed., Rahway, NJ, Merck & Co.,
    pp. 1238-1239

SOLVENTS

CARBON TETRACHLORIDE

This substance was considered by a previous IARC Working Group, in
December 1971 (IARC, 1972).   Since that time new data have become
available, and these have been incorporated into the monograph and taken
into account in the present evaluation.

A review on carbon tetrachloride is available (Mercier, 1977).

1.   Chemical and Physical Data

1.1   Synonyms and trade names

Chem. Abstr. Services Reg. No.:   56-23-5

Chem. Abstr. Name: Tetrachloromethane

Synonyms: Carbona; carbon chloride; carbon tet; methane
tetrachloride; perchloromethane; tetrachlorocarbon

Trade names: Benzinoform; Fasciolin; Flukoids; Freon 10;
Halon 104; Necatorina; Necatorine; Tetrafinol; Tetraform;
Tetrasol; Univerm; Vermoestricid

1.2   Structural and molecular formulae and molecular weight

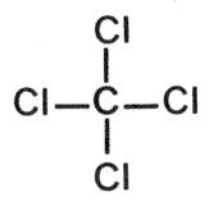

$$Cl-\overset{\displaystyle Cl}{\underset{\displaystyle Cl}{\overset{|}{\underset{|}{C}}}}-Cl$$

CCl_4 Mol. wt: 153.8

1.3   Chemical and physical properties of the pure substance

From Hawley (1977), unless otherwise specified

(a)   Description: Colourless liquid

(b)   Boiling-point: 76.7°C

(c)   Freezing-point: -23°C

(d) Density: d_4^{25} 1.585

(e) Refractive index: n_D^{20} 1.4607

(f) Spectroscopy data: λ_{vap} < 200 nm; infra-red and mass spectral data have been tabulated (Grasselli & Ritchey, 1975).

(g) Solubility: Miscible with ethanol, diethyl ether, chloroform, benzene, solvent naphtha and most fixed and volatile oils; insoluble in water

(h) Volatility: Vapour pressure is 91.3 mm at 20°C.

(i) Stability: Decomposes to phosgene in presence of limited quantity of water at 250°C (Hardie, 1964); noncombustible

(j) Reactivity: When dry, nonreactive with commonly used construction metals (iron and nickel); reacts slowly with copper and lead; reacts, sometimes explosively, with aluminium and its alloys; reduced to chloroform with zinc and acid; forms telomers with ethylene and vinyl compounds under pressure in the presence of a peroxide initiator (Hardie, 1964)

(k) Conversion factor: 1 ppm in air is equivalent to 6.3 mg/m^3.

1.4 Technical products and impurities

Carbon tetrachloride is available in the US in technical and chemically pure grades. Typical specifications for the technical grade are as follows: specific gravity (25/25°C), 1.588-1.590; acidity (as hydrogen chloride), 5 mg/kg max; residue, 5 mg/kg max; cloud-point, -10°C max; chlorides, none; free halogen, none; residual odour, none; and distillation range, 1°C including 76.7°C.

In Japan, technical-grade carbon tetrachloride has a purity of 99.9%; it may contain other chlorinated hydrocarbon impurities.

2. Production, Use, Occurrence and Analysis

2.1 Production and use

A review article on carbon tetrachloride has been published (Hardie, 1964).

(a) Production

Carbon tetrachloride was prepared in 1839 by Regnault, by chlorinating chloroform. Dumas prepared it shortly thereafter by chlorinating methane. In 1843, Kolbe produced carbon tetrachloride by reacting carbon disulphide with chlorine (Hardie, 1964).

Carbon tetrachloride is produced commercially in the US by 6 companies using the following processes: (1) as a coproduct with tetrachloroethylene, by the chlorination of short-chain hydrocarbons or their partially chlorinated derivatives; (2) by the chlorination of methane; and (3) by the chlorination of carbon disulphide. Six plants use the first method, two plants use the second method, and one plant uses the third method. As much as 50% of US capacity is based on co-production with tetrachloroethylene, which involves the use primarily of propane and propylene as raw materials.

In western Europe, carbon tetrachloride is produced primarily by the chlorination of propylene.

In Japan, 62% of carbon tetrachloride is produced by the chlorination of methane, and 32% is obtained as a coproduct of tetrachloroethylene production.

Production of carbon tetrachloride on a large scale in the US began in about 1907. By 1914, production was about 4.5 million kg annually (Hardie, 1964); and in 1976, US production reached 390 million kg (US International Trade Commission, 1977). In 1976, US imports of carbon tetrachloride amounted to 3.2 million kg, with 66.1% from the Federal Republic of Germany, 33.5% from Canada and 0.4% from at least one other country (US Department of Commerce, 1977a). The US exported a total of 7 million kg carbon tetrachloride in 1976, to the following countries (percent of total exports): Japan (48), The Netherlands (29), Mexico (17), and at least two other countries (6) (US Department of Commerce, 1977b).

Production of carbon tetrachloride in western Europe is more than 320 million kg annually. France and the Federal Republic of Germany are the major producing countries (more than 100 million kg per year); Benelux, Italy, Spain and the UK are intermediate producers (10-100 million kg per year); and Austria, Scandinavia and Switzerland are

minor producing countries (less than 100 thousand kg per year).
Annual production of carbon tetrachloride in eastern Europe is 5-100
million kg.

Carbon tetrachloride has been produced commercially in Japan since
1946.   In 1977, 7 companies produced an estimated 51.5 million kg;
imports amounted to 2.5 million kg and exports were 200 thousand kg.

(b) Use

In 1975, carbon tetrachloride was used in the US as follows:
for synthesis of dichlorofluoromethane (Fluorocarbon 12), 57%;   for
synthesis of trichlorofluoromethane (Fluorocarbon 11), 34%;   and miscellaneous uses, 9%, including its use as a fumigant.   Fluorocarbons
11 and 12 are produced by the liquid-phase reaction of carbon tetrachloride with anhydrous hydrogen fluoride in the presence of an antimony halide catalyst.   The degree of fluorination can be varied by
changing conditions of temperature, pressure and fluoride concentration.

Miscellaneous applications for carbon tetrachloride include use in
solvents, grain fumigants, pesticides (used in a mixture with carbon
disulphide and as a raw material in the manufacture of other agricultural chemicals) and in the formulation of petrol additives.

Carbon tetrachloride was formerly used as a solvent (spot remover)
domestically, but its use in this way in the US was banned by the US
Food and Drug Administration as of 11 November, 1970 (US Environmental
Protection Agency, 1970).   It has also been used as a vermidical agent
in human medicine (Von Oettingen, 1964).

In 1975, an estimated 9.1 million kg carbon tetrachloride were
used in the US as a fumigant for commodities and buildings.   In 1977,
a total of 3.1 thousand kg carbon tetrachloride were used as a pesticide
in California on a variety of grain crops, and in structures (California
Department of Food & Agriculture, 1978).

In Europe, carbon tetrachloride is used primarily in the production
of fluorocarbons (90%) and as a solvent (10%).   In Japan in 1977, 87%
was used for the synthesis of fluorocarbons and 13% for solvent and
miscellaneous uses.

Carbon tetrachloride was evaluated by the 1971 Joint Meeting of
the FAO Working Party of Experts on Pesticide Residues and the WHO
Expert Committee on Pesticide Residues.   The following residue levels
were recommended for use as guidelines: in raw cereals, at point of
entry into a country or when supplied for milling, provided that the
commodity is freely exposed to air for a period of at least 24 hrs
after fumigation and before sampling, 50 mg/kg (ppm);   in milled cereal
products that are to be subjected to baking or cooking, 10 mg/kg (ppm);

in bread and other cooked cereal products, 0.05 mg/kg (i.e., at or about the limit of determination) (WHO, 1972).

Carbon tetrachloride is exempted from the requirement of a tolerance for residues when used as a fumigant for barley, corn, oats, popcorn, rice, rye, sorghum and wheat (US Environmental Protection Agency, 1976). An exemption from a tolerance is granted when it appears that the total quantity of the pesticide chemical in or on all raw agricultural commodities for which it is of current or prevailing use will involve no hazard to public health.

Carbon tetrachloride is presently registered for use as an insecticide in the US for fumigation of barley, corn, oats, rice, rye, sorghum and wheat, and for agricultural premises, including grain bins and granaries (US Environmental Protection Agency, 1971). However, it was scheduled to have a rebuttable presumption against registration (RPAR) (see General Remarks on Substances Considered, p. 31) issued in 1977 on the basis of carcinogenicity (Anon., 1976); this has not yet been issued.

Permissible levels of carbon tetrachloride in the working environment have been established in various countries. The US Occupational Safety and Health Administration's health standards require that an employee's exposure to carbon tetrachloride at no time exceed a time-weighted average of 65 mg/m^3 (10 ppm) in any 8-hr shift of a 40-hr work week (US Occupational Safety & Health Administration, 1977). The corresponding standard in the Federal Republic of Germany and Sweden is also 65 mg/m^3, and in the German Democratic Republic and Czechoslovakia, 50 mg/m^3; the ceiling concentration in the USSR is 20 mg/m^3 (Winell, 1975).

In February 1976, the US National Institute for Occupational Safety and Health recommended that occupational exposure to carbon tetrachloride not exceed 12.6 mg/m^3 (2 ppm), determined as a time-weighted average exposure for up to a 10-hr work day in a 40-hr work week (National Institute for Occupational Safety & Health, 1976).

2.2 Occurrence

Carbon tetrachloride is formed in the troposphere by solar-induced photochemical reactions of chlorinated alkenes (Singh et al., 1975). Its occurrence in the US environment has been reviewed (Johns, 1976).

(a) Air

Air samples taken at 42 locations in the US contained an average concentration of 1.4 µg/m^3 (0.22 ppb) carbon tetrachloride. Of 4 halocarbons measured, carbon tetrachloride showed the least variation in concentration, with more than 86% of all measurements falling within the range 0.6-1.9 µg/m^3 (0.1-0.3 ppb) (Simonds *et al.*, 1974).

Maximum levels of carbon tetrachloride found in the atmosphere ranged from 0.9-113 µg/m^3 (0.14-18 ppb); minimum levels, 0.3-1.3 µg/m^3 (0.05-0.20 ppb); and mean levels, 0.6-10.3 µg/m^3 (0.09-1.63 ppb) (Lillian *et al.*, 1975). In 3 locations, atmospheric concentrations of carbon tetrachloride ranged from 0.4-0.7 µg/m^3 (0.07-0.11 ppb), 0.56-0.63 µg/m^3 (0.09-0.10 ppb) and 0.4-0.5 µg/m^3 (0.07-0.08 ppb) (Hanst *et al.*, 1975).

Carbon tetrachloride was detected in a rural atmosphere at a level of 756 ng/m^3 (120 ppt) (Grimsrud & Rasmussen, 1975). Levels of carbon tetrachloride determined in other rural air samples ranged from 500-700 ng/m^3 (80-100 ppt) (Russell & Shadoff, 1977).

The ambient air in a Japanese town was sampled at 26 sites on 3 or 4 days of every month from May 1974 to April 1975: the annual average concentration of carbon tetrachloride was 8.8 µg/m^3 (1.4 ppb). The distribution of carbon tetrachloride in the atmosphere was found to correlate with the location of chemical factories (Ohta *et al.*, 1976).

Atmospheric concentrations of carbon tetrachloride at ground level measured at sites in the northern and southern hemispheres were 700 ng/m^3 (111 ppt) and 434 ng/m^3 (68.9 ppt), respectively (Cox *et al.*, 1976).

Formation of carbon tetrachloride in the troposphere by solar-induced photochemical reactions of chlorinated alkenes was studied experimentally by simulated tropospheric irradiations of synthetic mixtures of tetrachloroethylene in air. It was found that tetrachloroethylene photodecomposition leads to an average formation of about 8% by weight carbon tetrachloride. The relatively uniform global concentrations, significant atmospheric loading and almost exclusive use of carbon tetrachloride for fluorocarbon synthesis had led to earlier speculation that there was a natural source of carbon tetrachloride. This study shows, however, that tetrachloroethylene (found at several locations in relatively large concentrations) could account for a significant percentage of atmospheric carbon tetrachloride (Singh *et al.*, 1975).

(b) Water

In a summary of the frequency of reports of the occurrence of organic compounds in water, it was indicated that carbon tetrachloride has been found in rivers, lakes, raw-water, finished drinking-water, effluent water from commercial manufacturing sources and sewage treatment plant effluent water taken from 43 sites in the US and Europe (Shackelford & Keith, 1976).

Carbon tetrachloride has been detected in a lake, and in subterranean (0.5-6 ng/l) and tap (5 ng/l) water (Eurocop-Cost, 1976).

A National Organics Reconnaissance Survey performed by the US
Environmental Protection Agency in 1975 reported levels of carbon tetrachloride in 80 water supplies distributed over various regions of the US,
representing a wide variety of raw-water sources and treatment techniques.
Carbon tetrachloride was detected in 12.5% of finished waters, up to a
level of 4 µg/l (Symons *et al.*, 1975).

Carbon tetrachloride was found in 8/10 water supply utilities (Safe
Drinking Water Committee, 1977) and in the drinking-water of 2 cities
(Saunders *et al.*, 1975).

Carbon tetrachloride, benzene and dichloroethane were detected
together in river water at the entrance to a water treatment facility,
at the clarifier effluent stage of the water-treatment process, and in
finished water, at total relative concentrations of 12.27:3.26:36.61
(Dowty *et al.*, 1975a,b).

Periods of high agricultural runoff have been associated with peak
concentrations of halomethanes, including carbon tetrachloride, due to
increased turbidity of the raw water (Morris & Johnson, 1976).

In a survey sampling 172 stations of bay-water, the maximum concentration of carbon tetrachloride was 2.4 µg/l and the average concentration of combined 1,1,1-trichloroethane and carbon tetrachloride was
0.25 µg/l (Pearson & McConnell, 1975).

Carbon tetrachloride was identified as a major constituent of organic
compounds found in a river (Zuercher & Giger, 1976).

(c) Food and drink

Carbon tetrachloride, in combination with ethylene dibromide and
ethylene dichloride, has been applied to wheat stored in paper laminate
bins; concentrations of carbon tetrachloride gas were greatest at the
bottoms of the bins. Carbon tetrachloride residues in the wheat varied,
depending on bin location and contact time, from 3.2-72.6 mg/kg.
Residues on bran and middlings derived from the treated wheat ranged from
0.2-2.23 mg/kg; in bread made from the wheat, residues ranged from 0-
0.04 mg/kg (Berck, 1974).

The following concentrations of carbon tetrachloride were found in
foodstuffs in the UK in 1973: dairy produce, 0.2-14 µg/kg; meat, 7-9
µg/kg; oils and fats, 0.7-18 µg/kg; beverages, 0.2-6 µg/kg; and fruits
and vegetables, 3-8 µg/kg (McConnell *et al.*, 1975).

(d) Animals

Five species of fish and 3 species of molluscs were collected from
relatively clean sea-water. Concentrations in the various organs ranged
from 2-114 µg/kg (dry-weight basis) in molluscs and from 3-209 µg/kg

(dry-weight basis) in fish.   The relative concentrations in organs of
the fish were: brain > gill > liver > muscle (Dickson & Riley, 1976).

(e)   Occupational exposure

A 1974 National Occupational Hazard Survey estimated that workers
exposed to carbon tetrachloride are primarily those at blast furnaces and
steel mills, in the air transportation industry, and in motor vehicle and
telephone and telegraph equipment manufacturing (National Institute for
Occupational Safety & Health, 1977a).

2.3 Analysis

Gas chromatographic methods to collect and determine halocarbons,
including carbon tetrachloride, in the ambient air (Appleby, 1976) and
sampling and analytical methods for trace determination of carbon tetrachloride in water (Bertsch et al., 1975) have been reviewed.   Table 1
lists methods used for the analysis of carbon tetrachloride in environmental samples.

The efficiency of charcoal for trapping carbon tetrachloride from
air has been studied collaboratively (Reckner & Sachdev, 1975).

Other analytical methods to isolate and identify carbon tetrachloride include use of gas-phase coulometry (Lillian & Singh, 1974;
Seto et al., 1977) and ultra-violet spectrometry (Ellison & Wallbank,
1974).

3.   Biological Data Relevant to the Evaluation
of Carcinogenic Risk to Humans

3.1 Carcinogenicity studies in animals

(a)   Oral administration

Mouse: Strain A mice of both sexes, $2\frac{1}{2}$–3 months of age at the
beginning of treatment, were given oral doses of 0.1, 0.2, 0.4, 0.8 and
1.6 ml/kg bw (0.16, 0.32, 0.64, 1.28 and 2.5 g/kg bw) carbon tetrachloride in olive oil; the interval between consecutive doses was 1–5
days; each animal received 30 doses.   The experiment was terminated
at 150 days.   No hepatomas were seen in the group given 30 doses of
1.6 ml/kg bw over a period of 30 days, whereas a significant number of
hepatomas was observed in all groups that received 30 doses of 0.1 ml/kg
bw or more over a period of 90 days or more (Eschenbrenner & Miller,
1944).

Groups of 50 male and 50 female B6C3F1 hybrid mice, 5 weeks of age,
received carbon tetrachloride as a 2–5% solution in corn oil by oral

TABLE 1. METHODS FOR THE ANALYSIS OF CARBON TETRACHLORIDE

SAMPLE TYPE	ANALYTICAL METHOD			
	EXTRACTION/CLEAN-UP	DETECTION	LIMIT OF DETECTION	REFERENCE
Formulations				
Encapsulated liquids and cough syrups	Transfer to ethanol, dilute as appropriate, transfer to separator containing 10% sucrose solution and carbon disulphide	IR		Horwitz (1975)
Capsules and drugs	Heat under pressure with alcoholic potassium hydroxide to dechlorinate	Titration		Horwitz (1970)
Air				
Ambient	Trap in pyridine, add aqueous solution of sodium hydroxide, allow colour to develop	Colorimetry at 525 nm	157 mg/m^3	Gage et al. (1962)
Ambient	Trap in Drechsel flask fitted with rubber septum, sample with gas syringe	GC/ECD	0.2 µg/m^3	Bureau International Technique des Solvants Chlorés (1976)
Ambient	Trap in glass container, inject on GC column	GC/ECD		Ohta et al. (1976)
Ambient	Trap by cryogenic method, vaporize into second trap, analyse	IR		Hanst et al. (1975)
Rural	Trap on porous polymer, desorb by heating, retrap in line on GC column	GC/ECD GC/MS confirmation	190-800 ng/m^3	Russell & Shadoff (1977)
Workplace	Trap on charcoal, desorb (carbon disulphide), extract	GC/FID	Range of application: 65-299 mg/m^3	National Institute for Occupational Safety & Health (1977b)
Atmosphere	Trap on polymer, desorb by heating, retrap in line on GC column	GC/MS		Dowty et al. (1975a,b)
Atmosphere	Inject directly	GC/MS	30 ng/m^3	Grimsrud & Rasmussen (1975)

TABLE 1. METHODS FOR THE ANALYSIS OF CARBON TETRACHLORIDE (continued)

SAMPLE TYPE	ANALYTICAL METHOD			
	EXTRACTION/CLEAN-UP	DETECTION	LIMIT OF DETECTION	REFERENCE
Water				
Sea and fresh water	Extract (pentane), dry	GC/ECD	25 ng/kg	Bureau International Technique des Solvants Chlorés (1976)
River	Cool to 4°C, extract (pentane)	GC/FID GC/ECD	10 µg/l 10 ng/l	Dietz & Traud (1973)
Drinking-water	Inject directly	GC/ECD	0.1 µg/l	Nicholson et al. (1977)
Sediments	Wash (water), cool to 4°C, extract (pentane)	GC/FID GC/ECD	10 µg/l 10 ng/l	Dietz & Traud (1973)
Food				
Cereals and other foodstuffs	Extract (acetone-water, aceto-nitrile-water), dry	GC/ECD, FID	0.1 mg/kg	Heuser & Scudamore (1969)
Cereals	Extract (acetone-water)	GC/FID, ECD		Heuser & Scudamore (1968)
Grains	3 possible extraction methods: sweep co-distillation, steam distillation, acid reflux	GC/ECD	0.1 mg/kg	Malone (1969)
Grains	Grind in dry ice, boil in acid, trap volatile fumigant in cold solvent	GC/ECD	40 µg/kg	Malone (1970)
Biological				
Blood	Put in sealed tube, equilibrate in water bath (27°C) for 30 min, head-space analysis	GC/FID		Premel-Cabic et al. (1974)
Plasma	Adsorb on polymer, desorb by heating, retrap in line on GC column	GC/MS		Dowty et al. (1975a)

Abbreviations: IR - infra-red spectroscopy; GC/FID - gas chromatography/flame-ionization detection; ECD - electron capture detection; MS - mass spectrometry

gavage 5 times weekly at dose levels of 1250 and 2500 mg/kg bw for 78 weeks. Pooled control (77 males and 80 females) and matched controls, (18 males and 18 females) were treated with corn oil only. The experiment was terminated 90-92 weeks from the start. Hepatocellular carcinomas developed in nearly all treated mice: 49/49 and 47/48 male, 40/40 and 43/45 female mice given low and high dose levels, respectively, compared with 5/77 male and 1/80 female pooled controls and 3/18 and 1/18 matched controls. In this experiment, carbon tetrachloride was used as a positive control (National Cancer Institute, 1976; Weisburger, 1977).

Groups of male C3H mice, 2 months old, received doses of 0.2, 0.4 and 1.6 g/kg bw carbon tetrachloride in corn oil intragastrically 3 times weekly for 10 weeks. The experiment was terminated 150 days after the first treatment, at which time 8/30, 18/60 and 6/30 treated animals and 18/30 vehicle controls were still alive. Hepatomas developed in 5, 4 and 1 mice; the number of hepatomas per animal varied from 1-6. No hepatomas were seen in 28 untreated controls or in 18 vehicle controls (Kiplinger & Kensler, 1963).

Rat: In an experiment in which carbon tetrachloride was used as a positive control, groups of 50 male and 50 female 45-day-old Osborne-Mendel rats were treated 5 times weekly by gavage with carbon tetrachloride in corn oil for 78 weeks. Males received 47 and 94 mg/kg bw, and females 80 and 160 mg/kg bw. Surviving animals were then fed a control diet and killed at 110 weeks. Hepatocellular carcinomas occurred in 2/49 and 2/50 males, compared with 0/20 matched controls [$P > 0.05$]; neoplastic nodules of the liver occurred in 9 and 3 males treated with the low and high doses. In females, hepatocellular carcinomas occurred in 4/50 and 2/49 rats, compared with 1/20 in matched controls [$P > 0.05$]; neoplastic nodules of the liver were found in 11 and 9 treated females, and in 1 female control. Among pooled controls, 1/99 males and 0/98 females had hepatocellular carcinomas and 0/99 males and 2/98 females had neoplastic nodules of the liver (National Cancer Institute, 1976; Weisburger, 1977).

Hamster: Ten 12 week-old Syrian golden hamsters of each sex received 30 weekly doses of 6.25-12.5 µl (10-20 mg) carbon tetrachloride in 5% corn oil solution. All 5 animals of each sex that survived 10 or more weeks after the end of treatment had liver-cell carcinomas (Della Porta et al., 1961) [The Working Group noted that no data on controls were reported].

Trout: Rainbow trout were given diets containing 3200 and 12,800 mg/kg diet carbon tetrachloride. Four out of 44 animals given the lower dose level and 3/34 given the higher dose level developed hepatomas after 20 months, whereas no tumours were found in the controls (Halver, 1967).

(b) Inhalation and/or intratracheal administration

Rat: A group of albino rats (sex unspecified) that had inhaled carbon tetrachloride (dose and schedule unspecified) daily for 7 months were killed 2-10 months after the end of treatment.   Among 30 survivors, 12 had 'adenocirrhosis' and 10 had liver nodules measuring up to 1 cm, diagnosed histologically as early or established liver carcinomas (Costa *et al.*, 1963) [The Working Group noted that no controls were used in this study].

(c) Subcutaneous and/or intramuscular administration

Rat: A group of 49 male Wistar rats weighing about 120 g received 2-3 ml/kg bw (3.2-4.8 g/kg bw) carbon tetrachloride in olive oil twice weekly for 25-35 weeks and were killed 4-78 weeks after the end of treatment; hepatomas (malignant, according to the author, but degree of malignancy not specified) were found in 2 animals (Kawasaki, 1965) [The Working Group noted that no controls were used in this study].

In a study in which 12-week-old male rats were given s.c. injections of 1.3 ml/kg bw (2 g/kg bw) of a 50% solution of carbon tetrachloride in corn oil twice weekly, 4/12 Wistar rats, 8/13 Osborne-Mendel rats and 12/15 Japanese rats that survived 68 or more weeks had hepatocellular carcinomas.   No liver tumours were found in 12 control rats of each strain (Reuber & Glover, 1970).   In an earlier experiment on groups of 10-14 Buffalo male and female rats, 4, 12, 24 and 52 weeks old, in which the same schedule of treatment was used, a low yield of hepatomas was observed (Reuber & Glover, 1967).

Thirty white female rats, 5-6 months old at the start of the experiment, received twice weekly s.c. injections of 1 ml/kg bw (1.6 g/kg bw) carbon tetrachloride for 2 years.   Eight rats developed mammary adenocarcinomas, the first of which appeared 13 months after the beginning of treatment; 3 of these rats also had fibroadenomas of the mammary glands; 1 rat developed only a mammary fibroadenoma.   No mammary tumours were observed in an untreated control group of 15 rats (Alpert *et al.*, 1972).

(d) Other experimental systems

Intrarectal administration: Twenty-five C3H male mice received biweekly intrarectal administrations of 0.1 ml of a 40% solution of carbon tetrachloride in olive oil for 20-26 weeks and were killed 1-37 weeks later.   A total of 13 mice had liver tumours, described as nodular hyperplasia.   No such tumours developed in 10 olive-oil-treated control mice (Confer & Stenger, 1965).

(e) Combined administration with other agents   [These studies were not carried out to test carbon tetrachloride for carcinogenic activity]

Administration of a single dose of N-nitrosobutylurea to mice treated 24 hrs earlier with a single dose of carbon tetrachloride resulted in an increased incidence of hepatomas and leukaemia, as compared with mice treated with N-nitrosobutylurea alone (Yokoro et al., 1973). An increased incidence of liver and kidney tumours was observed in mice treated with a single dose of N-nitrosodiethylamine 24 or 48 hrs after a single injection of carbon tetrachloride (Pound, 1978).

(C57L x A)F1 mice that had received a single whole-body exposure to fast neutrons (165-306 rad) received a single s.c. injection of carbon tetrachloride (0.15 ml of a 40% solution in sesame oil) 2-18 months later. The frequency of hepatomas was increased from 19-61%. No hepatomas appeared in controls given carbon tetrachloride only (Cole & Nowell, 1964). Similar findings were reported by Curtis & Tilley (1972).

Administration of a single dose of N-nitrosodimethylamine to rats treated 24 hrs earlier with a single dose of carbon tetrachloride resulted in an increased incidence of liver and kidney tumours, as compared with corresponding controls (Pound et al., 1973a). An increased incidence of hepatomas and a shortening of the latent period of tumour induction were observed in rats that received a single dose of aflatoxin followed by chronic administration of carbon tetrachloride (Lemmonier et al., 1974).

Carbon tetrachloride promoted the hepatocarcinogenesis induced by 3'-methyl-4-dimethylaminoazobenzene in female Donryu rats (Kanematsu, 1976).

3.2 Other relevant biological data

(a) Experimental systems

Toxic effects

The single oral LD_{50} of carbon tetrachloride in rats is 2.92 g/kg bw (Klaassen & Plaa, 1969; Smyth et al., 1970); that in mice is 12.1-14.4 g/kg bw (Dybing & Dybing, 1946); and that in dogs 2.3 g/kg bw (Klaassen & Plaa, 1967).   The i.p. LD_{50} in mice is 4.1 g/kg bw (Klaassen & Plaa, 1966); the s.c. LD_{50} in mice is 30.4 g/kg bw (Plaa et al., 1958).   The s.c. LD_{33} in cats is 4.8 g/kg bw (Cantarow et al., 1938).

The minimal lethal i.v. dose of carbon tetrachloride in dogs was 125 mg/kg bw (Barsoum & Saad, 1934).   Single exposures to 315 mg/m^3 (50 ppm) carbon tetrachloride vapour for 7 hrs had no adverse effect

upon male rats (Adams *et al.*, 1952); however, alterations in liver
biochemistry can be produced by oral doses of carbon tetrachloride as
small as 15.4 mg/kg bw (Rechnagel & Ghoshal, 1966).

Variations in data on acute toxicity may be due to different
observation times (1-10 days). High doses kill animals by central
nervous depression within hours; smaller and subnarcotic doses produce
death by liver damage after several days.

After 40-150 exposures to carbon tetrachloride vapour for 7 hrs/
day over about 200 days, toxic effects were seen with 315 mg/m^3 (50 ppm)
in rabbits and guinea-pigs and with 100 ppm in rats and monkeys.
Adverse effects included increased liver weight, moderate fatty
degeneration and cirrhosis; slight effects were seen with 25 ppm
(Adams *et al.*, 1952).

In rats, an i.g. dose of 3.8 g/kg bw carbon tetrachloride greatly
reduced *N*-nitrosodimethylamine-demethylase activity in the liver for
42-72 hrs but did not alter the activity of this enzyme in the kidney
(Pound *et al.*, 1973b).

Changes have been observed in mammalian liver cells following
administration of carbon tetrachloride: diene conjugation of the poly-
enoic fatty acids of the endoplasmic membrane, lipid peroxidation,
scission of carbon chains, covalent binding of carbon tetrachloride
metabolites to cellular constituents, triglyceride accumulation,
membrane damage, leakage of enzymes, fatty degeneration and centrilobular necrosis (Recknagel, 1967; Recknagel & Glende, 1973; Smuckler,
1976; Uehleke *et al.*, 1977).

The influence of a number of chemicals on various parameters of
carbon tetrachloride toxicity has been reviewed by Suriyachan &
Thithapandha (1977). Induction or inhibition of hepatic drug metabolism
altered the toxicity of carbon tetrachloride (Cignoli & Castro, 1971;
Garner & McLean, 1969; Pani *et al.*, 1973; Seawright & McLean, 1967;
Uehleke, 1977; Uehleke & Werner, 1975).

Embryotoxicity and teratogenicity

Increased foetal mortality was observed in pregnant mice given
single doses of 150 mg/animal carbon tetrachloride in a 40% oily
solution during the last part of pregnancy. The adverse effect was
more pronounced after i.p. than after s.c. administration. Cause of
death was suggested to be failure of peripheral circulation, mainly due
to foetal liver damage. Moreover, circulatory disturbances and necroses
were found in the placentas, which probably also contributed to the death
of the foetuses (Roschlau & Rodenkirchen, 1969).

The foetuses of rats exposed for 7 hrs/day on days 6-15 of gestation to concentrations of 1890 and 6300 mg/m^3 (300 and 1000 ppm) carbon tetrachloride in air showed retarded development (Schwetz *et al.*, 1974).

Absorption, distribution and excretion

Carbon tetrachloride is absorbed rapidly after ingestion, inhalation or application to injured skin (Von Oettingen, 1964).

After oral administration of carbon tetrachloride to rats, blood and liver concentrations increased during the following 90 min and then decreased continuously (Recknagel & Litteria, 1960). I.g. administration to rats of 4.4 mg/kg bw carbon tetrachloride produced peak liver concentrations after 4 hrs and highest blood levels after 2 hrs. The elimination rate was 7.6% per hr from liver and 2.5% per hr from blood (Nachtomi & Alumot, 1972).

After dogs were exposed by inhalation to 94.5 g/m^3 (15,000 ppm) carbon tetrachloride in air, blood and liver concentrations were comparable (Von Oettingen, 1964). The highest concentrations of carbon tetrachloride in monkeys exposed to 315 mg/m^3 (50 ppm) of ^{14}C-carbon tetrachloride for 140-340 min were found in fat, liver, bone marrow, blood, brain and kidney. Approximately 50% of the retained amount was exhaled unchanged; some labelled material was exhaled after 20 days (McCollister *et al.*, 1951).

Cutaneous absorption of 7.2 g/m^3 (1150 ppm) ^{14}C-labelled carbon tetrachloride vapours by a monkey produced blood levels of 0.3 mg/l after 270 min (McCollister *et al.*, 1951).

Metabolism

The toxicity of carbon tetrachloride results from its biotransformation. In monkeys, 11% of a ^{14}C-labelled dose of carbon tetrachloride was exhaled as $^{14}CO_2$ over 18 hrs (McCollister *et al.*, 1951). In dogs, chloroform was identified among the expired compounds (Butler, 1961). Liver microsomes metabolize carbon tetrachloride to CO_2 (Rubinstein & Kanics, 1964); this reaction is increased both *in vivo* and with liver microsomes after pretreatment of the animals with phenobarbital or DDT (Garner & McLean, 1969; Seawright & McLean, 1967).

Lipid peroxidation, presumably initiated by a free-radical metabolite of carbon tetrachloride (Butler, 1961), seems to be the most important factor in carbon tetrachloride-induced liver toxicity (Glende *et al.*, 1976; Ghoshal & Recknagel, 1965; Recknagel, 1967; Recknagel & Glende, 1973; Recknagel & Ghoshal, 1966; Slater, 1966). Similar events may be responsible for extrahepatic tissue damage (Von Oettingen, 1964) in lung (Chen *et al.*, 1977), kidney (Von Oettingen, 1964), testes

(Chatterjee, 1966), adrenals (Castro *et al.*, 1972) and placenta (Tsirel'nikov & Tsirel'nikova, 1976).

Carbon tetrachloride binds to cytochrome P450 in hepatic microsomes. It may also destroy P450 by lipid peroxidation (Glende *et al.*, 1976; Sasame *et al.*, 1968; Smuckler *et al.*, 1967).

Binding to macromolecules

The irreversible (covalent) binding of hepatic macromolecules with carbon and chlorine from carbon tetrachloride (^{14}C or ^{36}Cl) suggests that its toxic action on the liver is mediated by a chemical attack of carbon tetrachloride cleavage products on lipids and proteins, preferentially of the endoplasmic reticulum (Cessi *et al.*, 1966; Gordis, 1969; Rao & Recknagel, 1969; Reynolds, 1967).

Less than 0.2% radioactivity was found in ribosomal RNA or nuclear DNA from rats dosed with ^{14}C-labelled carbon tetrachloride (Reynolds, 1967), or in ribosomal RNA from microsomes taken from phenobarbital-treated rats and rabbits and incubated with carbon tetrachloride (Uehleke & Werner, 1975); however, radioactivity was bound to soluble nucleotides (Harders *et al.*, 1976). Diaz Gomez & Castro (1978) claim that radioactivity of ^{14}C-tetrachloride binds to nuclear DNA in rats and mice.

Mutagenicity and other related short-term tests

In plate tests with *Salmonella typhimurium* TA100, TA1535 and TA1538, carbon tetrachloride was non-mutagenic both in the presence and absence of a microsomal activation system (McCann & Ames, 1976; McCann *et al.*, 1975; Uehleke *et al.*, 1977). It was also negative with *Escherichia coli* K12 (Uehleke *et al.*, 1976). However, it has been claimed that it interacts with cellular macromolecules (including DNA) of mammalian cells both *in vivo* and *in vitro* if the animals (rats and mice) have been pretreated with 3-methylcholanthrene (Rocchi *et al.*, 1973).

(b) Humans

Numerous poisonings and fatalities have occurred due to accidental or suicidal ingestion of carbon tetrachloride or from its medical use; the majority of cases resulted from the inhalation of carbon tetrachloride vapours used as a solvent or dry-cleaning agent (Von Oettingen, 1964). The major pathological changes are seen in liver and kidney.

Death has been reported after ingestion of as little as 1.5 ml; some patients have been known to survive after swallowing more than 100 ml. When inhaled, it may cause central nervous system depression, pulmonary oedema, alveolitis and fatal cardiac arrhythmias (Bagnasco *et al.*, 1978).

Renal failure due to carbon tetrachloride is increased by the consumption of alcohol (New *et al.*, 1962).

After exposure of male volunteers to 315 mg/m^3 (49 ppm) carbon tetrachloride vapours in air during 70 min or to 63 mg/m^3 (10 ppm) for 180 min, concentrations in the expired air were 11 mg/m^3 (1.7 ppm) and 4.4 mg/m^3 (0.7 ppm) after 1 hr; these decreased exponentially (Stewart *et al.*, 1961). Carbon tetrachloride could be detected 450 hrs after the accidental intake of a large quantity (Stewart *et al.*, 1963).

After 30 min immersion of one thumb in carbon tetrachloride, volunteers exhaled concentrations of 3 mg/m^3 (0.64 ppm); expiration half-time was approximately 2 hrs (Stewart & Dodd, 1964).

3.3 Case reports and epidemiological studies

Cases of liver cancer have been reported in humans several years after carbon tetrachloride poisoning. Johnstone (1948) reported the case of a woman who developed nodular cirrhosis of the liver followed by cancer of the liver, and who died 3 years after first exposure. She had suffered from periodic jaundice for 5 years before exposure to carbon tetrachloride. Simler *et al.* (1964) reported that a fireman who was acutely intoxicated by carbon tetrachloride developed cirrhosis and an 'epithelioma' of the liver 4 years after exposure.

Tracey & Sherlock (1968) reported a hepatocellular carcinoma with concomitant fibrosis in a 59-year-old man 7 years after acute poisoning with carbon tetrachloride during a short (a few days) exposure to the compound used for cleaning his rug.

4. Summary of Data Reported and Evaluation

4.1 Experimental data

Carbon tetrachloride was tested in several experiments in mice by oral and intrarectal administration and in rats by oral and subcutaneous administration and by inhalation exposure; it was also tested in one experiment in hamsters and one in trout by oral administration. In various strains of mice, it produced liver tumours, including hepatocellular carcinomas. In various strains of rats, it produced benign and malignant liver tumours; and in one experiment with subcutaneous injection, an increased incidence of mammary adenocarcinoams was observed. In hamsters and trout, increased incidences of liver tumours were observed; however, these studies were considered to be inadequate.

Carbon tetrachloride is foetotoxic. It was not mutagenic in bacteria.

4.2 Human data[1]

No epidemiological studies were available to the Working Group.
Three case reports were available describing the appearance of liver
tumours associated with cirrhosis following exposure to carbon tetrachloride. In one of the cases, a single, high-level exposure was thought
to have occurred; in another, exposure was limited to a period of a few
days.

The extensive production and widespread use of carbon tetrachloride
indicate that human exposure occurs. This is confirmed by many reports
of its occurrence in the general environment and of numerous poisonings
and fatalities due to this compound.

4.3 Evaluation

There is *sufficient evidence* that carbon tetrachloride is carcinogenic in experimental animals. There are suggestive case reports of
liver cancer in humans. In the absence of adequate data in humans, it
is reasonable, for practical purposes, to regard carbon tetrachloride as
if it presented a carcinogenic risk to humans.

---

[1]Subsequent to the meeting of the Working Group, the Secretariat
became aware of a study of 330 deceased laundry and dry-cleaning workers
who had been exposed to carbon tetrachloride, trichloroethylene and
tetrachloroethylene. An excess of lung, cervical and skin cancers and
a slight excess of leukaemias and liver cancers were observed (Blair
et al., 1979).

5. References

Adams, E.M., Spencer, H.C., Rowe, V.K., McCollister, D.D. & Irish, D.D.
    (1952) Vapor toxicity of carbon tetrachloride determined by
    experiments on laboratory animals. AMA Arch. ind. Hyg., 6, 50-66

Alpert, A.E., Arkhangelsky, A.V., Lunts, A.M. & Panina, N.P. (1972)
    Experimental hepatopathies and carcinoma of the breast in rats (Russ.).
    Bjull. Eksp. Biol. Med., 74, 78-81

Anon. (1976) New RPAR decision schedule drafted; chemicals grouped
    by use. Pestic. Tox. chem. News, 15 December, pp. 24-25

Appleby, A. (1976) Atmospheric Freons and Halogenated Compounds,
    EPA-600/3-76-108, Research Triangle Park, NC, US Environmental Protection
    Agency, pp. 54-105, 325-336

Bagnasco, F.M., Stringer, B. & Muslim, A.M. (1978) Carbon tetrachloride
    poisoning. Radiographic findings. NY State J. Med., 78, 646-647

Barsoum, G.S. & Saad, K. (1934) Relative toxicity of certain chlorine
    derivatives of the aliphatic series. Q. J. Pharm. Pharmacol., 7,
    205-214

Berck, B. (1974) Fumigant residues of carbon tetrachloride, ethylene
    dichloride, and ethylene dibromide in wheat, flour, bran, middlings,
    and bread. J. agric. Food Chem., 22, 977-984

Bertsch, W., Anderson, E. & Holzer, G. (1975) Trace.analysis of organic
    volatiles in water by gas chromatography-mass spectrometry with
    glass capillary columns. J. Chromatogr., 112, 701-718

Blair, A., Decoufle, P. & Grauman, D. (1979) Causes of death among
    laundry and dry cleaning workers. Am. J. Publ. Health, 69, 508-511

Bureau International Technique des Solvants Chlorés (1976)
    Standardization of methods for the determination of traces of some
    volatile chlorinated aliphatic hydrocarbons in air and water by gas
    chromatography. Anal. chim. acta, 82, 1-17

Butler, T.C. (1961) Reduction of carbon tetrachloride in vivo and
    reduction of carbon tetrachloride and chloroform in vitro by
    tissues and tissue constituents. J. Pharmacol. exp. Ther., 134,
    311-319

California Department of Food & Agriculture (1978) Pesticide Use
    Report, Annual 1977, Sacramento, CA, pp. 25-26

Cantarow, A., Stewart, H.L. & Morgan, D.R. (1938) Experimental
    carbon tetrachloride poisoning in the cat. I. The influence of
    calcium administration. J. Pharmacol. exp. Ther., 63, 153-172

Castro, J.A., Díaz Gómez, M.I., de Ferreyra, E.C., de Castro, C.R.,
    D'Acosta, N. & de Fenos, O.M. (1972) Carbon tetrachloride effect
    on rat liver and adrenals related to their mixed-function oxygenase
    content. Biochem. biophys. Res. Commun., 47, 315-321

Cessi, C., Colombini, C. & Mameli, L. (1966) The reaction of liver
    proteins with a metabolite of carbon tetrachloride. Biochem. J.,
    101, 46c-47c

Chatterjee, A. (1966) Testicular degeneration in rats by carbon
    tetrachloride intoxication. Experientia, 22, 395-396

Chen, W.-J., Chi, E.Y. & Smuckler, E.A. (1977) Carbon tetrachloride-
    induced changes in mixed function oxidases and microsomal
    cytochromes in the rat lung. Lab. Invest., 36, 388-394

Cignoli, E.V. & Castro, J.A. (1971) Effect of inhibitors of drug
    metabolizing enzymes on carbon tetrachloride hepatotoxicity.
    Toxicol. appl. Pharmacol., 18, 625-637

Cole, L.J. & Nowell, P.C. (1964) Accelerated induction of hepatomas in
    fast neutron-irradiated mice injected with carbon tetrachloride.
    Ann. NY Acad. Sci., 114, 259-267

Confer, D.B. & Stenger, R.J. (1965) Tumors of the liver in C3H mice
    after longterm carbon tetrachloride administration. A light and
    electron microscopic study. Am. J. Path., 46, 19a

Costa, A., Weber, G., Bartoloni St Omer, F. & Campana, G. (1963)
    Experimental cancer of carbon tetrachloride in the rat (Ital.).
    Arch. De Vecchi Anat. pat., 39, 303-356

Cox, R.A., Derwent, R.G., Eggleton, A.E.J. & Lovelock, J.E. (1976)
    Photochemical oxidation of halocarbons in the troposphere.
    Atmos. Environ., 10, 305-308

Curtis, H.J. & Tilley, J. (1972) The role of mutations in liver tumor
    induction in mice. Radiat. Res., 50, 539-542

Della Porta, Terracini, B. & Shubik, P. (1961) Induction with carbon
    tetrachloride of liver-cell carcinomas in hamsters. J. natl Cancer
    Inst., 26, 855-863

Díaz Gómez, M.I. & Castro, J.A. (1978) Covalent binding of carbon
    tetrachloride metabolites to liver nuclear DNA, proteins, and lipids
    (Abstract no. 223). Toxicol. appl. Pharmacol., 45, 315

Dickson, A.G. & Riley, J.P. (1976) The distribution of short-chain
    halogenated aliphatic hydrocarbons in some marine organisms.
    Marine Poll. Bull., 7, 167-169

Dietz, F. & Traud, J. (1973) Gas chromatographic determination of low-
    molecular-weight chlorohydrocarbons in water samples and sediments
    (Germ.). Vom Wasser, 41, 137-155 [Chem. Abstr., 81, 54214p]

Dowty, B., Carlisle, D., Laseter, J.L. & Storer, J. (1975a) Halogenated
    hydrocarbons in New Orleans drinking water and blood plasma.
    Science, 187, 75-77

Dowty, B.J., Carlisle, D.R. & Laseter, J.L. (1975b) New Orleans drinking
    water sources tested by gas chromatography-mass spectrometry.
    Environ. Sci. Technol., 9, 762-765

Dybing, F. & Dybing, O. (1946) The toxic effect of tetrachloromethane
    and tetrachlorethylene in oily solution. Acta pharmacol., 2,
    223-226

Ellison, W.K. & Wallbank, T.E. (1974) Solvents in sewage and industrial
    waste waters. Identification and determination. Water Pollut.
    Control, 73, 656-672 [Chem. Abstr., 82, 102823f]

Eschenbrenner, A.B. & Miller, E. (1944) Studies on hepatomas. I.
    Size and spacing of multiple doses in the induction of carbon
    tetrachloride hepatomas. J. natl Cancer Inst., 4, 385-388

Eurocop-Cost (1976) A Comprehensive List of Polluting Substances
    Which Have Been Identified in Various Fresh Waters, Effluent
    Discharges, Aquatic Animals and Plants, and Bottom Sediments,
    2nd ed., EUCO/MDU/73/76, XII/476/76, Luxembourg, Commission of the
    European Communities, p. 29

Gage, J.C., Strafford, N. & Truhaut, R. (1962) Methods for the
    Determination of Toxic Substances in Air, International Union of
    Pure & Applied Chemistry, London, Butterworths, pp. 24.1-24.2

Garner, R.C. & McLean, A.E.M. (1969) Increased susceptibility to
    carbon tetrachloride poisoning in the rat after pretreatment with
    oral phenobarbitone. Biochem. Pharmacol., 18, 645-650

Ghoshal, A.K. & Recknagel, R.O. (1965) Positive evidence of
    acceleration of lipoperoxidation in rat liver by carbon tetra-
    chloride: in vitro experiments. Life Sci., 4, 1521-1530

Glende, E.A., Jr, Hruszkewycz, A.M. & Recknagel, R.O. (1976) Critical
    role of lipid peroxidation in carbon tetrachloride-induced loss
    of aminopyrine demethylase, cytochrome P-450 and glucose 6-phospha-
    tase. Biochem. Pharmacol., 25, 2163-2170

Gordis, E. (1969) Lipid metabolites of carbon tetrachloride. J. clin. Invest., 48, 203-209

Grasselli, J.G. & Ritchey, W.M., eds (1975) CRC Atlas of Spectral Data and Physical Constants for Organic Compounds, 2nd ed., Vol. III, Cleveland, OH, Chemical Rubber Co., p. 599

Grimsrud, E.P. & Rasmussen, R.A. (1975) Survey and analysis of halo-carbons in the atmosphere by gas chromatography-mass spectrometry. Atmos. Environ., 9, 1014-1017

Halver, J.E. (1967) Crystalline aflatoxin and other vectors for trout hepatoma. US Fish Wild. Serv. Res. Rep., 70, 78-102

Hanst, P.L., Spiller, L.L., Watts, D.M., Spence, J.W. & Miller, M.F (1975) Infrared measurement of fluorocarbons, carbon tetrachloride, carbonyl sulfide, and other atmospheric trace gases. J. Air Pollut. Control Assoc., 25, 1220-1226

Harders, I., Kunz, W., Uehleke, H. & Werner, B. (1976) Irreversible binding of $^{14}CCl_4$-metabolites to reduced phosphorpyridine-nucleotides in vivo and in vitro (Abstract No. 257). Arch. Pharmacol. (Suppl.), 293, R65

Hardie, D.W.F. (1964) Chlorocarbons and chlorohydrocarbons. Carbon tetrachloride. In: Kirk, R.E. & Othmer, D.F., eds, Encyclopedia of Chemical Technology, 2nd ed., Vol. 5, New York, John Wiley & Sons, pp. 128-139

Hawley, G.G., ed. (1977) The Condensed Chemical Dictionary, 9th ed., New York, Van Nostrand-Reinhold, p. 165

Heuser, S.G. & Scudamore, K.A. (1968) Methods, apparatus: new product research, process development and design. Chem. Ind., 24 August, pp. 1154-1157

Heuser, S.G. & Scudamore, K. A. (1969) Determination of fumigant residues in cereals and other foodstuffs: a multi-detection scheme for gas chromatography of solvent extracts. J. Sci. Food Agric., 20, 566-572

Horwitz, W., ed. (1970) Official Methods of Analysis of the Association of Official Analytical Chemists, 11th ed., Washington DC, Association of Official Analytical Chemists, pp. 680-682

Horwitz, W., ed. (1975) Official Methods of Analysis of the Association of Official Analytical Chemists, 12th ed., Washington DC, Association of Official Analytical Chemists, pp. 91, 658-660

IARC (1972) IARC Monographs on the Evaluation of Carcinogenic Risk
    of Chemicals to Man, 1, Lyon, pp. 53-60

Johns, R. (1976) Air Pollution Assessment of Carbon Tetrachloride,
    PB 256 732, Springfield, VA, National Technical Information Service

Johnstone, R.T. (1948) Occupational Medicine and Industrial Hygiene
    St Louis, MO, C.V. Mosby Company, p. 157

Kanematsu, T. (1976) Promoting effect of carbon tetrachloride on azo-dye
    hepatocarcinogenesis in rats. Fukuoka Igaku Zasshi, 67, 134-145

Kawasaki, H. (1965) Development of tumor in the course of spontaneous
    restoration of carbon tetrachloride induced cirrhosis of the liver
    in rats. Kurume med. J., 12, 37-42

Kiplinger, G.F. & Kensler, C.J. (1963) Failure of phenoxybenzamine to
    prevent formation of hepatomas after chronic carbon tetrachloride
    administration. J. natl Cancer Inst., 30, 837-843

Klaassen, C.D. & Plaa, G.L. (1966) Relative effects of various chlorinated
    hydrocarbons on liver and kidney function in mice. Toxicol. appl.
    Pharmacol., 9, 139-151

Klaassen, C.D. & Plaa, G.L. (1967) Relative effects of various chlorinated
    hydrocarbons on liver and kidney function in dogs. Toxicol. appl.
    Pharmacol., 10, 119-131

Klaassen, C.D. & Plaa, G.L. (1969) Comparison of the biochemical
    alterations elicited in livers from rats treated with carbon
    tetrachloride, chloroform, 1,1,2-trichloroethane and 1,1,1-
    trichloroethane. Biochem. Pharmacol., 18, 2019-2027

Lemonnier, F.J., Scotto, J.M. & Thuong-Trieu, C. (1974) Disturbances
    in tryptophan metabolism after a single dose of aflatoxin B_1
    and chronic intoxication with carbon tetrachloride. J. natl Cancer
    Inst., 53, 745-749

Lillian, D. & Singh, H.B. (1974) Absolute determination of atmospheric
    halocarbons by gas phase coulometry. Anal. Chem., 46, 1060-1063

Lillian, D., Singh, H.B., Appleby, A., Lobban, L., Arnts, R., Gumpert, R.,
    Hague, R., Toomey, J., Kazazis, J., Antell, M., Hansen, D. & Scott,
    B. (1975) Atmospheric fates of halogenated compounds. Environ.
    Sci. Tech., 9, 1042-1048

Malone, B. (1969) Analysis of grains for multiple residues of organic
    fumigants. J. Assoc. off. anal. Chem., 52, 800-805

Malone, B. (1970) Method for determining multiple residues of organic
    fumigants in cereal grains. J. Assoc. off. anal. Chem., 53, 742-
    746

McCann, J. & Ames, B.N. (1976) Detection of carcinogens as mutagens in
    the *Salmonella*/microsome test: assay of 300 chemicals: discussion.
    Proc. natl Acad. Sci. (Wash.), 73, 950–954

McCann, J., Choi, E., Yamasaki, E. & Ames, B.N. (1975) Detection of
    carcinogens as mutagens in the *Salmonella*/microsome test: assay
    of 300 chemicals. Proc. natl Acad. Sci. (Wash.), 72, 5135–5139

McCollister, D.D., Beamer, W.H., Atchison, G.J. & Spencer, H.C. (1951)
    The absorption, distribution and elimination of radioactive
    carbon tetrachloride by monkeys upon exposure to low vapor
    concentrations. J. Pharmacol. exp. Ther., 102, 112–124

McConnell, G., Ferguson, D.M. & Pearson, C.R. (1975) Chlorinated
    hydrocarbons and the environment. Endeavour, 34, 13–18

Mercier, M.C. (1977) Criteria (Exposure/Effect Relationships) for
    Organochlorine Solvents, Doc. V/F/177-4, Luxembourg, Commission
    of the European Communities, pp. 59–93

Morris, R.L. & Johnson, L.G. (1976) Agricultural runoff as a source
    of halomethanes in drinking water. J. Am. Water Works Assoc.,
    September, pp. 492–494

Nachtomi, E. & Alumot, E. (1972) Comparison of ethylene dibromide
    and carbon tetrachloride toxicity in rats and chicks: blood and
    liver levels; lipid peroxidation. Exp. mol. Pathol., 16, 71–78

National Cancer Institute (1976) Report on Carcinogenesis Bioassay of
    Chloroform, Bethesda, MD, Carcinogenesis Program, Division of Cancer
    Cause & Prevention

National Institute for Occupational Safety & Health (1976)
    Criteria document: recommendations for a carbon tetrachloride
    standard. Occup. Saf. Health Rep., 5, 1247–1253

National Institute for Occupational Safety & Health (1977a)
    National Occupational Hazard Survey, Vol. III, Survey Analyses and
    Supplemental Tables, Cincinnati, OH, US Department of Health, Education,
    & Welfare, pp. 444, 2539–2547

National Institute for Occupational Safety & Health (1977b)
    NIOSH Manual of Analytical Methods, 2nd ed., Part II, Standards
    Completion Program Validated Methods, Vol. 3, Method S314,
    DHEW (NIOSH), Publ. No. 77-157-B, Washington DC, US Government
    Printing Office, pp. S314-1–S314-9

New, P.S., Lubash, G.D., Scherr, L. & Rubin, A.L. (1962) Acute renal
    failure associated with carbon tetrachloride intoxication.
    J. Am. med. Assoc., 181, 903–906

Nicholson, A.A., Meresz, O. & Lemyk, B. (1977) Determination of free
    and total potential haloforms in drinking water. Anal. Chem., 49,
    814-819

Ohta, T., Morita, M. & Mizoguchi, I. (1976) Local distribution of
    chlorinated hydrocarbons in the ambient air in Tokyo. Atmos.
    Environ., 10, 557-560

Pani, P., Torrielli, M.V., Gabriel, L. & Gravela, E. (1973)
    Further observation on the effects of 3-methylcholanthrene and
    phenobarbital on carbon tetrachloride hepatotoxicity.
    Exp. mol. Pathol., 19, 15-22

Pearson, C.R. & McConnell, G. (1975) Chlorinated C_1 and C_2 hydrocarbons
    in the marine environment. Proc. R. Soc. Lond. B., 189, 305-332

Plaa, G.L., Evans, E.A. & Hine, C.H. (1958) Relative hepatotoxicity
    of seven halogenated hydrocarbons. J. Pharmacol. exp. Ther.,
    123, 224-229

Pound, A.W. (1978) Influence of carbon tetrachloride on induction of
    tumours of the liver and kidneys in mice by nitrosamines.
    Br. J. Cancer, 37, 67-75

Pound, A.W., Lawson, T.A. & Horn, L. (1973a) Increased carcinogenic
    action of dimethylnitrosamine after prior administration of
    carbon tetrachloride. Br. J. Cancer, 27, 451-459

Pound, A.W., Horn, L. & Lawson, T.A. (1973b) Decreased toxicity of
    dimethylnitrosamine in rats after treatment with carbon
    tetrachloride. Pathology, 5, 233-242

Premel-Cabic, A., Cailleux, A. & Allain, P. (1974) A gas chromatographic
    assay of fifteen volatile organic solvents in blood (Fr.) Clin.
    chim. acta , 56, 5-11

Rao, K.S. & Recknagel, R.O. (1969) Early incorporation of carbon-
    labeled carbon tetrachloride into rat liver particulate lipids
    and proteins. Exp. mol. Pathol., 10, 219-228

Recknagel, R.O. (1967) Carbon tetrachloride hepatoxicity. Pharmacol.
    Rev., 19, 145-208

Recknagel, R.O. & Ghoshal, A.K. (1966) Lipoperoxidation as a vector
    in carbon tetrachloride hepatotoxicity. Lab. Invest., 15, 132-148

Recknagel, R.O. & Glende, E.A., Jr (1973) Carbon tetrachloride
    hepatotoxicity: an example of lethal cleavage. CRC Crit. Rev.
    Toxicol., 2, 263-297

Recknagel, R.O. & Litteria, M. (1960) Biochemical changes in carbon tetrachloride fatty liver. Concentration of carbon tetrachloride in liver and blood. Am. J. Pathol., 36, 521-531

Reckner, L.R. & Sachdev, J. (1975) Collaborative Testing of Activated Charcoal Sampling Tubes for Seven Organic Solvents, National Institute for Occupational Safety & Health, Contract No. HSM 99-72-98. Available from Washington DC, US Government Printing Office, pp. 1.0, 2-1-2-4, 3-1-3-6

Reuber, M.D. & Glover, E.L. (1967) Hyperplastic and early neoplastic lesions of the liver in Buffalo strain rats of various ages given subcutaneous carbon tetrachloride. J. natl Cancer Inst., 38, 891-899

Reuber, M.D. & Glover, E.L. (1970) Cirrhosis and carcinoma of the liver in male rats given subcutaneous carbon tetrachloride. J. natl Cancer Inst., 44, 419-427

Reynolds, E.S. (1967) Liver parenchymal cell injury. IV. Pattern of incorporation of carbon and chlorine from carbon tetrachloride into chemical constituents of liver in vivo. J. Pharmacol. exp. Ther., 155, 117-126

Rocchi, P., Prodi, G., Grilli, S. & Ferreri, A.M. (1973) In vivo and in vitro binding of carbon tetrachloride with nucleic acids and proteins in rat and mouse liver. Int. J. Cancer, 11, 419-425

Roschlau, G. & Rodenkirchen, H. (1969) Histological examination of the diaplacental action of carbon tetrachloride and allyl alcohol in mice embryos (Germ.). Exp. Path., 3, 255-263

Rubinstein, D. & Kanics, L. (1964) The conversion of carbon tetrachloride and chloroform to carbon dioxide by rat liver homogenates. Can. J. Biochem., 42, 1577-1585

Russell, J.W. & Shadoff, L.A. (1977) The sampling and determination of halocarbons in ambient air using concentration on porous polymer. J. Chromatogr., 134, 375-384

Safe Drinking Water Committee (1977) Drinking Water and Health, Washington DC, National Academy of Sciences, p. 703

Sasame, H.A., Castro, J.A. & Gillette, J.R. (1968) Studies on the destruction of liver microsomal cytochrome P-450 by carbon tetrachloride administration. Biochem. Pharmacol., 17, 1759-1768

Saunders, R.A., Blachly, C.H., Kovacina, T.A., Lamontagne, R.A., Swinnerton, J.W. & Saalfeld, F.E. (1975)   Identification of volatile organic contaminants in Washington, D.C. municipal water.   Water Res., 9, 1143-1145

Schwetz, B.A., Leong, B.K.J. & Gehring, P.J. (1974)   Embryo- and feto-toxicity of inhaled carbon tetrachloride, 1,1-dichloroethane and methyl ethyl ketone in rats.   Toxicol. appl. Pharmacol., 28, 452-464

Seawright, A.A. & McLean, A.E.M. (1967)   The effect of diet on carbon tetrachloride metabolism.   Biochem. J., 105, 1055-1060

Seto, H., Akiyama, K. & Mizoguchi, I. (1977)   An application of gas-phase coulometry for determination of atmospheric halocarbons (Jap.).   Taiki Osen Kenkyu, 11, 214-218 [Chem. Abstr., 87, 122112e]

Shackelford, W.M. & Keith, L.H. (1976)   Frequency of Organic Compounds Identified in Water, EPA-600/4-76-062, Athens, GA, US Environmental Protection Agency, pp. 163-164

Simler, M., Maurer, M. & Mandard, J.C. (1964)   Liver cancer after cirrhosis due to carbon tetrachloride (Fr.).   Strasbourg méd., 15, 910-918

Simmonds, P.G., Kerrin, S.L., Lovelock, J.E. & Shair, F.H. (1974)   Distribution of atmospheric halocarbons in the air over the Los Angeles Basin.   Atmos. Environ., 8, 209-216

Singh, B.H., Lillian, D., Appleby, A. & Lobban, L. (1975)   Atmospheric formation of carbon tetrachloride from tetrachloroethylene.   Environ. Lett., 10, 253-256

Slater, T.F. (1966)   Necrogenic action of carbon tetrachloride in the rat: a speculative mechanism based on activation.   Nature (Lond.), 209, 36-40

Smuckler, E.A. (1976)   Structural and functional changes in acute liver injury.   Environ. Health Perspect., 15, 13-25

Smuckler, E.A., Arrhenius, E. & Hultin, T. (1967)   Alterations in micro-somal electron transport, oxidative N-demethylation and azo-dye cleavage in carbon tetrachloride and dimethylnitrosamine-induced liver injury.   Biochem. J., 103, 55-64

Smyth, H.F., Jr, Weil, C.S., West, J.S. & Carpenter, C.P. (1970)   An exploration of joint toxic action.   II. Equitoxic versus equivolume mixtures.   Toxicol. appl. Pharmacol., 17, 498-503

Stewart, R.D. & Dodd, H.C. (1964)   Absorption of carbon tetrachloride, trichloroethylene, tetrachloroethylene, methylene chloride, and 1,1,1-trichloroethane through the human skin.   Am. ind. Hyg. Assoc. J., 25, 439-446

Stewart, R.D., Gay, H.H., Erley, D.S., Hake, C.L. & Peterson, J.E. (1961) Human exposure to carbon tetrachloride vapor. Relationship of expired air concentration to exposure and toxicity. J. occup. Med., 3, 586-590

Stewart, R.D., Boettner, E.A., Southworth, R.R. & Cerny, J.C. (1963) Acute carbon tetrachloride intoxication. J. Am. med. Assoc., 183, 994-997

Suriyachan, D. & Thithapandha, A. (1977) Modification of carbon tetrachloride hepatotoxicity by chemicals. Toxicol. appl. Pharmacol., 41, 369-376

Symons, J.M., Bellar, T.A., Carswell, J.K., De Marco, J., Kropp, K.L., Robeck, G.G., Seeger, D.R., Slocum, C.J., Smith, B.L. & Stevens, A.A. (1975) National Organics Reconnaissance Survey for halogenated organics. J. Am. Water Works Assoc., November, pp. 634-647

Tracey, J.P. & Sherlock, P. (1968) Hepatoma following carbon tetra-chloride poisoning. NY State J. Med., 68, 2202-2204

Tsirel'nikov, N.I. & Tsirel'nikova, T.G. (1976) Morphohistochemical study of the rat placenta after exposure to carbon tetrachloride at different stages of pregnancy. Byull. eksp. Biol. Med., 82, 1007-1009

Uehleke, H. (1977) Binding of haloalkanes to liver microsomes. In: Jollow, D.J., Kocsis, J.J., Snyder, R. & Vainio, H., eds, Biological Reactive Intermediates, Formation, Toxicity, and Inactivation, New York, Plenum, pp. 431-445

Uehleke, H. & Werner, T. (1975) A comparative study on the irreversible binding of labeled halothane trichlorofluoromethane, chloroform, and carbon tetrachloride to hepatic protein and lipids in vitro and in vivo. Arch. Toxikol., 34, 289-308

Uehleke, H., Greim, H., Krämer, M. & Werner, T. (1976) Covalent binding of haloalkanes to liver constituents, but absence of mutagenicity on bacteria in a metabolizing test system (Abstract No. 25). Mutat. Res., 38, 114

Uehleke, H., Werner, T., Greim, H. & Krämer, M. (1977) Metabolic activation of haloalkanes and tests in vitro for mutagenicity. Xenobiotica, 7, 393-400

US Department of Commerce (1977a) US Imports for Consumption and General Imports, TSUSA Commodity by Country of Origin, FT 246/Annual 1976, Washington DC, US Government Printing Office, p. 230

US Department of Commerce (1977b)   US Exports, Schedule B Commodity by
    Country, FT 410/December 1976, Washington DC, US Government Printing
    Office, p. 2-85

US Environmental Protection Agency (1970)   Carbon tetrachloride; findings
    of fact and conclusions and final order regarding classification as
    banned hazardous substances.   Part 191.   Fed. Regist., 35, 13198-
    13205

US Environmental Protection Agency (1971)   EPA Compendium of Registered
    Pesticides, Washington DC, US Government Printing Office, p. III-C-11

US Environmental Protection Agency (1976)   Protection of environment.
    Carbon tetrachloride; exemption from the requirement of a tolerance.
    US Code Fed. Regul., Title 40, part 180.1005, p. 379

US International Trade Commission (1977)   Synthetic Organic Chemicals,
    US Production and Sales, 1976, USITC Publication 833, Washington DC,
    US Government Printing Office, p. 302

US Occupational Safety & Health Administration (1977)   Air contaminants.
    US Code Fed. Regul., Title 29, part 1910.1000, p. 26

Von Oettingen, W.F. (1964)   The Halogenated Hydrocarbons of Industrial
    and Toxicological Importance, Amsterdam, Elsevier, pp. 107-170

Weisburger, E.K. (1977)   Carcinogenicity studies on halogenated hydro-
    carbons.   Environ. Health Perspect., 21, 7-16

WHO (1972)   1971 Evaluations of some pesticide residues in food.
    World Health Organ. Pestic. Residues Ser., No. 1, pp. 259-265

Winell, M. (1975)   An international comparison of hygienic standards
    for chemicals in the work environment.   Ambio, 4, 34-36

Yokoro, K., Takizawa, S., Kawamura, Y., Nakano, M. & Kawase, A. (1973)
    Multicarcinogenicity of N-nitrosobutylurea in mice and rats as
    demonstrated by host conditioning.   Gann, 64, 193-196

Zuercher, F. & Giger, W. (1976)   Volatile organic trace components in
    the Glatt [river] (Germ.).   Vom Wasser, 47, 37-55 [Chem. Abstr.,
    87, 58231p]

CHLOROFORM

This substance was considered by a previous Working Group, in December 1971 (IARC, 1972). Since that time new data have become available, and these have been incorporated into the monograph and taken into consideration in the present evaluation.

Three reviews on chloroform, including a literature collection, are available (Berkowitz, 1978; Mercier, 1977; Winslow & Gerstner, 1977).

1. Chemical and Physical Data

1.1 Synonyms and trade names

Chem. Abstr. Services Reg. No.: 67-66-3

Chem. Abstr. Name: Trichloromethane

Synonyms: Formyl trichloride; methane trichloride; methenyl chloride; methenyl trichloride; methyl trichloride; trichloroform

Trade names: Freon 20; R 20; R 20 [refrigerant]

1.2 Structural and molecular formulae and molecular weight

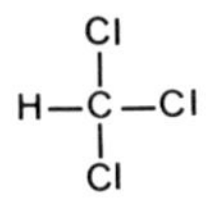

$$H-\overset{\textstyle Cl}{\underset{\textstyle Cl}{\overset{|}{\underset{|}{C}}}}-Cl$$

CHCl$_3$ Mol. wt: 119.4

1.3 Chemical and physical properties of the pure substance

From Hawley (1977), unless otherwise specified

(a) Description: Clear, colourless liquid

(b) Boiling-point: 61.2°C

(c) Freezing-point: -63.5°C

(d) Density: d_{20}^{20} 1.485

(e) Spectroscopy data: $\lambda_{vap} < 200$ nm; infra-red, nuclear magnetic resonance and mass spectral data have been tabulated (Grasselli & Ritchey, 1975).

(f) Refractive index: n_D^{25} 1.4422

(g) Solubility: Miscible with ethanol, diethyl ether, benzene, solvent naphtha and fixed and volatile oils; slightly soluble in water (0.822 g/100 g water at 20°C) (Hardie, 1964)

(h) Volatility: Vapour pressure is 200 mm at 25.9°C (Perry & Chilton, 1973).

(i) Stability: Decomposes slowly on prolonged exposure to sunlight in the presence or absence of air, and in the dark when air is present (Hardie, 1964).

(j) Reactivity: Oxidized by strong oxidizing agents such as chromic acid, with formation of phosgene and chlorine gas; reacts readily with halogens or halogenating agents, forming various products depending on the reactants and reaction conditions; reacts with primary amines to form isonitriles; reacts with phenols in alkaline solution, forming hydroxy-substituted aromatic aldehydes (Hardie, 1964)

(k) Conversion factor: 1 ppm in air is equivalent to approximately 4.9 mg/m^3.

1.4 Technical products and impurities

Typical specifications for National Formulary grade chloroform are as follows: boiling-range, 59.8-71.3°C (760 mm); acidity, as hydrogen chloride, 0.0002% max; specific gravity at 25/25°C, 1.474-1.478; residue on evaporation, 0.0013% max; and stabilizer, 0.5-1.0% ethanol by volume.

Technical-grade chloroform has the following specifications: boiling-range, 59.8-61.3°C (760 mm); acidity, as hydrogen chloride, 0.002% max; specific gravity at 25/25°C, 1.476-1.480; residue on evaporation, 0.0007% max; moisture, 0.0150% max; and stabilizer, 0.5-1.0% ethanol by volume.

The following impurities have been detected in chloroform: bromo-chloromethane, bromodichloroethane, bromodichloromethane, carbon tetra-chloride (see monograph, p. 371), dibromodichloroethane, dibromodichloro-methane, 1,1-dichloroethane, 1,2-dichloroethane (see monograph, p. 429), vinylidene chloride (see IARC, 1978a), *cis*-1,2-dichloroethene, *trans*-1,2-dichloroethylene, dichloromethane (see monograph, p. 449), diethyl carbonate, ethylbenzene, 2-methoxyethanol, nitromethane, pyridine, 1,1,2,2-tetra-chloroethane (see monograph, p. 477), trichloroethylene (see monograph, p. 545), *meta*-xylene, *ortho*-xylene and *para*-xylene.

N-Nitrosomorpholine was found in 4/10 batches of analytical grade chloroform, at levels of 2-376 µg/1 (Eisenbrand *et al.*, 1978; IARC, 1978b).

In Japan, chloroform has a minimum purity of 99.95% and may contain water and chlorinated hydrocarbons as impurities.

2. Production, Use, Occurrence and Analysis

2.1 Production and use

(a) Production

Chloroform was prepared, almost simultaneously in 1831, by Liebig (by the action of alkali on chloral) and by Soubeirain (by treating bleaching powder with ethanol or acetone) (Hardie, 1964). It is current-ly manufactured in the US by hydrochlorination of methanol or by chlori-nation of methane. All chloroform production in Japan and western Europe is by chlorination of methane.

Although one US manufacturer began chloroform production in 1903, by reduction of carbon tetrachloride, commercial production was not reported until 1922 (US Tariff Commission, 1923). Immediately prior to World War II, total combined annual output of the US and the UK was 1-1.5 million kg (Hardie, 1964). In 1976, 5 US producers reported a total production of 133 million kg (US International Trade Commission, 1977). Preliminary data indicated that US production in 1977 was 137 million kg (US International Trade Commission, 1978). US imports in 1976 amounted to 503 thousand kg, 99% of which was from Spain (US Department of Commerce, 1977a); 8.8 million kg were exported to the following countries (percent of total exports): The Netherlands (37), Canada (23), Brazil (19), Mexico (12), Argentina (5) and at least one other country (4) (US Department of Commerce, 1977b).

Annual production of chloroform in eastern Europe is estimated to be 10-50 million kg, and that in western Europe 50-100 million kg. Benelux, the Federal Republic of Germany, France and the UK are the major producing regions; and Austria, Italy, Scandinavia, Spain and Switzer-land are minor producers.

Chloroform has been produced commercially in Japan since 1950.   In 1976, 4 companies produced an estimated 20 million kg, and exports were negligible.

The estimated world production of chloroform in 1973 was 245 million kg (Pearson & McConnell, 1975).

(b) Use

Use of chloroform in the US in 1974 was as follows: synthesis of chlorodifluoromethane (Fluorocarbon 22) for use in refrigerants and propellants, 51.3%; synthesis of Fluorocarbon 22 for use in plastics, 24%; and miscellaneous uses, 24,7%.

In 1976, US production of Fluorocarbon 22 amounted to 77.1 million kg (US International Trade Commission, 1977).   In 1973, 40.4 million kg Fluorocarbon 22 were used for air conditioning and refrigeration purposes. It is used in residential and commercial unit air conditioners, heat pumps, centrifrugal chillers and motor vehicle air conditioners (US Department of Commerce, 1975).   Fluorocarbon 22 is pyrolysed to produce polytetrafluoroethylene (see IARC, 1978c), the major volume fluoroplastic. Fluorocarbon 22 is also used to foam plastics, although Fluorocarbons 11 and 12 are most commonly used for this purpose (US Department of Commerce, 1975).

Miscellaneous uses of chloroform have been in drugs and cosmetics (including toothpastes), in the extraction and purification of penicillin and other antibiotics, in the solvent extraction of vitamins and flavours, in grain fumigants, as a general solvent (e.g., for adhesives, resins and pesticides) and as an intermediate in the preparation of dyes, drugs and pesticides.

Chloroform was first employed medically as an orally administered stimulant and as an inhalant for treatment of asthma; it was first used as an anaesthetic in obstetrics in 1847.   Before World War II, chloro- form was still being used primarily as an anaesthetic and in pharmaceutical preparations; but by 1964, only about 10% was so used (Hardie, 1964).

In western Europe, chloroform is used primarily in the synthesis of Fluorocarbon 22.   In Japan, in 1976, 80% was used as a refrigerant and 20% for solvent uses.

In April 1976, the US Food and Drug Administration (FDA) listed approximately 1900 human drug products that contained chloroform.   These included cough syrups, expectorants, antihistamines, liniments and decongestants (US Food & Drug Administration, 1976a).   The FDA banned the use of chloroform as an ingredient (active or inactive) in human drug and cosmetic products as of 29 July, 1976.   However, any drug product containing chloroform in residual amounts from its use as a processing

solvent in manufacture or as a by-product from the synthesis of an
ingredient is not considered to contain chloroform as an ingredient (US
Food & Drug Administration, 1976b).

Chloroform is registered for use in the US as an insecticidal
fumigant on stored barley, corn, oats, popcorn, rice, rye, sorghum and
wheat (US Environmental Protection Agency, 1971). In 1971, farmers
used approximately 51 thousand kg chloroform for fumigant purposes.
Chloroform is exempted from the requirement of a tolerance for residues
on agricultural commodities when used as a solvent and when used as a
fumigant after harvest for the following grains: barley, corn, oats,
popcorn, rice, rye, sorghum and wheat (US Environmental Protection
Agency, 1976a).

A notice of rebuttable presumption against registration and continued
registration (RPAR) (see General Remarks on Substances Considered,
p. 31) of pesticide products containing chloroform was issued by the
US Environmental Protection Agency on 6 April, 1976 (US Environmental
Protection Agency, 1976b). The future use of chloroform in agriculture
in the US depends largely on the outcome of these actions.

The US Occupational Safety and Health Administration's health
standards require that an employee's exposure to chloroform at no time
exceed 240 mg/m^3 (50 ppm) (US Occupational Safety & Health Administration,
1978). On 9 June 1976, the US National Institute for Occupational
Safety and Health recommended that occupational exposure to chloroform
be controlled so that no employees be exposed to chloroform in excess of
9.78 mg/m^3 (2 ppm) in air as determined by a 1-hr air sample (National
Institute for Occupational Safety & Health, 1976).

2.2 Occurrence

Chloroform may be formed in the troposphere by solar-induced
photochemical reactions of trichloroethylene (Appleby et $al.$, 1976).

(a) Air

Maximum levels of chloroform found in the atmosphere at any one
location ranged from < 0.05-73.5 µg/m^3 (< 0.01-15 ppb); minimum levels
were all less than 0.05 µg/m^3 (0.01 ppb); and mean levels, 0.045-5 µg/m^3
(0.009-1.03 ppb) (Lillian et $al.$, 1975). Background concentrations of
atmospheric chloroform, defined numerically as the average of the lower
50% of data points, were determined for two sites as 100 and 130 ng/m^3
(Singh et $al.$, 1977).

Chloroform was detected in rural atmospheres at levels of 100 ng/m^3
(Grimsrud & Rasmussen, 1975) and 100-180 ng/m^3 (Russell & Shadoff, 1977).

Atmospheric concentrations of chloroform at ground level at sites in the northern and southern hemispheres were 130 ng/m^3 and < 15 ng/m^3, respectively (Cox *et al.*, 1976).

Chloroform has been detected as a photochemical product in simulated ambient air containing trichloroethylene. It is suggested that a portion of the total atmospheric content of chloroform may result from tropospheric irradiation of trichloroethylene in air (Appleby *et al.*, 1976).

(b) Water

The occurrence and formation of chloroform in drinking-water have been reviewed (Bellar *et al.*, 1974; Morris & McKay, 1975).

Chloroform has been found in rivers, lakes, ground-water, commercial effluent water and sewage treatment plant effluent water at nearly 100 US and European locations (Shackelford & Keith, 1976). It has been detected in tap-water in the US and Czechoslovakia in concentrations ranging from 1.7-910 μg/l, and in waste-water discharges from the treatment of sewage and industrial wastes in concentrations ranging from 7.1-12.1 μg/l (Eurocop-Cost, 1976).

In 1975, a National Organics Reconnaissance Survey measured levels of chloroform in 80 US water supplies distributed over various regions of the US and representing a wide variety of raw-water sources and treatment techniques. Chloroform was present in raw water at 49 locations, in concentrations of < 1 μg/l, with the exception of one source that was receiving chlorinated raw water. All of the finished waters tested contained chloroform in concentrations ranging from < 0.1-311 μg/l (Symons *et al.*, 1975).

Chloroform was found at concentrations of 47-92 μg/l in drinking-water at 4 locations (Kleopfer, 1976), at about 5 μg/l at another location (Saunders *et al.*, 1975) and in 2 other locations (Bertsch *et al.*, 1975).

It was detected in river water at the entrance to a water treatment facility, in the clarifier effluent stage of the water treatment process and in the finished water, at relative concentrations of 1.17:1.87:8.73 (Dowty *et al.*, 1975).

Periods of high agricultural runoff have been found to be associated with peaks in chloroform concentrations, due to the increased turbidity of the raw water (Morris & Johnson, 1976).

Chloroform has been detected in drinking-water in Japan; the concentration at one site was 18-36 μg/l and was reportedly related to the chlorine dosing rate at the water purification plant and to the types of residual chlorine present (Kajino, 1977; Morita, 1976).

The maximum concentration of chloroform found in a survey sampling bay-water at 172 stations was 1 µg/l (Pearson & McConnell, 1975).

(c)   Food

Residues of a fumigant mixture of carbon disulphide, carbon tetrachloride, chloroform and trichloroethylene were determined in cereals aired at 17°C and 30°C.   Initial chloroform residues in barley aired at the two temperatures were 123 and 132 mg/kg. After 60 days, residues had disappeared from that aired at 17°C but were still present at 16 mg/kg in that aired at 30°C.   Initial residues in corn were 189 and 224 mg/kg; after 60 days they had disappeared at 17° but were still present at 16 mg/kg at 30°C.   Initial residues in sorghum were 176 mg/kg at 17°C and 178 mg/kg at 30°C; after 25 days, residues had disappeared at 17°C, but they were still present at 22 mg/kg after 60 days at 30°C (Alumot & Bielorai, 1969).

The following concentrations of chloroform were found in foodstuffs in the UK in 1973: dairy produce, 1.4-33 mg/kg; meat, 1-4 mg/kg; oils and fats, 2-10 mg/kg; beverages, 0.4-18 mg/kg; and fruits and vegetables, 2-18 mg/kg (McConnell *et al.*, 1975).

(d)   Marine organisms

Concentrations of chloroform in 5 species of fish and 3 species of molluscs collected from relatively clean sea-water ranged from 56-1040 µg/kg (dry-weight basis) in the various organs of molluscs and from 7-851 µg/kg (dry-weight basis) in fish. Relative concentrations in the organs of fish were found to be: brain > gill > liver > muscle (Dickson & Riley, 1976).

(e)   Humans

Chloroform has been detected in post-mortem human tissue samples, at levels of 1-68 µg/kg (wet tissue) (McConnell *et al.*, 1975). In expired air, traces to 11 µg/hr/subject have been found (Conkle *et al.*, 1975).

(f)   Occupational exposure

A 1974 National Occupational Hazard Survey noted that workers primarily exposed to chloroform were those in hospitals, department stores and in the biological products, internal combustion engine and building paper and board industries (National Institute for Occupational Safety & Health, 1977a).

2.3 Analysis

Analytical methods to determine chloroform in environmental samples, mostly based on chromatographic techniques, have been reviewed (Fishbein, 1973; National Institute for Occupational Safety & Health, 1974).

Methods of analysis used for the analysis of chloroform in environmental samples are listed in Table 1.

A number of comparative studies on analytical techniques have been undertaken. An Official First Action method for determining volatile denaturants, including chloroform, in ethanol used in flavours (Horwitz, 1970, 1975) was studied collaboratively by 6 laboratories. Chloroform was determined by gas chromatography with flame ionization detection in alcoholic solution by 10 different collaborators (Martin & Figert, 1974). The initial results of a collaborative study by 15 US laboratories on chloroform in workplace air involved collection on activated charcoal at 4 levels, ranging from 12-485 mg/m^3 (2.4-98.6 ppm), with analysis by gas chromatography (Reckner & Sachdev, 1975).

In one study, the efficiency of the removal of organic compounds, including chloroform, from aqueous solution by gas stripping, adsorption on polymeric adosrbant, thermal desorption and analysis by gas chromatography with flame ionization detection at the μg/l (ppb) level has been described (Kuo *et al.*, 1977).

Sparging of drinking-water to strip organic pollutants was compared with extraction by carbon tetrachloride or nitrobenzene. No pollutants were found by solvent extraction, but the inert gas technique resulted in the identification of a number of organic compounds, including chloroform, at a concentration of 0.91 μg/l (ppb) (Novak *et al.*, 1973).

Gas chromatography combined with infra-red and ultra-violet spectroscopy has been used to detect and identify immiscible solvents, including chloroform, in industrial waste waters, sewage and sludges (Ellison & Wallbank, 1974).

Ambient air sampling and analysis has been carried out by gas chromatography, with levels of detection of 0.3 μg/m^3 (0.06 ppb) (Lillian *et al.*, 1976). Chloroform has also been determined in ambient air using gas chromatography/mass spectrometry, with a limit of detection of 250 ng/m^3 (5 ppt) (Grimsrud & Rasmussen, 1975).

3. Biological Data Relevant to the Evaluation of Carcinogenic Risk to Humans

3.1 Carcinogenicity studies in animals

(a) Oral administration

Mouse: Groups of 5 A mice of each sex, 3 months old at the beginning of the experiment, were given 30 oral doses of 0.1, 0.2, 0.4, 0.8 or 1.6 ml/kg bw (0.15-2.4 g/kg bw) chloroform in olive oil at 4-day intervals.

TABLE 1. METHODS FOR THE ANALYSIS OF CHLOROFORM

SAMPLE TYPE	ANALYTICAL METHOD EXTRACTION/CLEAN-UP	DETECTION	LIMIT OF DETECTION	REFERENCE
Formulations				
Drugs	Heat under pressure with ethanolic potassium hydroxide to dechlorinate	Titration (Volhard)		Horwitz (1970, 1975)
Capsules & cough syrups	Mix contents with ethanol, add 10% sucrose solution, extract (carbon disulphide)	IR		Horwitz (1975)
Air				
	Trap on charcoal, extract (carbon disulphide)	GC/FID	Working range, 99.8-416 mg/m^3	National Institute for Occupational Safety & Health (1977b)
	Trap in pyridine, add sodium hydroxide solution, heat	Spectrophotometry (525 nm)	340 mg/m^3 (75 ppm) (v/v 20°C/760 mm)	Gage et al. (1962)
	Trap on charcoal or chromosorb 101, desorb by heating, retrap in line on GC column	GC/FID	Working range, 0.2-200 mg/m^3 (40 ppb-40 ppm)	Parkes et al. (1976)
Environmental air & stacks	Trap on porous polymer (Tenax), desorb by heating, retrap in line on GC column	GC/FID, ECD		Parsons & Mitzner (1975)
Ambient	Trap in Drechsel flask fitted with rubber septum, sample with gas syringe	GC/ECD	1.5 μg/m^3	Bureau International Technique des Solvants Chlorés (1976)
Water				
Drinking-water	Inject directly Sparge (carrier gas, helium), retrap on GC column	GC/ECD GC/Hall	1 μg/l 0.1 μg/l	Nicholson et al. (1977)
Drinking-water	Extract (tetralin)	GC/FID GC/MS	0.04 μg/l	Keith et al. (1976)
Drinking-water	Trap on adsorbant, desorb by heating, retrap in line on GC column	GC/MS	0.1 μg/l	Coleman et al. (1976)

TABLE 1. METHODS FOR THE ANALYSIS OF CHLOROFORM (continued)

SAMPLE TYPE	EXTRACTION/CLEAN-UP	DETECTION	LIMIT OF DETECTION	REFERENCE
Drinking-water	Inject directly	GC/ECD	< 1 µg/l	Hammarstrand (1976)
Drinking-water	Inject directly	GC/MS	0.1 µg/l	Fujii (1977)
Drinking, natural or effluent water	Cool to 4°C, extract (pentane)	GC/FID GC/ECD		Dietz & Traud (1973)
Drinking, natural or effluent water	Add sodium chloride, extract (methylcyclohexane)	GC/ECD	< 1 µg/l	Mieure (1977); Richard & Junk (1977)
Surface and drinking-water	Headspace analysis	GC/ECD	0.1 µg/l	Kaiser & Oliver (1976) Rook et al. (1975)
Municipal, artesian, de-ionized, charcoal-filtered water	Sparge (helium), trap on para-2,6-diphenylphenylene oxide, desorb by heating, retrap in line on GC	GC/MS	0.1 µg/l	Dowty et al. (1975)
Sea- and fresh-water	Extract (pentane), dry	GC/ECD	80 ng/l	Bureau International Technique des Solvants Chlorés (1976)
Food	Extract (acetone-water or aceto-nitrile-water), decant, add sodium chloride	GC/ECD GC/FID	0.1 mg/kg	Heuser & Scudamore (1969); Thompson et al. (1974a)
	Extract (acetone-water)	GC		
Biological				
Blood	Headspace analysis	GC/FID	1.5 mg/l	Premel-Cabic et al. (1974)
Blood	Shake, centrifuge	GC/FID	Working range, 10-500 mg/l	Poobalasingam (1976)

Abbreviations: IR - infra-red spectrometry; GC/FID - gas chromatography/flame-ionization detection; UV - ultra-violet spectrometry; ECD - electron capture detection; Hall - Hall conductivity detection; MS - mass spectrometry

Survivors were killed 1 month after the last treatment.   All females at
the 3 highest doses and all males at the 3 highest doses died early in
the experiment.   Nonmetastasizing hepatomas and cirrhosis were found in
all surviving females given 0.8 or 0.4 ml/kg bw per dose.   No hepatomas
were observed in those at the two lowest dose levels or in the controls
(Eschenbrenner & Miller, 1945).

A group of 24 XVII/G mice (sex unspecified), 3 months old at the
start of treatment, were administered 0.1 ml of a 40% oily solution of
chloroform by stomach tube twice weekly for 6 months.   Of 5 animals
that survived 297 days, 3 developed hepatomas (Rudali, 1967) [The
Working Group noted that no data on controls were reported].

Groups of 50 male and 50 female B6C3F1 mice, 5 weeks of age,
received a 2-5% solution of chloroform (USP grade) in corn oil by
gavage 5 times weekly for 78 weeks.   The initial dose levels for males
were 100 and 200 mg/kg bw, and those for females 200 and 400 mg/kg bw.
These doses were increased after 18 weeks to 150 and 300 mg/kg bw for
males and 250 and 500 mg/kg bw for females, so that the average levels
were 138 and 277 mg/kg bw for males and 238 and 477 mg/kg bw for females.
Pooled control groups, consisting of 77 male and 80 female mice, and
matched control groups, consisting of 20 males and 20 females, were
treated with corn oil only.   The experiment was terminated at 92-93
weeks.   The incidence of hepatocellular carcinomas in all treated groups
of mice was statistically significant (P < 0.001) when compared with
that in controls (see Table 2) (National Cancer Institute, 1976).

Rat: Groups of 50 male and 50 female Osborne-Mendel rats, 52 days
old, received a 10% solution of chloroform (USP grade) in corn oil by
gavage 5 times weekly.   Males were given doses of 90 and 180 mg/kg bw for
78 weeks; female rats started on dose levels of 125 and 250 mg/kg bw, but
these were lowered to 90 and 180 mg/kg bw after 22 weeks, giving an
average level of 100 and 200 mg/kg bw for the study.   Pooled control
groups of 100 males and 100 females and matched control groups of 20
males and 20 females were treated with the vehicle only.   The experiment
was terminated at 111 weeks.   The incidence of kidney epithelial tumours
in male rats was statistically greater (P=0.0016) than that in controls
(see Table 2) (National Cancer Institute, 1976).

(b) Subcutaneous and/or intramuscular administration

Newborn mouse: An unspecified number of (C57 x DBA2 F1) mice
received subcutaneously either a single dose of 200 µg chloroform in
0.02 ml arachis oil when less than 24 hrs old or 8 daily doses of 200 µg
during the first week of life.   They were killed when 77-80 weeks old.
It was reported that no evidence of carcinogenicity was obtained (Roe *et
al*., 1968) [The Working Group noted the inadequate reporting of the
experiment].

TABLE 2. TUMOUR INCIDENCES IN MICE AND RATS GIVEN GRADED DOSES OF CHLOROFORM BY GAVAGE

SPECIES	DOSE (mg/kg bw) INITIAL	DOSE (mg/kg bw) FINAL	SEX	NUMBER OF ANIMALS	NUMBER OF TUMOUR-BEARING ANIMALS/ NUMBER OF ANIMALS EXAMINED HISTOLOGICALLY KIDNEY	LIVER	THYROID[a]
B6C3F1 mice	100	150[b]	M	50	1/50	18/50[c]	0/48
	200	250	F	50	0/45	36/45[c]	0/41
	200	300	M	50	2/45	44/45[c]	0/43
	400	500	F	50	0/40	39/41[c]	0/36
Matched controls Corn oil			M	20	1/18	1/18[c]	0/17
			F	20	0/20	0/20	0/20
Pooled controls Corn oil			M	77	1/77	5/77[e]	0/77
			F	80	0/80	1/80	0/80
Osborne-Mendel rats	90	90	M	50	4/50[d]	0/50	3/49[f]
	125	90[e]	F	50	0/49	0/49	8/49[f]
	180	180[e]	M	50	12/50[g]	1/50[c]	4/48
	250	180[e]	F	50	2/48	0/48	10/46[h]
Matched controls Corn oil			M	20	0/19	0/19	4/19
			F	20	0/20	0/20	1/19
Pooled controls Corn oil			M	100	0/99	1/99[c]	8/99
			F	100	0/98	0/98	1/98

[a] No biological significance attached to findings
[b] Dosage increased to final levels after 18 weeks
[c] Carcinomas
[d] 2 carcinomas + 2 adenomas
[e] Dosage reduced to final levels after 22 weeks
[f] 7 adenomas + 1 carcinoma
[g] 10 carcinomas + 3 adenomas
[h] 7 adenomas + 3 carcinomas

(c) Intraperitoneal administration

Mouse: Groups of 20 male A/St mice, 6-8 weeks old, were given
thrice weekly i.p. injections of 80, 200 or 400 mg/kg bw chloroform in
tricaprylin for 8 weeks, except for those given the highest dose, which
received only 2 injections per week. All survivors were killed 24 weeks
after the first injection. No increase in the incidence of lung tumours
was observed in comparison with tricaprylin-injected controls (Theiss
et al., 1977) [The Working Group noted the limitations of a negative
result obtained in this test system; see also General Remarks on the
Substances Considered, p. 34].

3.2 Other relevant biological data

(a) Experimental systems

Toxic effects

The acute toxicity of chloroform is species-, strain-, sex- and
age-dependent. Thus, the acute oral LD_{50}s in young and older adult
male Sprague-Dawley rats are 1336 and 1188 mg/kg bw, whereas in 14-day-
old animals it is 445 mg/kg bw (Kimura et al., 1971). The single oral
LD_{50} in male mice varied from 120 mg/kg bw in DBA/2J mice to 490 mg/kg
bw in C57BL/6J mice (Hill et al., 1975).

Males of many mouse strains are susceptible to renal tubular
necrosis, whereas females are not similarly affected. The response
to chloroform increased with age of the mice. Strains C3H, $C3H_f$, A
and HR were susceptible, and strains C57BL, C57L, C57BR/cd and ST
resistant, to exposure (Deringer et al., 1953).

Liver damage was the cause of death of rats and mice after acute
administration of chloroform (Brown et al., 1974a; Doyle et al., 1967).
An early dilatation of the granular endoplasmic reticulum, with detach-
ment of the ribosomes, was observed in the livers of treated rats
(Scholler, 1968). In rats, rabbits and guinea-pigs exposed to 125, 250
or 425 mg/m^3 (25, 50 or 85 ppm) chloroform in air, and in dogs exposed
to 25 ppm, for 7 hrs/day on 5 days/week for 6 months, histopathological
alterations in the liver and kidney, higher mortality and changes in
organ weights were observed; centrilobular granular degeneration was
seen in rat liver. These effects appeared to be reversible in rats
given only 25 ppm (Torkelson et al., 1976).

Embryotoxicity and teratogenicity

Doses of 20, 50 or 126 mg/kg bw/day were given to rats on days 6-15
of gestation, and 20, 35 or 50 mg/kg bw/day to rabbits on days 6-18 of
gestation; reduced birth weights were observed with the highest dose
levels in both species. There was no evidence of teratogenicity in
either species with any dose level (Thompson et al., 1974b).

Rats were exposed to subanaesthetic doses of chloroform: 150, 500 and 1500 mg/m^3 (30, 100 and 300 ppm), in air by inhalation for 7 hrs per day on days 6-15 of gestation.   The 100 ppm dose caused a low incidence of acaudate foetuses with imperforate anuses.   All doses of chloroform were foetotoxic and retarded development (Schwetz et al., 1974).

It was reported in an abstract that chloroform caused increased foetal mortality and decreased foetal weight, but no teratogenic effects were observed when pregnant rats were exposed to 20.1 ± 1.2 g/m^3 during days 7-14 of gestation (Dilley et al., 1977).

Absorption, distribution, excretion and metabolism

Chloroform is rapidly absorbed and distributed to all organs, with relatively high concentrations in nervous tissue (Von Oettingen, 1964). After intraduodenal injection of ^{14}C-chloroform to rats, 70% of the chloroform was found unchanged in the expired air and 4% as ^{14}CO$_2$ during 24 hrs.   At least 75% of the radioactivity was excreted in the expired air in 18 hrs; the liver and, to a much lesser extent, the kidney were the main organs in which CO$_2$ was formed (Paul & Rubinstein, 1963). Male mice had the greatest amounts of radioactivity in the kidney, while female mice had more radioactivity in the liver (Taylor et al., 1974).

The metabolism of chloroform has been reviewed (Charlesworth, 1976; Hathway, 1974).   When ^{14}C-chloroform was administered orally to mice rats and monkeys, radioactivity was found in expired air.   Most of the dose was excreted unchanged by monkeys, as ^{14}CO$_2$ by mice, and as both by rats.   Three metabolites were detected in the urine of rats and mice, one of which was identified as urea (Brown et al., 1974b; Taylor et al., 1974).

Various treatments that affect hepatic drug-metabolizing enzymes alter the hepatotoxicity of chloroform, indicating that a metabolite of chloroform may be responsible for the liver necrosis (McLean, 1970; Scholler, 1970).   After administration of ^{14}C-chloroform, there was extensive covalent ^{14}C-binding to liver and kidney proteins; this paralleled the extent of necrosis in control and treated mice (Ilett et al., 1973).   In similar experiments, binding in the kidneys of mice of two strains was related to their susceptibility to kidney lesions (Vesell et al., 1976).   Other factors, such as the availability of glutathione (Brown et al., 1974a), concentration of cytochrome P450 and oxygen tension (Sipes et al., 1977; Uehleke & Werner, 1975) affected the extent of covalent binding and of hepatic centrilobular damage.

In phenobarbital-treated rats, liver necrosis was observed only with doses of chloroform high enough to decrease levels of reduced glutathione in liver (Docks & Krishna, 1976).   In vitro, covalent binding of radioactivity from ^{14}C-chloroform to microsomal macromolecules is inhibited by cysteine (Pohl *et al.*, 1977).   The finding of 2-oxo-thiazolidine-4-carboxylic acid in incubates was strong evidence for formation of phosgene: the reactive metabolite phosgene is formed by mixed-function oxidation of chloroform to trichloromethanol following dehydrochlorination (Mansuy *et al.*, 1977; Pohl *et al.*, 1977, 1979).

Mutagenicity and other related short-term tests
_____

In assays with *Salmonella typhimurium* TA1535 and TA1538 and with *Escherichia coli* K12, chloroform was not mutagenic in the presence of microsomal preparations from mouse, rabbit or rat liver (Uehleke *et al.*, 1976, 1977).

(b)   Humans
_____ _____

Chloroform exposure has repeatedly been fatal to man.   Rapid death was attributed to cardiac arrest and delayed death to liver and kidney damage (Challen *et al.*, 1958; Matsuki & Zsigmond, 1974). Symptoms of chloroform exposure include respiratory depression, coma, renal damage and liver damage as measured by elevated serum enzyme levels (Storms, 1973).   In 8 volunteers, 20-68% of an oral dose of 500 mg ^{13}C-chloroform was expired unchanged in the air; in 2 subjects, 48-50% of the dose was eliminated in the expired air as $^{13}CO_2$ (Fry *et al.*, 1972).   Blood concentrations and kinetics of chloroform after anaesthesia were described by Smith *et al.* (1973).

For the occurrence of chloroform in human tissues, see section 2.2 (e).

3.3   Case reports and epidemiological studies[1]
_____

Hepatomegaly was demonstrated in 17/68 workers exposed regularly to chloroform for 1-4 years, in 5/39 workers with past exposure to chloroform, in 2/23 workers with hepatitis but no exposure to chloroform (positive controls) and in 2/164 workers with no hepatitis and no exposure to chloroform.   Of the 17 cases with hepatomegaly, 4 had toxic hepatitis and 14 had fatty degeneration of the liver.   No liver cancers were found (Bomski *et al.*, 1967) [The Working Group noted that this study is uninformative with regard to the carcinogenicity of chloroform, due to small numbers, disproportionate number of current employees and short follow-up time since first exposure].

_____

[1]The Working Group was aware of a mortality study in progress on anaesthetists employed when chloroform was in use as an anaesthetic (IARC, 1978d).

4. Summary of Data Reported and Evaluation

4.1 Experimental data[1]

Chloroform was tested in three experiments in mice and in one in rats by oral administration. It produced hepatomas and hepatocellular carcinomas in mice, malignant kidney tumours in male rats and tumours of the thyroid in female rats. Chloroform was also tested in one experiment by subcutaneous injection and in one by intraperitoneal injection in mice: these experiments were considered to be inadequate.

Chloroform is foetotoxic; it was not mutagenic in the bacterial systems tested.

---

[1]Subsequent to the meeting of the Working Group, the Secretariat became aware of the results of 3 studies, in which mice, rats and dogs were administered toothpaste containing chloroform by gavage or in gelatin capsules on 6 days per week for 80 weeks (mice and rats) or $7\frac{1}{2}$ years (dogs), followed by observation periods ranging from 15-24 weeks. No treatment-related increase in the incidence of tumours was observed in rats receiving 60 mg/kg bw/day chloroform (Palmer *et al.*, 1979) or in dogs receiving 15 or 30 mg/kg bw/day (Heywood *et al.*, 1979).   In mice, benign and malignant tumours of the kidney occurred in 8/38 male ICI mice administered 60 mg/kg bw/day chloroform, but no such tumours occurred in females given that dose, or in males and females receiving 17 mg/kg bw/day or in controls.   In a second experiment in mice, 7 benign and 2 malignant tumours of the kidney occurred among 49 male CFLP (ICI-redefined) mice given 60 mg/kg bw/day chloroform in toothpaste base compared with 6 benign kidney tumours among 237 male mice given the toothpaste base without chloroform.   In a third experiment, groups of C57BL, CBA, CF/1 or ICI male mice received 60 mg/kg bw/day chloroform in toothpaste base or toothpaste base alone; 2 additional groups of male ICI mice received 60 mg/kg bw/day chloroform in arachis oil or arachis oil alone.   Two benign and 3 malignant tumours of the kidney occurred among 47 ICI male mice given chloroform in toothpaste base, and 3 benign and 9 malignant tumours of the kidney occurred among 48 ICI male mice given chloroform in arachis oil.   One benign tumour of the kidney occurred in each group of respective controls.   No kidney tumours occurred in treated C57BL or CBA mice; and no increased incidence of malignant kidney tumours was seen in CF/1 male mice (1/48 treated and 2/45 controls) (Roe *et al.*, 1979).

4.2 Human data

No case reports or epidemiological studies were available to the Working Group.

The past use of chloroform as an anaesthetic and its present use in drugs and cosmetic products, as an insecticidal fumigant and as an industrial solvent indicate that widespread human exposure occurs. This is confirmed by many reports of its presence in air, water and foods.

4.3 Evaluation

There is *sufficient evidence* that chloroform is carcinogenic in mice and rats.   In the absence of adequate data in humans, it is reasonable, for practical purposes, to regard chloroform as if it presented a carcinogenic risk to humans.

5. References

Alumot, E. & Bielorai, R. (1969) Residues of fumigant mixture in cereals
    fumigated and aired at two different temperatures. J. agric. Food
    Chem., 12, 869-870

Appleby, A., Kazazis, J., Lillian, D. & Singh, H.B. (1976) Atmospheric
    formation of chloroform from trichloroethylene. J. environ. Sci.
    Health, A11, 711-715

Bellar, T.A., Litchenberg, J.J. & Kroner, R.C. (1974) The Occurrence of
    Organohalides in Chlorinated Drinking Waters, EPA-670/4-74-008,
    Washington DC, US Government Printing Office

Berkowitz, J.B. (1978) Literature Review - Problem Definition Studies
    on Selected Chemicals, Chloroform, Contract No. DAMD17-77-C-7037,
    Monthly Progress Report 10, Cambridge, MA, Arthur D. Little Inc.

Bertsch, W., Anderson, E. & Holzer, G. (1975) Trace analysis of organic
    volatiles in water by gas chromatography-mass spectrometry with glass
    capillary columns. J. Chromatogr., 112, 701-718

Bomski, H., Sobolewska, A. & Strakowski, A. (1967) Toxic damage of the liver
    by chloroform in chemical industry workers (Germ.). Arch. Gewerbepathol
    Gewerbehyg., 24, 127-134

Brown, B.R., Jr, Sipes, I.G. & Sagalyn, A.M. (1974a) Mechanisms of acute
    hepatic toxicity: chloroform, halothane and glutathione. Anesthesiolog
    41, 554-561

Brown, D.M., Langley, P.F., Smith, D., & Taylor, D.C. (1974b) Metabolism
    of chloroform. I. The metabolism of [^{14}C] chloroform by different
    species. Xenobiotica, 4, 151-163

Bureau International Technique des Solvants Chlorés (1976) Standard-
    ization of methods for the determination of traces of some volatile
    chlorinated aliphatic hydrocarbons in air and water by gas chromato-
    graphy. Anal. chim. acta, 82, 1-17

Challen, P.J.R., Hickish, D.E. & Bedford, J. (1958) Chronic chloroform
    intoxication. Br. J. ind. Med., 15, 243-249

Charlesworth, F.A. (1976) Patterns of chloroform metabolism. Food
    Cosmet. Toxicol., 14, 59-60

Coleman, W.E., Lingg, R.D., Melton, R.G. & Kopfler, F.G. (1976) The
    occurrence of volatile organics in five drinking water supplies using
    gas chromatography mass spectrometry. In: Keith, L.H., ed., Identi-
    fication and Analysis of Organic Pollutants of Water, Ann Arbor, MI,
    Ann Arbor Science, pp. 305-327

Conkle, J.P., Camp, B.J. & Welch, B.E. (1975) Trace composition of human respiratory gas. Arch. environ. Health, 30, 290-295

Cox, R.A., Derwent, R.G., Eggleton, A.E.J. & Lovelock, J.E. (1976) Photochemical oxidation of halocarbons in the troposphere. Atmos. Environ., 10, 305-308

Deringer, M.K., Dunn, T.B. & Heston, W.E. (1953) Results of exposure of strain C3H mice to chloroform. Proc. Soc. exp. Biol. NY, 83, 474-478

Dickson, A.G. & Riley, J.P. (1976) The distribution of short-chain halogenated aliphatic hydrocarbons in some marine organisms. Marine Pollut. Bull., 7, 167-169

Dietz, F. & Traud, J. (1973) Gas chromatographic determination of low-molecular-weight chlorohydrocarbons in water samples and sediments (Germ.). Vom Wasser, 41, 137-155 [Chem. Abstr., 81, 54214p]

Dilley, J.V., Chernoff, N., Kay, D., Winslow, N. & Newell, G.W. (1977) Inhalation teratology studies of five chemicals in rats (Abstract No. 154). Toxicol. appl. Pharmacol., 41, 196

Docks, E.L. & Krishna, G. (1976) The role of glutathione in chloroform-induced hepatotoxicity. Exp. mol. Path., 24, 13-22

Dowty, B.J., Carlisle, D.R. & Laseter, J.L. (1975) New Orleans drinking water sources tested by gas chromatography-mass spectrometry. Occurrence and origin of aromatics and halogenated aliphatic hydrocarbons. Environ. Sci. Technol., 9, 762-765

Doyle, R.E., Woodard, J.C., Lewis, A.L. & Moreland, A.F. (1967) Mortality in Swiss mice exposed to chloroform. J. Am. Vet. med. Assoc., 151, 930-934

Eisenbrand, G., Spiegelhalder, B., Janzowski, C., Kann, J. & Preussmann, R. (1978) Volatile and non-volatile N-nitroso compounds in foods and other environmental media. In: Walker, E.A., Castegñaro, M., Griciute, L. & Lyle, R.E., eds, Environmental Aspects of N-Nitroso Compounds (IARC Scientific Publications No. 19), Lyon, pp. 311-324

Ellison, W.K. & Wallbank, T.E. (1974) Solvents in sewage and industrial waste waters. Identification and determination. Water Pollut. Control, 73, 656-672 [Chem. Abstr., 82, 102823f]

Eschenbrenner, A.B. & Miller, E. (1945) Induction of hepatomas in mice by repeated oral administration of chloroform, with observations on sex differences. J. natl Cancer Inst., 5, 251-255

Eurocop-Cost (1976) A Comprehensive List of Polluting Substances Which
    Have Been Identified in Various Fresh Waters, Effluent Discharges,
    Aquatic Animals and Plants, and Bottom Sediments, 2nd Ed., EUCO/MDU/
    73/76, XII/476/76, Luxembourg, Commission of the European Communities,
    p. 31

Fishbein, L. (1973) Chromatography of Environmental Hazards, Vol. II,
    Metals, Gaseous and Industrial Pollutants, New York, Elsevier, pp.
    471-472, 489-490

Fry, B.J., Taylor, T. & Hathway, D.E. (1972) Pulmonary elimination of
    chloroform and its metabolite in man. Arch. int. Pharmacodyn., 196,
    98-111

Fujii, T. (1977) Direct aqueous injection gas chromatography-mass spectro-
    metry for analysis of organohalides in water at concentrations below
    the parts per billion level. J. Chromatogr., 139, 297-302

Gage, J.C., Strafford, N. & Truhaut, R. (1962) Methods for the Determinati
    of Toxic Substances in Air, International Union of Pure & Applied
    Chemistry, London, Butterworths, pp. 25.1-25.2

Grasselli, J.G. & Ritchey, W.M., eds (1975) CRC Atlas of Spectral Data and
    Physical Constants for Organic Compounds, 2nd ed., Vol. III, Cleveland
    OH, Chemical Rubber Co., p. 600

Grimsrud, E.P. & Rasmussen, R.A. (1975) Survey and analysis of halocarbons
    in the atmosphere by gas chromatography-mass spectrometry. Atmos.
    Environ., 9, 1014-1017

Hammarstrand, K. (1976) Chloroform in drinking water. Varian Instrum.
    Appl., 10, 2-4

Hardie, D.W.F. (1964) Chlorocarbons and Chlorohydrocarbons. Chloroform.
    In: Kirk, R.E. & Othmer, D.F., eds, Encyclopedia of Chemical
    Technology, 2nd ed., Vol. 5, New York, John Wiley & Sons, pp. 119-127

Hathway, D.E. (1974) Chemical, biochemical and toxicological differences
    between carbon tetrachloride and chloroform. A critical review of
    recent investigations of these compounds in mammals. Arzneimittel-
    Forsch., 24, 173-176

Hawley, G.G., ed. (1977) The Condensed Chemical Dictionary, 9th ed., New
    York, Van Nostrand-Reinhold, p. 197

Heuser, S.G. & Scudamore, K.A. (1969) Determination of fumigant residues
    in cereals and other foodstuffs: a multi-detection scheme for gas
    chromatography of solvent extracts. J. Sci. Food Agric., 20, 566-572

Heywood, R., Sortwell, R.J., Noel, P.R.B., Street, A.E., Prentice, D.E., Roe, F.J.C., Wardsworth, P.F., Worden, A.N. & Van Abbé, N.J. (1979) Safety evaluation of toothpaste containing chloroform. III. Long-term study in beagle dogs. J. environ. Pathol. Toxicol., 2, 835-851

Hill, R.N., Clemens, T.L., Liu, D.K., Vesell, E.S. & Johnson, W.D. (1975) Genetic control of chloroform toxicity in mice. Science, 190, 159-161

Horwitz, W., ed. (1970 Official Methods of Analysis of the Association of Official Analytical Chemists, 11th ed., Washington DC, Association of Official Analytical Chemists, pp. 680-682; 3rd Supplement, pp. 472-473

Horwitz, W., ed. (1975) Official Methods of Analysis of the Association of Official Analytical Chemists, 12th ed., Washington DC, Association of Official Analytical Chemists, pp. 658-660

IARC (1972) IARC Monographs on the Evaluation of Carcinogenic Risk of Chemicals to Man, 1, Lyon, pp. 61-65

IARC (1978a) IARC Monographs on the Evaluation of the Carcinogenic Risk of Chemicals to Humans, 19, Some Monomers, Plastics and Synthetic Elastomers, and Acrolein, Lyon, pp. 439-459

IARC (1978b) IARC Monographs on the Evaluation of the Carcinogenic Risk of Chemicals to Humans, 17, Some N-Nitroso Compounds, Lyon, p. 264

IARC (1978c) IARC Monographs on the Evaluation of the Carcinogenic Risk of Chemicals to Humans, 19, Some Monomers, Plastics and Synthetic Elastomers, and Acrolein, Lyon, pp. 285-301

IARC (1978d) Directory of On-going Research in Cancer Epidemiology, 1978 (IARC Scientific Publications No. 26), Lyon, Abstract No. 802, pp. 303-304

Ilett, K.F., Reid, W.D., Sipes, I.G. & Krishna, G. (1973) Chloroform toxicity in mice: correlation of renal and hepatic necrosis with covalent binding of metabolites to tissue macromolecules. Exp. mol. Path., 19, 215-229

Kaiser, K.L.E. & Oliver, B.G. (1976) Determination of volatile halogenated hydrocarbons in water by gas chromatography. Anal. Chem., 48, 2207-2209

Kajino, M. (1977) Formation of chloroform during chlorination of drinking water (Jap.). Osaka-shi Suidokyoku Komobu Suishitsu Shikensho Chosa Hokoku narabini Shiken Seiseki, 27, 1-4 [Chem. Abstr., 88, 27631k]

Keith, L.H., Garrison, A.W., Allen, F.R., Carter, M.H., Floyd, T.L., Pope, J.D. & Thruston, A.D., Jr (1976) Identification of organic compounds in drinking water from thirteen US cities. In: Keith, L.H., ed., Identification and Analysis of Organic Pollutants of Water, Ann Arbor, MI, Ann Arbor Science, pp. 329-373

Kimura, E.T., Ebert, D.M. & Dodge, P.W. (1971) Acute toxicity and limits of solvent residue for sixteen organic solvents. Toxicol. appl. Pharmacol. 19, 699-704

Kleopfer, R.D. (1976) Analysis of drinking water for organic compounds. In: Keith, L.H., ed., Identification and Analysis of Organic Pollutants of Water, Ann Arbor, MI, Ann Arbor Science, pp. 399-416

Kuo, P.P.K., Chian, E.S.K., DeWalle, F.B. & Kim, J.H. (1977) Gas stripping, sorption, and thermal desorption procedures for preconcentrating volatile polar water-soluble organics from water samples for analysis by gas chromatography. Anal. Chem., 49, 1023-1029

Lillian, D., Singh, H.B., Appleby, A., Lobban, L., Arnts, R., Gumpert, R., Hague, R., Toomey, J., Kazazis, J., Antell, M., Hansen, D. & Scott, B. (1975) Atmospheric fates of halogenated compounds. Environ. Sci. Technol., 9, 1042-1048

Lillian, D., Singh, H.B. & Appleby, A. (1976) Gas chromatographic analysis of ambient halogenated compounds. J. Air Pollut. Control Assoc., 26, 141-143

Mansuy, D., Beaune, P., Cresteil, T., Lange, M. & Leroux, J.-P. (1977) Evidence for phosgene formation during liver micromal oxidation of chloroform. Biochem. biophys. Res. Comm., 79, 513-517

Martin, G.E. & Figert, D.M. (1974) Gas-solid chromatographic determination of volatile denaturants in ethanol solution. J. Assoc. off. anal. Chem., 57, 148-152

Matsuki, A. & Zsigmond, E.K. (1974) The first fatal case of chloroform anaesthesia in the United States. Anesth. Analg., 53, 152-154

McConnell, G., Ferguson, D.M. & Pearson, C.R. (1975) Chlorinated hydro-carbons and the environment. Endeavor, 34, 13-18

McLean, A.E.M. (1970) The effect of protein deficiency and microsomal enzyme induction by DDT and phenobarbitone on the acute toxicity of chloroform and a pyrrolizidine alkaloid, retrorsine. Br. J. exp. Path., 51, 317-321

Mercier, M. (1977) Criteria (Exposure/Effect Relationships) for Organo-chlorine Solvents, Doc. V/F/177-4, Luxembourg, Commission of the European Communities, pp. 30-58

Mieure, J.P. (1977) A rapid and sensitive method for determining volatile organohalides in water. J. Am. Water Works Assoc., 69, 60-62

Morita, M. (1976) Chlorination and chlorinated organic materials (Jap.). Yosui To Haisui, 18, 143-149 [Chem. Abstr., 85, 148872m]

Morris, J.C. & McKay, G. (1975) Formation of Halogenated Organics by Chlorination of Water Supplies (A Review), EPA-600/1-75-002, Washington DC, US Government Printing Office

Morris, R.L. & Johnson, L.G. (1976) Agricultural runoff as a source of halomethanes in drinking water. J. Am. Water Works Assoc., September, pp. 492-494

National Cancer Institute (1976) Report on Carcinogenesis Bioassay of Chloroform, Bethesda, MD, Carcinogenesis Program, Division of Cancer Cause and Prevention

National Institute for Occupational Safety & Health (1974) Criteria for a Recommended Standard .... Occupational Exposure to Chloroform, Washington DC, US Government Printing Office, pp. 60-67, 82-102

National Institute for Occupational Safety & Health (1976) NIOSH revises standard recommendations, cites carcinogenic hazards of substance. Occup. Saf. Health Rep., 6, 63

National Institute for Occupational Safety & Health (1977a) National Occupational Hazard Survey, Vol. III, Survey Analyses and Supplemental Tables, Cincinnati, OH, US Department of Health, Education & Welfare, pp. 2864-2866

National Institute for Occupational Safety & Health (1977b) NIOSH Manual of Analytical Methods, 2nd ed., Part II, Standards Completion Program Validated Methods, Vol. 3, Method S351, DHEW (NIOSH) Publ. No. 77-157-B, Washington DC, US Government Printing Office, pp. S351-1 - S351-9

Nicholson, A.A., Meresz, O. & Lemyk, B. (1977) Determination of free and total potential haloforms in drinking water. Anal. Chem., 49, 814-819

Novák, J., Žlutický, J., Kubelka, V. & Mostecký, J. (1973) Analysis of organic constituents present in drinking water. J. Chromatogr., 76, 45-50

Palmer, A.K., Street, A.E., Roe, F.J.C., Worden, A.N. & Van Abbé, N.J. (1979) Safety evaluation of toothpaste containing chloroform. II. Long term studies in rats. J. environ. Pathol. Toxicol., 2, 821-833

Parkes, D.G., Ganz, C.R., Polinsky, A. & Schulze, J. (1976) A simple gas chromatographic method for the analysis of trace organics in ambient air. Am. Ind. Hyg. Assoc. J., 37, 165-172

Parsons, J.S. & Mitzner, S. (1975) Gas chromatographic method for concentration and analysis of traces of industrial organic pollutants in environmental air and stacks. Environ. Sci. Tech., 9, 1053-1058

Paul, B.B. & Rubinstein, D. (1963) Metabolism of carbon tetrachloride and chloroform by the rat. J. Pharmacol. exp. Ther., 141, 141-148

Pearson, C.R. & McConnell, G. (1975) Chlorinated C_1 and C_2 hydrocarbons in the marine environment. Proc. R. Soc. Lond. B., 189, 305-332

Perry, R.H. & Chilton, C.H., eds (1973) Chemical Engineers' Handbook, 5th ed., New York, McGraw-Hill, p. 3-51

Pohl, L.R., Bhooshan, B., Whittaker, N.F. & Krishna, G. (1977) Phosgene: a metabolite of chloroform. Biochem. biophys. Res. Comm., 79, 684-691

Pohl, L.R., Bhooshan, B. & Krishna, G. (1979) Mechanism of the metabolic activation of chloroform. Toxicol. appl. Pharmacol (in press)

Poobalasingam, N, (1976) Analysis of chloroform in blood. Br. J. Anaesth., 48, 953-956

Premel-Cabic, A., Cailleux, A. & Allain, P. (1974) A gas chromatographic assay of fifteen volatile organic solvents in blood (Fr.). Clin. chim. acta, 56, 5-11

Reckner, L.R. & Sachdev, J. (1975) Collaborative Testing of Activated Charcoal Sampling Tubes for Seven Organic Solvents, National Institute for Occupational Safety & Health, DHEW (NIOSH) Contract No. HSM 99-72-98, Washington DC, US Government Printing Office, pp. 1.0, 2-1-2-4, 3-1-3-6

Richard, J.J. & Junk, G.A. (1977) Liquid extraction for the rapid determination of halomethanes in water. J. Am. Water Works Assoc., 69, 62-64

Roe, F.J.C., Carter, R.L. & Mitchley, B.C.V. (1968) Test of chloroform and 8-hydroxyquinoline for carcinogenicity using newborn mice. Br. Emp. Cancer Campgn, 46, 13

Roe, F.J.C., Palmer, A.K., Worden, A.N. & Van Abbé, N.J. (1979) Safety evaluation of toothpaste containing chloroform. I. Long term studies in mice. J. environ. Pathol. Toxicol., 2, 799-819

Rook, J.J., Meijers, A.P., Gras, A.A. & Noordsij, A. (1975) Headspace analysis of volatile trace compounds in the Rhine (Germ.). Vom Wasser, 44, 23-30 [Chem. Abstr., 86, 60313q]

Rudali, G. (1967) Oncogenic activity of some halogenated hydrocarbons used in therapeutics (Fr.). UICC Monogr. Ser., 7, 138-143

Russell, J.W. & Shadoff, L.A. (1977) The sampling and determination of halocarbons in ambient air using concentration on porous polymer. J. Chromatogr., 134, 375-384

Saunders, R.A., Blachly, C.H., Kovacina, T.A., Lamontagne, R.A., Swinnerton, J.W. & Saalfeld, F.E. (1975) Identification of volatile organic contaminants in Washington DC municipal water. Water Res., 9, 1143-1145

Scholler, K.L. (1968) Electron-microscopic and autoradiographic studies on the effect of halothane and chloroform on liver cells. Acta anaesthesiol. scand., Suppl. 32, 15

Scholler, K.L. (1970) Modification of the effects of chloroform on the rat liver. Br. J. Anaesth., 42, 603-605

Schwetz, B.A., Leong, B.K.J. & Gehring, P.J. (1974) Embryo- and feto-toxicity of inhaled chloroform in rats. Toxicol. appl. Pharmacol., 28, 442-451

Shackelford, W.M. & Keith, L.H. (1976) Frequency of Organic Compounds Identified in Water, EPA-600/4-76-062, Athens, GA, US Environmental Protection Agency, pp. 165-168

Singh, H.B., Salas, L.J. & Cavanagh, L.A. (1977) Distribution, sources and sinks of atmospheric halogenated compounds. J. Air Poll. Control Assoc., 27, 332-336

Sipes, I.G., Krishna, G. & Gillette, J.R. (1977) Bioactivation of carbon tetrachloride, chloroform and bromotrichloromethane: role of cytochrome P-450. Life Sci., 20, 1541-1548

Smith, A.A., Volpitto, P.P., Gramling, Z.W., DeVore, M.B. & Glassman, A.B. (1973) Chloroform, halothane, and regional anesthesia: a comparative study. Anesth. Analg., 52, 1-11

Storms, W.W. (1973) Chloroform parties. J. Am. med. Assoc., 225, 160

Symons, J.M., Bellar, T.A., Carswell, J.K., DeMarco, J., Kropp, K.L., Robeck, G.G., Seeger, D.R., Slocum, C.J., Smith, B.L. & Stevens, A.A. (1975) National Organics Reconnaissance Survey for Halogenated Organics. J. Am. Water Works Assoc., November, pp. 634-647

Taylor, D.C., Brown, D.M., Keeble, R. & Langley, P.F. (1974) Metabolism of chloroform. II. A sex difference in the metabolism of [^{14}C] chloroform in mice. Xenobiotica, 4, 165-174

Theiss, J.C., Stoner, G.D., Shimkin, M.B. & Weisburger, E.K. (1977) Test for carcinogenicity of organic contaminants of United States drinking waters by pulmonary tumor response in strain A mice. Cancer Res., 37, 2717-2720

Thompson, R.H., Fishwick, F.B., Green M., Grevenstuck, W.B.F., Harris, A.H., Harts, H.V., Heuser, S.G., Hoodless, R.A., Scudamore, K.A. et al. (1974a) Determination of residues of volatile fumigants in grain. Analyst (Lond.), 99, 570-576 [Chem. Abstr., 82, 96532s]

Thompson, D.J., Warner, S.D. & Robinson, V.B. (1974b) Teratology studies on orally administered chloroform in the rat and rabbit. Toxicol. appl. Pharmacol., 29, 348-357

Torkelson, T.R., Oyen, F. & Rowe, V.K. (1976) The toxicity of chloroform as determined by single and repeated exposure of laboratory animals. Am. Ind. Hyg. Assoc. J., 37, 697-705

Uehleke, H. & Werner, T. (1975) A comparative study on the irreversible binding of labeled halothane trichlorofluoromethane, chloroform, and carbon tetrachloride to hepatic protein and lipids in vitro and in vivo. Arch. Toxicol., 34, 289-308

Uehleke, H., Greim, H., Krämer, M. & Werner, T. (1976) Covalent binding of haloalkanes to liver constituents, but absence of mutagenicity on bacteria in a metabolizing test system (Abstract no. 25). Mutat. Res., 38, 114

Uehleke, H., Werner, T., Greim, H. & Krämer, M. (1977) Metabolic activation of haloalkanes and tests in vitro for mutagenicity. Xenobiotica, 7, 393-400

US Department of Commerce (1975) Bureau of Domestic Commerce, Staff Study: Economic Significance of Fluorocarbons, Washington DC, Office of Business Research & Analysis, pp. 50-51, 66-67, 70, 72, 81-83, 86, 127, 169-174

US Department of Commerce (1977a) US Imports for Consumption and General Imports, TSUSA Commodity by Country of Origin, FT 246/Annual 1976, Bureau of the Census, Washington DC, US Government Printing Office, p. 230

US Department of Commerce (1977b) US Exports, Schedule B, Commodity by Country, FT 410/December 1976, Washington DC, US Government Printing Office, p. 2-85

US Environmental Protection Agency (1971) EPA Compendium of Registered Pesticides, Washington DC, US Government Printing Office, p. III-C-19

US Environmental Protection Agency (1976a) Protection of environment. US Code Fed. Regul., Title 40, part 180.1001, pp. 371, 380

US Environmental Protection Agency (1976b) Extension of period for submission of rebuttal evidence and comments with regard to presumption against registration and continued registration of pesticide products containing chloroform (trichloromethane). Fed. Regist., 41, 22297

US Food & Drug Administration (1976a) Human Drugs Containing Chloroform, April, 635.000, Rockville, MD

US Food & Drug Administration (1976b) Chloroform as an ingredient of human drug and cosmetic products. Fed. Regist., 41, 26842-26845

US International Trade Commission (1977) Synthetic Organic Chemicals, US Production and Sales, 1976, USITC Publication 833, Washington DC, US Government Printing Office, pp. 182, 302, 331

US International Trade Commission (1978) Preliminary Report on US Production of Selected Synthetic Organic Chemicals (Including Synthetic Plastics and Resin Materials) Preliminary Totals, 1977, Series C/P-78-1, Washington DC, US Government Printing Office, p.3

US Occupational Safety & Health Administration (1978) Air contaminants. US Code Fed. Regul., Title 29, part 1910.1000, pp. 612-614

US Tariff Commission (1923) Census of Dyes and Other Synthetic Organic Chemicals, 1922, Tariff Information Series No. 31, Washington DC, US Government Printing Office, pp. 112, 118-120

Vesell, E.S., Lang, C.M., White, W.J., Passananti, G.T., Hill, R.N., Clemens, T.L., Liu, D.K. & Johnson, W.D. (1976) Environmental and genetic factors affecting the response of laboratory animals to drugs. Fed. Proc., 35, 1125-1132

Von Oettingen, W.E. (1964) The Halogenated Hydrocarbons of Industrial and Toxicological Importance, New York, Elsevier, pp. 77-81, 95-101

Winslow, S.G. & Gerstner, H.B. (1977) Health Aspects of Chloroform - A Review and An Abstracted Literature Collection 1907 to 1977, ORNL/TIRC-77/4, Oak Ridge, TN, Oak Ridge National Laboratory

1,2-DICHLOROETHANE

1. Chemical and Physical Data

1.1 Synonyms and trade names

Chem. Abstr. Services Reg. No.: 107-06-2

Chem. Abstr. Name: 1,2-Dichloroethane

Synonyms: 1,2-Bichloroethane; α,β-dichloroethane; sym-dichloroethane; dichloroethylene; EDC; ENT 1,656; ethylene chloride; ethylene dichloride; glycol dichloride

Trade names: Brocide; Dutch liquid; Dutch oil; Freon 150

1.2 Structural and molecular formulae and molecular weight

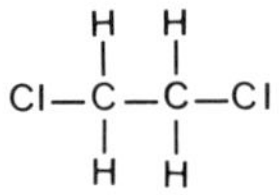

$$Cl\!-\!\overset{\displaystyle H}{\underset{\displaystyle H}{C}}\!-\!\overset{\displaystyle H}{\underset{\displaystyle H}{C}}\!-\!Cl$$

$C_2H_4Cl_2$ Mol. wt: 98.9

1.3 Chemical and physical properties of the pure substance

From Hardie (1964), unless otherwise specified

(a) Description: Clear, colourless, oily liquid (Hawley, 1971; Patterson *et al.*, 1976)

(b) Boiling-point: 83.5°C

(c) Melting-point: -35.4°C

(d) Density: d^{20} 1.253

(e) Refractive index: n_D^{20} 1.4449

(f) Spectroscopy data: Infra-red, Raman, nuclear magnetic resonance and mass spectral data have been tabulated (Grasselli & Ritchey, 1975).

(g) Solubility: Slightly soluble in water (0.869 g/100 ml at
     20°C); soluble in most organic solvents

(h) Volatility: Vapour pressure is 64 mm at 20°C.

(i) Vapour density: 3.4 (air = 1) (National Fire Protection
     Association, 1972)

(j) Stability: Stable at ordinary temperatures when dry; at
     > 600°C, decomposes to vinyl chloride (see IARC, 1979a),
     hydrogen chloride and acetylene. In the presence of air,
     moisture and light, at ordinary temperatures, darkens in
     colour. Resistant to oxidation (Hawley, 1971)

(k) Reactivity: Can be hydrolysed to ethylene glycol in the
     presence of water at 160-175°C, 15 atm, or in the presence of
     alkali at 140-250°C, 40 atm.   Both chlorine atoms are reactive.
     Does not corrode metal (Hawley, 1971)

(l) Conversion factor: 1 ppm in air is equivalent to 4 mg/m^3.

1.4 Technical products and impurities

1,2-Dichloroethane is available in drums or tank cars as technical
and spectrophotometric grades (Hawley, 1971).   One manufacturer's
specifications for a technical-grade product are as follows: water,
0.03% max; alkalinity (as NaOH) 0.0005% max; acidity (as HCl) 0.0002%
max; free halogens, none; residue on evaporation, 0.01% max; boiling-
range at 760 mm, within a 1.5°C range including 83.5°C.

1,2-Dichloroethane produced in Japan is reported to contain polychlorinated ethanes as impurities.

When used as a fumigant, 1,2-dichloroethane is usually mixed with
carbon tetrachloride in a ratio of 3:1 to reduce the fire hazard (Martin
& Worthing, 1977).

2. Production, Use, Occurrence and Analysis

A review article on 1,2-dichloroethane has been published (Hardie, 1964).

(a) Production and use

1,2-Dichloroethane was the first chlorinated hydrocarbon to be synthesized: it was first produced in 1795 by the chlorination of ethylene by Delman *et al*. (Prager *et al*., 1918). Since late 1970, all of the 1,2-dichloroethane produced in the US has been made by the chlorination or oxychlorination (a catalysed reaction with air and hydrogen chloride) of ethylene (Approximately 3.17 kg of 1,2-dichloro-ethane are produced per kg of ethylene consumed). It is currently produced primarily by chlorination, but an increasing percentage is being produced by oxychlorination. 1,2-Dichloroethane has also been produced as a by-product in the chlorohydrin process for the manufacture of ethylene oxide, which involves the conversion of ethylene to ethylene chlorohydrin by reacting it with hypochlorous acid; the chlorohydrin is converted to the oxide by dehydrochlorination with slaked lime (Approximately 0.1 kg of 1,2-dichloroethane may be produced for each kg of ethylene oxide). Ethylene oxide is no longer produced by this method in the US.

In Japan, all commercial production of 1,2-dichloroethane is based upon the chlorination of ethylene.

Commercial production of 1,2-dichloroethane in the US was first reported in 1922 (US Tariff Commission, 1923). In 1976, 13 US producers reported a total production of 3600 million kg (US International Trade Commission, 1977); however, this is likely to be an underestimate, since some 1,2-dichloroethane that is produced is not separated (and therefore not reported) by some producers. US exports in 1976 amounted to 208 million kg (US Department of Commerce, 1977); imports are not reported separately but are believed to be negligible in all years except 1974, when an estimated 34 million kg were imported.

1,2-Dichloroethane is produced at an annual rate in excess of 100 million kg in the Benelux countries, the Federal Republic of Germany, France, Italy, the UK, Scandinavia, Spain, and eastern Europe. Austria and Switzerland each produce less than 100 thousand kg annually.

1,2-Dichloroethane was first produced commercially in Japan in 1965. In 1976, 18 producers reported a total production of 1800 million kg; imports were 89 million kg, and no exports were reported.

(b) Use

Use of 1,2-dichloroethane in the US in 1976 was as follows:
production of vinyl chloride, 81.6%; production of 1,1,1-trichloro-
ethane, 3.3%; production of ethyleneamines, 2.8%; production of tetrachloroethylene, 2.3%; production of trichloroethylene, 2.0%; as a
lead scavenger, 1.9%; production of vinylidene chloride, 1.8%; miscellaneous applications, 0.1%; and exports, 4.2%.

About 4000 million kg 1,2-dichloroethane were used in the US for
the production of vinyl chloride in 1976.   About 96% of the vinyl
chloride made in that year was used for the production of vinyl chloride
homopolymer and copolymer resins.   The remainder was used for the
production of 1,1,1-trichloroethane and as a comonomer with vinylidene
chloride in the production of resins (For more detailed information on
the uses of vinyl chloride and polyvinyl chloride, see IARC 1979a).

In 1976, 165 million kg 1,2-dichloroethane were used in the US in
the production of 1,1,1-trichloroethane (For information on the uses
of 1,1,1-trichloroethane, see monograph, p. 515); approximately 139
million kg were used to make ethyleneamines; 115 million kg were used
for the production of tetrachloroethylene (For information on the uses
of tetrachloroethylene, see monograph, p. 491); 99 million kg were used
for the production of trichloroethylene (For information on the uses of
trichloroethylene, see monograph, p. 545); and 89 million kg were used
for the production of vinylidene chloride (For information on the uses
of vinylidene chloride, see IARC, 1979b).

1,2-Dichloroethane is used as a lead-scavenging agent in petrol to
transform the combustion products of lead alkyls to more easily vapour-
ized forms.   It is a major ingredient of many petrol antiknock mixtures.
About 92 million kg were used for this purpose in the US in 1976.

Miscellaneous applications for 1,2-dichloroethane, which consumed
7.3 million kg in 1976, include: various solvent applications; use as
a fumigant for grain, upholstery and carpets; and as a chemical intermediate for the manufacture of polysulphide elastomers and ethylene-
imine.

No data on its use in Europe were available.

In Japan, 90% of 1,2-dichloroethane is used for the production of
vinyl chloride and 10% as an industrial solvent and a chemical intermediate.

1,2-Dichloroethane is registered for agricultural use in the US in
various formulations with other fumigants for the postharvest fumigation
of grain and for use in orchards, agricultural premises and mushroom
houses (US Environmental Protection Agency, 1969).

This substance was evaluated at the 1971 Joint Meeting of the FAO Working Party of Experts on Pesticide Residues and the WHO Expert Committee on Pesticide Residues. It was noted that there is little direct information on the amount of residues appearing in commercial samples or in food reaching the consumer; however, the following residue levels were recommended as guidelines: in raw cereals at point of entry into a country or when supplied for milling, provided that the commodity is freely exposed to air for a period of at least 24 hrs after fumigation before sampling, 50 mg/kg; in milled cereal products that are to be subjected to baking or cooking, 10 mg/kg; in bread and other cooked cereal products, 0.1 mg/kg (WHO, 1972).

In the US, 1,2-dichloroethane is exempted from the requirement of a tolerance when used as a fumigant after harvest for the following grains: barley, corn, oats, popcorn, rice, rye, sorghum and wheat (US Environmental Protection Agency, 1976). The basis for this exemption and similar exemptions in Australia and Canada is that no hazard will remain when the food reaches the consumer (WHO, 1972).

1,2-Dichloroethane has been cited by the US Environmental Protection Agency as a candidate for action through the rebuttable presumption against registration (RPAR) (see General Remarks on Substances Considered, p. 31) process because of possible carcinogenicity and mutagenicity (Anon., 1978a).

The US Occupational Safety and Health Administration's health standards for air contaminants require that an employee's exposure to 1,2-dichloroethane not exceed 200 mg/m^3 (50 ppm) in the workplace air in any 8-hr work shift of a 40-hr work week (US Occupational Safety & Health Administration, 1977). In April 1976, the US National Institute for Occupational Safety and Health recommended that occupational exposure to ethylene dichloride not exceed 20 mg/m^3 (5 ppm), determined as a time-weighted average exposure for up to a 10-hr work day in a 40-hr work week, and 60 mg/m^3 (15 ppm) as a peak concentration (National Institute for Occupational Safety & Health, 1976a). That Institute has recently proposed that these values be lowered to 1 ppm and 2 ppm, respectively (Anon., 1978b).

2.2 Occurrence

1,2-Dichloroethane is not known to occur as a natural product.

(a) Air

Chlorinated hydrocarbons, including 1,2-dichloroethane, have been detected in urban air at levels of 0.04-38 µg/m^3 (0.01-9.4 ppb) (Okuno *et al.*, 1974). A level of 300 µg/m^3 has been detected near a vinyl chloride plant (Kretzschmar *et al.*, 1976).

In 1974, total annual US emissions of 1,2-dichloroethane to the ambient air were estimated to have been 74 million kg (representing about 1.8% of total reported production). The individual sources of these emissions were: (1) manufacture of end-products, primarily vinyl chloride, 38.6 million kg; (2) manufacture of 1,2-dichloroethane, 26.3 million kg; (3) use as a solvent, 6.4 million kg; and (4) storage and distribution, 2.7 million kg (Patterson *et al.*, 1976).

(b) Water

As part of a US Environmental Protection Agency study, the National Organics Reconnaissance Survey for Halogenated Organics sampled finished drinking-water supplies in 80 US cities. 1,2-Dichloroethane was found in the waters of 28 cities at level of 0-6 µg/l (Symons *et al.*, 1975).

In a more recent study, surface water samples taken near heavily industrialized sites across the US were examined for all contaminants present. Levels of 1,2-dichloroethane greater than 1 µg/l were detected at 53 of 204 sites (Ewing *et al.*, 1977).

1,2-Dichloroethane has also been detected in: (1) tap-water, at levels of 8 µg/l and 61 mg/l; (2) river-water, at a level of 0.7 µg/l (Eurocop-Cost, 1976); (3) raw and finished drinking-water (Shackelford & Keith, 1976); and (4) tap-water in Japan, at a level of 0.9 µg/l (Fujii, 1977).

(c) Humans

1,2-Dichloroethane has been found in expired air at levels of 0-0.8 µg/hr (Conkle *et al.*, 1975).

(d) Occupational exposure

A 1974 National Occupational Hazard Survey estimated that workers primarily exposed to 1,2-dichloroethane were those in hospitals, blast furnaces, steel mills and air transportation industries (National Institute for Occupational Safety & Health, 1977a).

(e) Other

1,2-Dichloroethane has been detected in waste products that had been dumped in the North Sea from vinyl chloride production plants in Europe (Jensen *et al.*, 1975).

2.3 Analysis

Methods used for the analysis of 1,2-dichloroethane in environmental samples are listed in Table 1.

TABLE 1. METHODS FOR THE ANALYSIS OF 1,2-DICHLOROETHANE

SAMPLE TYPE	ANALYTICAL METHOD			
	EXTRACTION/CLEAN-UP	DETECTION	LIMIT OF DETECTION	REFERENCE
Formulations				
Fumigant mixtures	Inject directly	GC		Horwitz (1975)
Air	Trap on activated charcoal or porous polymer packing (Chromosorb 101), desorb by heating, retrap in line on GC column	GC/FID	Working range, 160 µg/m³-160 mg/m³(40 ppb-40 ppm)	Parkes et al. (1976)
	Trap on porous polymer (Tenax), desorb by heating, retrap in line on GC column	GC/FID		Parsons & Mitzner (1975)
	Trap in pyridine, add sodium hydroxide solution, heat	Spectrophotometry (415 nm)	400 mg/m³ (100 ppm) (v/v, 20°C, 760 mm)	Gage et al. (1962)
	Trap on charcoal, extract (carbon disulphide)	GC/FID	Working range, 195-819 mg/m³	National Institute for Occupational Safety & Health (1977b)
	Direct	Laser absorption spectroscopy, 9-11 nm	Alone: 944 mg/m³ (236 ppm); in gas mixture: 4000 mg/m³ (1000 ppm)	Green & Steinfeld (1976)
	Direct	Photoionization MS	28 mg/m³ (7 ppm)	Driscoll & Warneck (1973)
Water				
Drinking-water	Inject directly	GC/ECD	90 µg/l	Nicholson et al. (1977)
	Sparge (helium), retrap on GC column	GC/Hall	0.2 µg/l	Nicholson et al. (1977)

TABLE 1. METHODS FOR THE ANALYSIS OF 1,2-DICHLOROETHANE (continued)

SAMPLE TYPE	ANALYTICAL METHOD			
	EXTRACTION/CLEAN-UP	DETECTION	LIMIT OF DETECTION	REFERENCE
Municipal, artesian deionized, charcoal filtered water	Sparge (helium), trap on *para*-2,6-diphenyl phenylene oxide, desorb by heating, retrap in line on GC column	GC/MS		Dowty *et al.* (1975)
Drinking-water	Sparge (helium), trap on adsorbant, desorb by heating, retrap in line on GC column	GC, microcoulometry (halide-specific mode)	0.1 µg/l	Symons *et al.* (1975)
Food				
Grains	Grind in dry ice, boil in acid, trap volatile fumigant in cold solvents	GC/ECD	4 mg/kg	Malone (1969, 1970)
Spice oleoresins	Dilute (ethanol), add internal standard (1,2-dichloropropane)	GC, microcoulometry		Horwitz (1975)

Abbreviations: GC - gas chromatography; FID - flame-ionization detection; ECD - electron capture detection; MS - mass spectrometry; Hall - Hall conductivity detection

A collaborative study was carried out to determine the efficiency of activated charcoal as a trapping agent for organic vapours in air (Reckner & Sachdev, 1975).

3. Biological Data Relevant to the Evaluation of Carcinogenic Risk to Humans

3.1 Carcinogenicity studies in animals[1]

(a) Oral administration

Mouse: Groups of 50 male and 50 female 5 week-old B6C3F1 mice were administered technical-grade 1,2-dichloroethane in corn oil by gavage on 5 consecutive days per week for 78 weeks. High-dose males received 150 mg/kg bw/day for 8 weeks and then 200 mg/kg bw/day for 70 weeks, followed by 13 weeks without treatment. High-dose females received 250 mg/kg bw/day for 8 weeks, 400 mg/kg bw/day for 3 weeks and 300 mg/kg bw for 67 weeks, followed by 13 weeks without treatment. Low-dose males received 75 mg/kg bw/day for 8 weeks and 100 mg/kg bw/day for 70 weeks, followed by 12 weeks without treatment. Low-dose females received 125 mg/kg bw/day for 8 weeks, 200 mg/kg bw/day for 3 weeks and 150 mg/kg bw/day for 67 weeks, followed by 13 weeks without treatment. The time-weighted average doses were 195 and 299 mg/kg bw/day for high-dose males and females and 97 and 149 mg/kg bw/day for low-dose males and females. A group of 20 male and 20 female mice that received corn oil alone served as matched vehicle controls. Another group of 60 male and 60 female mice that received the same vehicle served as pooled vehicle controls. Of high-dose males, 50% survived at least 84 weeks, and 42% survived until the end of the study; 72% (36/50) of high-dose female mice died between weeks 60 and 80. In the low-dose groups, 52% (26/50) of males survived less than 74 weeks, and 68% (34/50) of females survived until the end of the study. In the vehicle control groups, 55% (11/20) of males and 80% (16/20) of females survived until the end of the study. Almost all organs, and any tissue containing visible lesions, were examined histologically. The numbers of animals with tumours and the total numbers of tumours were significantly greater in male and female mice treated with the higher dose level, and in female mice treated with the low dose, than in controls. Increased incidences of the following neoplasms were observed: mammary adenocarcinomas, uterine adenocarcinomas, endometrial stromal neoplasms of the uterus, and squamous-cell carcinomas of the forestomach in females; lung adenomas and malignant histiocytic lymphomas in males and females; and hepato-cellular carcinomas in male mice (see Table 2). A group of 20 male

---

[1]The Working Group was aware of studies in progress to assess the carcinogenicity of 1,2-dichloroethane by skin application in mice and by oral administration in rats (IARC, 1978).

TABLE 2. ORAL ADMINISTRATION OF 1,2-DICHLOROETHANE TO MICE AND RATS

GROUP	NO. OF ANIMALS EXAMINED HISTO-PATHOLOGICALLY	NO. OF ANIMALS WITH TUMOURS	TOTAL NO. OF TUMOURS	HEPATOCELLULAR CARCINOMAS	MALIGNANT HISTIO-CYSTIC LYMPHOMAS	LUNG ADENOMAS + CARCINOMAS	FORESTOMACH SQUAMOUS-CELL CARCINOMAS	S.C. FIBROSARCOMAS	MAMMARY ADENOCARCINOMAS AND FIBROSARCOMAS	UTERINE ADENOCARCINOMAS	UTERINE ENDOMETRIAL STROMAL SARCOMAS	HAEMANGIOSARCOMAS (SEVERAL ORGANS)
Mice												
Males												
Pooled vehicle controls	59	–	–	4	–	0	1	1	–	–	–	0
Matched vehicle controls	19	4	4	1	0	0	1	0	–	–	–	0
Low-dose	46	15	17	6	8	1	1	0	–	–	–	0
High-dose	47	28	40	12	5	15	2	4	–	–	–	0
Females												
Pooled vehicle controls	60	–	–	–	–	2	1	–	0	1	0	0
Matched vehicle controls	20	6	7	1	2	1	1	0	0	0	0	0
Low-dose	50	33	43	0	10	7	2	0	9	3	2	0
High-dose	48	29	43	1	2	15[a]	5	0	7	4	3	0
Rats												
Males												
Pooled vehicle controls	60	–	–	0	0	0	0	0	–	0	0	1
Matched vehicle controls	20	4	4	0	0	0	0	0	1	0	0	0
Low-dose	50	20	31	0	0	0	3	0	2	0	0	11
High-dose	50	20	39	0	0	0	9	0	0	0	0	7
Females												
Pooled vehicle controls	59	–	–	0	0	0	–	0	6	0	0	–
Matched vehicle controls	20	7	9	0	0	0	0	0	0	0	0	0
Low-dose	50	24	39	0	0	0	1	0	15[b]	0	0	5
High-dose	50	33	47	0	0	0	0	0	24[b]	0	0	4

a 1 mouse had 1 adenoma and 1 adenocarcinoma
b 2 rats had 1 fibroadenoma and 1 adenocarcinoma

and 20 female untreated matched controls was included, but it was not considered in the statistical analyses of tumour incidence (National Cancer Institute, 1978).

Rat: Groups of 50 male and 50 female Osborne Mendel rats, 9 weeks old, were administered technical-grade 1,2-dichloroethane in corn oil by gavage on 5 consecutive days per week for 78 weeks. High and low doses were 100 and 50 mg/kg bw/day for 7 weeks, 150 and 75 mg/kg bw/day for 10 weeks, and 100 and 50 mg/kg bw/day for 18 weeks, respectively, followed by cycles of 1 treatment-free week and 4 weeks under treatment with the same doses (100 and 50 mg/kg bw/day) for 43 weeks (34 weeks under treatment and 9 treatment-free weeks). The time-weighted average doses were 95 and 47 mg/kg bw/day for high- and low-dose males and females. A group of 20 male and 20 female rats received corn oil alone and were used as matched vehicle controls; another group of 60 male and 60 female rats received the same vehicle and were used as the pooled vehicle control group. The last high-dose male rat died during week 23 of the observation period following administration of the chemical, and the last high-dose female rat died during week 15 of the observation period. Low-dose rats were observed for 32 weeks after administration. Mortality was increased in the high-dose groups: 50% of males were dead by week 55 and 50% of females by week 57; by week 75, 84% of males and 80% of females were dead. In the low-dose group, 52% of the males survived over 82 weeks, and 50% of the females survived over 85 weeks. All treated and control animals were examined histologically. The total number of tumours was significantly greater than that in controls only in female rats treated with the high dose; however, a significant increase in the number of squamous-cell carcinomas of the forestomach in male rats and of mammary gland adenocarcinomas and fibroadenomas in female rats treated with the high dose was observed. An increase in the incidence of haemangiosarcomas in animals of both sexes was also noted, but it was statistically significant only in males (see Table 2). A group of 20 male and 20 female untreated matched controls was included, but it was not considered in the statistical analyses of tumour incidence (National Cancer Institute, 1978).

(b) Intraperitoneal administration

Mouse: Groups of 20 male A/St mice, 6-8 weeks old, were given thrice weekly i.p. injections of 20, 40 or 100 mg/kg bw 1,2-dichloro-ethane in tricaprylin for 8 weeks. All survivors were killed 24 weeks after the first injection. No significant increase in the incidence of lung tumours was observed compared with that in tricaprylin-treated controls (Theiss et al., 1977) [The Working Group noted the limitations of a negative result obtained with this test system; see also General Remarks on Substances Considered, p. 34].

3.2 Other relevant biological data

(a) Experimental systems

The toxicity and metabolism of 1,2-dichloroethane have been reviewed (WHO, 1970; National Institute for Occupational Safety & Health, 1976b; Von Oettingen, 1964).

Toxic effects

The single oral LD_{50} in rats is 700 mg/kg bw (McCollister *et al.*, 1956); the inhalational LD_{50} in rats is 4000 mg/m^3 (1000 ppm) in air for a 4-hr exposure (Carpenter *et al.*, 1949).   Rats exposed to various concentrations in air showed central nervous system depression, anaesthesia and coma (Von Oettingen, 1964).   Acute exposure caused disseminated haemorrhagic lesions, mainly in the liver; chronic exposure caused degeneration of the liver and tubular damage and necrosis of the kidneys (McCollister *et al.*, 1956).   Necrosis of the corneal endothelium was seen in dogs after s.c. injection of 1,2-dichloroethane (Kuwabara *et al.*, 1968).

No data on the embryotoxicity or teratogenicity of 1,2-dichloroethane were available.

Absorption, distribution, excretion and metabolism

Following i.p. injection of 50-170 mg/kg bw ^{14}C-1,2-dichloroethane to mice, 10-42% was expired unchanged or 12-15% as CO_2, depending upon the dose; most of the remainder was excreted in the urine, primarily as chloroacetic acid, *S*-carboxymethylcysteine and thiodiacetic acid. The metabolism of 1,2-dichloroethane to chloroacetic acid proceeds possibly *via* chloroacetaldehyde to 2-chloroethanol (Yllner, 1971). Little dechlorination of 1,2-dichloroethane was found to occur in rat and rabbit liver preparations *in vitro* (Bray *et al.*, 1952; Van Dyke & Wineman, 1971).

Studies *in vitro* and in isolated perfused rat liver indicate that 1,2-dichloroethane, in the presence of glutathione and rat liver cytosol or glutathione-*S*-transferases A and C, forms a chemically reactive sulphur-half mustard intermediate.   It has been proposed that the active compound is *S*-chloroethyl glutathione (Rannug & Beije, 1979; Rannug *et al.*, 1978).

The similarity of the toxic effects of ethylene chlorohydrin (2-chloroethanol) and 1,2-dichloroethane (Ambrose, 1950; Hayes *et al.*, 1973; Miller *et al.*, 1970) suggests that poisoning by 1,2-dichloroethane is due at least in part to its metabolic products.

Mutagenicity and other related short-term tests

1,2-Dichloroethane is mutagenic in *Salmonella typhimurium* TA1530, TA1535 and TA100, presumably causing base-pair substitution mutations (Bignami *et al.*, 1977; Brem *et al.*, 1974; McCann *et al.*, 1975; Rannug *et al.*, 1978); the mutagenic effect was enhanced by addition of cytosol and glutathione (Rannug *et al.*, 1978; Rannug & Beije, 1979). It was ineffective in inducing somatic crossing-over and non-disjunction in *Aspergillus nidulans* (Bignami *et al.*, 1977).

Ehrenberg *et al.* (1974) reported an increase in mutation frequency in barley (*Hordeum vulgare*) when kernels were treated for 24 hrs at 20°C with 30.3 mM 1,2-dichloroethane. It caused no chromosome breaks in *Allium* root tips or in human lymphocytes, nor did it induce lysogeny in *Escherichia coli* K39 (λ) (Kristoffersson, 1974).

1,2-Dichloroethane induced sex-linked recessive lethals in *Drosophila melanogaster* when larvae or adult males were treated; the frequency of these mutations was dose related (Rapoport, 1960). Exposure of virgin *Drosophila melanogaster* females to 1,2-dichloroethane vapours in air (7 mg in a 1.5-litre dessicator for 4 or 8 hours) led to an increase in the frequency of sex-linked recessive lethals; an increase in the frequency of sex-chromosome non-disjunction was seen after the 8-hr treatment (Shakarnis, 1969). In a subsequent study using a radioresistant stock of *Drosophila melanogaster* and treatment for up to 6 hrs with 10 ml of a 0.07% solution of 1,2-dichloroethane in the gas phase, Shakarnis (1970) confirmed the effect of the compound in inducing sex-linked recessive lethals; non-disjunction was not observed, however.

Chloroacetaldehyde, a postulated metabolite of 1,2-dichloroethane, is mutagenic in *Salmonella typhimurium* TA100 (McCann *et al.*, 1975; see IARC, 1979c).

(b) Humans

The toxic effects of 1,2-dichloroethane in humans have been reviewed recently. Deaths due to ingestion and inhalation of the solvent have been attributed to circulatory and respiratory failure (National Institute for Occupational Safety & Health, 1976b).

In many cases of acute poisoning, hyperaemia and haemorrhagic lesions have been observed throughout the body; Martin *et al.* (1968) attributed these to a reduction in the level of blood clotting factors and to thrombocytopenia.

Repeated exposures to 1,2-dichloroethane in the occupational environment have been associated with anorexia, nausea, abdominal pain, irritation of the mucous membranes, dysfunction of liver and kidney and neurological disorders (Byers, 1943; Delplace *et al.*, 1962; Watrous, 1947).

3.3 Case reports and epidemiological studies

No data were available to the Working Group.

4. Summary of Data Reported and Evaluation

4.1 Experimental data

1,2-Dichloroethane was tested in one experiment in mice and in one in rats by oral administration. In mice, it produced benign and malignant tumours of the lung and malignant lymphomas in animals of both sexes, hepatocellular carcinomas in males and mammary and uterine adenocarcinomas in females. In rats, it produced carcinomas of the forestomach in male animals, benign and malignant mammary tumours in females and haemangiosarcomas in animals of both sexes. It was inadequately tested by intraperitoneal administration in mice.

1,2-Dichloroethane is mutagenic in *Salmonella typhimurium*, *Drosophila melanogaster* and *Hordeum vulgare*. It can form a reactive chloroethyl sulphide intermediate in the presence of rat liver enzymes.

4.2 Human data

No case reports or epidemiological studies were available to the Working Group.

The extensive production of 1,2-dichloroethane and its use as a lead scavenging agent in petrol, as a fumigant and as a chemical intermediate suggest that widespread human exposure occurs. This is confirmed by many reports of its occurrence in the general and working environments.

4.3 Evaluation

There is *sufficient evidence* that 1,2-dichloroethane is carcinogenic in mice and rats. In the absence of adequate data in humans, it is reasonable, for practical purposes, to regard 1,2-dichloroethane as if it presented a carcinogenic risk to humans.

5. References

Ambrose, A.M. (1950) Toxicological studies of compounds investigated for use as inhibitors of biological processes. II. Toxicity of ethylene chlorohydrin. Arch. ind. Hyg. occup. Med., 2, 591-597

Anon. (1978a)   OPP draft notice lists pesticides accepted, rejected as RPAR candidates. Pestic. Tox. Chem. News, 6, 3-5

Anon. (1978b) NIOSH for lower ethylene dichloride limits. Chem. Eng. News, 6 October, p. 17

Bignami, M., Cardamone, G., Comba, P., Ortali, V.A., Morpurgo, G. & Carere, A. (1977)   Relationship between chemical structure and mutagenic activity in some pesticides: the use of *Salmonella typhimurium* and *Aspergillus nidulans* (Abstract no. 79). Mutat. Res., 46, 243-244

Bray, H.G., Thorpe, W.V. & Vallance, D.K. (1952) The liberation of chloride ions from organic chloro compounds by tissue extracts. Biochem. J., 51, 193-201

Brem, H., Stein, A.B. & Rosenkranz, H.S. (1974) The mutagenicity and DNA-modifying effect of haloalkanes. Cancer Res., 34, 2576-2579

Byers, D.H. (1943) Chlorinated solvents in common wartime use. Ind. Med., 12, 440-443

Carpenter, J., Smyth, H.F., Jr & Pozzani, V.C. (1949)   The assay of acute vapor toxicity, and the grading and interpretation of results on 96 chemical compounds. J. ind. Hyg. Toxicol., 31, 343-346

Conkle, J.P., Camp, B.J. & Welch, B.E. (1975) Trace composition of human respiratory gas. Arch. environ. Health, 30, 290-295

Delplace, Y., Cavigneaux, A. & Cabasson, G. (1962) Occupational diseases due to methylene chloride and dichloroethane (Fr.). Arch. Mal. prof., 23, 816-817

Dowty, B.J., Carlisle, D.R. & Laseter, J.L. (1975) New Orleans drinking water sources tested by gas chromatography-mass spectrometry. Occurrence and origin of aromatics and halogenated aliphatic hydrocarbons. Environ. Sci. Technol., 9, 762-765

Driscoll, J.N. & Warneck, P. (1973) The analysis of ppm levels of gases in air by photoionization mass spectrometry. J. Air Poll. Control Assoc., 23, 858-863

Ehrenberg, L., Osterman-Golkar, S., Singh, D. & Lundqvist, U. (1974)   On the reaction kinetics and mutagenic activity of methylating and β-halogenoethylating gasoline additives.   Radiat. Bot., 15, 185-194

Eurocop-Cost (1976)   A Comprehensive List of Polluting Substances Which Have Been Identified in Various Fresh Waters, Effluent Discharges, Aquatic Animals and Plants, and Bottom Sediments, 2nd ed., EUCO/MDU/ 73/76, XII/476/76, Luxembourg, Commission of the European Communities, p. 41

Ewing, B.B., Chian, E.S.K., Cook, J.C., Evans, C.A., Hopke, P.K. & Perkins, E.G. (1977)   Monitoring to Detect Previously Unrecognized Pollutants in Surface Waters, EPA-560/6-77-015, Washington DC, US Environmental Protection Agency, pp. 63-64, 73

Fujii, T. (1977)   Direct aqueous injection gas chromatography-mass spectrometry for analysis of organohalides in water at concentrations below the parts per billion level.   J. Chromatogr., 139, 297-302

Gage, J.C., Strafford, N. & Truhaut, R. (1962)   Methods for the Determination of Toxic Substances in Air, International Union of Pure & Applied Chemistry, London, Butterworths, pp. 27.1-27.2

Grasselli, J.G. & Ritchey, W.M., eds (1975)   CRC Atlas of Spectral Data and Physical Constants for Organic Compounds, 2nd ed., Vol. III, Cleveland, OH, Chemical Rubber Co., p. 249

Green, B.D. & Steinfeld, J.I. (1976)   Laser absorption spectroscopy: method for monitoring complex trace gas mixtures.   Environ. Sci. Technol., 10, 1134-1139

Hardie, D.W.F. (1964)   Chlorocarbons and chlorohydrocarbons.   1,2-Dichloroethane.   In: Kirk, R.E. & Othmer, D.F., eds, Encyclopedia of Chemical Technology, 2nd ed., Vol. 5, New York, John Wiley & Sons, pp. 149-154

Hawley, G.G., ed. (1971)   The Condensed Chemical Dictionary, 8th ed., New York, Van Nostrand-Reinhold, p. 364

Hayes, F.D., Short, R.D. & Gibson, J.E. (1973)   Differential toxicity of monochloroacetate, monofluoroacetate and monoiodoacetate in rats. Toxicol. appl. Pharmacol., 26, 93-102

Horwitz, W., ed. (1975)   Official Methods of Analysis of the Association of Official Analytical Chemists, 12th ed., Washington DC, Association of Official Analytical Chemists, pp. 91, 383

IARC (1978)   Information Bulletin on the Survey of Chemicals Being Tested for Carcinogenicity, No. 7, Lyon, p. 276

IARC (1979a)   IARC Monographs on the Evaluation of the Carcinogenic Risk of Chemicals to Humans, 19, Some Monomers, Plastics and Synthetic Elastomers, and Acrolein, Lyon, pp. 377-438

IARC (1979b)   IARC Monographs on the Evaluation of the Carcinogenic Risk of Chemicals to Humans, 19, Some Monomers, Plastics and Synthetic Elastomers, and Acrolein, Lyon, pp. 439-459

IARC (1979c)   IARC Monographs on the Evaluation of the Carcinogenic Risk of Chemicals to Humans, 19, Some Monomers, Plastics and Synthetic Elastomers, and Acrolein, Lyon, p. 396

Jensen, S., Lange, R., Berge, G., Palmork, K.H. & Renberg, L. (1975) On the chemistry of EDC-tar and its biological significance in the sea.   Proc. R. Soc. Lond. B, 189, 333-346

Kretzschmar, J.G., Peperstraete, H. & Rymen, T. (1976)   Air pollution in and around Tessenderlo [The Netherlands] (Neth.).   Extern, 5, 147-178

Kristoffersson, U. (1974)   Genetic effects of some gasoline additives (Abstract).   Hereditas, 78, 319

Kuwabara, T., Quevedo, A.R. & Cogan, D.C. (1968)   An experimental study of dichloroethane poisoning.   Arch. Ophthal., 79, 321-330

Malone, B. (1969)   Analysis of grains for multiple residues of organic fumigants.   J. Assoc. off. anal. Chem., 52, 800-805

Malone, B. (1970)   Method for determining multiple residues of organic fumigants in cereal grains.   J. Assoc. off. anal. Chem., 53, 742-746

Martin, G., Knorpp, K., Huth, K., Heinrich, F. & Mittermayer, D. (1968) Clinical features, pathogenesis and management of dichloroethane poisoning (Germ.).   Dtsch. med. Wschr., 93, 2002 [Translation in: Germ. Med. Mth. (1969), 14, 62-67]

Martin, H. & Worthing, C.R., eds (1977)   Pesticide Manual, 5th ed., Malvern, Worcestershire, British Crop Protection Council, p. 251

McCann, J., Simmon, V., Streitzieser, D. & Ames, B.N. (1975)   Mutagenicity of chloroacetaldehyde, a possible metabolic product of 1,2-dichloroethane (ethylene dichloride), chloroethanol (ethylene chlorohydrin), vinyl chloride, and cyclophosphamide.   Proc. natl Acad. Sci. (Wash.), 72, 3190-3193

McCollister, D.D., Hollingsworth, R.L., Oyen, F. & Rowe, V.K. (1956) Comparative inhalation toxicity of fumigant mixtures.   Individual and joint effects of ethylene dichloride, carbon tetrachloride and ethylene dibromide.   Arch. ind. Health., 13, 1-7

Miller, V., Dobbs, R.J. & Jacobs, S.I. (1970)   Ethylene chlorohydrin intoxication with fatality.   Arch. Dis. Child., 45, 589-590

National Cancer Institute (1978) Bioassay of 1,2-Dichloroethane for Possible Carcinogenicity (Technical Report Series No. 55), DHEW Publication No. (NIH) 78-1361, Washington, DC, US Department of Health, Education, & Welfare

National Fire Protection Association (1972) Fire Protection Guide on Hazardous Materials, 4th ed., Boston, MA, p. 325M-78

National Institute for Occupational Safety & Health (1976a) Criteria document recommendations for an ethylene dichloride standard. US Occup. Saf. Health Rep., 5, 1552-1557

National Institute for Occupational Safety & Health (1976b) Criteria for a Recommended Standard. Occupational Exposure to Ethylene Dichloride (1,2-Dichloroethane), DHEW Publication No. (NIOSH) 76-139, Washington DC, US Government Printing Office

National Institute for Occupational Safety & Health (1977a) National Occupational Hazard Survey, Vol. III, Survey Analyses and Supplemental Tables, Draft, Cincinnati, OH, p. 445, 3,832-3,841

National Institute for Occupational Safety & Health (1977b) NIOSH Manual of Analytical Methods, Part II, Standards Completion Program Validated Methods, Vol. 2, Method S122, DHEW (NIOSH) Publication No. 77-157-B, Washington DC, US Government Printing Office, pp. S122-1 - S122-9

Nicholson, A.A., Meresz, O. & Lemyk, B. (1977) Determination of free and total potential haloform in drinking water. Anal. Chem., 49, 814-819

Okuno, T., Tsuji, M., Shintani, Y. & Watanabe, H. (1974) Gas chromatography of chlorinated hydrocarbon in urban air (Jap.). Hyogo-ken Kogai Kenkyusho Kenkyu Hokoku, 6, 1-6 [Chem. Abstr., 87, 72564f]

Parkes, D.G., Ganz, C.C., Polinsky, A. & Schulze, J. (1976) A simple gas chromatographic method for the analysis of trace organics in ambient air. Am. ind. Hyg. Assoc. J., 37, 165-173

Parsons, J.S. & Mitzner, S. (1975) Gas chromatographic method for concentration and analysis of traces of industrial organic pollutants in environmental air and stacks. Environ. Sci. Technol., 9, 1053-1058

Patterson, R.M., Bornstein, M.I. & Garshick, E. (1976) Assessment of Ethylene Dichloride as a Potential Air Pollution Problem, Vol. III, Research Triangle Park, NC, US Environmental Protection Agency, Contract No. 68-02-1337. Available from Springfield, VA, National Technical Information Service, No. PB-258 355

Prager, B., Jacobson, P., Schmidt, P. & Stern, D., eds (1918)
    Beilsteins Handbuch der Organichen Chemie, 4th ed., Vol. 1,
    System No. 8, Berlin, Springer, p. 84

Rannug, U. & Beije, B. (1979) The mutagenic effect of 1,2-dichloroethane
    on *Salmonella typhimurium*. II. Activation by the isolated perfused
    rat liver. Chem.-biol. Interact., 24, 265-285

Rannug, U., Sundvall, A. & Ramel, C. (1978) The mutagenic effect of
    1,2-dichloroethane on *Salmonella typhimurium*. I. Activation through
    conjugation with glutathion *in vitro*. Chem.-biol. Interact., 20, 1-16

Rapoport, I.A. (1960) The reaction of genic proteins with 1,2-dichloro-
    ethane (Russ.). Dokl. Akad. Nauk SSR, 134, 1214-1217 [Translation
    in Dokl. Biol. Sci. (1960), 134, 745-747]

Reckner, L.R. & Sachdev, J. (1975) Collaborative Testing of Activated
    Charcoal Sampling Tubes for Seven Organic Solvents, DHEW (NIOSH)
    Publication No. 75-184, Washington DC, US Government Printing
    Office, pp. 1.0, 2-1-2-4, 3-1-3-6

Shackelford, W.M. & Keith, L.H. (1976) Frequency of Organic Compounds
    Identified in Water, EPA-600/4-76-062, Athens, GA, US Environmental
    Protection Agency, p. 134

Shakarnis, V.F. (1969) 1,2-Dichloroethane induced chromosome non-
    disjunction and recessive sex-linked lethal mutation in *Drosophila
    melanogaster* (Russ.). Genetika, 5, 89-95

Shakarnis, V.F. (1970) Effect of 1,2-dichloroethane on chromosome
    non-disjunction and recessive sex-linked lethals in a radio-
    resistant strain of *Drosophila melanogaster* (Russ.). Vestn.
    Leningrad Univ. Ser. Biol., 25, 153-156

Symons, J.M., Bellar, T.A., Carswell, J.K., DeMarco, J., Kropp, K.L.,
    Robeck, G.G., Seeger, D.R., Slocum, C.J., Smith, B.L. &
    Stevens, A.A. (1975) National organics reconnaissance survey for
    halogenated organics. J. Am. Water Works Assoc., 67, 634-647

Theiss, J.C., Stoner, G.D., Shimkin, M.B. & Weisburger, E.K. (1977)
    Test for carcinogenicity of organic contaminants of United States
    drinking water by pulmonary tumor response in strain A mice.
    Cancer Res., 37, 2717-2720

US Department of Commerce (1977) US Exports, Schedule B Commodity
    Groupings, Schedule B Commodity by Country, FT 410/December,
    Bureau of the Census, Washington DC, US Government Printing Office,
    p. 2-85

US Environmental Protection Agency (1969) EPA Compendium of Registered Pesticides, Washington DC, US Government Printing Office, pp. III-E-10.1-III-E-10.2

US Environmental Protection Agency (1976) Protection of environment. US Code Fed. Regul., Title 40, part 180.1007, p. 222

US International Trade Commission (1977) Synthetic Organic Chemicals, US Production and Sales, 1976, USITC Publication 833, Washington DC, US Government Printing Office, pp. 302, 331

US Occupational Safety & Health Administration (1977) Air contaminants. US Code Fed. Regul., Title 29, part 1910.1000, p. 28

US Tariff Commission (1923) Census of Dyes and Other Synthetic Organic Chemicals 1922, Tariff Information Series No. 31, Washington DC, US Government Printing Office, Table 6

Van Dyke, R.A. & Wineman, C.G. (1971) Enzymatic dechlorination. Dechlorination of chloroethanes and propanes in vitro. Biochem. Pharmacol., 20, 463-470

Von Oettingen, W.F. (1964) The Halogenated Hydrocarbons of Industrial and Toxicological Importance, Amsterdam, Elsevier, pp. 186-197

Watrous, R.M. (1947) Health hazards of the pharmaceutical industry. Br. J. ind. Med., 4, 111-125

WHO (1970) Toxicological evaluation of some extraction solvents and certain other substances. WHO/Food/Add/70. 39, pp. 91-93

WHO (1972) 1971 evaluations of some pesticide residues in food. WHO Pestic. Residue Ser., No. 1, pp. 276-279, 325-328

Yllner, S. (1971) Metabolism of 1,2-dichloroethane-^{14}C in the mouse. Acta pharmacol. toxicol., 30, 257-265

DICHLOROMETHANE

Two reviews on dichloromethane are available (Berkowitz, 1978; Mercier, 1977).

1. Chemical and Physical Data

1.1 Synonyms and trade names

Chem. Abstr. Services Reg. No.: 75-09-2

Chem. Abstr. Name: Dichloromethane

Synonyms: Methane dichloride; methylene bichloride; methylene chloride; methylene dichloride

Trade names: Aerothene MM; Freon 30; Narkotil; Solaesthin; Solmethine

1.2 Structural and molecular formulae and molecular weight

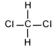

CH_2Cl_2 Mol. wt: 84.9

1.3 Chemical and physical properties of the pure substance

From Hawley (1977), unless otherwise specified

(a) Description: Colourless liquid

(b) Boiling-point: 40.1°C

(c) Freezing-point: -97°C

(d) Density: d_4^{15} 1.335

(e) Refractive index: n_D^{20} 1.4244

(f) Spectroscopy data: λ_{vap} < 200 nm; infra-red, nuclear magnetic resonance and mass spectral data have been tabulated (Grasselli & Ritchey, 1975).

(g) Solubility: Soluble in water (2 g/100 g water at 20°C), phenols, aldehydes, ketones, glacial acetic acid, triethyl phosphate, acetoacetic ester, formamide and cyclohexylamine; miscible in all proportions with commercial chlorinated solvents, diethyl ether and ethanol (Hardie, 1964).

(h) Volatility: Vapour pressure is 400 mm at 24.1°C (Perry & Chilton, 1973).

(i) Stability: Nonflammable and nonexplosive in air; no appreciable decomposition at room temperature when in contact with common metals.   Prolonged heating with water at 180°C results in formation of formic acid, methyl chloride, methanol, hydrochloric acid and some carbon monoxide (Hardie, 1964)

(j) Reactivity: Reacts at normal temperatures with aluminium and alloys of potassium and sodium; at elevated temperatures in contact with water, it corrodes iron, some stainless steels, copper, nickel and certain other metals and alloys; readily chlorinated to chloroform and carbon tetrachloride in the presence of chlorination catalysts (Hardie, 1964)

(k) Conversion factor: 1 ppm in air is equivalent to 3.5 mg/m^3.

1.4 Technical products and impurities

In the US, standard grade dichloromethane has the following typical specifications: a clear, water-white liquid, free of suspended matter; specific gravity, 25°C/25°C, 1.319-1.323; acidity, 5 mg/kg max; non-volatile residue, 10 mg/kg max; free halogen, none; and a 100% distill-ation range of 39.5-40.5°C.

Commercial grades of dichloromethane may contain 0.0001-1% of added stabilizers, such as phenol, hydroquinone, *para*-cresol, resorcinol, thymol, 1-naphthol or amines.   A representative commercial sample contains not more than the following impurities: water, 200 mg/kg; acid (as HCl), 5 mg/kg; and chloroform, 2500 mg/kg (Hardie, 1964).

In Japan, dichloromethane has a purity of 99-100%.

2. Production, Use, Occurrence and Analysis

2.1 Production and use

(a) Production

Dichloromethane was first prepared in 1840 by Regnault by chlorinating methyl chloride in sunlight (Hardie, 1964).   It is currently produced commercially in the US either by: (1) chlorination of methyl chloride (which is obtained from reaction of methanol and hydrogen chloride) or (2) by direct chlorination of methane.   Approximately 65% of that produced in 1976 involved the chlorination of methyl chloride, in which chloroform and carbon tetrachloride are obtained as coproducts.

In Japan, approximately 73% of dichloromethane is produced by chlorination of methane and about 27% by chlorination of methyl chloride.

Commercial production of dichloromethane in the US was first reported in 1934 (US Tariff Commission, 1936).   In 1976, 5 US companies reported a total production of 244 million kg (US International Trade Commission, 1977).   Imports in that year were 19.1 million kg, with 47.9% from the Federal Republic of Germany, 31.2% from Belgium, 10.6% from Japan, 7.6% from The Netherlands and 2.7% from France (US Department of Commerce, 1977a).   Exports were 38.2 million kg, to the following countries (percent of total exports): The Netherlands (33.6), Canada (25.3), Mexico (8.4), Brazil (7.9), Japan (6.1), Republic of South Africa (6.1), Australia (5.4), Venezuela (3.0), Sweden (1.2) and at least 5 other countries (30) (US Department of Commerce, 1977b).

Dichloromethane is believed to be produced in the following European countries (number of producers): Belgium (1), the Federal Republic of Germany (3), France (4), Italy (2), The Netherlands (3), Spain (1), and the UK (1).

It has been produced commercially in Japan since about 1944.   In 1976, 4 companies produced an estimated 24.6 million, and 3 million kg were exported.

(b) Use

In 1976, dichloromethane was used in the US as follows: paint removers, 44%; solvents (degreasing), 25%; aerosol propellants, 19%; and other applications, 12%.

Of all organic paint removers, those based on dichloromethane are the most widely used (Downing, 1967).   Typical paint-stripping compositions that have dichloromethane as the major component may also contain paraffins, glacial acetic acid, formic acid, alcohols, acetone and a sulphonated detergent (Hardie, 1964).

Dichloromethane is used for degreasing engine parts in the motor transportation, railway and aircraft industries (Gosselin *et al.*, 1976). It is a component of diphase chlorinated solvents, the upper phase of which is water to reduce evaporation of the dichloromethane (Spring, 1967). With other chlorinated solvents, dichloromethane is replacing trichloro-ethylene for use in metal degreasing because of restrictions concerning photochemically reactive materials and, more recently, concern about the carcinogenicity of trichloroethylene (Anon., 1976).

Aerosol applications for dichloromethane include insecticides, hair sprays, shampoos, paints and others. It has been predicted that use as aerosols, as replacements for fluorocarbons, could become the second most important market for dichloromethane (Anon., 1976).

Miscellaneous applications of dichloromethane include use as a solvent in certain pharmaceutical applications and in the extraction of naturally-occurring heat-sensitive substances, such as edible fats, cocoa, butter, caffeine and the beer flavouring in hops. It is also used as a solvent in the manufacture of photographic film and synthetic fibre (Hardie, 1964), as a component of fire-extinguishing compositions and as an insecticidal fumigant. Virtually all caffeine extraction for the production of decaffeinated coffee in the US is now carried out with dichloromethane instead of trichloroethylene.

No data on its use in Europe were available.

In 1976, it was used in Japan as follows: solvent, 40%; blowing agent for urethane, 20%; paint remover, 18%; and other 22%.

Dichloromethane is registered for use in the US as an insecticide for commodity fumigation of a variety of grains (US Environmental Protection Agency, 1969); and an estimated 45.4 thousand kg dichloromethane were used in 1975 in the US as a commodity and space fumigant. It is exempted from the requirement of a tolerance for residues when used as a fumigant after harvest for barley, corn, oats, popcorn, rice, rye, sorghum and wheat and for the postharvest fumigation of citrus fruits (US Environmental Protection Agency, 1976).

The US Food and Drug Administration (FDA) permits the presence of dichloromethane in the following foods: (1) in spice oleoresins as a residue after spice extraction, at a level no greater than 30 mg/kg; (2) in hops extract, at a level no greater than 2.2%; and (3) in coffee as a residue from its use as a solvent in caffeine extraction, at a level no greater than 10 mg/kg. The FDA also allows its use in adhesives and in the production of polycarbonate resins intended for use in producing, manufacturing, packaging, processing, preparing or holding food (US Food & Drug Administration, 1977).

Permissible levels of dichloromethane in the working environment have been established in various countries.   The US Occupational Safety and Health Administration's health standards require that an employee's exposure to dichloromethane at no time exceed 1740 mg/m^3 (500 ppm) in any 8-hr work shift of a 40-hr work week, with an acceptable ceiling concentration of 3500 mg/m^3 (1000 ppm), and not exceed 7000 mg/m^3 (2000 ppm) for more than 5 min in any 2 hrs (US Occupational Safety & Health Administration, 1977).   The 8-hr time-weighted average value in The Federal Republic of Germany is 1750 mg/m^3 (500 ppm);   in the German Democratic Republic and Czechoslovakia, 500 mg/m^3 (144 ppm);   and in Sweden, 350 mg/m^3 (100 ppm).   The acceptable ceiling concentration in the USSR is 50 mg/m^3 (14 ppm) (Winell, 1975).

The US National Institute for Occupational Safety and Health has recommended that occupational exposure to dichloromethane not exceed 261 mg/m^3 (75 ppm), determined as a time-weighted average for up to a 10-hr work day of a 40-hr work week, in the absence of exposure to carbon monoxide above a time-weighted average of 31.5 mg/m^3 (9 ppm) for up to a 10-hr work day (National Institute for Occupational Safety & Health, 1976).

2.2   Occurrence

Dichloromethane is formed during the chlorination of water.

(a)   Air

Dichloromethane was one of 12 chlorinated hydrocarbons detected in urban air, at levels of 0.035-32.9 µg/m^3 (0.01-9.4 ppb) (Okuno *et al.*, 1974);   it has been detected at levels of < 17.5 ng/m^3 (5 ppt) in rural air samples (Grimsrud & Rasmussen, 1975).   A level of 121 ng/m^3 (35 ppt) was detected in the troposphere (Cox *et al.*, 1976).   It has also been detected in air in which cigarette smoke was present (Holzer *et al.*, 1976).

(b)   Water

Dichloromethane is formed during the chlorination of water.   A survey in the US indicated that 1% of raw-water supplies and 8% of finished-water supplies contained it, with a mean concentration in finished water of < 1 µg/l.   Nine out of 10 US water supplies surveyed in one study contained dichloromethane;   the highest concentration was 1.6 µg/l (Safe Drinking Water Committee, 1977).   Dichloromethane was detected in the municipal drinking-water in 2 locations at a level of < 5 µg/l, and in bottled water (Dowty *et al.*, 1975;   Saunders *et al.*, 1975).   In another location, dichloromethane was detected in drinking-water at a level of 0.3 µg/l (Fujii, 1977).

The concentrations of dichloromethane detected at various stages of treatment in a sewage-treatment plant were 8.2 µg/l in the influent before treatment, 2.9 µg/l in the effluent before chlorination and 3.4 µg/l in the effluent after chlorination (Bellar *et al.*, 1974).

Published reports of the detection of dichloromethane in river and lake water as well as in effluent from paper mills and chemical and latex manufacturing plants at various US locations have been tabulated (Shackelford & Keith, 1976).

(c) Humans

Dichloromethane was detected in the expired air of 5/8 male human subjects at levels of 0.12-340 µg/hr (Conkle *et al.*, 1975).

(d) Occupational exposure

On the basis of health hazard evaluations of various US companies conducted in 1973 and 1974, dichloromethane exposure concentrations in a variety of jobs were as follows (in ppm): servicing diesel engines, 11 ppm; spray-painting booths, 1-74 ppm; chemical plant, 0-5520 ppm, 8-hr time-weighted average, 875 ppm; plastic tank construction, a few ppm; ski manufacture, 0-36 ppm; cleaning foam heads, 3-29 ppm; cleaning nozzles in plastics manufacture, 5-37 ppm (National Institute for Occupational Safety & Health, 1976).

In a 1973 study of occupational exposure to propellants used in hair spray in a hairdresser's in Wilmington, DE, it was determined that beauticians were exposed to a daily mean background concentration of < $3.5-7$ mg/m^3 (< 1-2 ppm) dichloromethane. Air samples taken 1-2 min after a hairdresser had completed spraying a hair-do contained 3.5-455 mg/m^3 (1-130 ppm) dichloromethane (Hoffman, 1973).

(e) Other

Dichloromethane was detected in 15/17 spice oleoresins from one manufacturer and in 3 from another as follows (mg/kg): allspice (68), black pepper (23), capsicum (31 and 4), cassia (83), celery (33), cinnamon (24), coriander (24), ginger (10 and 7), marjoram (48), nutmeg (63), paprika (14), rosemary (41), sage (29), thyme (36) and turmeric (59 and 1) (Page & Kennedy, 1975).

2.3 Analysis

The collection of dichloromethane from air, using silica gel, activated charcoal, porous polymer beads and liquids, and its analysis, using colorimetry, gas chromatography, infra-red spectrometry and photo-detector analysis, have been reviewed (National Institute for Occupational Safety & Health, 1976).

Methods used for the analysis of dichloromethane in environmental samples are listed in Table 1.

Gas chromatography-mass spectrometric methods have been proposed to determine dichloromethane in air and water (Coleman *et al.*, 1976; Grimsrud & Rasmussen, 1975).   Other methods include the use of gas chromatography-thermal conductivity detection (Naumova & Belova, 1976), colorimetry (Tyras & Blochowicz, 1974) and photoionization-mass spectrometry (Driscoll & Warneck, 1973).

3.   Biological Data Relevant to the Evaluation
of Carcinogenic Risk to Humans

3.1 Carcinogenicity studies in animals[1]

Intraperitoneal administration

Mouse: Groups of 20 male A/St mice, 6-8 weeks old, received reagent-grade dichloromethane in tricaprylin at doses of 160, 400 and 800 mg/kg bw (found in preliminary toxicity tests to be the maximum tolerated dose, i.e., that tolerated by all of 5 mice that received 6 i.p. injections over a 2-week period).   Each dose was injected intraperitoneally thrice weekly for a total of 16-17 injections (total doses, 2720, 6800 and 12,800 mg/kg bw in the respective groups).   After 24 weeks, 18, 5 and 12 animals in the three groups were still alive; these were killed and their lungs examined for tumours and compared with 15 survivors out of 20 vehicle-treated controls.   In the treated mice, 0.9, 0.8 and 0.5 lung tumours per mouse were observed, which were not significantly different from the 0.27 observed in controls injected with tricaprylin (Theiss *et al.*, 1977) [The Working Group noted the poor survival of treated animals and the limitations of negative results obtained with this test system; see also General Remarks on Substances Considered, p. 34].

3.2 Other relevant biological data

(a) Experimental systems

Toxic effects

The LD_{50} by i.p. injection in mice is 2000 mg/kg bw (Klaassen & Plaa, 1966); the LC_{50} by inhalation in mice is 56 g/m^3 (16,200 ppm) (Svirbely *et al.*, 1947).

---

[1]The Working Group was aware of studies in progress to assess the carcinogenicity of dichloromethane in rats and hamsters by inhalation, and in mice and rats by oral administration (IARC, 1978a).

TABLE 1. METHODS FOR THE ANALYSIS OF DICHLOROMETHANE

SAMPLE TYPE	ANALYTICAL METHOD			
	EXTRACTION/CLEAN-UP	DETECTION	LIMIT OF DETECTION	REFERENCE
Formulations				
Hair-spray aerosol	Analyse directly	GC/TCD		Schubert & Ketel (1972)
Air				
Workplace	Trap on charcoal, extract (carbon disulphide)	GC/FID	Working range, 1700-7100 mg/m^3	National Institute for Occupational Safety & Health (1977)
	Inject sample directly, using diglycerol as GC stationary phase	GC/MS	0.7 µg/m^3 (0.2 ppb)	Fujii (1977)
	Inject directly	GC/FID	10 mg/m^3	Kuptsova et al. (1976)
Standard mixtures in air	Adsorb on Chromosorb 101, desorb by heating, retrap in line on GC column	GC/ECD	14 µg/m^3-35 mg/m^3 (0.4 ppb-40 ppm; v/v)	Parkes et al. (1976)
Industrial discharge to atmosphere	Trap in evacuated glass pipette containing glacial acetic acid, react with alkali and pyridine	Spectrophotometry 530 nm		Prikhod'ko et al. (1974)
Water	Remove organics by heating under a stream of helium, adsorb on poly-para-diphenyl phenylene oxide, desorb by heating, trap in line on GC column	GC/MS		Dowty et al. (1975)
	Transfer volatile to gaseous phase by bubbling nitrogen through sample, concentrate	GC/FID GC/microcoulometry	0.1 µg/l	Bellar et al. (1974)
Chlorinated drinking-water	Gas strip volatile, trap on Tenax-GC, desorb by heating, retrap in line on GC column	GC/FID	ppb range	Kuo et al. (1977)
	Cool to 4°C, extract (pentane)	GC/FID GC/ECD	1-10 mg/l	Dietz & Traud (1973)

TABLE 1. METHODS FOR THE ANALYSIS OF DICHLOROMETHANE (continued)

SAMPLE TYPE	ANALYTICAL METHOD			REFERENCE
	EXTRACTION/CLEAN-UP	DETECTION	LIMIT OF DETECTION	
Chlorinated drinking-water	Sparge, trap in line on GC column	GC/Hall	0.1 µg/l	Nicholson *et al.* (1977)
Soil				
Sediments	Mix with water, cool to 4°C, extract (pentane)	GC/FID		Dietz & Traud (1973)
Food				
Spice oleoresins	Vacuum distill (toluene), wash (water)	GC/ECD	1 mg/kg	Page & Kennedy (1975)
Biological				
Blood	Equilibrate with air in closed vessel, inject directly	GC/FID		Premel-Cabic *et al.* (1974)
Blood	Weigh capsule containing sample, break in line, vaporize, flush onto column with carrier gas	GC/FID	1 mg/kg	Laham & Potvin (1976)

Abbreviations: GC/TCD - gas chromatography/thermal conductivity detection; FID - flame-ionization detection; MS - mass spectrometry; ECD - electron capture detection; Hall - Hall conductivity detection

Dichloromethane affects mainly the central nervous system (National Institute for Occupational Safety & Health, 1976); hepatotoxic effects were observed in mice only with single lethal doses (Gehring, 1968). No renal dysfunction was detected in mice; slight calcification of the tubules was seen in dogs (Klaassen & Plaa, 1966, 1967). In mice, continuous inhalation of 17.5 g/m^3 (5000 ppm) caused swelling of the rough endoplasmic reticulum, transient severe fatty changes in the liver and necrosis in isolated hepatocytes (Weinstein et al., 1972).

Embryotoxicity and teratogenicity

Groups of rats and mice were exposed by inhalation for 7 hrs daily on days 6-15 of gestation to 4.4 g/m^3 in air (1250 ppm) dichloromethane; no effects were observed on the average number of implantation sites per litter, litter size, incidence of foetal resorptions, foetal sex ratios or foetal body measurements. No treatment-related increase in the incidence of skeletal or visceral malformations was observed (Schwetz et al., 1975).

Absorption, distribution, excretion and metabolism

The highest levels of radioactivity in rats following exposure by inhalation to 1935 mg/m^3 ^{14}C-dichloromethane were found in the fat, liver, kidney and adrenals. Two hours after exposure, the concentration in fat **had** decreased by more than 90% and the concentration in liver by 25% (Carlsson & Hultengren, 1975).

In vivo and in vitro studies indicate that dichloromethane is metabolized to CO (Carlsson & Hultengren, 1975; Fodor et al., 1973; Kubic et al., 1974) by microsomal mono-oxygenase(s) (Hogan et al., 1976).

Mutagenicity and other related short-term tests

Dichloromethane was mutagenic in Salmonella typhimurium TA100 and TA98, both in the presence and absence of a liver microsomal activation system (Jongen et al., 1978).

(b) Humans

Fatalities have been associated with acute or prolonged exposure to dichloromethane (Moskowitz & Shapiro, 1952; Stewart & Hake, 1976). It acts primarily on the central nervous system (National Institute for Occupational Safety & Health, 1976), causing narcosis (Irish, 1963). Long-term occupational exposure to dichloromethane causes damage to the liver and central nervous system (Hanke et al., 1974; Weiss, 1967).

After a 2-hr exposure, about 50% of inhaled dichloromethane is taken up into the bloodstream (Astrand, 1975); it is also absorbed through the skin (Steward & Dodd, 1964).   It is eliminated mainly in expired air (Riley *et al.*, 1966).

Inhalation of 0.18-3.5 g/m^3 (500-1000 ppm) in air for 1-2 hrs resulted in the formation of significant amounts of carboxyhaemoglobin (Stewart & Hake, 1976; Stewart *et al.*, 1972).

3.3 Case reports and epidemiological studies[1]

No case reports or adequate epidemiological studies were available to the Working Group.

4.   Summary of Data Reported and Evaluation

4.1 Experimental data

Dichloromethane was tested in only one experiment in male mice by intraperitoneal injection.   This experiment was considered to be inadequate, although the results suggested an increased incidence of lung tumours.

Dichloromethane is mutagenic in *Salmonella typhimurium*.

4.2 Human data

No case reports or epidemiological studies were available to the Working Group.

The extensive production and use of dichloromethane mainly as a solvent over the past several decades and its recovery from air and drinking-water indicate that widespread human exposure occurs.

4.3 Evaluation

The available data do not permit an evaluation of the carcinogenicity of dichloromethane to be made.

---

[1]The Working Group was aware of a **retrospective** cohort **study** in progress on workers employed in a fibre production process using dichloromethane as a solvent (IARC, 1978b).

5. References

Anon. (1976) Chemical briefs: methylene chloride. Chem. Purch., October, pp. 39-40

Astrand, I. (1975) Uptake of solvents in the blood and tissues of man. A review. Scand. J. Work. Environ. Health., 1, 199-218

Bellar, T.A., Lichtenberg, J.J. & Kroner, R.C. (1974) The occurrence of organohalides in chlorinated drinking waters. J. Am. Water Works Assoc., 66, 703-706

Berkowitz, J.B. (1978) Literature Review - Problem Definition Studies on Selected Chemicals, Appendix B, Methylene Chloride, Cambridge, MA, Arthur D. Little, Inc., pp. 58-105

Carlsson, A. & Hultengren, M. (1975) Exposure to methylene chloride. III. Metabolism of ^{14}C-labelled methylene chloride in rat. Scand. J. Work. Environ. Health, 1, 104-108

Coleman, W.E., Lingg, R.D., Melton, R.G. & Kopfler, F.C. (1976) The occurrence of volatile organics in five drinking water supplies using gas chromatography/mass spectrometry. In: Keith, L.H., ed., Identification and Analysis of Organic Pollutants in Water, Ann Arbor, MI, Ann Arbor Science, pp. 305-327

Conkle, J.P., Camp, B.J. & Welch, B.E. (1975) Trace composition of human respiratory gas. Arch. environ. Health, 30, 290-295

Cox, R.A., Derwent, R.G., Eggleton, A.E.J. & Lovelock, J.E. (1976) Photochemical oxidation of halocarbons in the troposphere. Atmos. Environ., 10, 305-308

Dietz, F. & Traud, J. (1973) Gas chromatographic determination of low-molecular-weight chlorohydrocarbons in water samples and sediments (Germ.). Vom Wasser, 41, 137-155

Downing, R.S. (1967) Paint and varnish removers. In: Kirk, R.E. & Othmer, D.F., eds, Encyclopedia of Chemical Technology, 2nd ed., Vol. 14, New York, John Wiley & Sons, pp. 485-493

Dowty, B.J., Carlisle, D.R. & Laseter, J.L. (1975) New Orleans drinking water sources tested by gas chromatography-mass spectrometry. Occurrence and origin of aromatics and halogenated aliphatic hydrocarbons. Environ. Sci. Technol., 9, 762-765

Driscoll, J.N. & Warneck, P. (1973) The analysis of ppm levels of gases in air by photoionization mass spectrometry. J. Air Pollut. Control Assoc., 23, 858-863

Fodor, G.G., Prajsnar, D. & Schlipköter, H.-W. (1973)   Endogenous
    formation of CO from incorporated halogenated hydrocarbons of the
    methane series (Germ.).   Staub-Reinhalt. Luft, 33, 258-259

Fujii, T. (1977) · Direct aqueous injection gas chromatography-mass
    spectrometry for analysis of organohalides in water at concentrations
    below the parts per billion level.   J. Chromatogr., 139, 297-302

Gehring, P.J. (1968)   Hepatotoxic potency of various chlorinated hydro-
    carbon vapours relative to their narcotic and lethal potencies in
    mice.   Toxicol. appl. Pharmacol., 13, 287-298

Gosselin, R.E., Hodge, H.C., Smith, R.P. & Gleason, M.N. (1976)
    Clinical Toxicology of Commercial Products, 4th ed., Baltimore, MD,
    Williams & Wilkins Co., pp. 97, 108, 111

Grasselli, J.G. & Ritchey, W.M., eds (1975)   CRC Atlas of Spectral Data
    and Physical Constants for Organic Compounds, 2nd ed., Vol. III,
    Cleveland, OH, Chemical Rubber Co., p. 594

Grimsrud, E.P. & Rasmussen, R.A. (1975)   Survey and analysis of halocarbons
    in the atmosphere by gas chromatography-mass spectrometry.   Atmos.
    Environ., 9, 1014-1017

Hanke, C., Ruppe, K. & Otto, J. (1974)   Results of the study of the toxic
    action of dichloromethane in floor layers (Germ.).   Z. Ges. Hyg.,
    20, 81-84

Hardie, D.W.F. (1964)   Chlorocarbons and chlorohydrocarbons. Methylene
    chloride.   In: Kirk, R.E. & Othmer, D.F., eds, Encyclopedia of
    Chemical Technology, 2nd ed., Vol. 5, New York, John Wiley & Sons,
    pp. 111-119

Hawley, G.G., ed. (1977)   The Condensed Chemical Dictionary, 9th ed.,
    New York, Van Nostrand-Reinhold, p. 567

Hoffman, C.S., Jr (1973)   Beauty salon air quality measurements.
    Cosmet. Toiletries Fragrance Assoc. Cosmet. J., 5, 16-21

Hogan, G.K., Smith, R.G. & Cornish, H.H. (1976)   Studies on the micro-
    somal conversion of dichloromethane to carbon monoxide (Abstract
    No. 49).   Toxicol. appl. Pharmacol., 37, 112

Holzer, G., Oró, J. & Bertsch, W.. (1976)   Gas chromatographic-mass
    spectrometric evaluation of exhaled tobacco smoke.   J. Chromatogr.,
    126, 771-785

IARC (1978a)   Information Bulletin on the Survey of Chemicals Being
    Tested for Carcinogenicity, No. 7, Lyon, pp. 255, 270

IARC (1978b) Directory of On-Going Research in Cancer Epidemiology, 1978 (IARC Scientific Publications No. 26), Lyon, p. 330 (Abstract no. 873)

Irish, D.D. (1963) Halogenated hydrocarbons. I. Aliphatic. In: Patty, F.A., ed., Industrial Hygiene and Toxicology, Vol. II, 2nd ed., New York, Interscience, pp. 1257-1259

Jongen, W.M.F., Alink, G.M. & Koeman, J.H. (1978) Mutagenic effect of dichloromethane on Salmonella typhimurium. Mutat. Res., 56, 245-248

Klaassen, C.D. & Plaa, G.L. (1966) Relative effects of various chlorinated hydrocarbons on liver and kidney function in mice. Toxicol. appl. Pharmacol., 9, 139-151

Klaassen, C.D. & Plaa, G.L. (1967) Relative effects of various chlorinated hydrocarbons on liver and kidney function in dogs. Toxicol. appl. Pharmacol., 10, 119-131

Kubic, V.L., Anders, M.W., Engel, R.R., Barlow, C.H. & Caughey, W.S. (1974) Metabolism of dihalomethanes to carbon monoxide. I. In vivo studies. Drug Metab. Disp., 2, 53-57

Kuo, P.P.K., Chian, E.S.K., DeWalle, F.B. & Kim, J.H. (1977) Gas stripping, sorption and thermal desorption procedures for pre-concentrating volatile polar water-soluble organics from water samples for analysis by gas chromatography. Anal. Chem., 49, 1023-1029

Kuptsova, G.A., Shapovalov, V.E. & Ryazanov, K.D. (1976) Gas-liquid chromatographic determination of chlorinated hydrocarbons in air (Russ.). Gig. Sanit., 4, 61-62 [Chem. Abstr., 85, 181618f]

Laham, S. & Potvin, M. (1976) Microdetermination of dichloromethane in blood with a syringeless gas chromatographic injection system. Chemosphere, 6, 403-411

Mercier, M. (1977) Criteria (Exposure/Effect Relationships) for Organochlorine Solvents, Doc. V/F/177-4, Luxembourg, Commission of the European Communities, pp. 1-29

Moskowitz, S. & Shapiro, H. (1952) Fatal exposure to methylene chloride vapor. AMA Arch. ind. Hyg. occup. Med., 6, 116-123

National Institute for Occupational Safety & Health (1976) Criteria for a recommended Standard ... Occupational Exposure to Methylene Chloride, HEW Publication No. (NIOSH) 76-138, Washington DC, US Government Printing Office

National Institute for Occupational Safety & Health (1977) NIOSH Manual of Analytical Methods, 2nd ed., Part II, Standards Completion Program Validated Methods, Vol. 3, Method No. S329, Washington DC, US Government Printing Office, pp. S329-1-S329-9

Naumova, L.K. & Belova, Z.A. (1976) Gas chromatographic method of determining methylene chloride in air mixtures (Russ.). Metody Anal. Krontrolya Prozvod. Khim. Prom-sti., 2, 1-2 [Chem. Abstr., 85, 112235s]

Nicholson, A.A., Meresz, O. & Lemyk, B. (1977) Determination of free and total potential haloforms in drinking water. Anal. Chem., 49, 814-819

Okuno, T., Tsuji, M., Shintani, Y. & Watanabe, H. (1974) Gas chromatography of chlorinated hydrocarbon in urban air (Jap.). Hyogo-ken Kogai Kenkyusho Kenkyu Hokoku, 6, 1-6 [Chem. Abstr., 87, 72564f]

Page, B.D. & Kennedy, B.P.C. (1975) Determination of methylene chloride, ethylene dichloride, and trichloroethylene as solvent residues in spice oleoresins, using vacuum distillation and electron capture gas chromatography. J. Assoc. off. anal. Chem., 58, 1062-1068

Parkes, D.G., Ganz, C.R., Polinsky, A. & Schulze, J. (1976) A simple gas chromatographic method for the analysis of trace organics in ambient air. Am. ind. Hyg. Assoc. J., 37, 165-173

Perry, R.H. & Chilton, C.H., eds (1973) Chemical Engineers' Handbook, 5th ed., New York, McGraw-Hill, p. 3-57

Premel-Cabic, A., Cailleux, A. & Allain, P. (1974) Gas chromatographic assay of fifteen volatile organic solvents in blood (Fr.). Clin. chim. acta, 56, 5-11

Prikhod'ko, L.S., Pashneva, R.A. & Fedorina, L.V. (1974) Determination of methylene chloride in industrial discharges into the atmosphere (Russ.). Khim. -Farm. Zh., 8, 56-58 [Chem. Abstr., 81, 158174s]

Riley, E.C., Fassett, D.W. & Sutton, W.L. (1966) Methylene chloride vapor in expired air of human subjects. Am. ind. Hyg. Assoc., 27, 341-348

Safe Drinking Water Committee (1977) Drinking Water and Health, Washington DC, National Academy of Sciences, p. 743

Saunders, R.A., Blachly, C.H., Kovacina, T.A., Lamontagne, R.A., Swinnerton, J.W. & Saalfeld, F.E. (1975) Identification of volatile organic contaminants in Washington DC municipal water. Water Res., 9, 1143-1145

Schubert, R. & Ketel, L. (1972) Gas chromatographic determination of methylene chloride in aerosol hair sprays. J. Soc. Cosmet. Chem., 23, 115-124

Schwetz, B.A., Leong, B.K.J. & Gehring, P.J. (1975) The effect of maternally inhaled trichloroethylene, perchloroethylene, methyl chloroform, and methylene chloride on embryonal and fetal development in mice and rats. Toxicol. appl. Pharmacol., 32, 84-96

Shackelford, W.M. & Keith, L.H. (1976) Frequency of Organic Compounds Identified in Water, EPA-600/4-76-062, Athens, GA, US Environmental Protection Agency, pp. 158-161

Spring, S. (1967) Metal surface treatments. In: Kirk, R.E. & Othmer, D.F., eds, Encyclopedia of Chemical Technology, 2n ed., Vol. 13, New York, John Wiley & Sons, pp. 285,292

Stewart, R.D. & Dodd, H.C. (1964) Absorption of carbon tetrachloride, trichloroethylene, tetrachloroethylene, methylene chloride, and 1,1,1-trichloroethane through the human skin. Am. ind. Hyg. Assoc. J., 25, 439-446

Stewart, R.D. & Hake, C.L. (1976) Paint-remover hazard. J. Am. med. Assoc., 235, 398-401

Stewart, R.D., Fisher, T.N., Hosko, M.J., Peterson, J.E., Baretta, E.D. & Dodd, H.C. (1972) Carboxyhemoglobin elevation after exposure to dichloromethane. Science, 176, 295-296

Svirbely, J.L., Highman, B., Alford, W.C. & Von Oettingen, W.F. (1947) The toxicity and narcotic action of mono-chloro-mono-bromo-methane with special reference to inorganic and volatile bromide in blood, urine and brain. J. ind. Hyg. Toxicol., 29, 382-389

Theiss, J.C., Stoner, G.D., Shimkin, M.B. & Weisburger, E.K. (1977) Test for carcinogenicity of organic contaminants of United States drinking waters by pulmonary tumor response in strain A mice. Cancer Res., 37, 2717-2720

Tyras, H. & Blochowicz, A. (1974) Modification of a spectrophotometric method for assaying methylene chloride in the air (Pol.). Bromatol. Chem. Toksykol., 7, 409-413 [Chem. Abstr., 82, 102533m]

US Department of Commerce (1977a) US Imports for Consumption and General Imports, TSUSA Commodity by Country of Origin, FT246/Annual 1976, Bureau of the Census, Washington DC, US Government Printing Office, p. 230

US Department of Commerce (1977b) US Exports, Schedule B, Commodity by Country, FT 410/December 1976, Bureau of the Census, Washington DC, US Government Printing Office, p. 2-85

US Environmental Protection Agency (1969) EPA Compendium of Registered Pesticides, Vol. III, Washington DC, US Government Printing Office, P. III-M-14

US Environmental Protection Agency (1976) Protection of environment. US Code Fed. Regul., Title 40, part 180.1010, p. 380

US Food & Drug Administration (1977) Food and drugs. US Code Fed. Regul., Title 21, parts 173.255, 175.105, 177.1580, pp. 430, 438, 443, 527-528

US International Trade Commission (1977) Synthetic Organic Chemicals, US Production and Sales, 1976, USITC Publication 833, Washington DC, US Printing Office, pp. 302, 331

US Occupational Safety & Health Administration (1977) Air contaminants. US Code Fed. Regul., Title 29, part 1910.1000, p. 28

US Tariff Commission (1936) Dyes and Other Synthetic Organic Chemicals in the US, 1934, Report No. 101, Second Series, Washington DC, US Government Printing Office, p. 66

Weinstein, R.S., Boyd, D.D. & Back, K.C. (1972) Effects of continuous inhalation of dichloromethane in the mouse: morphologic and functional observations. Toxicol. appl. Pharmacol., 23, 660-679

Weiss, G. (1967) Toxic encephalosis due to occupational exposure to methylene chloride (Germ.). Zbl. Arbeitsmed. Arbestschutz, 17, 282-285

Winell, M. (1975) An international comparison of hygienic standards for chemicals in the work environment. Ambio, 4, 34-36

HEXACHLOROETHANE

1. Chemical and Physical Data

1.1 Synonyms and trade names

Chem. Abstr. Services Reg. No.:   67-72-1

Chem. Abstr. Name: Hexachloroethane

Synonyms: Carbon hexachloride; hexachloroethane; 1,1,1,2,2,2-hexachloroethane; hexachloroethylene; perchloroethane

Trade names: Avlothane; Distokal; Distopan; Distopin; Egitol; Falkitol; Fasciolin; Mottenhexe; Phenohep

1.2 Structural and molecular formulae and molecular weight

$$Cl-\underset{\underset{Cl}{|}}{\overset{\overset{Cl}{|}}{C}}-\underset{\underset{Cl}{|}}{\overset{\overset{Cl}{|}}{C}}-Cl$$

C_2Cl_6 Mol. wt: 236.7

1.3 Chemical and physical properties of the pure substance

From Weast (1976), unless otherwise specified

(a) Description: Colourless crystals with a camphor-like odour (Hawley, 1977)

(b) Boiling-point: 185°C (sublimes) (Hawley, 1977)

(c) Melting-point: 186.8-187.4°C (sealed tube)

(d) Spectroscopy data: Infra-red, Raman and mass spectral data have been tabulated (Grasselli & Ritchey, 1975).

(e) Solubility: Insoluble in water, soluble in ethanol, diethyl ether, benzene, chloroform and oils (Windholz, 1976)

(f) Volatility: Vapour pressure is 1 mm at 32.7°C (Perry & Chilton, 1973).

(g) Stability: Nonflammable (Hardie, 1964); at temperatures > 185°C, may give carbon tetrachloride and tetrachloroethylene (van Oss, 1972)

(h) Reactivity: Generally inert chemically (Hardie, 1964)

1.4 Technical products and impurities

The specifications for technical hexachloroethane produced in Japan are as follows: melting-point, 184-187°C; purity, 98.5% min; water content, 0.03% max; ash, 0.05% max; acid (as HCl), 0.01% max.

2. Production, Use, Occurrence and Analysis

2.1 Production and use

(a) Production

Hexachloroethane was prepared by heating carbon tetrachloride with copper powder to 120°C (Prager et al., 1918). The commercial process of manufacture is the chlorination of tetrachloroethylene in the presence of ferric chloride at 100-140°C (Hardie, 1964).

Hexachloroethane was first produced commercially in the US in 1921 (US Tariff Commission, 1922); it was last reported in the US in 1967, when one company reported production of an undisclosed amount (see preamble, p. 16) (US Tariff Commission, 1969). US imports of hexachloroethane in 1976 were 730 thousand kg, with 380 thousand kg from the UK and 350 thousand kg from France (US Department of Commerce, 1977).

Annual production by one company in Spain is estimated to be 700 thousand kg, 500 thousand kg of which are exported.

Hexachloroethane was first produced commercially in Japan in 1955. Annual production of 300-500 thousand kg by one company continued until 1975, when it was discontinued. Japanese requirements for the chemical, which have been relatively constant in recent years, have since been filled by imports, which amounted to about 300 thousand kg in 1976. Formulations containing the chemical are also believed to have been imported.

(b) Use

Hexachloroethane is used in the US in the following applications:
(1) as a constituent of candles and grenades for the generation of
'smoke' or 'fog'; (2) a degassing agent for magnesium; (3) a component
of extreme pressure lubricants; (4) an ignition suppressant in combus-
tible liquids; (5) a moth repellent; (6) a plasticizer for cellulose
esters; (7) an anthelminthic in veterinary medicine; (8) an accelerator
in rubber; (9) a retardant in fermentation processes; (10) a component
of submarine paints; (11) an additive to fire-extinguishing fluids; and
(12) as a constituent of various fungicidal and insecticidal formulations.
With the possible exception of use for smoke generation, only limited
quantities of hexachloroethane are used in these applications (Hardie,
1964).

Smoke is produced by igniting a mixture of hexachloroethane and zinc
dust; fairly volatile zinc chloride is evolved which then condenses in
the form of smoke (Van Oss, 1972).

The US Occupational Safety and Health Administration's health
standards for exposure to air contaminants require that an employee's
exposure to hexachloroethane not exceed an 8-hr time-weighted average
of 10 mg/m^3 (1 ppm) in the working atmosphere in any 8-hr work shift of
a 40-hr work week (US Occupational Safety & Health Administration,
1977).

No data on its use in Europe were available.

The major use of hexachloroethane in Japan is for degassing in the
aluminium casting industry. Small amounts are also used for smoke
generation.

2.2 Occurrence

Hexachloroethane is not known to occur as a natural product.

(a) Water

Hexachloroethane has been found in 1 river-water sample, 8 samples
of finished drinking-water, and in the effluent water from 1 chemical
plant and 1 chlorinated sewage treatment plant in the US (Shackelford &
Keith, 1976). It has been detected in river-water and tap-water, at
a level of 4.4 µg/l, and in the effluent from a US chemical plant, at
a level of 8.4 µg/l (Eurocop-Cost, 1976). It was detected in only one
sample of surface waters collected from 204 sites near heavily industrialized areas (Ewing et al., 1977).

Hexachloroethane has also been detected in effluent waters from
kraft paper mills, at levels of < 1 µg/l (Keith, 1976) and in drinking-

TABLE 1.   METHODS FOR THE ANALYSIS OF HEXACHLORETHANE

SAMPLE TYPE	ANALYTICAL METHOD			REFERENCE
	EXTRACTION/CLEAN-UP	DETECTION	LIMIT OF DETECTION	
Air	Adsorb on charcoal, extract (carbon disulphide)	GC/FID	Useful range, 5-25 mg/m³	National Institute for Occupational Safety & Health (1977b)
Water				
Sea and fresh-water	Extract (pentane), dry, inject aliquot	GC/ECD	Useful range, 0.01-10 µg/l	Bureau International Technique des Solvants Chlorés (1976)
Waste-water	Separate neutral and acidic compounds, extract alkaline solution (chloroform)	GC/FID		Keith (1976)
Drinking-water	Extract (tetralin or chloroform)	GC/FID GC/MS	0.04 µg/l	Keith et al. (1976)
Tap-water	Adjust pH and dechlorinate, drain on XAD2 macroreticular resin, elute with ether, collect and dry eluant	GC/MS		Suffet et al. (1976)
Surface-water	Sample at 60°C, strip (nitrogen gas), trap on Tenax GC, desorb by heating, retrap in line on GC column	GC/MS	1 µg/l	Ewing et al. (1977)
Water	Standard solutions in water only	UV at 240 nm	Useful range, 5-25 mg/l	Simonov et al. (1971)

Abbreviations: GC/ECD - gas chromatography/electron capture detection;   FID - flame-ionization detection;   MS - mass spectrometry;   UV - ultra-violet spectrometry

water in 4 of 13 cities sampled, at levels of 0.03-4.3 µg/l (Keith *et al.*, 1976).

(b) Occupational exposure

A 1974 National Occupational Hazard Survey indicated that workers primarily exposed to hexachloroethane are those in paperboard mills (National Institute for Occupational Safety & Health, 1977a).

2.3 Analysis

Methods used for the analysis of hexachloroethane in environmental samples are listed in Table 1.

3. Biological Data Relevant to the Evaluation

of Carcinogenic Risk to Humans

3.1 Carcinogenicity studies in animals

Oral administration

Mouse: Groups of 50 male and 50 female 5-week-old B6C3F1 mice were administered a solution of technical-grade hexachloroethane (purity 98%) in corn oil by gavage on 5 consecutive days a week for 78 weeks. High- and low-dose animals received 1000 and 500 mg/kg bw/day; after 8 weeks, these doses were increased to 1200 and 600 mg/kg bw/day, respectively, and these were maintained for the remaining 70 weeks. The time-weighted average doses were 1179 and 590 mg/kg bw/day, respectively. Animals were killed and necropsied 13 weeks after the last dose. Groups of 20 male and 20 female mice that served as vehicle controls were given corn oil alone for 78 weeks and killed after 90 weeks; another group of 20 male and 20 female untreated control mice were also killed after 90 weeks. In males, survival was unexpectedly low in control and low-dose animals: only 5/20 of the vehicle controls, 1/20 of the untreated controls and 7/50 of the low-dose mice survived until the end of the test, compared with 29/50 of the high-dose mice. In females, 34/50 high-dose, 40/50 low-dose, 16/20 vehicle controls and 17/20 untreated controls survived until the end of the test. The numbers of tumour-bearing animals/animals examined histopathologically were: in males, 3/17 untreated controls, 4/20 vehicle controls, 17/50 low-dose and 34/49 high-dose animals; in females, 5/18 untreated controls, 8/20 vehicle controls, 32/50 low-dose and 26/49 high-dose animals. A significant increase was observed in the incidence of hepatocellular carcinomas: in males examined histologically, 1/18 untreated controls, 3/20 vehicle controls (3/19 lived for more than 41 weeks), 15/50 low-dose animals (15/46 lived for more than 41 weeks) and 31/49 high-dose animals (31/48 lived for more than 41 weeks). In females examined histologically, the respective incidences of hepatocellular carcinomas were: 0/18 untreated controls, 2/20 vehicle controls, 20/50 low-dose and 15/49 high-dose animals (National Cancer Institute, 1978).

Rat: Groups of 50 male and 50 female 7-week-old Osborne-Mendel rats were administered technical-grade hexachloroethane in corn oil by gavage on 5 consecutive days a week. High- and low-dose animals received 500 and 250 mg/kg bw/day for 22 weeks, followed by 11 cycles of 4 weeks of treatment and 1 week treatment-free. The animals were then maintained for a further 34 weeks on a standard diet without treatment. Time-weighted average doses were 423 and 212 mg/kg bw/day, respectively. Groups of 20 animals of each sex used as vehicle controls were administered corn oil alone; groups of 20 males and 20 females served as untreated controls. In males, 38% of the high-dose and 48% of the low-dose animals lived for more than 90 weeks; and 16% of high-dose and 20% of low-dose animals survived until the end of test, compared with 48% of high-dose and 54% of low-dose females. The numbers of animals with tumours/animals examined histopathologically were: in males, 10/20 untreated controls, 9/20 vehicle controls, 17/49 low-dose and 11/50 high-dose animals; in females, 15/20 untreated controls, 14/20 vehicle controls, 33/50 low-dose and 20/49 high-dose animals. Kidney tumours were observed in 6 males and 1 female given the low dose and in 3 females given the high dose, compared with 1 in male vehicle controls and 2 in untreated female controls (National Cancer Institute, 1978).

3.2 Other relevant biological data

(a) Experimental systems

The i.p. LD_{50} of hexachloroethane in mice is 4.5 mg/kg bw; maximal lethality was observed after 4 days (Baganz et al., 1961).

Hexachloroethane depresses the central nervous system (Bywater, 1955) and causes hepatic dysfunction and damage (Fowler, 1969). A single oral dose of 2.5 g/kg bw reduces hepatic microsomal mono-oxygenase activities in rats by 50% (Vainio et al., 1976).

Orally administered hexachloroethane is absorbed and appears rapidly in the systemic circulation. It is distributed widely throughout the body, the highest concentrations being found in fat, the lowest in muscle (Fowler, 1969).

When 500 mg/kg ^{14}C-hexachloroethane were fed to rabbits, only 5% of the radioactivity was excreted in the urine after 3 days, as di- and trichloroethanol, mono-, di- and trichloroacetic acid and oxalic acid. Between 14 and 24% of the dose was expired unchanged or as CO_2, tetrachloroethylene and 1,1,2,2-tetrachloroethane; the rest was retained in the carcass (Jondorf et al., 1957). In sheep, a small portion of the dose was excreted in the bile (Fowler, 1969). Dechlorination occurs in homogenates of rabbit liver (Bray *et al.*, 1952). Formation of pentachloroethane and tetrachloroethylene was observed in sheep and in slices of sheep liver (Fowler, 1969).

No data on the embryotoxicity, teratogenicity or mutagenicity of hexachloroethane were available.

(b) Humans

No data were available to the Working Group.

3.3 Case reports and epidemiological studies

No data were available to the Working Group.

4. Summary of Data Reported and Evaluation

4.1 Experimental data

Hexachloroethane was tested in one experiment in mice and in one in rats by oral administration. In mice, it produced malignant liver tumours in males and females. In rats, no statistically significant excess of tumours was observed; however, a few renal tumours, rarely seen in untreated animals, were found.

4.2 Human data

No case reports or epidemiological studies were available to the Working Group.

The production and many uses of hexachloroethane for over 50 years, and its occurrence in water and air, indicate that human exposure occurs.

4.3 Evaluation

There is *limited evidence* that hexachloroethane is carcinogenic in experimental animals.

5. References

Baganz, H., Perkow, W., Lim, G.T. & Meyer, F. (1961)   Studies on the
    toxicity of alkylated and chlorinated ethanes and ethenes (Germ.).
    Arzneimittel-Forsch., 11, 902-905

Bray, H.G., Thorpe, W.V. & Vallance, D.K. (1952)   The liberation of
    chloride ions from organic chloro compounds by tissue extracts.
    Biochem. J., 51, 193-201

Bureau International Technique des Solvants Chlorés (1976)   Standardization
    of methods for the determination of traces of some volatile
    chlorinated aliphatic hydrocarbons in air and water by gas
    chromatography. Anal. chem. acta, 82, 1-17

Bywater, H.E. (1955)   The toxicity of hexachloroethane. Vet. Rec.,
    67, 382

Eurocop-Cost (1976)   A Comprehensive List of Polluting Substances Which
    Have Been Identified in Various Fresh Water, Effluent Discharges,
    Aquatic Animals and Plants, and Bottom Sediments, 2nd ed., EUCO/
    MDU/73/76, XII/476/76, Luxembourg, Commission of the European
    Communities, p. 48

Ewing, B.B., Chian, E.S.K., Cook, J.C., Evans, C.A., Hopke, P.K. & Perkins,
    E.G. (1977)   Monitoring to Detect Previously Unrecognized Pollutants
    in Surface Waters, EPA-560/6-77-015, Washington DC, US Environmental
    Protection Agency. Available from Springfield, VA, National Technical
    Information Service, No. PB273 34g, pp. 1, 35-68

Fowler, J.S.K. (1969)   Some hepatotoxic actions of hexachloroethane and
    its metabolites in sheep. Br. J. Pharmacol., 35, 530-542

Grasselli, J.G. & Ritchey, W.M., eds (1975)   CRC Atlas of Spectral Data
    and Physical Constants for Organic Compounds, 2nd ed., Vol. III,
    Cleveland, OH, Chemical Rubber Co., p. 256

Hardie, D.W.F. (1964)   Chlorocarbons and chlorohydrocarbons. Hexachloro-
    ethane. In: Kirk, R.E. & Othmer, D.F., eds, Encyclopedia of
    Chemical Technology, 2nd ed. Vol. 5, New York, John Wiley & Sons,
    pp. 166-170

Hawley, G.G., ed (1977)   The Condensed Chemical Dictionary, 9th ed.,
    New York, Van Nostrand-Reinhold, p. 437

Jondorf, W.R., Parke, D.V. & Williams, R.T. (1957)   The metabolism of
    [^{14}C] hexachloroethane. Biochem. J., 65, 14P-15P

Keith, L.H. (1976) Identification of organic compounds in unbleached
    treated kraft paper mill wastewaters. Environ. Sci. Technol., 10,
    555-564

Keith, L.H., Garrison, A.W., Allen, F.R., Carter, M.H., Floyd, T.L.,
    Pope, J.D. & Thruston, A.D., Jr (1976) Identification of organic
    compounds in drinking water from thirteen US cities. In: Keith,
    L.H., ed., Identification and Analysis of Organic Pollutants in
    Water, Ann Arbor, MI, Ann Arbor Science, pp. 329-373

National Cancer Institute (1978) Bioassay of Hexachloroethane for
    Possible Carcinogenicity (Technical Report Series No. 68), DHEW
    Publication No. (NIH) 78-1318, Washington DC, US Department of Health,
    Education, & Welfare

National Institute for Occupational Safety & Health (1977a) National
    Occupational Hazard Survey, Vol. III, Survey Analyses and Supplemental
    Tables, Cincinnati, OH, p. 5,582

National Institute for Occupational Safety & Health (1977b) NIOSH
    Manual of Analytical Methods, 2nd ed., Part II, Standards Completion
    Program Validated Methods, Vol. 2, Method No. S101, DHEW (NIOSH)
    Pub. No. 77-157-B, Washington DC, US Government Printing Office, pp.
    S101-1-S101-8

van Oss, J.F. (1972) Chemical Technology: An Encyclopedic Treatment,
    Vol. 4, New York, Barnes & Noble, p. 204

Perry, R.H. & Chilton, C.H., eds (1973) Chemical Engineers' Handbook,
    5th ed., New York, McGraw-Hill, p. 3-56

Prager, B., Jacobson, P., Schmidt, P. & Stern, D., eds (1918) Beilsteins
    Handbuch der Organischen Chemie, 4th ed., Vol. 1, Syst. No. 8,
    Berlin, Springer, p. 87

Shackelford, W.M. & Keith, L.H. (1976) Frequency of Organic Compounds
    Identified in Water, EPA-600/4-76-062, Athens, GA, US Environmental
    Protection Agency, p. 119

Simonov, V.D., Popova, L.N. & Shamsutdinov, T.M. (1971) Spectrophotometric
    determination of perchlorinated hydrocarbons in water (Russ.). Dokl
    Neftekhim. Sekts., Bashkir. Respub. Pravl., Vses. Khim. Obshchest.,
    (6), 357-361 [Chem. Abstr., 78, 47526b]

Suffet, I.H., Brenner, L. & Radziul, J.V. (1976) GC/MS identification
    of trace organic compounds in Philadelphia waters. In: Keith, L.H.,
    ed., Identification and Analysis of Organic Pollutants in Water,
    Ann Arbor, MI, Ann Arbor Science, pp. 375-397

US Department of Commerce (1977) US Imports for Consumption and General Imports, TSUSA Commodity by Country of Origin, FT246/Annual 1976, Bureau of the Census, Washington DC, US Government Printing Office, p. 230

US Occupational Safety & Health Administration (1977) Air contaminants. US Code Fed. Regul., Title 29, part 1910.1000, p. 27

US Tariff Commission (1922) Census of Dyes and other Synthetic Organic Chemicals, 1921, Tariff Information Series No. 26, Washington DC, US Government Printing Office, p. 150

US Tariff Commission (1969) Synthetic Organic Chemicals, US Production and Sales, 1967, TC Publication 295, Washington DC, US Government Printing Office, p. 188

Vainio, H., Parkki, M.G. & Marniemi, J. (1976) Effects of aliphatic chlorohydrocarbons on drug-metabolizing enzymes in rat liver *in vivo*. Xenobiotica, 6, 599–604

Weast, R.C., ed. (1976) CRC Handbook of Chemistry and Physics, 57th ed., Cleveland, OH, Chemical Rubber Co., p. C-293

Windholz, M., ed. (1976) The Merck Index, 9th ed., Rahway, NJ, Merck & Co., p. 612

1,1,2,2-TETRACHLOROETHANE

1. Chemical and Physical Data

1.1 Synonyms and trade names

Chem. Abstr. Services Reg. No.: 79-34-5

Chem. Abstr. Name: 1,1,2,2-Tetrachloroethane

Synonyms: Acetylene tetrachloride; dichloro-2,2-dichloroethane; tetrachloroethane; sym-tetrachloroethane

Trade names: Acetosal; Bonoform; Cellon; Westron

1.2 Structural and molecular formulae and molecular weight

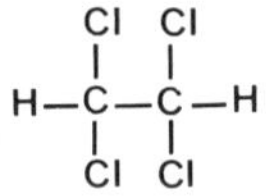

$$\begin{array}{c} \quad Cl \quad Cl \\ \quad | \quad | \\ H-C-C-H \\ \quad | \quad | \\ \quad Cl \quad Cl \end{array}$$

$C_2H_2Cl_4$ Mol. wt: 167.9

1.3 Chemical and physical properties of the pure substance

From National Institute for Occupational Safety & Health (1976), unless otherwise specified

(a) Description: Colourless, corrosive liquid with a chloroform-like odour (Hawley, 1977)

(b) Boiling-point: 146.3°C

(c) Melting-point: -36°C

(d) Density: d_4^{20} 1.596

(e) Spectroscopy data: Infra-red, Raman, nuclear magnetic resonance and mass spectral data have been tabulated (Grasselli & Ritchey, 1975).

(f) Refractive index: n_D^{25} 1.4918 (Hawley, 1977)

(g) Solubility: Sparingly soluble in water (0.29 g/100 ml at
     25°C); soluble in methanol, ethanol, benzene, diethyl ether,
     petroleum ether, carbon tetrachloride, chloroform, carbon
     disulphide, dimethylformamide and oils (Windholz, 1976)

(h) Volatility: Vapour pressure is 5 mm at 21°C.

(i) Vapour density: 5.79 (air = 1)

(j) Stability: Nonflammable (Hawley, 1977).   In the absence of
     air, moisture and light, it is stable, even at high temper-
     atures.   When exposed to air, it degrades slowly to tri-
     chloroethylene and traces of phosgene (Hardie, 1964).

(k) Reactivity: Unaffected by strong acids at ordinary and
     moderate temperatures, but converted to glyoxal sulphate by
     fuming sulphuric acid.   In weak alkali, trichloroethylene is
     produced, and in strong alkali, explosive dichloroacetylene
     is formed.   Metals, in the presence of steam, convert it to
     1,2-dichloroethylene (Hardie, 1964).

(l) Conversion factor: 1 ppm in air is equivalent to 6.87 mg/m^3.

1.4 Technical products and impurities

No data were available to the Working Group.

2. Production, Use, Occurrence and Analysis

2.1 Production and use

(a) Production

1,1,2,2-Tetrachloroethane was first prepared in 1869 by Bethelot
and Jungfleisch (Hardie, 1964) by the reaction of acetylene with
excess antimony pentachloride (Prager *et al.*, 1918).   It is produced
commercially by the reaction of acetylene with chlorine.   Other patented
processes involve the chlorination of 1,2-dichloroethylene and the two-
stage chlorination of 1,2-dichloroethane (Hardie, 1964).

Commercial production of 1,1,2,2-tetrachloroethane in the US was
first reported in 1921 (US Tariff Commission, 1922).   For many years,
large quantities of this chemical were produced and consumed captively in

the production of trichloroethylene, but separate production data were never reported; however, an estimated 222 million kg 1,1,2,2-tetra-chloroethane were produced in the US in 1967 for this purpose. This figure is believed to have decreased to about 17 million kg by 1974, and in 1976, only one US company reported the production of an undisclosed amount (see preamble, p. 16) (US International Trade Commission, 1977).

No data on its production in Europe were available. It is not produced commercially in Japan. Two companies in Canada and one in Argentina produce 1,1,2,2-tetrachloroethane as an intermediate in the manufacture of trichloroethylene.

(b) Use

The principal use for 1,1,2,2-tetrachloroethane is as an intermediate in the production of trichloroethylene from acetylene. Other relatively minor uses are as an insecticide and as a solvent (Hardie, 1964).

In 1967, an estimated 85% (189 million kg) of the total 222 million kg trichloroethylene produced in the US was made *via* 1,1,2,2-tetrachloroethane as an intermediate. By 1974, however, the amount had decreased to about 8% (17 million kg) of the total 217 million kg produced.

1,1,2,2-Tetrachloroethane is registered by the US Environmental Protection Agency as a mothproofing agent for textiles. Its use as a fumigant for control of white fly in greenhouses (Hardie, 1964) and as a grain fumigant (van Oss, 1972) has been reported, but these uses are not currently registered in the US.

Miscellaneous uses, based on its solvent properties, include extraction of ruthenium compounds from aqueous solutions and use as a reaction solvent for chlorination reactions (Hardie, 1964).

No data on its use in Europe and Japan were available.

The US Occupational Safety and Health Administration's health standards for exposure to air contaminants require that an employee's exposure to 1,1,2,2-tetrachloroethane not exceed an 8-hr time-weighted average of 35 mg/m^3 (approx. 5 ppm) in the working atmosphere during any 8-hr work shift of a 40-hr work week (US Occupational Safety & Health Administration, 1977). The corresponding standard in the Federal Republic of Germany is 7 mg/m^3 (1 ppm) and in the German Democratic Republic, 10 mg/m^3 (1.5 ppm); the acceptable ceiling concentration in the USSR is 5 mg/m^3 (0.7 ppm) (Winell, 1975).

In early 1977, the US National Institute for Occupational Safety and Health recommended that occupational exposure to 1,1,2,2-tetrachloro-

ethane be controlled so that no employee is exposed to the chemical at
a concentration greater than 6.87 mg/m^3 (1 ppm) of air by volume,
determined as a time-weighted average concentration in the workplace air,
for up to a 10-hr work day in a 40-hr work week (National Institute for
Occupational Safety & Health, 1977a).

2.2 Occurrence

1,1,2,2-Tetrachloroethane is not known to occur as a natural
product.

(a) Air

Various chlorinated hydrocarbons, including 1,1,2,2-tetrachloroethane,
have been detected in urban atmospheres in Japan, at levels of 0.07-64 µg/
m^3 (0.01-9.4 ppb) (Okuno *et al.*, 1974).

(b) Water

1,1,2,2-Tetrachloroethane has been found in 3 samples of finished
drinking-water and in samples of effluent from 3 chemical plants and
one sewage treatment plant in the US (Shackelford & Keith, 1976).   It
has been detected in tap-water, at a level of 0.11 µg/l, and in effluent
from a chemical production plant, at a level of 2.2 mg/l.   An unspecified
isomer of tetrachloroethane has been determined in tap-water at a level
of 0.01 µg/l (Eurocop-Cost, 1976).

(c) Food

Tetrachloroethane (unspecified isomer) has been detected in the
volatile flavour components of boiled beef (MacLeod & Coppock, 1976).

(d) Occupational exposure

Occupational exposure to 1,1,2,2-tetrachloroethane in the US, Japan,
India, Italy and Czechoslovakia has been reviewed (National Institute for
Occupational Safety & Health, 1976).

A 1974 National Occupational Hazard Survey estimated that workers
primarily exposed to 1,1,2,2-tetrachloroethane are those in the toiletry
preparations, industrial controls and electric service industries
(National Institute for Occupational Safety & Health, 1977b).

(e) Other

1,1,2,2-Tetrachloroethane has been detected in vinyl chloride waste
products dumped into the North Sea (Jensen *et al.*, 1975), and an
unspecified isomer has been detected in commercial solvent cleaners used
in the electronics industry (Lin *et al.*, 1975).

2.3 Analysis

Sampling and analytical methods to determine 1,1,2,2-tetrachloro-
ethane in the environment have been reviewed (National Institute for
Occupational Safety & Health, 1976).   Methods used for the analysis
of 1,1,2,2-tetrachloroethane in environmental samples are listed in
Table 1.

3. Biological Data Relevant to the Evaluation
of Carcinogenic Risk to Humans

3.1 Carcinogenicity studies in animals

(a) Oral administration

Mouse: Groups of 50 male and 50 female 5-week-old B6C3F1 hybrid
mice were administered technical-grade 1,1,2,2-tetrachloroethane in
corn oil by gavage on 5 days per week.   Initially, high-dose animals
received 200 mg/kg bw/day, and low-dose animals received 100 mg/kg bw/
day;   however, after 18 weeks these doses were increased to 300 and
150 mg/kg bw/day, respectively.   Test animals were maintained at these
levels for 3 weeks, followed by 5 weeks at 400 and 200 mg/kg bw/day and
52 weeks at 300 and 150 mg/kg bw/day.   The measured, time-weighted
average doses were 142 (low-dose) and 284 (high-dose) mg/kg bw/day.
Animals were killed and necropsied 12 weeks after the last dose.   Groups
of 20 male and 20 female mice that served as matched controls were given
corn oil alone for 78 weeks and killed after 91 weeks;   another group
of 20 male and 20 female control mice were fed the standard diet for
90 weeks.   By 90 weeks, only 1 male that received the high dose was
still alive, whereas 34% of females lived to that time.   Histopathology
was performed on all organ systems in 98% or more of animals entered into
the experiment.   In males, hepatocellular carcinomas occurred in 2/19
untreated controls, in 1/18 vehicle-treated controls, in 13/50 low-dose
animals and in 44/49 high-dose animals;   in females, the respective
incidences were 0/19, 0/20, 30/48 and 43/47 (National Cancer Institute,
1978).

Rat: Groups of 50 male and 50 female 7-week-old Osborne-Mendel
rats were administered technical-grade 1,1,2,2-tetrachloroethane in
corn oil by gavage on 5 days per week.   High-dose animals received
100 mg/kg bw/day;   in males, this was increased after 14 weeks to 130 mg/
kg bw/day for 18 weeks followed by 9 cycles of 4 weeks at this dose and
1 week treatment-free for 45 weeks (total, 78 weeks);   in females, the
dose was reduced after 25 weeks to 80 mg/kg bw/day for 7 weeks followed
by the cyclic treatment at this dose level for 45 weeks.   Low-dose
males received 50 mg/kg bw/day for 14 weeks and 65 mg/kg bw for 64 weeks;
females received 50 mg/kg bw/day for 25 weeks and 40 mg/kg bw/day for
53 weeks.   All groups were then maintained for a further 32 weeks on a

TABLE 1. METHODS FOR THE ANALYSIS OF 1,1,2,2-TETRACHLOROETHANE

SAMPLE TYPE	ANALYTICAL METHOD			
	EXTRACTION/CLEAN-UP	DETECTION	LIMIT OF DETECTION	REFERENCE
Air				
	Trap on charcoal, extract (carbon disulphide)	GC/FID	Useful range, 16-70 mg/m^3	National Institute for Occupational Safety & Health (1977c)
Ambient	Trap in Drechsel flask fitted with rubber septum, sample with gas syringe	GC/ECD		Bureau International Technique des Solvants Chlorés (1976)
Water				
	Cool in water, extract (pentane)	GC/FID GC/ECD	0.01-0.1 mg/l 0.01-0.1 mg/l	Dietz & Traud (1973)
Drinking-water	Inject directly	GC/ECD	7 µg/l	Nicholson et al. (1977)
Drinking-water	Adjust pH, dechlorinate, adsorb on ionic exchangers, elute ether, or liquid-liquid extraction, or headspace sampling	GC/MS		Suffet et al. (1976)
Drinking-water	Extract (pentane), dry	GC/ECD	0.035 µg/l	Bureau International Technique des Solvants Chlorés (1976)
Sediments				
	Cool sample at 4°C, mix with water, extract (pentane)	GC/FID GC/ECD	0.01-0.1 mg/l 0.01-0.1 µg/l	Dietz & Traud (1973)

Abbreviations: GC/FID - gas chromatography/flame-ionization detection; ECD - electron capture detection; MS - mass spectrometry

standard diet without treatment.   Time-weighted average doses were 62 mg/kg bw/day and 108 mg/kg bw/day in males and 43 and 76 mg/kg bw/day in females.   Groups of 20 animals of each sex used as matched controls were administered corn oil alone;   groups of 20 males and 20 females served as untreated controls.   Weight gain was consistently lower in high-dose groups than in low-dose and control groups;   and 50% of high-dose males, 40% of high-dose females, 50% of low-dose males and 58% of low-dose females lived for more than 105 weeks.   Histopathology of all organ systems was performed on 98% or more of the animals entered into the study.   The incidences of tumours in treated and vehicle control rats were not significantly different for any tumour type;   however, 2 of 49 males treated with the high dose developed hepatocellular carcinomas and another had a neoplastic nodule of the liver (time of appearance unspecified), compared with 0/20 vehicle controls (National Cancer Institute, 1978).

(b)   Intraperitoneal administration

Mouse: Groups of 20 male A/St mice, 6-8 weeks old, were given thrice weekly i.p. injections of 1,1,2,2-tetrachloroethane in tricaprylin at doses of 80 mg/kg bw (5 injections), 200 mg/kg bw (18 injections) or 400 mg/kg bw (16 injections).   All survivors (10, 15 and 5 at the 3 doses, respectively) were killed 24 weeks after the first injection. The average numbers of lung tumours per mouse were 0.3, 0.5 and 1.0, which were not significantly different from the 0.27 observed in tricaprylin-injected controls (Theiss *et al.*, 1977) [The Working Group noted the poor survival of treated animals and the limitations of a negative result obtained with this test system;   see also General Remarks on Substances Considered, p. 34].

3.2   Other relevant biological data

(a)   Experimental systems

Toxic effects

The oral LD_{50} of 1,1,2,2-tetrachloroethane in rats is 250 mg/kg bw (Gohlke *et al.*, 1977);   the i.p. LD_{50} in mice is 820 mg/kg bw (Takeuchi, 1966).

In dogs and mice, the compound causes central nervous system depression and is highly hepatotoxic (Bolman & Mann, 1931;   Plaa *et al.*, 1958;   Tomokuni, 1969).   Marked changes in lipid and adenosine triphosphate levels were observed in the livers of mice after 3 hrs' exposure by inhalation to 41 mg/m^3 (600 ppm) 1,1,2,2-tetrachloroethane in air;   the changes were similar to those caused by carbon tetrachloride (Tomokuni, 1969).   A single oral dose of 437 mg/kg bw to rats reduced hepatic benzo[*a*]pyrene-hydroxylase and *para*-nitroanisole-*O*-demethylase levels by 50% after 24 hrs;   uridine 5'-diphosphate-glucuronyltransferase activity was reduced to a lesser extent (Vainio *et al.*, 1976).

Embryotoxicity and teratogenicity

Treatment of AB-Jena and DBA mice with 300-400 mg/kg bw/day tetra-chloroethane during organogenesis produced embryotoxic effects and a low incidence of malformations (exencephaly, cleft palate, anophthalmia, fused ribs and vertebrae). The effects were related to dose and period of treatment (Schmidt, 1976).

Absorption, distribution, excretion and metabolism

^{14}C-1,1,2,2-Tetrachloroethane injected intraperitoneally to mice is metabolized rapidly: less than 4% was expired unchanged, half of the dose was expired as CO_2 and minute amounts as tri- and tetrachloroethylene. About 30% was excreted in the urine, and 16% remained in the body. The urin contained di- and trichloroacetic acid, trichloroethanol, oxalic acid and small amounts of glyoxylic acid and urea. About 50% of the radioactivity in the urine was unaccounted for. The author (Yllner, 1971) concluded that 1,1,2,2-tetrachloroethane is metabolized as follows:

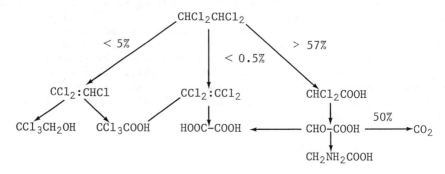

Mutagenicity and other related short-term tests

1,1,2,2-Tetrachloroethane was mutagenic in *Salmonella typhimurium* strains TA1530 and TA1535, showing a linear increase in reversion frequency with increasing concentration; negative results were obtained in strain TA1538. It also inhibited the growth of DNA polymerase-deficient (*pol A⁻*) *Escherichia coli*; the ratio of the areas of inhibition of *pol A⁻*:*pol A⁺* was 1.88 with a concentration of 10 µl/plate (Brem *et al.*, 1974).

(b) Humans

The toxicity of 1,1,2,2-tetrachloroethane has been reviewed (Browning, 1953; Lobo-Mendonça, 1963; National Institute for Occupational Safety & Health, 1976). Numerous deaths due to its ingestion,

inhalation and cutaneous absorption have been recorded.   The solvent
affects primarily the central nervous system and the liver and caused
polyneuritis and paralysis (Browning, 1953; Hamilton & Hardie, 1974).
Of 380 workers exposed to the solvent 133 (35%) exhibited tremor and
other nervous symptoms (Lobo-Mendonça, 1963).   Accidental and occupational exposure produced liver damage, ranging from severe fatty degeneration to necrosis and acute atrophy, which was frequently fatal, and
gastrointestinal disorders; toxic effects were also observed in the
haematopoetic system (Horiguchi *et al.*, 1964; Lobo-Mendoça, 1963).

About 97% of inhaled 1,1,2,2-tetrachloroethane was retained in
the lungs 1 hr after exposure (Morgan *et al.*, 1970).

3.3 Case reports and epidemiological studies

No data were available to the Working Group.

4.   Summary of Data Reported and Evaluation

4.1 Experimental data

1,1,2,2-Tetrachloroethane was tested in one experiment in mice and
in one in rats by oral administration.   In male and female mice, it
produced hepatocellular carcinomas.   Although a few hepatocellular
carcinomas were observed in male rats, no significant increase in the
incidence of tumours was observed in animals of either sex.   The
compound was inadequately tested in one experiment in mice by intraperitoneal injection.

1,1,2,2-Tetrachloroethane is mutagenic in *Salmonella typhimurium*
and has teratogenic effects in mice.

4.2 Human data

No case reports or epidemiological studies were available to the
Working Group.

The extensive production of 1,1,2,2-tetrachloroethane, particularly
as an intermediate for other halogenated hydrocarbons, since the early
1920s indicates that exposure of both workers and the general population
occurs.   This is confirmed by reports of its occurrence in air, water
and certain industrial effluents.

4.3 Evaluation

There is *limited evidence* that 1,1,2,2-tetrachloroethane is carcinogenic in experimental animals.

5. References

Bollman, J.L. & Mann, F.C. (1931) Experimentally produced lesions of the liver. Ann. int. Med., 5, 699-712

Brem, H., Stein, A.B. & Rosenkranz, H.S. (1974) The mutagenicity and DNA-modifying effect of haloalkanes. Cancer Res., 34, 2576-2579

Browning, E. (1953) Toxicity of Industrial Organic Solvents, London, Her Majesty's Stationery Office, pp. 154-163

Bureau International Technique des Solvents Chlorés (1976) Standardization of methods for the determination of traces of some volatile chlorinated aliphatic hydrocarbons in air and water by gas chromatography. Anal. chim. acta, 82, 1-17

Dietz, F. & Traud, J. (1973) Gas chromatographic determination of low-molecular-weight chlorohydrocarbons in water samples and sediments (Germ.). Von Wasser, 41, 137-155 [Chem. Abstr., 81, 54214p]

Eurocop-Cost (1976) A Comprehensive List of Polluting Substances Which Have Been Identified in Various Fresh Waters, Effluent Discharges Aquatic Animals and Plants, and Bottom Sediments, 2nd ed., EUCO/ MDU/73/76, XII/476/76, Luxembourg, Commission of the European Communities, p. 53

Gohlke, R., Schmidt, P. & Bahmann, H. (1977) 1,1,2,2-Tetrachloroethane and heat-stress in animal experiments - morphological results (Germ.). Z. Ges. Hyg., 23, 278-282

Grasselli, J.G. & Ritchey, W.M., eds (1975) CRC Atlas of Spectral Data and Physical Constants for Organic Compounds, 2nd ed., Vol. III, Cleveland, OH, Chemical Rubber Co., p. 256

Hamilton, A. & Hardy, H.L. (1974) Industrial Toxicology, 3rd ed., Acton, MA, Publishing Sciences Group Inc., pp. 277-291

Hardie, D.W.F. (1964) Chlorocarbons and chlorohydrocarbons. 1,1,2,2- Tetrachloroethane. In: Kirk, R.E. & Othmer, D.F., eds, Encyclopedia of Chemical Technology, 2nd ed., Vol. 5, New York, John Wiley & Sons, pp. 159-164, 170

Hawley, G.G., ed. (1977) The Condensed Chemical Dictionary, 9th ed., New York, Van Nostrand-Reinhold, p. 845

Horiguchi, S., Morioka, S., Utsunomiya, T., Shinagawa, K. & Korenari, T. (1964) A survey of the actual conditions of artificial pearl factories with special reference to the work using tetrachlorethane (Jap.).

Jpn. J. ind. Health, 6, 251-256

Jensen, S., Lange, R., Berge, G., Palmork, K.H. & Renberg, L. (1975) On the chemistry of EDC-tar and its biological significance in the sea. Proc. R. Soc. Lond. B., 189, 333-346

Lin, L.-C., Wang, C.-B. & Hsieh, C.-C. (1975) Highly toxic substances found in local industrial removers by GC-MS spectrometry (Chin.). Hua Hsueh, 4, 123-125 [Chem. Abstr., 87, 10796z]

Lobo-Mendonça, R. (1963) Tetrachloroethane - a survey. Br. J. ind. Med., 20, 50-56

MacLeod, G. & Coppock, B.M. (1976) Volatile flavor components of beef boiled conventionally and by microwave radiation. J. agric. Food Chem., 24, 835-843

Morgan, A., Black, A. & Belcher, D.R. (1970) The excretion in breath of some aliphatic halogenated hydrocarbons following administration by inhalation. Ann. occup. Hyg., 13, 219-233

National Cancer Institute (1978) Bioassay of 1,1,2,2-Tetrachloroethane for Possible Carcinogenicity, DHEW Publication No. (NIOH) 78-827, Washington DC, US Department of Health Education, & Welfare

National Institute for Occupational Safety & Health (1976) Criteria for a Recommended Standard ... Occupational Exposure to 1,1,2,2-Tetrachloroethane, DHEW (NIOSH) Publication No. 77-121, Cincinnati, OH. Available from Washington DC, US Government Printing Office

National Institute for Occupational Safety & Health (1977a) Recommendations for workplace exposure to 1,1,2,2-tetrachloroethane. Occup. Saf. Health Rep., 3 March, pp. 1271-1278

National Institute for Occupational Safety & Health (1977b) National Occupational Hazard Survey, Vol. III, Survey Analyses and Supplemental Tables, DHEW, Cincinnati, OH, December, p. 11-236

National Institute for Occupational Safety & Health (1977c) NIOSH Manual of Analytical Methods, 2nd ed., Part II, Standards Completion Program Validated Methods, Vol. 2, Method S124, DHEW (NIOSH) Publication No. 77-157-B, Washington DC, US Government Printing Office, pp. S124-1-S124-8

Nicholson, A.A., Meresz, O. & Lemyk, B. (1977) Determination of free and total potential haloforms in drinking water. Anal. Chem., 49, 814-819

Okuno, T., Tsuji, M., Shintani, Y. & Watanabe, H. (1974) Gas chromatography of chlorinated hydrocarbon in urban air (Jap.). Hyogo-ken Kogai Kenkyusho Kenkyu Hokoku, 6, 1-6 [Chem. Abstr., 87, 72564f]

van Oss, J.F. (1972) Chemical Technology: An Encyclopedic Treatment,
    Vol. 4, New York, Barnes & Noble, p. 203

Plaa, G.L., Evans, E.A. & Hine, C.H. (1958)   Relative hepatotoxicity
    of seven halogenated hydrocarbons. J. Pharm. exp. Ther., 123,
    224-229

Prager, B., Jacobson, P., Schmidt, P. & Stern, D., eds (1918) Beilsteins
    Handbuch der Organischen Chemie, 4th ed., Vol. 1, Syst. No. 8,
    Berlin, Springer, p. 86

Schmidt, R. (1976) The embryotoxic and teratogenic effect of tetra-
    chloroethane - experimental investigations (Germ.). Biol. Rundschau,
    14, 220-223

Shackelford, W.M. & Keith, L.H. (1976)   Frequency of Organic Compounds
    Identified in Water, EPA-600/4-76-062, Athens, GA, US Environmental
    Protection Agency, p. 121

Suffet, I.H., Brenner, L. & Radziul, J.V. (1976)   GC/MS identification
    of trace organic compounds in Philadelphia waters. In: Keith,
    L.H., ed., Identification and Analysis of Organic Pollutants in
    Water, Ann Arbor, MI, Ann Arbor Science, pp. 375-397

Takeuchi, Y. (1966)   Experimental studies on the toxicity of 1,1,1,2-
    tetrachloroethane compared with 1,1,2,2-tetrachloroethane and
    1,1,1-trichloroethane (Jap.).   Jpn. J. ind. Health, 8, 371-374

Theiss, J.C., Stoner, G.D., Shimkin, M.B. & Weisburger, E.K. (1977)
    Test for carcinogenicity of organic contaminants of United States
    drinking waters by pulmonary tumor response in strain A mice.
    Cancer Res., 37, 2717-2720

Tomokuni, K. (1969)   Studies on hepatotoxicity induced by chlorinated
    hydrocarbons. Lipid and ATP metabolisms in the liver of mice
    exposed to 1,1,2,2-tetrachloroethane. Acta med. Okayama, 23,
    273-282

US International Trade Commission (1977)   Synthetic Organic Chemicals,
    US Production and Sales, 1976, US ITC Publication 833, Washington
    DC, US Government Printing Office, p. 331

US Occupational Safety & Health Administration (1977)   Air contaminants.
    US Code Fed. Regul., Title 29, part 1910.1000, p. 27

US Tariff Commission (1922) Census of Dyes and Other Synthetic Organic
    Chemicals, 1921, Tariff Information Series No. 26, Washington DC,
    US Government Printing Office, p. 151

Vainio, H., Parkki, M.G. & Marniemi, J. (1976)   Effects of aliphatic
    chlorohydrocarbons on drug-metabolizing enzymes in rat liver *in
    vivo*. Xenobiotica, 6, 599-604

Windholz, M., ed. (1976)   The Merck Index, 9th ed., Rahway, NJ, Merck
    & Co., p. 1184

Winell, M. (1975) An international comparison of hygienic standards
    for chemicals in the work environment. Ambio, 4, 34-36

Yllner, S. (1971) Metabolism of 1,1,2,2-tetrachloroethane-^{14}C in the
    mouse. Acta pharmacol. toxicol., 29, 499-512

TETRACHLOROETHYLENE

Two reviews on tetrachloroethylene are available (Berkowitz, 1979; National Institute for Occupational Safety & Health, 1976).

1. Chemical and Physical Data

1.1 Synonyms and trade names

Chem. Abstr. Services Reg. No.: 127-18-4

Chem. Abstr. Name: Tetrachloroethane

Synonyms: Carbon bichloride; carbon dichloride; ethylene tetrachloride; per; perc; perchlor; perchlorethylene; perchloroethylene; perk; tetrachlorethylene; 1,1,2,2-tetrachloroethylene

Trade names: Ankilostin; Antisal 1; Dee-Solv; Didakene; Dow-Per; ENT 1860; Fedal-Un; Nema; Perclene; Percosolv; Perklone; PerSec; Tetlen; Tetracap; Tetraleno; Tetravec; Tetroguer; Tetropil

1.2 Structural and molecular formulae and molecular weight

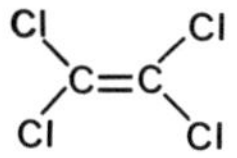

C_2Cl_4 Mol. wt: 165.8

1.3 Chemical and physical properties of the pure substance

From Hawley (1977), unless otherwise specified

(a) Description: Colourless liquid

(b) Boiling-point: 121°C

(c) Freezing-point: -22.4°C

(d) Density: d_{20}^{20} 1.625

(e) Refractive index: n_D^{25} 1.5029

(f) Spectroscopy data: Infra-red, Raman and mass spectral data have been tabulated (Grasselli & Ritchey, 1975).

(g) Solubility: Practically insoluble in water (0.015 g/100 ml water at 25°C) (Hardie, 1964); miscible with ethanol, diethyl ether and oils in all proportions

(h) Volatility: Vapour pressure is 20 mm at 26.3°C (Perry & Chilton, 1973).

(i) Stability: Nonflammable; decomposes slowly in contact with water to yield trichloroacetic and hydrochloric acids. At 700°C in contact with active carbon, it decomposes to hexachloroethane and hexachlorobenzene (Hardie, 1964).

(j) Reactivity: Oxidized by strong oxidizing agents (sulphuric and nitric acids, sulphur trioxide); reaction with excess hydrogen in the presence of reduced nickel catalyst produces total decomposition to hydrogen chloride and carbon (Hardie, 1964).

(k) Conversion factor: 1 ppm in air is equivalent to 6.78 mg/m^3.

1.4 Technical products and impurities

Tetrachloroethylene is available in the US in the following grades: purified, technical, USP, spectrophotometric (Hawley, 1977) and dry-cleaning. The technical and dry-cleaning grades both meet specifications for technical grade and differ only in the amount of stabilizer added to prevent decomposition. Stabilizers are believed to include amines or mixtures of epoxides and esters. Typical analysis of the commercial grades is as follows: appearance, clear and free of suspended matter; specific gravity, 20°C/20°C, 1.624; nonvolatile residue, 0.0003%; free chlorine, none; moisture, no cloud at -5°C; 100% distillation range, 120.8-121.6°C.

USP grade contains not less than 99.0% and no more than 99.5% tetrachloroethylene, the remainder consisting of ethanol; it is available in the US in 0.2, 0.5, 1.0, 2.5 and 5 ml capsules intended for internal drug use (US Pharmacopeial Convention, Inc., 1975).

In Japan, tetrachloroethylene is available as a technical product with the following specifications: nonvolatile matter, 0.002% max; acidity (as HCl), 0.0001% max; and pH, 6.8.

2. Production, Use, Occurrence and Analysis

2.1 Production and use

(a) Production

Tetrachloroethylene was first prepared in 1821 by Faraday by thermal decomposition of hexachloroethane (Hardie, 1964). The original commercial method of producing tetrachloroethylene involved a four-step process based on acetylene and chlorine as the raw materials. By July 1975, only one US plant with about 3% of total tetrachloroethylene capacity was using this process. Currently, the majority of tetrachloroethylene produced in the US is made by the oxyhydrochlorination, chlorination and/or dehydrochlorination of other hydrocarbons or chlorinated hydrocarbons. The raw materials include 1,2-dichloroethane (see monograph, p. 429), methane, ethane, propane, propylene, propylene dichloride and various other chlorinated materials such as 1,1,2-trichloroethane (see monograph, p. 533). An estimated 60% of the tetrachloroethylene produced in the US in 1974 was prepared from 1,2-dichloroethane, and about 40% from methane, ethane and propane.

In western Europe, tetrachloroethylene is produced by oxychlorination processes and by propylene chlorination.

In Japan, an estimated 60% of tetrachloroethylene is produced by chlorination of 1,2-dichloroethane and 40% by chlorination of methane and propane.

In 1972, worldwide demand for tetrachloroethylene was estimated to be 600 million kg.

It has been produced commercially in the US since 1925 (Hardie, 1964). In 1976, 9 US companies reported a total production of 304 million kg (US International Trade Commission, 1977). US imports in that year were 23.3 million kg, from the following countries (percent of total): France (34), Belgium (21), Italy (18), Japan (11), Canada (10), The Netherlands (4), and the Federal Republic of Germany (2) (US Department of Commerce, 1977a); exports were 22 million kg, and went to the following countries (percent of total): Mexico (38), the Federal Republic of Germany (18), The Netherlands (14), Belgium (9), Canada (5) and at least 5 other countries (16) (US Department of Commerce, 1977b).

Total annual production of tetrachloroethylene in western Europe is 250-500 million kg; the Federal Republic of Germany, France, Italy and the UK are the major producing countries, and Austria, Scandinavia, Spain, Switzerland and Benelux are minor producing regions. Annual production of tetrachloroethylene in eastern Europe is estimated to be 50-100 million kg.

Tetrachloroethylene has been produced commercially in Japan since 1952. In 1977, 8 companies produced an estimated 54.7 million kg; exports were 2.6 million kg in that year, none was imported.

(b) Use

In 1976, tetrachloroethylene was used in the US as follows: textile industry, 68%; industrial metal cleaning, 15%; chemical intermediate, 14%; and other applications, 3%.

Tetrachloroethylene is used in the textile industry for dry-cleaning and for processing and finishing. It is nonflammable, easily recoverable for reuse, does not hydrolyse appreciably, and can be used on all fabrics. In 1975, 70% of the dry-cleaners in the US used tetrachloroethylene, and it constituted over 65% of the total dry-cleaning solvent usage. In 1974, 18-27 million kg tetrachloroethylene were used for textile processing and finishing in the US.

It is used in both cold cleaning and vapour degreasing of metals; in 1974, about 80% of the total used in the US for metal cleaning was in vapour degreasing.

It is used as a chemical intermediate in the synthesis of Fluorocarbon 113 (1,1,2-trichloro-1,2,2-trifluoroethane), Fluorocarbon 114 (1,2-dichloro-1,1,2,2-tetrafluoroethane), Fluorocarbon 115 (chloropentafluoroethane), and Fluorocarbon 116 (hexafluoroethane).

Tetrachloroethylene is also used as a heat-exchange fluid, and as a drug against hookworms and some nematodes (National Institute for Occupational Safety & Health, 1978; US Pharmacopeial Convention, Inc., 1975).

In western Europe, use of tetrachloroethylene is as follows: dry-cleaning, 70-95%; metal cleaning and extraction, 5-15%; chemical intermediate, 0-10%; and other, 0-5%. Its use in Japan in 1977 was: dry-cleaning, 50%; metal cleaning, 21%; solvent and miscellaneous uses, 29%.

The US Occupational Safety and Health Administration's health standards for exposure to air contaminants require than an employee's exposure to tetrachloroethylene not exceed an 8-hr time-weighted average of 670 mg/m^3 (100 ppm) in the working atmosphere during an 8-hr work shift of a 40-hr work week (US Occupational Safety & Health Administration, 1977).   The corresponding standard in the Federal Republic of Germany is 670 mg/m^3;   in the German Democratic Republic, 300 mg/m^3; in Sweden, 200 mg/m^3;   and in Czechoslovakia, 250 mg/m^3;   the acceptable ceiling concentration in the USSR is 10 mg/m^3 (Winell, 1975).

2.2   Occurrence

Tetrachloroethylene is not known to occur as a natural product.

(a)   Air

About 85% of the tetrachloroethylene used annually in the US is lost to the atmosphere;   in 1974, this amount was estimated to be 250 million kg (Fuller, 1976).

Numerous US studies have reported tetrachloroethylene in air [concentrations in parts per trillion (ppt[1]), unless otherwise specified]: (1) in rural air in central Michigan (30-50) (Russell & Shadoff, 1977); (2) in locations in California, including Los Angeles (673.3), Palm Springs (278.1), Badger Pass (30.7), Menlo Park (201.9) (Singh, 1976), Stanford Hills (38.3), Point Reyes (43.1) (Singh *et al.*, 1977), Pasadena (1.3-4.2 ppb[2]), West San Gabriel Valley to Manhatten Beach (< 0.01-3.8 ppb) and the Los Angeles Basin (0.37-3.84 ppb) (Simmonds *et al.*, 1974); (3) in New Brunswick, New Jersey (0.5 ppb) (Lillian *et al.*, 1976); (4) in rural south-eastern Washington state (20) (Grimsrud & Rasmussen, 1975);   and (5) in various other locations (reported as mean concentrations), including Seagirt, New Jersey (0.32 ppb);   New York City, New York (4.5 ppb), Sandy Hook, New Jersey (0.39 ppb), Delaware City, Delaware (0.24 ppb), Baltimore, Maryland (0.18 ppb), Wilmington, Ohio (0.15 ppb), White Face Mountains, New York (0.07 ppb) and Bayonne, New Jersey (1.63 ppb) (Lillian *et al.*, 1975).

In a UK study, tetrachloroethylene was detected in the air at the following locations (ppb): Runcorn Works perimeter (15-40), Runcorn Heath (0.2-5), Liverpool/Manchester suburban area (< 0.1-10), Moel Famau, Flintshire (< 0.1-2.5), Rannoch Moor, Argyllshire (0.3-1), and Forest of Dean, Monmouthshire (3) (Pearson & McConnell, 1975).   In an air-sampling study conducted in central Exmoor and the moorlands of North Wales, tetrachloroethylene concentrations were found to range from 8-57 ng/m^3;   in air over the north-east Atlantic Ocean between Cap Blanc and Lands End 1-9 ng/m^3 were detected (Murray & Riley, 1973).   Tetrachloroethylene was also detected in the air over Adrigole, County Cork, Eire, at a level of 27.6 ppt (Cox *et al.*, 1976).

---

[1] 1 ppt in air is equivalent to 6.78 ng/m^3.
[2] 1 ppb in air is equivalent to 6.78 μg/m^3.

(b)   Water

Tetrachloroethylene may be formed in small quantities during chlorination of water: samples from 8 of 10 water utilities contained 0.07-0.46 µg/l (Safe Drinking Water Committee, 1977).   It has also been detected in the municipal drinking-water at a number of localities [Bertsch et al., 1975; (0.5 µg/l) Eurocop-Cost, 1976; (< 5 µg/l) Saunders et al., 1975].

Rainwater has been found to contain up to 0.15 µg/l tetrachloro-ethylene.   Average and maximum concentrations in sea-water were 0.12 µg/l and 2.6 µg/l and the maximum concentration in sediments 4.8 µg/l (Pearson & McConnell, 1975).   Surface water from the Atlantic Ocean contained 0.2-0.8 ng/l tetrachloroethylene (Murray & Riley, 1973). It has also been detected in rivers and in subterranean water (Dowty et al., 1975; Eurocop-Cost, 1976; Zürcher & Giger, 1976); and in commercial deionized charcoal-filtered water (Dowty et al., 1975).

Tetrachloroethylene was detected in the influent to a sewage treat-ment plant at a level of 6.2 µg/l, in the effluent before chlorination, at 3.9 µg/l, and in the effluent after chlorination, at 4.2 µg/l (Bellar et al., 1974).   It has also been detected in the effluents from chemical production plants, an oil refinery and textile plants and in lake water (Shackelford & Keith, 1976).

(c)   Food

Tetrachloroethylene has been detected in dairy produce (0.3-13 µg/ kg), meat (0.9-5 µg/kg), oils and fats (0.01-7 µg/kg), beverages (2-3 µg/kg), fruit and vegetables (0.7-2 µg/kg), fresh bread (1 µg/kg) (McConnell et al., 1975) and commercially available rendered fats and meat-and-bone meal (Ingr, 1976).

(d)   Marine organisms

Tetrachloroethylene residues were detected in specific organs of the following fish (concentrations expressed as µg/kg on a dry-weight basis): 3 species of molluscs (0-176), eel (1-43), cod (0-8), coalfish (0-6), dogfish (0-13), and bib (0-27) (Dickson & Riley, 1976).

In another study, tetrachloroethylene residues were reported as follows (concentrations expressed as µg/kg of wet tissue): in 14 species of invertebrates (0.05-15), 3 species of marine algae (13-20), 15 species of fish (0-41), the organs and eggs of 8 species of sea and freshwater birds (0.7-39), and the organs of 2 species of mammals (0-19) (Pearson & McConnell, 1975).

(e) Humans

Tetrachloroethylene has been detected in post-mortem human tissue samples, at levels of less than 0.5-29.2 µg/kg (wet tissue) (McConnell et al., 1975), and in expired air, at levels of 0.022-12 µg/hr/subject (Conkle et al., 1975).

(f) Occupational exposure

Tetrachloroethylene was detected in the air of industrial installations at a concentration of 2 mg/m^3 (0.3 ppm) (Kiparisova & Stepanenko, 1976). Concentrations measured in dry-cleaning plants varied from 20-300 mg/m^3 (3-45 ppm) (Engels et al., 1975).

2.3 Analysis

The determination of chlorinated hydrocarbons, including tetrachloroethylene, in ambient and alveolar air, workplace atmospheres, blood and urine has been reviewed (Walter et al., 1976). Methods used for the analysis of tetrachloroethylene in environmental samples are listed in Table 1.

Grimsrud & Rasmussen (1975) report that difficulty in removing tetrachloroethylene from the carrier gas system limits the value of gas chromatography/mass spectrometry methods. This method was used by Coleman et al. (1976) to quantify halocarbons, including tetrachloroethylene, in drinking-water.

Carbon dioxide laser absorption spectrometry can be used to detect tetrachloroethylene in prepared samples of air pollutants, with a limit of detection of 9.5 µg/m^3 (1.4 ppb) (Schnell & Fischer, 1975).

3. Biological Data Relevant to the Evaluation
of Carcinogenic Risk to Humans

3.1 Carcinogenicity studies in animals[1]

(a) Oral administration

Mouse: Groups of 50 male and 50 female B6C3F1 mice, approximately 5 weeks old at the beginning of treatment, were administered tetrachloroethylene (USP grade) in corn oil by gavage on 5 consecutive days per week for 78 weeks. High-dose males received 900 mg/kg bw/day for 11 weeks,

---

[1]The Working Group was aware of studies in progress to assess the carcinogenicity of tetrachloroethylene in mice and rats by oral administration and in mice by skin application (IARC, 1978a).

TABLE 1.   METHODS FOR THE ANALYSIS OF TETRACHLOROETHYLENE

| SAMPLE TYPE | ANALYTICAL METHOD | | | REFERENCE |
	EXTRACTION/CLEAN-UP	DETECTION	LIMIT OF DETECTION	
Formulations				
Encapsulated liquids	Dilute (ethanol)	IR		Horwitz (1975)
Cough syrups	Dilute (ethanol) if necessary	IR		Horwitz (1975)
Air				
Workplace	Sample on charcoal, extract (carbon disulphide)	GC/FID	Useful range, 655-2749 mg/m^3	National Institute for Occupational Safety & Health (1977)
Ambient	Determine directly Enrich	GC	15 mg/m^3 2.5 mg/m^3	Krynska et al. (1976)
Ambient	Trap on Chromosorb 101, desorb by heating, retrap in line on GC column	GC	3.4 µg/m^3 (0.5 ppb)	Parkes et al. (1976)
Ambient	Sample in Dreclusel flask fitted with rubber septum, sample with gas syringe	GC/ECD	1 µg/m^3	Bureau International Technique des Solvants Chlorés (1976)
Ambient	Sample on Porapak N, desorb by heating, retrap in line on GC column	GC/ECD, GC/MS	0.2 µg/m^3 (30 ppt)	Russell & Shadoff (1977)
Water				
Drinking- and sewage water	Bubble nitrogen through sample, concentrate	GC/FID; GC/MS	0.1 µg/l	Bellar et al. (1974)
Drinking-water	Extract (pentane), dry	GC/ECD	25 ng/l	Bureau International Technique des Solvants Chlorés (1976)
Drinking-water	Analyse directly	GC/ECD	0.5 µg/l	Nicholson et al. (1977)
Drinking-water	Analyse directly	GC/ECD	8 µg/l	Nicholson & Meresz (1975)

TABLE 1. METHODS FOR THE ANALYSIS OF TETRACHLOROETHYLENE (continued)

SAMPLE TYPE	ANALYTICAL METHOD			
	EXTRACTION/CLEAN-UP	DETECTION	LIMIT OF DETECTION	REFERENCE
Miscellaneous				
Oil and liquid paraffin	Heat sample, use headspace	GC/FID		Drexler & Osterkamp (1977)
Tobacco smoke	Trap on Tenax GC and Carbopack BHT coated with 5 and 25% OV-101 silicon fluid	GC/FID; GC/MS		Holzer *et al.* (1976)

Abbreviations: IR - infra-red spectrometry; GC/FID - gas chromatography/flame-ionization detection; ECD - electron capture detection; MS - mass spectrometry

1100 mg/kg bw/day for 67 weeks followed by 12 weeks without treatment; high-dose females received 600 mg/kg bw/day for 11 weeks and 800 mg/kg bw/day for 67 weeks.   Respective doses in low-dose animals were 450 and 550 mg/kg bw/day in males and 300 and 400 mg/kg bw/day in females. Time-weighted average doses were 536 and 1072 mg/kg bw/day in males and 386 and 772 mg/kg bw/day in females.   Groups of 20 male and 20 female mice were either untreated or received corn oil alone.   All surviving mice were killed 90 weeks after the start of the experiment.   The times at which 50% of animals were still alive were 90 weeks for control animals of both sexes, 78 weeks for low-dose males, 43 weeks for high-dose males, 62 weeks for low-dose females and 50 weeks for high-dose females. The shorter lifespan in treated animals was due to early toxicity and high incidences of hepatocellular carcinomas in animals of both sexes: hepatocellular carcinomas occurred in 2/17 untreated control males, 2/20 vehicle control males, 32/49 low-dose males and 27/48 high-dose males; in females, the respective incidences were 2/20, 0/20, 19/48 and 19/48.   Metastases were found in 1 untreated control male, in 3 low-dose males, in 1 low-dose female and in 1 high-dose female (National Cancer Institute, 1977).

Rat: Groups of 50 male and 50 female 7-week-old Osborne-Mendel rats were treated with tetrachloroethylene (USP grade) in corn oil by gavage on 5 days a week for 78 weeks.   High-dose animals received 1000-1400 mg/kg bw/day, and low-dose animals 500-700 mg/kg bw/day.   All surviving animals were then observed until 110 weeks after the start of treatment. The time-weighted average doses were 471 and 941 mg/kg bw/day in low- and high-dose males and 474 and 949 mg/kg bw/day in low- and high-dose females.   Dose-related mortality was observed in animals of both sexes after 30 weeks.   Groups of 20 male and 20 female untreated rats or vehicle-treated rats served as controls.   The times at which 50% of animals were still alive were 44 weeks for high-dose males, 66 weeks for high-dose females, 66 weeks for control groups, over 88 weeks for low-dose males and 102 weeks for low-dose females.   No increases in tumour incidences were observed.   Toxic nephropathy was observed in treated rats that died as early as week 20 (National Cancer Institute, 1977) [The Working Group noted the poor survival of treated animals].

(b) Inhalation and/or intratracheal administration

Rat: In a study reported as an abstract, groups of 96 male and 96 female Sprague-Dawley rats were exposed by inhalation to 2 or 4 g/m^3 (300 or 600 ppm) tetrachloroethylene in air for 6 hrs per day on 5 days a week for 12 months, followed by observation up to 30 months.   No statistically significant difference in tumour incidence between treated and control animals was found (Rampy *et al.*, 1977) [The Working Group noted the incomplete reporting of the experiment and the short duration of the exposure].

(c) Intraperitoneal administration

Mouse: Groups of 20 male A/St mice, 6-8 weeks old, were given thrice weekly i.p. injections of 80 mg/kg bw (14 injections), 200 mg/kg bw (24 injections) or 400 mg/kg bw (48 injections) tetrachloroethylene in tricaprylin. All survivors (15, 17, 18 mice in the three groups, respectively) were killed 24 weeks after the first injection. The average number of lung tumours per mouse was not increased compared with that in controls that received tricaprylin alone (Theiss *et al.*, 1977) [The Working Group noted the limitations of negative results obtained with this test system; see also General Remarks on Substances Considered, p. 34].

3.2 Other relevant biological data

(a) Experimental systems

Toxic effects

The toxic effects of tetrachloroethylene have been reviewed (Von Oettingen, 1964).

The oral LD_{50} of tetrachloroethylene in mice is 6.4-8 g/kg bw (Kohne, 1940), 8.85 and 10.8 g/kg bw; it was less toxic in oily solution than when undiluted (Dybing & Dybing, 1946). The inhalational LC_{50} in mice (4 hrs) is 35 g/m^3 (5200 ppm) (Friberg *et al.*, 1953), and the i.p. LD_{50} is 4.7 g/kg bw (Klaassen & Plaa, 1966). In rats, the oral LD_{50} is 13 g/kg bw (Smyth *et al.*, 1969). For rabbits, the minimum lethal dose (24 hrs) after s.c. injection is 2.2 g/kg bw; in dogs, the minimum lethal dose (30 min) after i.v. injection is 85 mg/kg bw (Barsoum & Saad, 1934). The i.p. LD_{50} in dogs is 3.5 g/kg bw (Klaassen & Plaa, 1967).

The minimal narcotic concentration of tetrachloroethylene for mice is 20 g/m^3 (2950 ppm) (Lazarew, 1929). Single exposure of rats to 13.6 g/m^3 (2000 ppm) for 5 hrs caused no loss of consciousness (Rowe *et al.*, 1952). Lamson *et al.* (1929) reported the narcotic concentration for dogs as 62 g/m^3 (9900 ppm).

Thirteen exposures to 17 g/m^3 (2500 ppm) tetrachloroethylene vapours for 7 hrs daily was fatal to the majority of rats (Rowe *et al.*, 1952). The average maximum tolerated oral dose of tetrachloroethylene over a period of 78 weeks was 941 mg/kg bw/day in male Osborne-Mendel rats, 949 mg/kg bw/day in females, 1072 mg/kg bw/day in male B6C3F1 mice, and 722 mg/kg bw/day in females (National Cancer Institute, 1977).

Repeated exposure to vapours has produced a variety of pathological changes in the liver, ranging from fatty degeneration to necrosis in rats, rabbits and guinea-pigs (Rowe *et al.*, 1952). Repeated exposure of male

Sprague-Dawley rats to 4 g/m^3 (600 ppm) vapour for 6 hrs/day on 5 days/ week for 12 months resulted in reversible toxic effects in the liver (Pegg et al., 1978).   Oral doses of 0.3 g/kg bw produced degenerative changes and extensive atrophy of the liver in dogs (Hall & Shillinger, 1925).

Oral doses of tetrachloroethylene have lesser effects on the kidney: only a nearly lethal dose (4 g/kg bw) caused swelling of the convoluted tubules and hydropic degeneration in male mice (Klaassen & Plaa, 1966; Plaa & Larson, 1965).   I.p. doses of 1.6-2.3 g/kg bw tetrachloroethylene caused slight calcification of the tubules of the kidneys in dogs (Klaassen & Plaa, 1967).

Embryotoxicity and teratogenicity

Groups of rats and mice were exposed by inhalation for 7 hrs daily on days 6-15 of gestation to 2 g/m^3 in air (300 ppm) tetrachloroethylene; no effects were observed on the average number of implantation sites per litter, litter size, incidence of foetal resorptions, foetal sex ratios or foetal body measurements.   No treatment-related increase in the incidence of skeletal or visceral malformations was observed (Schwetz et al., 1975).

Absorption, distribution, excretion and metabolism

Tetrachloroethylene is readily absorbed through the lungs and to some extent from the gastrointestinal tract (Von Oettingen, 1964). Fats and oils facilitate its absorption from the intestine after oral administration to dogs (Lamson et al., 1929).   Skin absorption of tetrachloroethylene in mice is low in relation to that of a series of chlorinated ethanes and ethylenes (Tsuruta, 1975).

The half-life of expiration of ^{36}Cl-labelled tetrachloroethylene in rats was about 7 hrs, regardless of dose or route of application (Pegg et al., 1978).

Mice excreted about 90% of an inhaled dose of 1300 mg/kg bw ^{14}C-labelled tetrachloroethylene: 70% in the expired air, 20% in the urine and < 0.5 % in the faeces.   The metabolites identified in the urine were trichloroacetic acid (52% of total urinary activity), oxalic acid (11%) and traces of dichloroacetic acid (Yllner, 1961).   In contrast, Daniel (1963) found only 2% of an oral dose of about 1000 mg/kg bw ^{36}Cl-tetrachloroethylene in the urine of rats; trichloroacetic acid (0.6%) and inorganic chloride were the only metabolites detected.

When ^{14}C-labelled tetrachloroethylene was administered to adult male rats by gavage or by inhalation, approximately 70% of the body burden was expired as unchanged compound, 26% as CO_2 in expired air and as nonvolatile metabolites in urine and faeces and 3-4% remained in the carcass (Pegg et al., 1978).

The hepatotoxicity of tetrachloroethylene was enhanced in rats treated with Aroclor 1254.   Pretreatment of rats with phenobarbital or Aroclor 1254 orally considerably increased the urinary excretion of trichloro compounds after oral administration of tetrachloroethylene in oil (Moslen et al., 1977).

In rat liver perfusion experiments, tetrachloroethylene was converted into trichloroacetic acid, the only metabolite detected (Bonse et al., 1975).

The presence of an epoxide intermediate (oxirane) has been proposed in the metabolism of tetrachloroethylene on the basis of its oxidative metabolism (Henschler & Bonse, 1977).

Mutagenicity and other related short-term tests

Results reported in an abstract suggest that tetrachloroethylene is mutagenic in plate tests in Salmonella typhimurium TA100.   In a host-mediated assay in mice, using Salmonella typhimurium TA1950, TA1951 and TA1952, there was a significant increase in the number of revertants with doses equivalent to the LD_{50} and to half the LD_{50}, but this was not dose-related (Černá & Kypěnová, 1977).

Tetrachloroethylene did not induce mutations to prototrophy at the gal, arg and nad loci in Escherichia coli K12 and had no effect on forward mutation frequency in the methyltryptophan resistance system at a nontoxic concentration of 0.9 mM (liquid tests) (Greim et al., 1975).

There was no induction of chromosomal aberrations in bone-marrow cells of mice that had received either single (half LD_{50}) or 5 daily i.p. injections (one-sixth LD_{50}) of the chemical (Černá & Kypěnová, 1977).

(b)   Humans

The effects of inhalation of various concentrations have been reviewed;   these include irritation of the mucous membranes, skin irritation (Von Oettingen, 1964) and lung oedema (Patel et al., 1977). The neurological effects of tetrachloroethylene on dry-cleaners have also been reviewed (Tuttle et al., 1977).

Chronic exposure to tetrachloroethylene vapours caused irritation of the respiratory tract, nausea, headache, sleeplessness, abdominal pains and constipation (Chmielewski et al., 1976;   Coler & Rossmiller, 1953;   Stewart et al., 1970;   Von Oettingen, 1964).   Pathological findings (liver cirrhosis, hepatitis and nephritis) are rare (Stewart, 1969).   Other reports of intoxications and fatalities due to tetrachloro- ethylene have been made (Eberhardt & Freundt, 1966;   Larsen et al.,

1977; Stewart, 1969; Trense & Zimmermann, 1969).   Therapeutic administration of tetrachloroethylene as an anthelminthic has occasionally
produced side effects (Von Oettingen, 1964).

A case of 'obstructive jaundice' in a 6-week old infant has been
attributed to tetrachloroethylene in breast milk.   During her pregnancy,
the mother had frequently visited her husband at his work place in a dry-
cleaning plant.   Liver function tests and serum transaminase levels in
the parents were normal (Bagnell & Ellenberger, 1977).

Tetrachloroethylene vapours and liquid can be absorbed through the
skin (Hake & Stewart, 1977; Stewart & Dodd, 1964) and through the lungs
(Stewart et al., 1961).   Inhaled tetrachloroethylene is excreted very
slowly: its biological half-life is 3-5 days, depending on the length
of exposure (Stewart et al., 1970).   The half-life of tetrachloroethylene
in alveolar air after dermal absorption of the liquid was approximately
8 hrs (Stewart & Dodd, 1964).   After exposure to 0.7 g/m^3 (100 ppm) in
air for 8 hrs, the concentrations in the alveolar air decreased exponentially, with an initial expiration half-life of 25-30 min (Fernandez
et al., 1976).   The total body half-life was calculated to be 71.5 hrs
(Guberan & Fernandez, 1974).

Inhalation of tetrachloroethylene is followed by a long-lasting
excretion of metabolites in the urine (Ikeda & Imamura, 1973).   Tetrachloroethylene is metabolized very slowly, and determination of its
urinary metabolites can therefore not be taken as a satisfactory measure
of exposure.   Male volunteers exposed to 0.6 g/m^3 (87 ppm) tetrachloroethylene vapours in air for 3 hrs excreted about 1.8% of the dose in the
urine as trichloroacetic acid in 67 hrs (Ogata et al., 1971).   At
concentrations well below 678 mg/m^3 (100 ppm), both trichloroacetic acid
and trichloroethanol concentrations in the urine reach a plateau (Ikeda,
1977).

Of 200 workers exposed to tetrachloroethylene vapours, 35% had more
than 10 mg/l trichloroacetic acid in their urine.   About half the
subjects with these levels of urinary trichloroacetic acid had some
symptoms of poisoning (Münzer & Heder, 1972).

3.3 Case reports and epidemiological studies[1]

No data were available to the Working Group.

_____

[1]The Working Group was aware of a mortality study in progress on
dry-cleaning workers exposed to tetrachloroethylene (IARC, 1978b).

4. Summary of Data Reported and Evaluation

4.1 Experimental data

Tetrachloroethylene was tested in one experiment in mice and in one in rats by oral administration. In mice, it produced hepatocellular carcinomas in animals of both sexes. The experiment in rats was considered to be inadequate. Tetrachloroethylene was also inadequately tested by inhalation exposure in rats and by intraperitoneal injection in mice.

Tetrachloroethylene was not mutagenic in *Escherichia coli* and was negative in cytogenetic tests in mice.

4.2 Human data[1]

No case reports or epidemiological studies were available to the Working Group.

The extensive production and use of tetrachloroethylene over the past several decades, particularly for dry-cleaning purposes, indicate that widespread human exposure occurs. This is confirmed by many reports of its occurrence in air, water, fish and food samples.

4.3 Evaluation

There is *limited evidence* that tetrachloroethylene is carcinogenic in mice.

---

[1]Subsequent to the meeting of the Working Group, the Secretariat became aware of a study of 330 deceased laundry and dry-cleaning workers who had been exposed to carbon tetrachloride, trichloroethylene and tetrachloroethylene. An excess of lung, cervical and skin cancers and a slight excess of leukaemias and liver cancers were observed (Blair *et al.*, 1979). In an abstract, Blair *et al.* (1978) described a clinical report of 5 cases of chronic lymphocytic leukaemia in a family that operated a dry-cleaning business.

5. References

Bagnell, P.C. & Ellenberger, H.A. (1977) Obstructive jaundice due to
    a chlorinated hydrocarbon in breast milk. Can. med. Assoc. J.,
    117, 1047-1048

Barsoum, G.S. & Saad, K. (1934)   Relative toxicity of certain chlorine
    derivatives of the aliphatic serie. Q. J. Pharm. Pharmacol., 7,
    205-214

Bellar, T.A., Lichtenberg, J.J. & Kroner, R.C. (1974) The Occurrence
    of Organohalides in Chlorinated Drinking Waters, EPA-670/4-74-008,
    Cincinnati, OH, US Environmental Protection Agency. Available from
    Springfield, VA, National Technical Information Service

Berkowitz, J.B. (1978)   Literature Review - Problem Definition Studies
    on Selected Chemicals, Tetrachloroethylene, Cambridge, MA, Arthur
    D. Little, Inc., pp. 10-57

Bertsch, W., Anderson, E. & Holzer, G. (1975)   Trace analysis of
    organic volatiles in water by gas chromatography-mass spectrometry
    with glass capillary columns. J. Chromatogr., 112, 701-718

Blair, A., Decoufle, P. & Grauman, D. (1978)   Mortality among laundry
    and dry cleaning workers (Abstract). Am. J. Epidemiol., 108, 238

Blair, A., Decoufle, P. & Grauman, D. (1979)   Causes of death among
    laundry and dry cleaning workers. Am. J. Publ. Health, 69, 508-
    511

Bonse, G., Urban, T., Reichert, D. & Henschler, D. (1975)   Chemical
    reactivity, metabolic oxirane formation and biological reactivity of
    chlorinated ethylenes in the isolated perfused rat liver preparation.
    Biochem. Pharmacol., 24, 1829-1834

Bureau International Technique des Solvents Chlorés (1976)
    Standardization of methods for the determination of traces of some
    volatile chlorinated aliphatic hydrocarbons in air and water by
    gas chromatography. Anal. chim. acta, 82, 1-17

Černá, M. & Kypěnová, H. (1977) Mutagenic activity of chloroethylenes
    analysed by screening system tests (Abstract No. 36). Mutat. Res.,
    46, 214-215

Chmielewski, J., Tomaszewski, R., Glombiowski, P., Kowalewski, W.,
    Kwiatkowski, S.R., Szczekocki, W. & Winnicka, A. (1976)   Clinical
    observations of the occupational exposure to tetrachloroethylene.
    Biul. Inst. Med. Morskiej, 27, 197-205

Coleman, W.E., Lingg, R.D., Melton, R.G. & Kopfler, F.C. (1976)   The occurrence of volatile organics in five drinking water supplies using gas chromatography/mass spectrometry.   In: Keith, L.H., ed., Identification and Analysis of Organic Pollutants in Water, Ann Arbor, MI, Ann Arbor Science, pp. 305-327

Coler, H.R. & Rossmiller, H.R. (1953) Tetrachloroethylene exposure in a small industry. AMA Arch. ind. Hyg., 8, 227-233

Conkle, J.P., Camp, B.J. & Welch, B.E. (1975)   Trace composition of human respiratory gas. Arch. environ. Health, 30, 290-295

Cox, R.A., Derwent, R.G., Eggleton, A.E.J. & Lovelock, J.E. (1976) Photochemical oxidation of halocarbons in the troposphere. Atmos. Environ., 10, 305-308

Daniel, J.W. (1963) The metabolism of ^{36}Cl-labelled trichloroethylene and tetrachloroethylene in the rat. Biochem. Pharmacol., 12, 795-802

Dickson, A.G. & Riley, J.P. (1976)   The distribution of short-chain halogenated aliphatic hydrocarbons in some marine organisms. Marine Biol. Pollut., 7, 167-169

Dowty, B.J., Carlisle, D.R. & Laseter, J.L. (1975) New Orleans drinking water sources tested by gas chromatography-mass spectrometry. Occurrence and origin of aromatics and halogenated aliphatic hydrocarbons. Environ. Sci. Technol., 9, 762-765

Drexler, H.-J. & Osterkamp, G. (1977)   Head-space analysis for the quantitative determination of trichloroethylene and tetrachloroethylene in oils and liquid paraffin. J. clin. Chem. clin. Biochem., 15, 431-432

Dybing, F. & Dybing, O. (1946)   The toxic effect of tetrachlormethane and tetrachlorethylene in oily solution. Acta pharmacol., 2, 223-226

Eberhardt, H. & Freundt, K.J. (1966)   Perchlorethylene poisoning (Germ.). Arch. Toxikol., 21, 338-351

Engels, L.H., Schuetz, A. & Wolf, D. (1975)   Perchloroethylene in dry cleaning. Polluant situation and technical prophylaxis (Germ.). Staub-Reinhalt. Luft, 35, 412-415 [Chem. Abstr., 84, 110939e]

Eurocop-Cost (1976)   A Comprehensive List of Polluting Substances Which Have Been Identified in Various Fresh Waters, Effluent Discharges, Aquatic Animals and Plants, and Bottom Sediments, 2nd ed., EUCO/MDU 73/76, XII/476/76, Luxembourg, Commission of the European Communities, pp. 53-54

Fernandez, J., Guberan, E. & Caperos, J. (1976)   Experimental human exposures to tetrachloroethylene vapor and elimination in breath after inhalation. Am. ind. Hyg. Assoc. J., 37, 143-150

Friberg, L., Kylin, B. & Nyström, A. (1953)   Toxicities of trichloro-ethylene and tetrachloroethylene and Fujiwara's pyridine-alkali reaction. Acta pharmacol. toxicol., 9, 303-312

Fuller, B.B. (1976)   Air Pollution Assessment of Tetrachloroethylene, Report No. MTR-7143, McLean, VA, Mitre Corp., p. 3. Available from Springfield, VA, National Technical Information Service

Grasselli, J.G. & Ritchey, W.M., eds (1975)   CRC Atlas of Spectral Data and Physical Constants for Organic Compounds, 2nd ed., Vol. III, Cleveland, OH, Chemical Rubber Co., p. 282

Greim, H., Bonse, G., Radwan, Z., Reichert, D. & Henschler, D. (1975) Mutagenicity in vitro and potential carcinogenicity of chlorinated ethylenes as a function of metabolic oxirane formation. Biochem. Pharmacol., 24, 2013-2017

Grimsrud, E.P. & Rasmussen, R.A. (1975)   Survey and analysis of halo-carbons in the atmosphere by gas chromatography-mass spectrometry. Atmos. Environ., 9, 1014-1017

Guberan, E. & Fernandez, J. (1974)   Control of industrial exposure to tetrachloroethylene by measuring alveolar concentrations: theoretical approach using a mathematical model. Br. J. ind. Med., 31, 159-167

Hake, C.L. & Stewart, R.D. (1977)   Human exposure to tetrachloroethylene: inhalation and skin contact. Environ. Health Perspect., 21, 231-238

Hall, M.C. & Shillinger, J.E. (1925)   Tetrachloroethylene, a new anthelmintic for worms in dogs. North Am. Vet., 9, 41-52

Hardie, D.W.F. (1964)   Chlorocarbons and chlorohydrocarbons. Tetra-chloroethylene. In: Kirk, R.E. & Othmer, D.F., eds, Encyclopedia of Chemical Technology, 2nd ed., Vol. 5, New York, John Wiley & Sons, pp. 195-203

Hawley, G.G., ed. (1977)   The Condensed Chemical Dictionary, 9th ed., New York, Van Nostrand-Reinhold, p. 660

Henschler, D. & Bonse, G. (1977)   Metabolic activation of chlorinated ethylenes: dependence of mutagenic effect on electrophilic reactivity of the metabolically formed epoxides. Arch. Toxikol., 39, 7-12

Holzer, G., Oró, J. & Bertsch, W. (1976)   Gas chromatographic-mass spectrometric evaluation of exhaled tobacco smoke.   J. Chromatogr., 126, 771-785

Horwitz, W., ed. (1975)   Official Methods of Analysis of the Association of Official Analytical Chemists, 12th ed., Washington DC, Association of Official Analytical Chemists, pp. 658-660

IARC (1978a)   Information Bulletin on the Survey of Chemicals Being Tested for Carcinogenicity, No. 7, Lyon, pp. 272-277

IARC (1978b)   Directory of On-Going Research in Cancer Epidemiology, 1978 (IARC Scientific Publications No. 26), Lyon, p. 286 (Abstract no. 753)

Ikeda, M. (1977)   Metabolism of trichloroethylene and tetrachloroethylene in human subjects.   Environ. Health Persp., 21, 239-245

Ikeda, M. & Imamura, T. (1973)   Biological half-life of trichloroethylene and tetrachloroethylene in human subjects.   Int. Arch. Arbeitsmed., 31, 209-224

Ingr, I. (1976)   Residues of perchloroethylene and gasoline in rendered fats and in feed meal (Czech.).   Vet. Med. (Prague), 21, 331-341 [Chem. Abstr., 86, 70192p]

Kiparisova, L.S. & Stepanenko, V.E. (1976)   Gas-chromatographic determination of some chlorinated hydrocarbons in the air of industrial installations (Russ.).   Gig. Sanit., 6, 54-55 [Chem. Abstr., 86, 8127t]

Klaassen, C.D. & Plaa, G.L. (1966)   Relative effects of various chlorinated hydrocarbons on liver and kidney function in mice.   Toxicol. appl. Pharmacol., 9, 139-151

Klaassen, C.D. & Plaa, G.L. (1967)   Relative effects of various chlorinated hydrocarbons on liver and kidney function in dogs.   Toxicol. appl. Pharmacol., 10, 119-131

Köhne, H. (1940)   Thesis, University of Hamburg (cited in Von Oettingen, 1964, p. 275)

Krynska, A., Grabowski, Z. & Posniak, M. (1976)   Determination of trichloroethylene, tetrachloroethylene and tetrachloroethane in air by gas chromatography (Pol.).   Pr. Cent. Inst. Ochr. Pr., 26, 293-306 [Chem. Abstr., 87, 140307b]

Lamson, P.D., Robbins, B.H. & Ward, C.B. (1929)   The pharmacology and toxicology of tetrachloroethylene.   Am. J. Hyg., 9, 430-444

Larsen, N.A., Nielsen, B. & Ravn-Nielsen, A. (1977) Poisoning with
    perchloroethylene. A risk of self-service dry-cleaning (Danish).
    Ugeskr. Laeg., 139, 270-275

Lazarew, N.W. (1929) Narcotic effect of vapours of chlorinated
    derivatives of methane, ethane and ethylene (Germ.). Naunyn
    Schmiedebeigs Arch. exp. Path. Pharmakol., 141, 19-24

Lillian, D., Singh, H.B., Appelby, A., Lobban, L., Arnts, R., Gumpert,
    R., Hague, R., Toomey, J., Kazazis, J., Antell, M., Hansen, D. &
    Scott, B. (1975) Atmospheric fates of halogenated compounds.
    Environ. Sci. Technol., 9, 1042-1048

Lillian, D., Singh, H.B. & Appleby, A. (1976) Gas chromatographic
    analysis of ambient halogenated compounds. J. Air Pollut. Control
    Assoc., 26, 141-143

McConnell, G., Ferguson, D.M. & Pearson, C.R. (1975) Chlorinated
    hydrocarbons and the environment. Endeavor, 34, 13-18

Moslen, M.T., Reynolds, E.S. & Szabo, S. (1977) Enhancement of the
    metabolism and hepatoxicity of trichloroethylene and perchloro-
    ethylene. Biochem. Pharmacol., 26, 369-375

Münzer, M. & Heder, K. (1972) Results of industrial-medical and
    technical examination of chemical purification operations (Germ.).
    Zbl. Arbeitsmed., 22, 133-138

Murray, A.J. & Riley, J.P. (1973) Occurrence of some chlorinated
    aliphatic hydrocarbons in the environment. Nature (Lond.), 242,
    37-38

National Cancer Institute (1977) Bioassay of Tetrachloroethylene for
    Possible Carcinogenicity (Technical Report Series No. 13) DHEW
    Publication No. (NIH) 77-813, Washington DC, US Department of
    Health, Education, & Welfare

National Institute for Occupational Safety & Health (1976) Criteria
    for a Recommended Standard ... Occupational Exposure to Tetra-
    chloroethylene (Perchloroethylene), DHEW Publication No. (NIOSH)
    76-185, Washington DC, US Department of Health, Education, and
    Welfare

National Institute for Occupational Safety & Health (1977) NIOSH Manual
    of Analytical Methods, 2nd ed., Part II, Standards Completion
    Program Validated Methods, Vol. 3, Method No. S335, Washington DC,
    US Government Printing Office, pp. S335-1-S335-9

National Institute for Occupational Safety & Health (1978) Current Intelligence Bulletin 20, Tetrachloroethylene (Perchloroethylene), Washington DC, US Government Printing Office, pp. 1-2

Nicholson, A.A. & Meresz, O. (1975) Analysis of volatile, halogenated organics in water by direct aqueous injection-gas chromatography. Bull. environ. Contam. Toxicol., 14, 453-456

Nicholson, A.A., Meresz, O. & Lemyk, B. (1977) Determination of free and total potential haloforms in drinking water. Anal. Chem., 49, 814-819

Ogata, M., Takatsuka, Y. & Tomokuni, K. (1971) Excretion of organic chlorine compounds in the urine of persons exposed to vapours of trichloroethylene and tetrachloroethylene. Br. J. ind. Med., 28, 386-391

Parkes, D.G., Ganz, C.R., Polinsky, A. & Schulze, J. (1976) A simple gas chromatographic method for the analysis of trace organics in ambient air. Am. ind. Hyg. Assoc. J., 37, 165-173

Patel, R., Janakiraman, N. & Towne, W.D. (1977) Pulmonary oedema due to tetrachloroethylene. Environ. Health Persp., 21, 247-249

Pearson, C.R. & McConnell, G. (1975) Chlorinated C_1 and C_2 hydrocarbons in the marine environment. Proc. R. Soc. Lond. B., 189, 305-332

Pegg, D.G., Zempel, J.A., Braun, W.H. & Gehring, P.J. (1978) Disposition of [^{14}C] tetrachloroethylene following oral and inhalation exposure in rats (Abstract no. 131). Toxicol. appl. Pharmacol., 45, 276-277

Perry, R.H. & Chilton, C.H., eds (1973) Chemical Engineers' Handbook, 5th ed., New York, McGraw-Hill, p. 3-59

Plaa, G.L. & Larson, R.E. (1965) Relative nephrotoxic properties of chlorinated methane, ethane and ethylene derivatives in mice. Toxicol. appl. Pharmacol., 7, 37-44

Rampy, L.W., Quast, J.F., Leong, B.K.J. & Gehring, P.J. (1977) Results of long-term inhalation toxicity studies on rats of 1,1,1-trichloroethane and perchloroethylene formulations (Abstract). In: International Congress on Toxicology, Toronto, Canada, 1977, p. 27

Rowe, V.K., McCollister, D.D., Spencer, H.C., Adams, E.M. & Irish, D.D. (1952) Vapor toxicity of tetrachloroethylene for laboratory animals and human subjects. AMA Arch. ind. Hyg. occup. Med., 5, 566-579

Russell, J.W. & Shadoff, L.A. (1977) The sampling and determination of halocarbons in ambient air using concentration on porous polymer. J. Chromatogr., 134, 375-384

Safe Drinking Water Committee (1977) Drinking Water and Health,
     Washington DC, National Academy of Sciences, p. 769

Saunders, R.A., Blachly, C.H., Kovacina, T.A., Lamontagne, R.A.,
     Swinnerton, J.W. & Saalfeld, F.E. (1975) Identification of
     volatile organic contaminants in Washington DC municipal water.
     Water Res., 9, 1143-1145

Schnell, W. & Fischer, G. (1975)   Carbon dioxide laser absorption
     coefficients of various air pollutants. Appl. Optics, 14, 2058-
     2059

Schwetz, B.A., Leong, B.K.J. & Gehring, P.J. (1975) The effect of
     maternally inhaled trichloroethylene, perchloroethylene, methyl
     chloroform, and methylene chloride on embryonal and fetal develop-
     ment in mice and rats. Toxicol. appl. Pharmacol., 32, 84-96

Shackelford, W.M. & Keith, L.H. (1976)   Frequency of Organic Compounds
     Identified in Water, EPA-600/4-76-062, Athens, GA, US Environmental
     Protection Agency, pp. 130-132

Simmonds, P.G., Kerrin, S.L., Lovelock, J.E. & Shair, F.H. (1974)
     Distribution of atmospheric halocarbons in the air over the Los
     Angeles Basin. Atmos. Environ., 8, 209-216

Singh, H.B. (1976) Phosgene in the ambient air. Nature (Lond.), 264,
     428-429

Singh, H.B., Salas, L.J. & Cavanagh, L.A. (1977) Distribution, sources
     and sinks of atmospheric halogenated compounds. J. Air Pollut.
     Control Assoc., 27, 332-336

Smyth, H.F., Jr, Weil, C.S., West, J.S. & Carpenter, C.P. (1969) An
     exploration of joint toxic action: twenty-seven industrial
     chemicals intubated in rats in all possible pairs. Toxicol. appl.
     Pharmacol., 14, 340-347

Stewart, R.D. (1969) Acute tetrachloroethylene intoxication. J. Am.
     med. Assoc., 208, 1490-1492

Stewart, R.D. & Dodd, H.C. (1964) Absorption of carbon tetrachloride,
     trichloroethylene, tetrachloroethylene, methylene chloride, and
     1,1,1-trichloroethane through the human skin. Am. ind. Hyg. Assoc.
     J., 25, 439-446

Stewart, R.D., Gay, H.H., Erley, D.S., Hake, C.L. & Schaffer, A.W. (1961)
     Human exposure to tetrachloroethylene vapor. Relationship of expired
     air and blood concentrations to exposure and toxicity. Arch. environ.
     Health, 2, 516-522

Stewart, R.D., Baretta, E.D., Dodd, H.C. & Torkelson, T.R. (1970)
Experimental human exposure to tetrachloroethylene. Arch. environ.
Health, 20, 224-229

Theiss, J.C., Stoner, G.D., Shimkin, M.B. & Weisburger, E.K. (1977)
Test for carcinogenicity of organic contaminants of United States
drinking waters by pulmonary tumor response in strain A mice.
Cancer Res., 37, 2717-2720

Trense, E. & Zimmermann, H. (1969) Fatal poisoning due to chronic
inhalation of perchlorethylene vapours (Germ.). Zbl. Arbeitsmed.,
19, 131-137

Tsuruta, H. (1975) Percutaneous absorption of organic solvents.
1. Comparative study of the in vivo percutaneous absorption of
chlorinated solvents in mice. Ind. Health., 13, 227-236

Tuttle, T.C., Wood, G.D., Grether, C.B., Johnson, B.L. & Xintaras, C.
(1977) A Behavioral and Neurological Evaluation of Dry-Cleaners
Exposed to Perchloroethylene, DHEW (NIOSH) Publication No. 77-214,
Cincinnati, OH, National Institute for Occupational Safety &
Health

US Department of Commerce (1977a) US Imports for Consumption and General
Imports, TSUSA Commodity by Country of Origin, FT 246/Annual 1976,
Washington DC, US Government Printing Office, p. 230

US Department of Commerce (1977b) US Exports, Schedule B Commodity by
Country, FT 410/December 1976, Washington DC, US Government Printing
Office, p. 2-85

US International Trade Commission (1977) Synthetic Organic Chemicals
US Production and Sales, 1976, USITC Publication 833, Washington
DC, US Government Printing Office, pp. 303, 331

US Occupational Safety & Health Administration (1977) Air contaminants.
US Code Fed. Regul., Title 29, part 1910.1000, pp. 59-60

US Pharmacopeial Convention, Inc. (1975) The United States Pharmacopeia,
19th Rev., Rockville, MD, pp. 496-497

Von Oettingen, W.F. (1964) The Halogenated Hydrocarbons of Industrial
and Toxicological Importance, Amsterdam, Elsevier, pp. 271-283

Walter, P., Craigmill, A., Villaume, J., Sweeney, S. & Miller, G.L.
(1976) Chlorinated Hydrocarbon Toxicity (1,1,1-Trichloroethane,
Trichloroethylene, and Tetrachloroethylene): a Monograph, CPSC-
BBSC-76-M1, Bethesda, MD, Consumer Product Safety Commission,
pp. 21-25

Winell, M. (1975) An international comparison of hygienic standards for chemicals in the work environment. Ambio, 4, 34-36

Yllner, S. (1961) Urinary metabolites of ^{14}C-tetrachloroethylene in mice. Nature (Lond.), 191, 820

Zürcher, F. & Giger, W. (1976) Volatile organic trace components in the Glatt [river] (Germ.). Vom Wasser, 47, 37-55 [Chem. Abstr., 87, 58231p]

1,1,1-TRICHLOROETHANE

One review on 1,1,1-trichloroethane is available (Mercier, 1977).

1.   Chemical and Physical Data

1.1 Synonyms and trade names

Chem. Abstr. Services Reg. No: 71-55-6

Chem. Abstr. Name: 1,1,1-Trichloroethane

Synonyms: Chloroethene; chlorotene; chlorothene; methyl chloroform; methyltrichloromethane; trichloroethane; α-trichloro-ethane

Trade names: Aerothene TT; Chlorten; Chlorothane NU; Chlorothene NU; Chlorothene VG; Inhibisol; α-T

1.2 Structural and molecular formulae and molecular weight

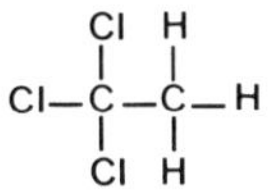

$$Cl-\overset{\displaystyle Cl}{\underset{\displaystyle Cl}{C}}-\overset{\displaystyle H}{\underset{\displaystyle H}{C}}-H$$

$C_2H_3Cl_3$ Mol. wt: 133.4

1.3 Chemical and physical properties of the pure substance

From Aviado *et al.* (1976), unless otherwise specified

(a) Description: Colourless liquid (Hardie, 1964)

(b) Boiling-point: 74.1°C

(c) Melting-point: -32.6°C (Hardie, 1964)

(d) Density: d^{25} 1.336

(e) Refractive index: n_D^{20} 1.4370 (Grasselli & Ritchey, 1975)

(f) Spectroscopy data: Infra-red, nuclear magnetic resonance and
     mass spectral data have been tabulated (Grasselli & Ritchey,
     1975).

(g) Solubility: Practically insoluble in water (0.03 g/100 g of
     water at 25°C); soluble in acetone, benzene, carbon tetra-
     chloride, methanol, diethyl ether and carbon disulphide

(h) Volatility: Vapour pressure is 103 mm at 20°C.

(i) Stability: Nonflammable; decomposes at high temperatures
     (> 360°C) or at ambient temperatures in the presence of water
     and metals, liberating hydrogen chloride; oxidized by
     atmospheric oxygen at high temperatures, forming phosgene
     (Hardie, 1964)

(j) Reactivity: Reacts with an aqueous suspension of calcium
     hydroxide, forming 1,1-dichloroethylene; reacts with chlorine
     in sunlight to give 1,1,1,2-tetrachloroethane and small
     quantities of penta- and hexachloroethane (Hardie, 1964)

(k) Conversion factor: 1 ppm in air is equivalent to 5.4 mg/m^3.

1.4 Technical products and impurities

1,1,1-Trichloroethane is available commercially in the US in
technical and solvent grades, which differ only in the amount of stabilizer added to prevent corrosion of metal parts. Stabilized grades
contain 3-8% stabilizer, such as nitromethane, N-methylpyrrole, 1,4-
dioxane, butylene oxide, 1,3-dioxolane and secondary butyl alcohols.
Typical specifications are as follows: a clear, water-white liquid;
specific gravity, 25°C/25°C, 1.300-1.320; nonvolatile residue, 0.001%
max; water content, 100 mg/kg max; acidity (as HCl), 0.001% max;
100% distillation range, 72-88°C; pH, 6.0-7.5; and acid acceptance
(as NaOH), 0.165% min.

Specifications for reagent grade 1,1,1-trichloroethane are as
follows; boiling-range of a 100 ml sample, the difference between
the temperature observed when 1 ml and 95 ml have distilled does not
exceed 16°C; specific gravity, 1.312-1.321; acidity (as HCl), 0.001%
max; residue on evaporation, 0.001% (US Pharmacopeial Convention,
Inc., 1975).

.Technical grade 1,1,1-trichloroethane available in Japan has the following specifications: distillation range, 70-88°C; acidity (as HCl), 0.001% max; nonvolatile matter, 0.001% max; moisture content, 0.01% max.

2. Production, Use, Occurrence and Analysis

2.1 Production and use

(a) Production

1,1,1-Trichloroethane was first prepared in 1840 by the reaction of chlorine with 1,1-dichloroethane (Prager *et al.*, 1918). It is produced commercially in the US by chlorination of vinyl chloride derived from 1,2-dichloroethane; hydrochlorination of vinylidene chloride derived from 1,2-dichloroethane; or thermal chlorination of ethane. Of the total US capacity for 1,1,1-trichloroethane manufacture, 90% is based on 1,2-dichloroethane-derived intermediates.

1,1,1-Trichloroethane is produced in Japan by chlorination of vinyl chloride.

Commercial production of 1,1,1-trichloroethane in the US was first reported in 1946 (US Tariff Commission, 1947). In 1976, total production by the 4 producing companies amounted to 287 million kg (US International Trade Commission, 1977); imports were negligible. US exports of 1,1,1-trichloroethane in 1974 were 32 million kg.

Total annual western European production of 1,1,1-trichloroethane is 120-200 million kg: the Federal Republic of Germany produces more than 100 million kg; France and the UK produce 10-50 million kg; and Austria, Benelux, Italy, Scandinavia, Spain and Switzerland each produce less than 100 thousand kg. Annual production in eastern Europe is estimated to be less than 100 thousand kg.

In 1976, 5 Japanese companies produced an estimated 60 million kg of 1,1,1-trichloroethane; exports were 5 million kg, and none was imported.

(b) Use

In 1974, use of 1,1,1-trichloroethane in the US was as follows: cold cleaning of metals, 37%; vapour degreasing, 34%; chemical intermediate for vinylidene chloride (see IARC, 1979), 23%; and other applications, 6%.

1,1,1-Trichloroethane is widely used as a cleaning solvent because of its nonflammability and solvent properties. It is used as a cold cleaning solvent for electric motors, generators, switchgear and electronic apparatus, and has also begun to compete with Fluorocarbon 113 (1,1,2-trichloro-1,2,2-trifluoroethane) in high-purity cleaning applications, such as missile parts, semiconductors and high-vacuum equipment.

Stabilized 1,1,1-trichloroethane (see section 1.4) protects against corrosion and is stable under conditions of vapour degreasing. Between 1971 and 1974, use of this compound for vapour degreasing grew at an average annual rate of 21%.

In 1974, approximately 47% of the vinylidine chloride produced in the US was derived from 1,1,1-trichloroethane (for information on uses of vinylidine chloride, see IARC, 1979).

The largest other use for 1,1,1-trichloroethane is in aerosols, in which it acts both as a vapour-pressure depressant (making it a good propellant) and as a solvent and carrier for many of the active ingredients used in aerosols. It has been estimated that 14 aerosol products and 45 nonaerosol products containing 10-100% 1,1,1-trichloro-ethane were available to US consumers in 1969 (Aviado et al., 1976).

Several million kg of 1,1,1-trichloroethane per year are used in adhesives as a resin solvent. It is also used as a lubricant carrier to inject graphite, grease and other lubricants; and it is used alone and in cutting oil formulations as a coolant and lubricant for drilling and tapping alloy and stainless steels. 1,1,1-Trichloroethane is also used to develop printed circuit boards and as a solvent in drain cleaners, shoe polishes, spot cleaners, insecticide formulations and printing inks. It is used in motion picture film cleaning, in stain repellents for upholstery fabrics, for wig cleaning, and in textile processing and finishing.

In western Europe, 1,1,1-trichloroethane is used as follows: vapour degreasing, 30%; cold cleaning of metals, 30%; solvent for manufactured products (such as adhesives), 30%; and other uses, 10%.

In 1976, 1,1,1-trichloroethane was used in Japan as follows: cleaning solvent for metals, 77%; spot removers, 10%, and other uses, 13%.

1,1,1-Trichloroethane is approved by the US Food and Drug Administration (FDA) as a constituent of adhesives used as components of articles intended for use in packaging, transporting or holding food (US Food and Drug Administration, 1977a). On 16 December, 1977, the FDA ruled that an approved new drug application is required, as of 16 January 1978, to market any aerosol drug product containing 1,1,1-trichloroethane and intended to be inhaled either directly or indirectly (US Food & Drug Administration, 1977b).

Also in the US, 1,1,1-trichloroethane is exempted from the requirement of a tolerance for residues: (1) when used as a solvent in pesticide formulations applied to growing crops and raw agricultural commodities after harvest; (2) when used as a solvent in pesticide formulations used on animals, when it comprises not more than 25% of the formulation; and (3) when used in the postharvest fumigation of citrus fruits (US Environmental Protection Agency, 1976).

The US Occupational Safety and Health Administration's standards for exposure to air contaminants require that an employee's exposure to 1,1,1-trichloroethane not exceed an 8-hr time-weighted average of 1900 mg/m^3 (350 ppm) in the workplace air in any 8-hr work shift of a 40-hr work week (US Occupational Safety & Health Administration, 1977). The corresponding standard in the Federal Republic of Germany is 1080 mg/m^3 (200 ppm); that in the German Democratic Republic and Czechoslovakia, 500 mg/m^3 (92 ppm); and that in Sweden, 540 mg/m^3 (100 ppm). In the USSR, the acceptable ceiling concentration is 20 mg/m^3 (3.7 ppm) (Winell, 1975).

2.2 Occurrence

1,1,1-Trichloroethane is not known to occur as a natural product.

(a) Air

1,1,1-Trichloroethane has been detected in air samples taken: (1) over the Los Angeles Basin, at an average concentration of 2 $\mu g/m^3$ (0.37 ppb[1]) (Simmonds et al., 1974); (2) in ambient air over New Brunswick, New Jersey, at a level of 4.5 $\mu g/m^3$ (0.83 ppb) (Lillian et al., 1976); (3) in air samples in Stanford Hills, California, at a level of 422 ng/m^3 (77.6 ppt[2]) (average), and Point Reyes, California, at a level of 492 ng/m^3 (90 ppt) (average) (Singh et al., 1977); (4) in rural air samples taken in central Michigan, at levels of 500-700 ng/m^3 (80-120 ppt) (Russell & Shadoff, 1977); (5) in rural air samples taken in southeastern Washington state, at a level of 545 ng/m^3 (100 ppt) (Grimsrud & Rasmussen, 1975); and (6) in the following locations (mean concentration in ppb): Seagirt, New Jersey (0.10); New York City, New York (0.61); Sandy Hook, New Jersey (0.15); Delaware City, Delaware (0.10); Baltimore, Maryland (0.12); Wilmington, Ohio (0.097); White Face Mountains, New York (0.067); and Bayonne, New Jersey (1.59) (Lillian et al., 1975).

1,1,1-Trichloroethane has also been detected in ambient air over Tokyo, at an average concentration of 4.3 $\mu g/m^3$ (0.8 ppb) (Ohta et al., 1976); in air in South Africa, at a level of 132 ng/m^3 (24.4 ppt); and in Eire, at a level of 350 ng/m^3 (64.8 ppt) (Cox et al., 1976).

[1] 1 ppb is equivalent to 5.4 $\mu g/m^3$ of air.
[2] 1 ppt is equivalent to 5.4 ng/m^3 of air.

In a UK study, 1,1,1-trichloroethane was detected in air at the following locations (in ppb): Runcorn Works perimeter (~ 16); Runcorn Heath (6.2-11); Liverpool/Manchester suburban area (< 0.1-6); Moel Famau, Flintshire (2-4); Rannoch Moor, Argyllshire (1-1.5); and Forest of Dean, Monmouthshire (2.8) (Pearson & McConnell, 1975).

(b) Water

1,1,1-Trichloroethane has been detected in finished drinking-water (Dowty *et al.*, 1975) and was one of 72 compounds found in the drinking-water supplies of 5 US cities (Coleman *et al.*, 1975).

Rainwater collected in UK was reported to contain up to 90 ng/l 1,1,1-trichloroethane, and municipal waters contained up to 300 ng/l combined carbon tetrachloride and 1,1,1-trichloroethane. The maximum concentration of 1,1,1-trichloroethane found in sea-water was 3.3 µg/l, and the average concentration in combination with carbon tetrachloride was 0.25 µg/l. Marine sediments contained up to 5 µg/kg 1,1,1-trichloroethane and carbon tetrachloride combined (Pearson & McConnell, 1975).

1,1,1-Trichloroethane has been measured in crude sewage at a level of 16.5 µg/l, in effluent from a biological treatment plant at a level of 9 µg/l, and in chlorinated biological effluent at a level of 8.5 µg/l (Eurocop-Cost, 1976).

(c) Food and drink

In a UK study of 12 food items, 1,1,1-trichloroethane residues were found in meat (3-6 µg/kg), oils and fats (5-10 µg/kg), tea (7 µg/kg), fruit and vegetables (1-4 µg/kg) and fresh bread (2 µg/kg) (McConnell *et al.*, 1975).

(d) Marine organisms

1,1,1-Trichloroethane was detected in the following marine organisms (concentration in µg/kg): 14 species of invertebrates (0.03-34); 3 species of algae (9.4-35, including carbon tetrachloride); in the flesh or organs of 9 species of fish (1-26) and 7 species of fish (0.7-47, including carbon tetrachloride); in the organs or eggs of 8 species of sea- and freshwater birds (1.1-43, including carbon tetrachloride); and in the organs of 2 species of mammals (0.3-30, including carbon tetrachloride) (Pearson & McConnell, 1975).

(e) Humans

1,1,1-Trichloroethane has been detected in human expired air, at levels of 0.03-140 µg/hr/subject (Conkle *et al.*, 1975).

2.3 Analysis

Analytical methods to determine halogenated hydrocarbons, including 1,1,1-trichloroethane, in air using gas chromatography and in blood and urine using infra-red spectrometry have been reviewed (Walter *et al.*, 1976). The identification and analysis of 1,1,1-trichloroethane in air, sewage sludge and paint using gas chromatography have also been reviewed (Franklin Institute Research Laboratories, 1975).

Methods used for the analysis of 1,1,1-trichloroethane in environmental samples are listed in Table 1.

Environmental air samples have been analysed by gas chromatography (Lillian *et al.*, 1976) or gas chromatography/mass spectrometry after trapping by a cryogenic technique (Tyson, 1975).

Laser absorption spectroscopy at 9-11 μm has been used to determine 1,1,1-trichloroethane in air samples either alone, with a limit of detection of 29 mg/m^3 (5.3 ppm), or in a mixture of gases, with a limit of detection of 50 mg/m^3 (9.2 ppm) (Green & Steinfeld, 1976).

3. Biological Data Relevant to the Evaluation
of Carcinogenic Risk to Humans

3.1 Carcinogenicity studies in animals[1]

(a) Oral administration

Mouse: Groups of 50 male and 50 female B6C3F1 mice, 5 weeks of age, were given technical-grade 1,1,1-trichloroethane containing about 3% *para*-dioxane and 2% minor impurities in corn oil by gavage on 5 days per week for 78 weeks. Initially, the high and low doses for both male and female mice were 4000 and 2000 mg/kg bw/day; during the 10th week of the study, these doses were increased to 5000 and 2500 mg/kg bw/day; at week 20 they were increased to 6000 and 3000 mg/kg bw/day and maintained at these levels to the end of the study. Time-weighted average doses for the high- and low-dose mice were 5615 and 2807 mg/kg bw/day, respectively. A group of 20 male and 20 female untreated mice were used as controls; no vehicle-control animals were used. In males, 10/20 of the matched controls, 21/50 of the low-dose group, and 25/50 of the high-dose group had died within 1 year after the start of the experiment; in females, the corresponding figures were 1/20, 9/50 and

---

[1]The Working Group was aware of studies in progress to assess the carcinogenicity of 1,1,1-trichloroethane in mice by i.p. injection and in mice and rats by oral administration (IARC, 1978).

TABLE 1. METHODS FOR THE ANALYSIS OF 1,1,1-TRICHLOROETHANE

ANALYTICAL METHOD

SAMPLE TYPE	EXTRACTION/CLEAN-UP	DETECTION	LIMIT OF DETECTION	REFERENCE
Formulations				
Aerosols	Analyse directly	GC/MS		Sheinin *et al.* (1975)
Air				
Workplace	Trap (charcoal), extract (carbon disulphide)	GC/FID	Working range, 904-3790 mg/m^3	National Institute for Occupational Safety & Health (1977)
Rural	Trap (porous polymer beads), desorb by heating, retrap in line on GC column	GC/ECD; GC/MS	Working range, 160-700 ng/m^3 (30-130 ppt)	Russell & Shadoff (1977)
Unspecified	Trap in Drechsel flask fitted with rubber septum, sample with gas syringe	GC/ECD	0.5 ng/l	Bureau International Technique des Solvants Chlorés (1976)
Water	Sparge (helium), trap on polymer column, desorb by heating, retrap in line on GC column	GC/MS		Coleman *et al.* (1976) Dowty *et al.* (1975)

Abbreviations: GC/FID - gas chromatography/flame-ionization detection; ECD - electron capture detection; MS - mass spectrometry

20/50.   At 90 weeks, 15 low-dose males, 11 high-dose males, 23 low-dose females and 13 high-dose females were still alive.   All animals were killed at 95 weeks.   Almost all organs, and all tissues with macroscopically visible lesions, were examined histologically.   Three out of 49 males in the high-dose group developed liver-cell adenomas and one a hepatocellular carcinoma.   No liver tumours occurred in controls (National Cancer Institute, 1977) [The Working Group noted the poor survival of the treated animals].

Rat: Groups of 50 male and 50 female Osborne-Mendel rats, 7 weeks of age, received technical-grade 1,1,1-trichloroethane containing 3% para-dioxane and 2% minor impurities in corn oil by gavage on 5 days a week for 78 weeks at two dose levels: 750 mg/kg bw/day and 1500 mg/kg bw/day.   A group of 20 male and 20 female untreated rats served as matched controls.   The animals were killed 110 weeks after the start of treatment.   Both males and females given the test chemical exhibited early mortality when compared with untreated controls: only 3% of treated rats survived to termination of the experiment.   A few tumours not considered to be related to treatment were observed (National Cancer Institute, 1977) [The Working Group noted the poor survival of the treated animals].

(b)   Inhalation and/or intratracheal administration

Rat: Results of a study reported as an abstract indicate that in groups of 96 male and 96 female Sprague-Dawley rats exposed to vapours of 9.5 and 4.7 g/m^3 (1750 and 875 ppm) 1,1,1-trichloroethane in air for 6 hrs per day on 5 days a week for 12 months, followed by observation up to 30 months, no increased incidence of tumours was observed (Rampy et al., 1977) [The Working Group noted the incomplete reporting of the experiment].

3.2 Other relevant biological data

(a) Experimental systems

Toxic effects

The toxicity of 1,1,1-trichloroethane has been reviewed (Aviado et al., 1976; Stewart, 1968).

The oral LD$_{50}$ of 1,1,1-trichloroethane in mice and rats is about 11 g/kg bw (Torkelson et al., 1958); the i.p. LD$_{50}$ in mice is 5 g/kg bw (Klaassen & Plaa, 1966).   After inhalation of 98 g/m^3 (18,000 ppm) for 3 hrs, 15/21 rats died (Adams et al., 1950).

1,1,1-Trichloroethane causes central nervous system depression in rats.   Liver damage has been reported in rats only after exposure to nearly lethal doses (Adams et al., 1950).   Continuous inhalation for

14 weeks caused hepatotoxicity in mice (McNutt *et al.*, 1975).   Inhalation of 1,1,1-trichloroethane was found to increase hepatic drug metabolism in rats (Lal *et al.*, 1969).

Embryotoxicity and teratogenicity

Groups of rats and mice were exposed by inhalation for 7 hrs daily on days 6-15 of gestation to 4.7 g/m^3 in air (875 ppm) 1,1,1-trichloroethane; no effects were observed on the average number of implantation sites per litter, litter size, incidence of foetal resorptions, foetal sex ratios or foetal body measurements.   No treatment-related increase in the incidence of skeletal or visceral malformations was observed (Schwetz *et al.*, 1975).

Absorption, distribution, excretion and metabolism

In mice and rats, 1,1,1-trichloroethane is absorbed through the lungs, gastrointestinal tract and skin (Stewart, 1968; Tsuruta, 1975). After inhalation in mice it was found in brain and kidney at approximately equal concentrations and in liver at higher concentrations (Holmberg *et al.*, 1977).   In rats, more than 98% of the absorbed dose was rapidly expired unchanged; 0.5% was converted to CO_2.   Much of the remainder was excreted as the glucuronide of 2,2,2-trichloroethanol in the urine (Hake *et al.*, 1960).   Small amounts of trichloroacetic acid were found in the urine of rats (Eben & Kimmerle, 1974).   Unlike 1,1,2,2-tetrachloroethane or the isomer 1,1,2-trichloroethane, 1,1,1-trichloroethane is not dechlorinated *in vitro* in the presence of hepatic microsomes, NADPH and O_2 (Van Dyke & Wineman, 1971).

Mutagenicity and other related short-term tests

1,1,1-Trichloroethane was mutagenic in *Salmonella typhimurium* strain TA100, with or without a microsomal activation system (Simmon *et al.*, 1977).

(b) Humans

At least 30 fatalities have been associated with exposure to 1,1,1-trichloroethane, mostly due to deliberate inhalation or to accidental occupational exposures.   Death was due to suffocation; the lungs showed acute oedema and congestion (Bass, 1970; Caplan *et al.*, 1976; Stahl *et al.*, 1969).   Exposure to 1.36-2.7 g/m^3 (250-500 ppm) of the solvent impairs psychophysiological functions (Gamberale & Hultengren, 1973). Generally, the toxic effects of 1,1,1-trichloroethane in humans are similar to those in animals (Stewart, 1968; Torkelson *et al.*, 1958).

1,1,1-Trichloroethane may be absorbed through the lungs, gastrointestinal tract or skin (Fukabori *et al.*, 1977; Stewart, 1968) and is excreted unchanged *via* the lungs for many hours after exposure

(Astrand *et al.*, 1973; Stewart *et al.*, 1961). A small percentage is metabolized to 2,2,2-trichloroethanol and trichloroacetic acid and excreted in the urine (Fukabori *et al.*, 1976; Seki *et al.*, 1975; Stewart, 1968).

3.3 Case reports and epidemiological studies

No data were available to the Working Group.

4. Summary of Data Reported and Evaluation

4.1 Experimental data

1,1,1-Trichloroethane was tested in one experiment in mice and in one in rats by oral administration and in one experiment by inhalation exposure in rats. Although a few liver tumours were observed in male mice, these experiments were considered to be inadequate.

1,1,1-Trichloroethane is mutagenic in *Salmonella typhimurium*.

4.2 Human data

No case reports or epidemiological studies were available to the Working Group.

The extensive production of this compound and its use as a chemical intermediate and in metal cleaning operations over several decades suggest that widespread human exposure occurs. This is confirmed by many reports of its occurrence in the general environment.

4.3 Evaluation

The available data do not permit an evaluation of the carcinogenicity of 1,1,1-trichloroethane to be made.

5. References

Adams, E.M., Spencer, H.C., Rowe, V.K. & Irish, D.D. (1950) Vapor
    toxicity of 1,1,1-trichloroethane (methylchloroform) determined
    by experiments on laboratory animals. Arch. ind. Hyg., 1, 225-236

Åstrand, I., Kilbom, Å., Wahlberg, I. & Övrum, P. (1973) Methylchloroform
    exposure. I. Concentration in alveolar air and blood at rest and
    during exercise. Work. environ. Health, 10, 69-81

Aviado, D.M., Zakhari, S., Simaan, J.A. & Ulsamer, A.G. (1976) Methyl
    Chloroform and Trichloroethylene in the Environment, Cleveland, OH,
    Chemical Rubber Co., pp. 1-44

Bass, M. (1970) Sudden sniffing death. J. Am. med. Assoc., 212, 2075-
    2079

Bureau International Technique des Solvants Chlorés (1976)
    Standardization of methods for the determination of traces of some
    volatile chlorinated aliphatic hydrocarbons in air and water by gas
    chromatography. Anal. chim. acta., 82, 1-17

Caplan, Y.H., Backer, R.C. & Whitaker, J.Q. (1976) 1,1,1-Trichloroethane:
    report of a fatal intoxication. Clin. Toxicol., 9, 69-74

Coleman, W.E., Lingg, R.D., Melton, R.G. & Kopfler, F.C. (1976) The
    occurrence of volatile organics in five drinking water supplies using
    gas chromatography/mass spectrometry. In: Keith, L.H., ed.,
    Identification and Analysis of Organic Pollutants in Water, Ann Arbor,
    MI, Ann Arbor Science, pp. 305-327

Conkle, J.P., Camp, B.J. & Welch, B.E. (1975) Trace composition of human
    respiratory gas. Arch. environ. Health, 30, 290-295

Cox, R.A., Derwent, R.G., Eggleton, A.E.J. & Lovelock, J.E. (1976)
    Photochemical oxidation of halocarbons in the troposphere. Atmos.
    Environ., 10, 305-308

Dowty, B.J., Carlisle, D.R. & Laseter, J.L. (1975) New Orleans drinking
    water sources tested by gas chromatography-mass spectrometry. Occurrence
    and origin of aromatics and halogenated aliphatic hydrocarbons.
    Environ. Sci. Technol., 9, 762-765

Eben, A. & Kimmerle, G. (1974) Metabolism, excretion and toxicology of
    methylchloroform in acute and subacute exposed rats. Arch. Toxikol.,
    31, 233-242

Eurocop-Cost (1976) A Comprehensive List of Polluting Substances Which
    Have Been Identified in Various Fresh Waters, Effluent Discharges,
    Aquatic Animals and Plants, and Bottom Sediments, 2nd ed., EUCO/MDU/
    73/76, XII/476/76, Luxembourg, Commission of the European Communities,
    p. 56

Franklin Institute Research Laboratories (1975) Preliminary Study of
    Selected Potential Environmental Contaminants - Optical Brighteners,
    Methyl Chloroform, Trichloroethylene, Tetrachloroethylene and Ion
    Exchange Resins, EPQ-560/2-75-002, Washington DC, US Environmental
    Protection Agency. Available from Springfield, VA, National Technical
    Information Service, No. PB243910, pp. 81-86, 123-128

Fukabori, S., Nakaaki, K., Yonemoto, J. & Tada, O. (1976) Cutaneous
    absorption of methyl chloroform   (Jpn). Rodo Kagaku, 52, 67-80
    [Chem. Abstr., 85, 14847y]

Fukabori, S., Nakaaki, K., Yonemoto, J. & Tada, O. (1977) On the cutaneous
    absorption of 1,1,1-trichloroethane (2). J. Sci. Lab., 53, 89-95

Gamberale, F. & Hultengren, M. (1973) Methylchloroform exposure. II.
    Psychophysiological functions. Work environ. Health., 10, 82-92

Gehring, P.J. (1968) Hepatotoxic potency of various chlorinated hydrocarbon
    vapours relative to their narcotic and lethal potencies in mice.
    Toxicol. appl. Pharmacol., 13, 287-298

Grasselli, J.G. & Ritchey, W.M., eds (1975) CRC Atlas of Spectral Data
    and Physical Constants for Organic Compounds, 2nd ed., Vol. III,
    Cleveland, OH, Chemical Rubber Co., p. 257

Green, B.D. & Steinfeld, J.I. (1976) Laser absorption spectroscopy: method
    for monitoring complex trace mixtures. Environ. Sci. Technol., 10,
    1134-1139

Grimsrud, E.P. & Rasmussen, R.A. (1975) Survey and analysis of halocarbons
    in the atmosphere by gas chromatography-mass spectrometry. Atmos.
    Environ., 9, 1014-1017

Hake, C.L., Waggoner, T.B., Robertson, D.N. & Rowe, V.K. (1960) The
    metabolism of 1,1,1-trichloroethane by the rat. Arch. environ. Health,
    1, 101-105

Hardie, D.W.F. (1964) Chlorocarbons and chlorohydrocarbons. 1,1,1-
    Trichloroethane. In: Kirk, R.E. & Othmer, D.F., eds, Encyclopedia
    of Chemical Technology, 2nd ed., Vol. 5, New York, John Wiley & Sons,
    pp. 154-157, 170

Holmberg, B., Jakobson, I. & Sigvardsson, K. (1977) A study on the
    distribution of methylchloroform and n-octane in the mouse during
    and after inhalation. Scand. J. Work environ. Health, 3, 43-52

IARC (1978)   Information Bulletin on the Survey of Chemicals Being
      Tested for Carcinogenicty, No. 7, Lyon, pp. 247, 272

IARC (1979)   IARC Monographs on the Evaluation of the Carcinogenic Risk
      to Humans, 19, Some Monomers, Plastics and Synthetic Elastomers, and
      Acrolein, Lyon, pp. 439-459

Klaassen, C.D. & Plaa, G.L. (1966)   Relative effects of various chlorinated
      hydrocarbons on liver and kidney function in mice.   Toxicol. appl.
      Pharmacol., 9, 139-151

Lal, H., Olshan, A., Puri, S., Shah, H.C. & Fuller, G.C. (1969)
      Enhancement of hepatic drug metabolism in rats after methyl-
      chloroform (MC) inhalation (Abstract no. 32).   Toxicol. appl.
      Pharmacol., 14, 625

Lillian, D., Singh, H.B., Appleby, A., Lobban, L., Arnts, R., Gumpert, R.,
      Hague, R., Toomey, J., Kazazis, J., Antell, M., Hansen, D. & Scott
      B. (1975)   Atmospheric fates of halogenated compounds.   Environ. Sci.
      Technol., 9, 1042-1048

Lillian, D., Singh, H.B. & Appleby, A. (1976)   Gas chromatographic analysis
      of ambient halogenated compounds.   J. Air Pollut. Control Assoc., 26,
      141-143

McConnell, G., Ferguson, D.M. & Pearson, C.R. (1975)   Chlorinated hyero-
      carbons and the environment.   Endeavor, 34, 13-18

McNutt, N.S., Amster, R.L., McConnell, E.E. & Morris, F. (1975)   Hepatic
      lesions in mice after continuous inhalation exposure to 1,1,1-
      trichloroethane.   Lab. Invest., 32, 642-654

Mercier, M. (1977)   Criteria (Exposure / Effect Relationships) for
      Organochlorine Solvents, Doc. V/F/177-4, Luxembourg, Commission of
      the European Communities, pp. 94-122

National Cancer Institute (1977)   Bioassay of 1,1,1-Trichloroethane for
      Possible Carcinogenicity (Technical Report Series No. 3), DHEW
      Publication No. (NIH) 77803, Washington DC, US Department of Health,
      Education, & Welfare

National Institute for Occupational Safety & Health (1977)   NIOSH
      Manual of Analytical Methods, 2nd ed., Part II, Standards Completion
      Program Validated Methods, Vol. 3,   Method S328, DHEW (NIOSH) Publica-
      tion No. 77-157-B, Washington DC, US Government Printing Office, pp.
      S328-1 - S328-9

Ohta, T., Morita, M. & Mizoguchi, I. (1976)   Local distribution of
      chlorinated hydrocarbons in the ambient air in Tokyo.   Atmos. Environ.,
      10, 557-560 [Chem. Abstr., 86, 59808y]

Pearson, C.R. & McConnell, G. (1975) Chlorinated C_1 and C_2 hydrocarbons in the marine environment. Proc. R. Soc. Lond. B., 189, 305-332

Prager, B., Jacobson, P., Schmidt, P. & Stern, D., eds (1918) Beilsteins Handbuch der Organischen Chemie, 4th ed., Vol. 1, Syst. No. 8, Berlin, Springer, p. 85

Rampy, L.W., Quast, J.F., Leong, B.K.J. & Gehring, P.J. (1977) Results of long-term inhalation toxicity studies on rats of 1,1,1-trichloroethane and perchloroethylene formulations (Abstract) In: Proceedings of the International Congress of Toxicology, Toronto, Canada, 1977, p. 27

Russell, J.W. & Shadoff, L.A. (1977) The sampling and determination of halocarbons in ambient air using concentration on porous polymer. J. Chromatogr., 134, 375-384

Schwetz, B.A., Leong, B.K.J. & Gehring, P.J. (1975) The effect of maternally inhaled trichloroethylene, perchloroethylene, methyl chloroform and methylene chloride on embryonal and fetal development in mice and rats. Toxicol. appl. Pharmacol., 32, 84-96

Seki, Y., Urashima, Y., Aikawa, H., Matsumura, H., Ichikawa, Y., Hiratsuka, F., Yoshioka, Y., Shimbo, S. & Ikeda, M. (1975) Trichloro-compounds in the urine of humans exposed to methyl chloroform at sub-threshold levels. Int. Arch. Arbeitsmed., 34, 39-49

Sheinin, E.B., Benson, W.R., Brannon, W.L. & Schwartzman, G. (1975) The analysis of pharmaceuticals by combined gas chromatography-mass spectrometry. I. The analysis of a medicated aerosol spray. J. Assoc. off. anal. Chem., 58, 530-540

Simmon, V.F., Kauhanen, K. & Tardiff, R.G. (1977) Mutagenic activity of chemicals identified in drinking water. In: Scott, D., Bridges, B.A. & Sobels, F.H., eds, Progress in Genetic Toxicology, Amsterdam, Elsevier/North Holland, pp. 249-258

Simmonds, P.G., Kerrin, S.L., Lovelock, J.E. & Shair, F.H. (1974) Distribution of atmospheric halocarbons in the air over the Los Angeles Basin. Atmos. Environ., 8, 209-216 [Chem. Abstr., 81, 28980r]

Singh, H.B., Salas, L.J. & Cavanagh, L.A. (1977) Distribution, sources and sinks of atmospheric halogenated compounds. J. Air Pollut. Control. Assoc., 27, 332-336

Stahl, C.J., Fatteh, A.V. & Dominguez, A.M. (1969) Trichloroethane poisoning: observations on the pathology and toxicology in six fatal cases. J. forensic Sci. Soc., 14, 393-397

Stewart, R.D. (1968) The toxicology of 1,1,1-trichloroethane. Ann. occup. Hyg., 11, 71-79

Stewart, R.D., Gay, H.H., Erley, D.S., Hake, C.L. & Schaffer, A.W. (1961)
   Human exposure to 1,1,1-trichloroethane vapor: relationship of
   expired air and blood concentrations to exposure and toxicity. Am.
   ind. Hyg. Assoc. J., 22, 252-262

Torkelson, T.R., Oyen, F., McCollister, D.D. & Rowe, V.K. (1958) Toxicity
   of 1,1,1-trichloroethane as determined on laboratory animals and
   human subjects. Am. ind. Hyg. Assoc. J., 19, 353-362

Tsuruta, H. (1975) Percutaneous absorption of organic solvents. I. Compara
   tive study of the *in vivo* percutaneous absorption of chlorinated solvents in mice. Ind. Health, 13, 227-236

Tyson, B.J. (1975) Chlorinated hydrocarbons in the atmosphere - analysis
   at the parts-per-trillion level by GC-MS. Anal. Lett., 8, 807-813

US Environmental Protection Agency (1976) Protection of environment.
   US Code Fed. Regul., Title 40, parts 180.1001, 180.1012,
   pp. 363, 369, 375-376, 379-380

US Food & Drug Administration (1977a) Food and drugs. US Code Fed.
   Regul., Title 21, part 175.105, pp. 438, 449

US Food & Drug Administration (1977b) Trichloroethane; status as a new
   drug in aerosolized drug products intended for inhalation. Fed.
   Regist., 42, 63386-63387

US International Trade Commission (1977) Synthetic Organic Chemicals, US
   Production and Sales, 1976, USITC Publication 833, Washington DC,
   US Government Printing Office, pp. 303, 332

US Occupational Safety & Health Administration (1977) Air contaminants.
   US Code Fed. Regul., Title 20, part. 1910.1000, p. 27

US Pharmacopeial Convention, Inc. (1975) The United States Pharmacopeia,
   19th Rev., Rockville, MD, p. 741

US Tariff Commission (1947) Synthetic Organic Chemicals, US Production
   and Sales, 1946, Report No. 159, Second Series, Washington DC, US
   Government Printing Office, p. 141

Van Dyke, R.A. & Wineman, C.G. (1971) Enzymatic dechlorination. Dechlorination of chloroethanes and propanes *in vitro*. Biochem. Pharmacol.,
   20, 463-470

Walter, P., Craigmill, A., Villaume, J., Sweeney, S. & Miller, G.L. (1976)
   Chlorinated Hydrocarbon Toxicity (1,1,1-Trichloroethane, Trichloroethylene, and Tetrachloroethylene): A Monograph. CPSC - BSC-76-M1,
   Washington DC, Consumer Product Safety Commission, pp. 21-25, 158,
   162, 164, 166

Winell, M. (1975) An international comparison of hygienic standards for chemicals in the work environment. _Ambio_, _4_, 34-36

1,1,2-TRICHLOROETHANE

1. Chemical and Physical Data

1.1 Synonyms and trade names

Chem. Abstr. Services Reg. No: 79-00-5

Chem. Abstr. Name: 1,1,2-Trichloroethane

Synonyms: Ethane trichloride; β-trichloroethane; 1,2,2-trichloro-ethane; vinyl trichloride

Trade name: β-T

1.2 Structural and molecular formulae and molecular weight

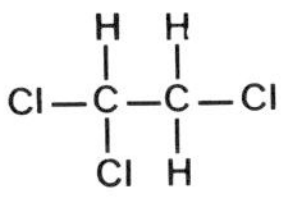

$$Cl-\underset{\underset{Cl}{|}}{\overset{\overset{H}{|}}{C}}-\underset{\underset{H}{|}}{\overset{\overset{H}{|}}{C}}-Cl$$

$C_2H_3Cl_3$ Mol. wt: 133.4

1.3 Chemical and physical properties of the pure substance

From Hardie (1964), unless otherwise specified

(a) Description: Colourless liquid

(b) Boiling-point: 113.5°C

(c) Melting-point: -37°C

(d) Density: d^{20} 1.4411

(e) Refractive index: n_D^{20} 1.47064

(f) Spectroscopy data: Infra-red, Raman, nuclear magnetic resonance and mass spectral data have been tabulated (Grasselli & Ritchey, 1975).

(g) Solubility: Soluble in water (0.45 g/100 ml water at 20°C);
     miscible with chlorinated solvents and soluble in other
     common organic solvents

(h) Volatility: Vapour pressure is 16.7 mm at 20°C.

(i) Stability: Stable in air at ordinary temperatures; in the
     absence of air or water it is stable up to about 110°C; in
     the presence of water, hydrolysis occurs at its boiling-point.

(j) Reactivity: Dehydrochlorinates to 1,1-dichloroethylene when
     heated with aqueous caustic soda; reaction with an aqueous
     lime suspension yields a mixture of 1,1- and 1,2-dichloro-
     ethylene; can be chlorinated in the vapour phase to 1,1,1,2-
     tetrachloroethane

(k) Conversion factor: 1 ppm in air is equivalent to 5.45 mg/m^3.

1.4 Technical products and impurities

In the US, 1,1,2-trichloroethane is available as a technical
grade product, which may be stabilized (identity of stabilizers unknown).
It typically meets the following specifications: a colourless liquid,
free of suspended matter and sediment; distillation range at 760 mm,
110.0-115.5°C; specific gravity, 25°C/25°C, 1.427-1.437; water
content, 200 mg/kg max; acidity (as HCl), 100 mg/kg max; and nonvolatile residue, 20 mg/kg max.

2. Production, Use, Occurrence and Analysis

2.1 Production and use

(a) Production

1,1,2-Trichloroethane was first prepared in about 1840 by Regnault
by the reaction of chloroethylene with antimony pentachloride (Hardie,
1964; Prager *et al.*, 1918).   It is produced in the US either by
reaction of acetylene gas with a mixture of hydrogen chloride and
chlorine in the presence of a catalyst or by chlorination of ethylene
followed by chlorination of the 1,2-dichloroethane intermediate.
Most 1,1,2-trichloroethane produced in the US is made by the chlorination of ethylene (Hardie, 1964).

In Japan, 1,1,2-trichloroethane is produced by chlorination of ethylene.

Commercial production of 1,1,2-trichloroethane in the US was first reported during 1941-1943 (US Tariff Commission, 1945). In 1976, only one US company reported commercial production of an undisclosed amount (see preamble, p. 16) (US International Trade Commission, 1977); however, an additional US company produces it as an intermediate in vinylidene chloride production. Data on US imports and exports were not available.

No data on its production in Europe were available. It has been produced commercially in Japan since 1951. In 1976, 3 companies produced approximately 36 million kg; none was imported or exported.

(b) Use

1,1,2-Trichloroethane is used in the US as an intermediate in the production of vinylidine chloride, as a solvent and as a component of adhesives.

An estimated 77 million kg vinylidene chloride (see IARC, 1979) were produced and isolated in the US in 1974, and approximately 53% of this was made from 1,1,2-trichloroethane. Vinylidene chloride is also produced by one US company as an unisolated chemical intermediate in the production of 1,1,1-trichloroethane; and in 1976, an estimated 50 million kg were produced from 1,1,2-trichloroethane.

A very little 1,1,2-trichloroethane is used as a solvent (Hardie, 1964).

No data on its use in Europe were available. In Japan, 1,1,2-trichloroethane is used captively in vinylidene chloride production.

1,1,2-Trichloroethane is approved by the US Food and Drug Administration as a constituent of adhesives used as components of articles intended for use in packaging, transporting or holding food (US Food & Drug Administration, 1977).

The US Occupational Safety and Health Administration's health standards for exposure to air contaminants require that an employee's exposure to 1,1,2-trichloroethane not exceed an 8-hr time-weighted average of 45 mg/m^3 (10 ppm) in the workplace air in any 8-hr work shift of a 40-hr work week (US Occupational Safety & Health Administration, 1977).

2.2 Occurrence

1,1,2-Trichloroethane is not known to occur as a natural product.

(a) Water

1,1,2-Trichloroethane was one of 72 compounds detected in drinking-water supplies sampled in 5 US cities (Coleman *et al.*, 1976). It has been detected in other drinking-water samples at levels of < 0.1-8.5 µg/l (Safe Drinking Water Committee, 1977) and 0.45 µg/l (Eurocop-Cost, 1976). It has also been detected in industrial effluent discharges, at a level of 5.4 mg/l (Eurocop-Cost, 1976).

In an estimated 75 million kg of chlorinated aliphatic hydrocarbons (also known as EDC-tar) formed as by-products during polyvinyl chloride production and dumped at sea, 1,1,2-trichloroethane constituted about 40% of the weight of one distillate (Rosenberg *et al.*, 1975).

(b) Occupational exposure

A 1974 National Occupational Hazard Survey indicated that workers primarily exposed to 1,1,2-trichloroethane were those in the blast furnace and steel mill, telephone communication, engineering and scientific instrument manufacturing industries (National Institute for Occupational Safety & Health, 1977a).

2.3 Analysis

A sampling and analytical method recommended by the US National Institute for Occupational Safety and Health for determining 1,1,2-trichloroethane in workplace atmospheres is based on collection on charcoal, desorption in carbon disulphide, followed by analysis by gas chromatography with flame ionization detection for a validated range of 26-111 mg/m^3 in air (National Institute for Occupational Safety & Health, 1977b).

Gas chromatography-mass spectrometry has been used to determine 1,1,2-trichloroethane in ambient air, with a limit of detection of 27 ng/m^3 (5 ppt) (Grimsrud & Rasmussen, 1975) and in drinking-water by sparging, trapping from the sparge gas and analysing from the trap in-line, with a limit of detection at the µg/l (ppb) level (Coleman *et al.*, 1976).

3. Biological Data Relevant to the Evaluation
of Carcinogenic Risk to Humans

3.1 Carcinogenicity studies in animals[1]

Oral administration

Mouse: Groups of 50 male and 50 female B6C3F1 mice, 5 weeks of
age, received technical-grade 1,1,2-trichloroethane in corn oil by
gavage on 5 consecutive days a week for 78 weeks. The experiment was
terminated after an additional 12 weeks of observation, at a total of
90 weeks. High-dose and low-dose animals received, respectively, 300
and 150 mg/kg bw/day for 8 weeks, and then 400 and 200 mg/kg bw/day for
70 weeks, followed by 12-13 weeks without treatment. The time-weighted
average doses were 390 and 195 mg/kg bw/day. Groups of 20 male and
20 female mice either received corn oil alone and served as matched
vehicle controls or remained untreated and served as matched untreated
controls. At least 50% of the male mice in each group were alive at
week 86; 50% of the female mice were still alive after 81, 58, 89 and
90 weeks in the high-dose, low-dose, vehicle control and untreated
control groups, respectively. The incidence of hepatocellular carcinomas was increased significantly ($P < 0.01$) in all treated groups: in
males, 2/17 (12%) untreated controls, 2/20 (10%) vehicle controls,
18/49 (37%) low-dose animals and 37/49 (76%) high-dose animals; in
females, 2/20 (10%) untreated controls, 0/20 vehicle controls, 16/48
(33%) low-dose animals and 40/45 (89%) high-dose animals. Adrenal
phaeochromocytomas were present in 8/48 (17%) high-dose males and in
12/43 (28%) high-dose females, but in no other groups (National Cancer
Institute, 1978).

Rat: Groups of 50 male and 50 female Osborne-Mendel rats, 6 weeks
old, received technical-grade 1,1,2-trichloroethane in corn oil by
gavage on 5 consecutive days a week for 78 weeks. High-dose and low-
dose groups received, respectively, 70 and 35 mg/kg bw/day for 20 weeks,
then 100 and 50 mg/kg bw/day for 58 weeks and were then left untreated
for the subsequent 34-35 weeks. The time-weighted average doses were
92 and 46 mg/kg bw/day. Groups of 20 male and 20 female rats either
received corn oil alone and served as matched vehicle controls or
remained untreated and served as untreated matched controls. At least
50% of the male rats in the high-dose, low-dose and untreated control
groups survived more than 96 weeks; 50% of females in the high-dose,
low-dose and untreated control groups survived more than 105 weeks.
Vehicle control groups had unexpectedly poor survival, with only 5%
(1/20) of males and 20% (4/20) of females still alive at the end of the

---

[1]The Working Group was aware of a completed but as yet unpublished
study in mice given 1,1,2-trichloroethane by i.p. injection (IARC, 1978).

study; the authors did not, therefore, include them in statistical
comparisons. No statistically significant increase in tumour incidence
was found, for any type of tumour, either in males or in females (see
Table 1) (National Cancer Institute, 1978).

3.2 Other relevant biological data

(a) Experimental systems

The oral LD_{50} of 1,1,2-trichloroethane in rats is 835 mg/kg bw
(Smyth *et al*., 1969); the i.p. LD_{50} in mice is 500 mg/kg bw (Klaassen
& Plaa, 1966).

1,1,2-Trichloroethane depresses the central nervous system, is
hepatotoxic and induces kidney damage in mice (Gehring, 1968; Klaassen
& Plaa, 1966; Plaa & Larson, 1965; Plaa *et al*., 1958). It is less
hepatotoxic than chloroform or carbon tetrachloride but more hepatotoxic than 1,1,1-trichloroethane, trichloroethylene or dichloromethane
(Gehring, 1968; Klaassen & Plaa, 1966). In mice, hepatic dysfunction
is observed at the LD_{10}; higher doses cause centrilobular necrosis
(Klaassen & Plaa, 1966). It is a skin irritant in guinea-pigs (Kronevi
et al., 1977).

No data on the embryotoxicity or teratogenicity of 1,1,2-trichloro-
ethane were available.

Following an i.p. dose of 0.1-0.2 g/kg bw ^{14}C-1,1,2-trichloroethane
to mice, 73-87% was found in the urine and 16-22% was expired (40%
unchanged and 60% as CO_2); 1-3% of the dose remained in the animal.
Three metabolites were identified in the urine: chloroacetic acid,
S-carboxymethylcysteine and thiodiacetic acid; small amounts of glycolic
acid, 2,2-dichloroethanol, 2,2,2-trichloroethanol, oxalic acid and trichloroacetic acid were also found, suggesting that the metabolism of
1,1,2-trichloroethane proceeds *via* the formation of chloroacetaldehyde
(Yllner, 1971).

The enzymic dechlorination of 1,1,2-trichloroethane *in vitro*
depends on the presence of hepatic microsomes, NADPH and oxygen and
was inducible by *in vivo* treatment with phenobarbital and benzo[*a*]-
pyrene (Van Dyke & Wineman, 1971).

1,1,2-Trichloroethane (20, 40 and 60 μmol/plate) was not mutagenic
in a plate assay with *Salmonella typhimurium* strain TA1535 with or without a microsomal activation system (Rannug *et al*., 1978).

(b) Humans

1,1,2-Trichloroethane has a narcotic action at low concentrations
and has an irritant effect on the eyes and the mucous membranes of the

TABLE 1. ORAL ADMINISTRATION OF 1,1,2-TRICHLOROETHANE TO RATS

GROUP	NO. OF ANIMALS EXAMINED	NO. OF ANIMALS WITH TUMOURS	TOTAL NO. OF TUMOURS	MAMMARY FIBROADENOMAS	MAMMARY ADENO-CARCINOMAS	PITUITARY ADENOMAS	ADRENAL ADENOMAS/CARCINOMAS AT ALL SITES	HAEMANGIOSARCOMAS	THYROID TUMOURS	KIDNEY HAMARTOMAS
Males										
Untreated controls	20	4	4	0	0	0	0	0	1	1
Vehicle controls	20	6	9	0	1	1	0	0	1	1
Low-dose	50	21	26	0	1	5	0	4	2	1
High-dose	50	11	14	1	1	1	1	1	0	0
Females										
Untreated controls	20	11	15	6	1	2	0	0	0	0
Vehicle controls	19	4	4	2	0	2	0	0	0	0
Low-dose	50	34	50	16	0	9	3	1	3	4
High-dose	50	22	28	9	4	5	1	0	1	1

respiratory tract.   When in contact with the skin it produces cracking
and erythema.   Long-term exposure to the vapour produces chronic gastric
symptoms, fat deposition in the kidneys and damage to the lungs (Hardie,
1964).

3.3 Case reports and epidemiological studies

No data were available to the Working Group.

4. Summary of Data Reported and Evaluation

4.1 Experimental data

1,1,2-Trichloroethane was tested in one experiment in mice and in
one in rats by oral administration.   It produced hepatocellular
carcinomas and adrenal phaeochromocytomas in mice of both sexes.   The
study in rats gave inconclusive results.

1,1,2-Trichloroethane was not mutagenic in *Salmonella typhimurium*.

4.2 Human data

No case reports or epidemiological studies were available to the
Working Group.

The extensive production of 1,1,2-trichloroethane over several
decades, primarily for use as an intermediate in the manufacture of
vinylidene chloride, indicates that occupational exposure occurs.
Reports of its occurrence in the environment indicate that the general
population is also exposed.

4.3 Evaluation

There is *limited evidence* that 1,1,2-trichloroethane is carcinogenic in mice.

5. References

Coleman, W.E., Lingg, R.D., Melton, R.G. & Kopfler, F.C. (1976) The
    occurrence of volatile organics in five drinking water supplies using
    gas chromatography/mass spectrometry. In: Keith, L.H., ed.,
    Identification and Analysis of Organic Pollutants in Water, Ann Arbor,
    MI, Ann Arbor Science, pp. 305-327

Eurocop-Cost (1976) A Comprehensive List of Polluting Substances Which
    Have Been Identified in Various Fresh Waters, Effluent Discharges,
    Aquatic Animals and Plants, and Bottom Sediments, 2nd ed., EUCO/MDU/73/
    76/, XII/476/76, Luxembourg, Commission of the European Communities,
    p. 56

Gehring, P.J. (1968) Hepatotoxic potency of various chlorinated hydrocarbon
    vapours relative to their narcotic and lethal potencies in mice.
    Toxicol. appl. Pharmacol., 13, 287-298

Grasselli, J.G. & Ritchey, W.M., eds (1975) CRC Atlas of Spectral Data
    and Physical Constants for Organic Compounds, 2nd ed., Vol. III,
    Cleveland, OH, Chemical Rubber Co., p. 257

Grimsrud, E.P. & Rasmussen, R.A. (1975) Survey and analysis of halocarbons
    in the atmosphere by gas chromatography-mass spectrometry. Atmos.
    Environ., 9, 1014-1017

Hardie, D.W.F. (1964) Chlorocarbons and chlorohydrocarbons. 1,1,2-Trichloro-
    ethane. In: Kirk, R.E. & Othmer, D.F., eds, Encyclopedia of Chemical
    Technology, 2nd ed., Vol. 5, New York, John Wiley & Sons, pp. 157-159,
    170

IARC (1978) Information Bulletin on the Survey of Chemicals Being
    Tested for Carcinogenicity, No. 7, Lyon, p. 247

IARC (1979) IARC Monographs on the Evaluation of the Carcinogenic Risk
    of Chemicals to Humans, 19, Some Monomers, Plastics and Synthetic Elas-
    tomers, and Acrolein, Lyon, pp. 439-459

Klaassen, C.D. & Plaa, G.L. (1966) Relative effects of various chlorinated
    hydrocarbons on liver and kidney function in mice. Toxicol. appl.
    Pharmacol., 9, 139-151

Kronevi, T., Wahlberg, J. & Holmberg, B. (1977) Morphological lesions in
    guinea pigs during skin exposure to 1,1,2-trichloroethane. Acta
    pharmacol. toxicol., 41, 298-305

National Cancer Institute (1978) Bioassay of 1,1,2-Trichloroethane for
    Possible Carcinogenicity (Technical Report Series No. 74), DHEW
    Publication No. (NIH) 78-1324, Washington DC, US Department of Health,
    Education, & Welfare

National Institute for Occupational Safety & Health (1977a) National
    Occupational Hazard Survey, Vol. III, Survey Analyses and
    Supplement Tables, Cincinnatti, OH, pp. 11,586 - 11,588

National Institute for Occupational Safety & Health (1977b) NIOSH
    Manual of Analytical Methods, 2nd ed., Part II, Standards Completion
    Program Validated Methods, Vol. 2, Method No. S134, DHEW (NIOSH))
    Publication No. 77-157-B, Washington DC, US Government Printing Office,
    pp. S134-1 - S134-9

Plaa, G.L. & Larson, R.E. (1965) Relative nephrotoxic properties of
    chlorinated methane, ethane, and ethylene derivatives in mice.
    Toxicol. appl. Pharmacol., 7, 37-44

Plaa, G.L., Evans, E.A. & Hine, G.H. (1958) Relative hepatotoxicity of
    seven halogenated hydrocarbons. J. Pharmacol. exp. Ther., 123, 224-
    229

Prager, B., Jacobson, P., Schmidt, P. & Stern, D., eds (1918) Beilsteins
    Handbuch der Organischen Chemie, 4th ed., Vol. 1, Syst. No. 8, Berlin,
    Springer, p. 85

Rannug, U., Sundvall, A. & Ramel, C. (1978) The mutagenic effect of 1,2-
    dichloroethane on Salmonella typhimurium. I. Activation through
    conjugation with glutathion in vitro. Chem.-biol. Interact., 20, 1-16

Rosenberg, R., Grahn, O. & Johansson, L. (1975) Toxic effects of aliphatic
    chlorinated by-products from vinyl chloride production on marine
    animals. Water Res., 9, 607-612

Safe Drinking Water Committee (1977) Drinking Water and Health, Washington
    DC, National Academy of Sciences, pp. 775-777

Smyth, H.F., Jr, Carpenter, C.P., Weil, C.S., Pozzani, U.S., Striegel, J.A.
    & Nycum, J.S. (1969) Range-finding toxicity data: list VII. Am.
    ind. Hyg. Assoc. J., 30, 470-476

US Food & Drug Administration (1977) Food and drugs. US Code Fed. Regul.,
    Title 21, part 175-165, pp. 438, 449

US International Trade Commission (1977) Synthetic Organic Chemicals, US
    Production and Sales, 1976, USITC Publication 833, Washington DC,
    US Government Printing Office, p. 332

US Occupational Safety & Health Administration (1977) Air contaminants.
    US Code Fed. Regul., Title 29, part 1910.1000, p. 27

US Tariff Commission (1945) Synthetic Organic Chemicals, US Production and
    Sales, 1941-43, Report No. 153, Second Series, Washington DC, US
    Government Printing Office, p. 131

Van Dyke, R.A. & Wineman, C.G. (1971) Enzymatic dechlorination. Dechlorination of chloroethanes and propanes *in vitro*. Biochem. Pharmacol., 20, 463-470

Yllner, S. (1971) Metabolism of 1,1,2-trichloroethane-1,2-^{14}C in the mouse. Acta pharmacol. toxicol., 30, 248-256

TRICHLOROETHYLENE

This compound was considered by a previous Working Group, in February 1976 (IARC, 1976a). Since that time new data have become available and these have been incorporated into the monograph and taken into account in the present evaluation.

Two reviews on trichloroethylene are available (Lyman, 1978; Mercier, 1977).

1. Chemical and Physical Data

1.1 Synonyms and trade names

Chem. Abstr. Services Reg. No.: 79-01-6

Chem. Abstr. Name: Trichloroethene

Synonyms: Acetylene trichloride; 1-chloro-2,2-dichloroethylene; 1,1-dichloro-2-chloroethylene; ethinyl trichloride; ethylene trichloride; TCE; Tri; trichlorethylene; 1,1,2-trichloroethylene

Trade names: Algylen; Anamenth; Benzinol; Blacosolv; Blancosolv; Cecolene; Chlorilen; Chlorylea; Chlorylen; Chorylen; Circosolv; Crawhaspol; Densinfluat; Dow-Tri; Dukeron; Fleck-Flip; Flock Flip; Fluate; Gemalgene; Germalgene; Lanadin; Lethurin; Narcogen; Narkogen; Narkosoid; Nialk; Perma-A-Chlor; Perm-A-Clor; Petzinol; Philex; Threthylen; Threthylene; Trethylene; Triad; Trial; Triasol; Trichloran; Trichloren; Triclene; Tri-Clene; Trielene; Trielin; Triklone; Trilen; Trilene; Triline; Trimar; Triol; TRI-plus; TRI-plus M; Vestrol; Vitran; Westrosol

1.2 Structural and molecular formulae and molecular weight

C_2HCl_3 Mol. wt: 131.4

1.3 Chemical and physical properties of the pure substance

From Weast (1976), unless otherwise specified

(a) Description: Colourless liquid (Irish, 1963)

(b) Boiling-point: 87°C

(c) Melting-point: -73°C

(d) Freezing-point: -86.8°C (Irish, 1963)

(e) Density: d_4^{20} 1.4642

(f) Refractive index: n_D^{20} 1.4773

(g) Spectroscopy data: λ_{vap} < 200 nm; infra-red, Raman, nuclear magnetic resonance and mass spectral data have been tabulated (Grasselli & Ritchey, 1975).

(h) Solubility: Miscible with water (0.1% w/v at 20°C) (Irish, 1963); miscible with acetone, ethanol, diethyl ether, chloroform and oils (Lloyd et al., 1975)

(i) Volatility: Vapour pressure is 77 mm at 25°C (Irish, 1963).

(j) Vapour density: 4.54 (air = 1) (Irish, 1963)

(k) Stability: Nonflammable; when pure and containing a stabilizer, it is stable in presence of air, moisture, light and in contact with metals up to 130°C. When heated with ozone, it decomposes rapidly into products such as hydrogen chloride, phosgene, carbon monoxide and chlorine peroxide. At 700°C and above, the vapour decomposes to give a mixture of dichloroethylene, tetrachloroethylene, carbon tetrachloride, chloroform and methyl chloride (Hardie, 1964). Upon contact with certain metals, high temperatures, open flame or ultra-violet light, it decomposes almost instantly to phosgene and/ or hydrogen chloride, chlorine and dichloroacetyl chloride. In the presence of alkali, trichloroethylene decomposes to highly toxic dichloroacetylene (US Occupational Safety & Health Administration, 1975).

(1) Reactivity: The most important reaction of trichloroethylene
     is its oxidative breakdown of atmospheric oxygen, greatly
     accelerated by elevation of temperature and exposure to light,
     especially ultra-violet; not hydrolysed by water under normal
     conditions; reacts with alkali under pressure at 150°C to
     produce glycolic acid and with sulphuric acid to give mono-
     chloroacetic acid (Hardie, 1964)

(m) Conversion factor: 1 ppm in air is equivalent to 5.37 mg/m^3.

1.4 Technical products and impurities

Trichloroethylene is available in the US in high-purity, electronic
USP, technical, metal degreasing and extraction grades (Hawley, 1971).
Typical analysis of a commercial grade is: boiling-range at 760 mm,
86.6-87.8°C; density, d_4^{15} 1.467-1.471; acidity (as HCl), 0.0005% max;
alkalinity (as NaOH), 0.001% max; no free halogen; residue on evaporation, 0.005 max; moisture content, not cloudy at -12°C.

Antioxidants, such as amines (0.001-0.01% or more) (Copelin, 1957)
or combinations of epoxides such as epichlorohydrin (see also IARC,
1976b) and esters (0.2-2% total) (Starks, 1956), are added to trichloroethylene.

Specifications for trichloroethylene produced in Japan are:
specific gravity (15°C/40°C), 1.4680; boiling-range, 86.5-88.2°C;
nonvolatile matter, 0.005% max; acid content (as HCl), 0.0002% max.

2. Production, Use, Occurrence and Analysis

2.1 Production and use

(a) Production

Trichloroethylene was prepared by Fischer in 1864 during experiments
on the reduction of hexachloroethane with hydrogen (Hardie, 1964). The
first commercial method for its preparation was the dehydrochlorination
of acetylene-derived 1,1,2,2-tetrachloroethane (see monograph, p. 477)
by reaction with calcium hydroxide or by gas-phase pyrolysis. Although
this method is still used today, over 90% of the trichloroethylene
produced in the US is prepared by the chlorination and dehydrochlorination of 1,2-dichloroethane (see monograph, p. 429). The same process
is used in Japan.

Trichloroethylene has been produced commercially in Austria and the UK since 1908, in Germany since 1910, in the US since 1925 (Hardie, 1964) and in Japan since 1935.   Production of trichloroethylene in the US in 1977 was 132 million kg (US International Trade Commission, 1977); output has been decreasing since 1970, when a reported 277 million kg were produced by 7 companies (US Tariff Commission, 1972), due primarily to legislation restricting the use and emissions of trichloroethylene and to the closing of 3 acetylene-based and 1 ethylene-based plants.

US exports of trichloroethylene in 1976 were 16 million kg, mostly to the Federal Republic of Germany (3.8 million kg), France (3.4 million kg), Mexico (2.1 million kg) and Brazil (2 million kg) (US Department of Commerce, 1977a).   US imports during that year totalled 7 million kg (US Department of Commerce, 1977b).

At least 9 companies in western Europe produce trichloroethylene, with a total production in excess of 200 million kg/year.   In at least 3 countries (the Federal Republic of Germany, France and the UK) annual production is estimated to exceed 50 million kg/year.   These countries and Italy import and export 10-50 million kg/year trichloroethylene. Annual production of trichloroethylene in eastern Europe is estimated to be more than 100 million kg.

In Japan, 4 companies produced 80 million kg trichloroethylene in 1976, compared with 106 million kg in 1972;   in 1976, 11 million kg trichloroethylene were exported.

(b) Use

Of the trichloroethylene produced in the US in 1977, 82% was used for vapour degreasing of fabricated metal parts, 15% was exported and the remainder (3%) was used in a variety of miscellaneous applications.

Trichloroethylene is widely used in vapour degreasing, since all of its physical and chemical properties fall within the limits required in such processes.   One disadvantage of trichloroethylene in this use is its high photochemical reactivity, which causes smog and led to restrictions on its use.   Since trichloroethylene decomposes rapidly upon exposure to high temperatures, open flame or ultra-violet light [see section 1.3 (k)], a proposed standard was issued by the US Occupational Safety and Health Administration on 20 October, 1975, which requires that operations involving high temperatures, open flames or ultra-violet light take place outside areas in which trichloroethylene vapours are present, unless such operations are appropriately shielded and ventilated (US Occupational Safety & Health Administration, 1975).

Miscellaneous applications of trichloroethylene include its use as a solvent in the textile industry;   as a solvent for adhesives and lubricants;   and as a low-temperature heat transfer fluid.   It has also been used as a component in several consumer products (e.g., spot removers, cleaning fluids for rugs) (Lloyd *et al.*, 1975).

A pharmaceutical grade of trichloroethylene is used as a general anaesthetic in surgical, dental and obstetrical procedures and as an analgesic in the treatment of trigeminal neuralgia.   It has been used as a disinfectant and detergent for skin, minor wounds and surgical instruments.   It has also been used on a variety of animals as a volatile anaesthetic.

The use of trichloroethylene as an extraction solvent (e.g., for use in the manufacture of decaffeinated coffee and for the extraction of spice oleoresins) was approved by the US Food and Drug Administration (FDA) for many years.   However, on 27 September 1977, the FDA proposed regulations prohibiting the use of trichloroethylene as a food additive, directly or indirectly.   Specific examples of practices to be prohibited include use in hop extraction, decaffeination of coffee, the isolation of spice oleoresins, adhesive coatings and components, and in vinyl chloride-hexene-1 copolymers.   Food containing any added or detectable level of trichloroethylene will be deemed to be adulterated when the final order has been issued.   On the same date, the FDA also proposed a regulation that any human drug containing trichloroethylene will be considered a new drug and will be deemed to be misbranded; under this regulation anaesthetics containing trichloroethylene would be banned.   It was also proposed to declare trichloroethylene a deleterious substance, thereby causing any cosmetic product containing it to be deemed adulterated under existing law.   The FDA also proposed a regulation prohibiting the use of trichloroethylene as an additive in animal and pet food;   such practices as the use of trichloroethylene for the extraction of oil-seed products would be prohibited.   The FDA also proposed an order prohibiting the use of trichloroethylene in animal drug products, such as its use as an inhalation anaesthetic, skin disinfectant and in detergents (US Food & Drug Administration, 1977).

No data on its use in Europe were available.   In 1977, trichloroethylene was used in Japan in metal cleaning (63%), solvent and other uses (23%) and exports (14%).

It was reported in May 1978 that trichloroethylene has been accepted by the US Environmental Protection Agency as a candidate for issuance of a notice of a rebuttable presumption against renewal of registration (RPAR) (see General Remarks on Substances Considered, p. 31) on the basis of its possible carcinogenicity (Anon., 1978).

The US Occupational Safety and Health Administration's health standards for exposure to air contaminants require that an employee's exposure to trichloroethylene not exceed an 8-hr time-weighted average of 535 mg/m^3 (100 ppm) in the working atmosphere in any 8-hr work shift of a 40-hr work week (US Occupational Safety & Health Administration, 1975). The corresponding standard in the Federal Republic of Germany is 260 mg/m^3, that in the German Democratic Republic and Czechoslovakia, 250 mg/m^3 and that in Sweden, 160 mg/m^3 (Winell, 1975).

It was proposed on 20 October 1975 that the maximum allowable concentration in the US be reduced from 1070 mg/m^3 (200 ppm) to 805 mg/m^3 (150 ppm) (US Occupational Safety & Health Administration, 1975). The maximum acceptable ceiling concentration in the USSR is 10 mg/m^3 (1.86 ppm) (Winell, 1975).

The US National Institute for Occupational Safety and Health has recently recommended that occupational exposure to halogenated anaesthetic agents, including trichloroethylene, be controlled so that no worker is exposed to concentrations greater than 10.7 mg/m^3 (2 ppm) (National Institute for Occupational Safety & Health, 1977b).

2.2 Occurrence

Trichloroethylene is not known to occur as a natural product. Its occurrence in air, water, soil and sediments, food, marine organisms and humans has been reviewed (Battelle Columbus Laboratories, 1977).

(a) Air

The US Environmental Protection Agency has estimated that approximately 60% of the total annual world production of trichloroethylene is released to the environment, with annual emissions of about 540 million kg to the atmosphere and 9.1 million kg to the ocean (Fuller, 1976). The dispersive uses of trichloroethylene (metal cleaning and solvent applications) have been estimated to result in annual emissions of 192 million kg in the US (Fuller, 1976) and 100 million kg in Japan (Ohta *et al.*, 1976).

The background ambient air concentration of trichloroethylene has been reported for several locations: (1) western Eire, levels of 80 ng/m^3 (15 ppt[1]); (2) over the North Atlantic, < 27 ng/m^3 (5 ppt) (Lovelock, 1974); (3) in a rural area, < 27 ng/m^3 (5 ppt) (Grimsrud & Rasmussen, 1975); (4) in the northern hemisphere, about 80 ng/m^3 (15 ppt); and (5) in the southern hemisphere, about 8 ng/m^3 (1.5 ppt) (Cox *et al.*, 1976).

Trichloroethylene has also been detected in ambient air: (1) in north-eastern US, at typical levels of 1 μg/m^3 (0.18 ppb[2]) in urban areas and < 0.1 μg/m^3 (0.02 ppb) in rural areas (Lillian *et al.*, 1975); (2) in Michigan, at levels of 150-500 ng/m^3 (30-90 ppt) (Russell & Shadoff,

---

[1]1 ppt in air is equivalent to 5.37 ng/m^3.
[2]1 ppb in air is equivalent to 5.37 μg/m^3.

1977);   (3) at 4 sites in California, at levels of 83-1670 ng/m^3
(15.6-310.8 ppt) (Singh, 1976);   (4) at 5 US land stations, at levels
ranging from 2-28 ng/m^3 (0.4-5.2 ppt);   (5) at 11 sea stations, at
levels ranging from 1-22 ng/m^3 (0.2-4 ppt) (Murray & Riley, 1973);
(6) in Tokyo, at 26 sites, at average levels of 6.4 µg/m^3 (1.2 ppb)
(Ohta *et al.*, 1976);   and (7) in Manchester, UK, at levels of 5.35-
343 µg/m^3 (1-64 ppb) (Pearson & McConnell, 1975).

(b) Water

Trichloroethylene has been found in 2 raw-water samples, 1 lake-water
sample, 10 finished drinking-water samples, 1 raw sewage sample, 5 rivers
and samples of effluent from 4 chemical plants and 4 sewage treatment
plants in the US (Shackelford & Keith, 1976).   It was detected in
samples of surface-water from 88/204 sites near heavily industrialized
areas, at levels > 1 µg/l (Ewing *et al.*, 1977).

Trichloroethylene has been detected in: (1) tap-water (Dowty *et
al.*, 1975);   (2) tap, lake, spring, and subterranean water, at levels
of 105, 38, 5 and 80 ng/l, respectively (Grob & Grob, 1974);   and (3)
effluent water from a chemical production plant, at a level of 0.2 mg/l
(Eurocop-Cost, 1976).

It has also been detected in: (1) a river, at a level of 25 µg/l
(Rook *et al.*, 1975);   (2) ground-water near waste deposits, at a level
of 100 µg/l (Kotzias *et al.*, 1975);   (3) the drinking-water of 5
cities, at levels of 0-0.5 µg/l (Coleman *et al.*, 1976);   and (4)
influent and effluent water from a sewage treatment plant, at levels of
8.6-40.4 µg/l (Bellar *et al.*, 1974).

(c) Soil and sediments

Concentrations of trichloroethylene in soil and sediment near
production and user sites in the US ranged from 0- > 100 µg/kg
(Battelle Columbus Laboratories, 1977).

(d) Food and drink

Trichloroethylene has been detected in the following foodstuffs
in the UK: dairy products (0.3-10 µg/kg), meat (12-22), oils and fats
(0-19), beverages (0-60) and fruits and vegetables (McConnell *et al.*,
1975).   Traces of trichloroethylene have also been found in edible
oils after extraction (Gracián & Martel, 1972).

(e) Marine organisms

Trichloroethylene has been detected in 3 species of mollusc at
levels of 0-250 ng/g, and in 5 species of fish at levels of 0-479 ng/g
(dry weight) (Dickson & Riley, 1976).

(f) Humans

Trichloroethylene has been detected in post-mortem human tissue samples, at levels of < 1-32 µg/kg (wet tissue) (McConnell *et al.*, 1975) and in human expired air, at levels of 0-3.9 µg/hr/subject (Conkle *et al.*, 1975).

It has been estimated that about 60,000 people are exposed annually to trichloroethylene as an anaesthetic (Fuller, 1976).

(g) Occupational exposure

Occupational exposure to trichloroethylene has been reviewed (National Institute for Occupational Safety & Health, 1973).

Trichloroethylene has been detected in the atmosphere of dry-cleaning plants (Babenko, 1974). Levels of 1076-43,000 mg/m^3 (200-8000 ppm) were found in a small factory (Kleinfeld & Tabershaw, 1954).

Concentrations of trichloroethylene vapour in a dial assembly workshop ranged from < 135 -> 538 mg/m^3 (25-100 ppm); those in the degreasing room were 800-1350 mg/m^3 (150-250 ppm) (Takamatsu, 1962).

The concentration to which surgeons and nurses were exposed in operating-rooms varied from 1.6-554 mg/m^3 (0.3-103 ppm) (Corbett, 1973). About 5000 medical, dental and hospital personnel are routinely exposed to trichloroethylene.

A 1974 National Occupational Hazard Survey indicated that workers primarily exposed to trichloroethylene are those in hospitals, in the aircraft manufacturing industry, in blast furnaces and in steel mills (National Institute for Occupational Safety & Health, 1977a).

(h) Other

Trichloroethylene has been detected as a trace impurity in helium (Schehl, 1973).

2.3 Analysis

A review of methods for the analysis of trichloroethylene in waste-treatment plant sludge was made by Camisa (1975). Analytical methods to determine trichloroethylene in air, oleoresins, blood and urine have also been reviewed (Kouer, 1975; Walter *et al.*, 1976).

Methods used for the analysis of trichloroethylene in environmental samples are listed in Table 1.

TABLE 1. METHODS FOR THE ANALYSIS OF TRICHLOROETHYLENE

SAMPLE TYPE	ANALYTICAL METHOD			
	EXTRACTION/CLEAN-UP	DETECTION	LIMIT OF DETECTION	REFERENCE
Formulations				
Cough syrups and encapsulated liquids	Transfer to ethanol, dilute as appropriate, transfer to separator containing 10% sucrose solution and carbon disulphide	IR		Horwitz (1975)
Air				
Workplace	Trap on charcoal, extract (carbon disulphide)	GC/FID	Useful range, 519-2176 mg/m^3	National Institute for Occupational Safety & Health (1977c)
Ambient	Trap in Drechsel flask fitted with rubber septum, sample with gas syringe	GC/ECD	1 µg/m^3	Bureau International Technique des Solvants Chlorés (1976)
Ambient	Analyse directly	GC/ECD	10 mg/m^3	Krynska et al. (1976)
Rural	Trap on porous polymer, desorb by heating, retrap in line on GC column	GC/ECD; GC/MS	160 ng/m^3 (30 ppt)	Russell & Shadoff (1977)
Atmosphere	Analyse directly	GC/MS	27 ng/m^3 (5 ppt)	Grimsrud & Rasmussen (1975)
Ambient	Analyse directly	Carbon dioxide laser	1.8 µg/m^3 (0.7 ppb)	Kreuzer et al. (1972)
Ambient	Analyse directly	Carbon dioxide laser	23 µg/m^3 (4.2 ppb)	Schnell & Fischer (1975)
Water				
Sea- and fresh-water	Extract (pentane), dry	GC/ECD	50 ng/l	Bureau International Technique des Solvants Chlorés (1976)
Waste-water	Extract (freon)	GC/FID	0.7 ng	Austern et al. (1975)
River water	Headspace analysis	GC/MS		Rook et al. (1975)

TABLE 1. METHODS FOR THE ANALYSIS OF TRICHLOROETHYLENE (continued)

SAMPLE TYPE	EXTRACTION/CLEAN-UP	ANALYTICAL METHOD		REFERENCE
		DETECTION	LIMIT OF DETECTION	
Drinking-water	Inject directly	GC/ECD	2 µg/l	Nicholson et al. (1977)
Tap-water	Inject directly	GC/MS	0.2 µg/l	Fujii (1977)
Food				
Spice oleoresins	Dilute with ethanol, add internal standard	GC/microcoulometry		Horwitz (1975)
Biological				
Blood	Analyse directly, using precolumn on GC and internal standard	GC/FID		Cole et al. (1975a,b)
Miscellaneous				
Oils and liquid paraffin	Headspace analysis	GC/FID	0.2 µg	Drexler & Osterkamp (1977)

Abbreviations: IR - infra-red spectrometry; GC/FID - gas chromatography/flame-ionization detection; ECD - electron capture detection; MS - mass spectrometry

Use of gas chromatography with electron capture detection to detect trichloroethylene residues in grain has been studied collaboratively by 8 European laboratories.   The limit of detection ranged from 0.005-0.2 mg/kg (Panel on Fumigant Residues in Grain, 1974).   Gas chromatography has also been used by Kuchinskii (1977) and Lillian *et al*. (1975).

A system to determine trichloroethylene in water is described by Ellison & Wallbank (1974).

3.   Biological Data Relevant to the Evaluation
of Carcinogenic Risk to Humans

3.1   Carcinogenicity studies in animals[1]

Oral administration

Mouse: Groups of 50 male and 50 female B6C3F1 hybrid mice, 5 weeks old, were administered 99% pure trichloroethylene, containing 0.19% 1,2-epoxybutane and 0.09% epichlorohydrin (see IARC, 1976b) in corn oil by gavage on 5 days a week for 78 weeks.   High-dose males received 2000-2400 mg/kg bw/day, and females 1400-1800 mg/kg bw/day;   low-dose males and females received 1000-1200 mg/kg bw/day and 700-900 mg/kg bw. All surviving animals were observed until they were 95 weeks of age. Time-weighted average doses were 1169 and 869 in low-dose males and females and 2339 and 1739 mg/kg bw/day in high-dose males and females. Groups of 20 male and 20 female mice served as vehicle-treated matched controls.   Survival was reduced in high-dose males and control males. Hepatocellular carcinomas occurred in 1/20 control males and 0/20 control females, in 26/50 low-dose males and 4/50 low-dose females, and in 31/48 high-dose males and 11/47 high-dose females.   Metastases of the liver-cell tumours to the lung were found in 7/98 treated males and in 1 control male.   The first hepatocellular carcinoma was observed in a mouse treated with the high dose of trichloroethylene which died during week 27. Lung tumours occurred in treated animals of both sexes: 5/50 (5 adenomas) in males and 4/50 (2 adenomas, 2 carcinomas) in females in the low-dose group, and 2/48 (1 adenoma, 1 carcinoma) in males and 7/47 (5 adenomas, 2 carcinomas) in females treated with the high dose of trichloroethylene.   Among controls, only one lung adenoma was reported in a

---

[1]The Working Group was aware of studies in progress to assess the carcinogenicity of trichloroethylene in mice by skin, subcutaneous and oral administration (IARC, 1978a) and of an inhalation study in rats and mice carried out under contract to the Manufacturing Chemist's Association (Toxicology Information Program, 1976).   Preliminary results of the inhalation study (Page & Arthur, 1978) indicate findings similar to those of the National Cancer Institute (1976).

female (National Cancer Institute, 1976) [The Working Group noted that the low-dose males and females also received 1 and 0.7 mg/kg bw/ day epichlorohydrin, and the high-dose males and females received 2.1 and 1.56 mg/kg bw/day epichlorohydrin].

Rat: Groups of 50 male and 50 female Osborne-Mendel rats, 7 weeks of age, received 99% pure trichloroethylene, containing 0.19% 1,2-epoxybutane and 0.09% epichlorohydrin (see IARC, 1976b) in corn oil by gavage on 5 days a week for 78 weeks.   High-dose animals received varying dose schedules of 1000-1500 mg/kg bw/day, and low-dose animals received 500-750 mg/kg bw/day.   All surviving animals were killed 110 weeks after the start of treatment. The time-weighted average doses were 549 and 1097 mg/kg bw/day.   A group of 20 male and 20 female vehicle-treated rats served as controls.   Of the males, 17/20 controls, 42/50 low-dose and 47/50 high-dose animals died before the end of the study; of the females, 12/20 controls, 35/48 low-dose animals and 37/50 high-dose animals died.   Median survival times were approximately 60 weeks for high-dose males, 85 weeks for low-dose males and 70 weeks for high- and low-dose females.   Of the males, 5/20 controls, 7/50 low-dose and 5/50 high-dose rats developed tumours; of the females, 7/20 controls, 12/48 low- and 12/50 high-dose rats developed tumours. No liver-cell tumours occurred; tumours that occurred in various other organs in treated and vehicle control animals were mainly reticulum-cell sarcomas, lymphosarcomas or malignant lymphomas, fibroadenomas of the mammary gland, haemangiosarcomas at various sites, follicular adenocarcinomas of the thyroid, chromophobe adenomas of the pituitary and renal hamartomas.   Toxic nephropathy was observed in rats of both sexes treated with high and low doses of trichloroethylene (National Cancer Institute, 1976) [The Working Group noted the poor survival of treated rats and that the low- and high-dose animals also received 0.5 and 1 mg/ kg bw/day epichlorohydrin].

In a preliminary report of a study in progress, groups of 30 male and 30 female Sprague Dawley rats, 13 weeks of age, were given 50 or 250 mg/kg bw trichloroethylene (purity unspecified) in olive oil by gavage 4-5 times per week for 52 weeks, followed by observation for life.   A group of 30 male and 30 female controls received olive oil alone.   Results were reported 76 weeks after the start of treatment, at which time 46 controls, 39 low-dose and 34 high-dose males and females combined of each group were still alive.   Among high-dose rats that died, 1 lymphoid leukaemia and 1 plasmocytoma were observed (minimum latent period, 38 weeks); 2 plasmocytomas occurred in low-dose animals that died (minimum latent period, 70 weeks).   No such tumours were found in controls (Maltoni & Maioli, 1977).

3.2 Other relevant biological data

(a) Experimental systems

Toxic effects

Wide variations in impurities and manufacturing processes of tri-chloroethylene produce inconsistencies in experimental toxicity tests (Defalque, 1961); in addition, pure trichloroethylene decomposes readily into highly toxic products. The extensive literature on the toxicity of trichloroethylene has been reviewed by Aviado *et al*. (1976), Browning (1965), Defalque (1961), the US Occupational Safety & Health Administration (1975), Lloyd *et al*. (1975), Von Oettingen (1964), Smith (1966) and Walter *et al*. (1976).

The oral LD_{50} in rats is 7.2 g/kg bw (Smyth *et al*., 1969) and in mice, 2.85 g/kg bw (Aviado *et al*., 1976). The i.p. LD_{50} in mice is 3.2 g/kg bw (Klaassen & Plaa, 1966) or 1.83 g/kg bw (Schumacher & Grandjean, 1960); that in dogs is 2.8 g/kg bw (Klaassen & Plaa, 1967). The lowest lethal i.v. dose for dogs is 150 mg/kg bw; in rabbits, the s.c. lethal dose is 1.8 g/kg bw (Barsoum & Saad, 1934).

The maximum concentrations of vapour that produced no toxic effects after exposure for 7 hrs daily on 5 days a week for 6 months were: rats and rabbits, 1076 mg/m^3 (200 ppm); guinea-pigs, 538 mg/m^3 (100 ppm); and monkeys, 2150 mg/m^3 (400 ppm) (Adams *et al*., 1951). Thirty expo-sures for 8 hrs daily on 5 days/week to 3825 mg/m^3 (700 ppm), or continuous exposure to 189 mg/m^3 (35 ppm) for 90 days caused no visible sign of toxicity in rats, dogs, monkeys, guinea-pigs or rabbits (Pren-dergast *et al*., 1967).

In 8 cats exposed to concentrations of 108 mg/m^3 of air (20 ppm) for 1-1.5 hrs per day for 4-6 months, centrilobular hepatitis, nephritis, hypertrophy of lymphoid glands and splenomegaly were observed (Mosinger & Fiorentini, 1955). In mice, trichloroethylene caused less damage to the kidneys and liver than did carbon tetrachloride or chloroform (Klaassen & Plaa, 1966).

In a chronic toxicity study, the maximal tolerated oral dose of industrial-grade trichloroethylene in Osborne-Mendel rats was 1100 mg/kg bw for animals of both sexes; that in B6C3F1 hybrid mice was 2340 mg/kg (males) and 1740 mg/kg (females) (National Cancer Institute, 1976).

Embryotoxicity and teratogenicity

Groups of rats and mice were exposed by inhalation for 7 hrs daily on days 6-15 of gestation to 1600 mg/m^3 in air (300 ppm) trichloroethylene; no effects were observed on the average number of implantation sites per litter, litter size, incidence of foetal resorptions, foetal sex ratios or foetal body measurements.   No treatment-related increased incidence in skeletal or visceral malformations was observed (Schwetz *et al.*, 1975).

Absorption, distribution, excretion and metabolism

A review is available (Piotrowski, 1977).

Following inhalation of trichloroethylene, none was detected in the blood or organs of rats (Kimmerle & Eben, 1973a).

Dogs exposed to trichloroethylene excreted trichloroacetic acid and the glucuronide of trichloroethanol in the urine (Barrett & Johnston, 1939; Butler, 1949).   When [36]Cl-trichloroethylene was given by gavage to rats, 10-20% of the dose was excreted in the urine as 1-5% trichloro-acetic acid and 10-15% trichloroethanol; 0-0.5% was excreted as tri-chloroethylene in the faeces and 72-85% as trichloroethylene in the expired air (Daniel, 1963).

The demonstration of the enzymic conversion of trichloroethylene to chloral by liver microsomes from rabbits, rats and dogs supports the suggestion of Powell (1945) that the trichloroethylene oxide intermediate rearranges into chloral hydrate (Byington & Leibman, 1965; Leibman, 1965).   Chloral was also isolated *in vitro* as an intramolecular re-arrangement product of trichloroethylene oxide; chloral is then in part reduced to trichloroethanol or oxidized to trichloroacetic acid (Bonse & Henschler, 1976; Bonse *et al.*, 1975).   Spectral evidence for the formation of trichloroethylene oxide (2,2,3-trichloro-oxirane) during incubation of trichloroethylene with metabolizing hepatic micro-somes was reported by Uehleke *et al.* (1977).

[14]C-Trichloroethylene is bound irreversibly to liver endoplasmic protein *in vivo* and *in vitro* (Allemand *et al.*, 1978; Bolt *et al.*, 1977; Uehleke & Poplawski-Tabarelli, 1977; Van Duuren & Banerjee, 1976); it is bound to exogenous DNA *in vitro* (Banerjee & Van Duuren, 1978). Binding is correlated with the activity of hepatic mixed-function oxidases (Uehleke & Poplawski-Tabarelli, 1977); thus, treatment of animals with inducers of hepatic mixed-function oxidases, such as phenobarbital, methylcholanthrene, Aroclor 1254 or hexachlorobenzene, increases the hepatotoxicity of trichloroethylene (Carlson, 1974; Moslen *et al.*, 1977a) and depletes hepatic glutathione (Moslen *et al.*, 1977b).

Mutagenicity and other related short-term tests

Trichloroethylene was mutagenic in *Escherichia coli* K12 and in *Salmonella typhimurium* TA100 (Greim *et al.*, 1975; Simon *et al.*, 1977) in the presence of a microsomal activation system.   In another assay with *Salmonella typhimurium* TA100, the pure compound was not mutagenic either in the presence or absence of rat liver microsomes; it was shown additionally that two of the impurities in a technical-grade sample of trichloroethylene, epichlorohydrin and 1,2-epoxybutane, were mutagenic in the absence of rat liver microsomes (Henschler *et al.*, 1977).

In *Saccharomyces cerevisiae* strain XV185-14C, trichloroethylene induced reverse mutations in the presence of mouse liver microsomes; the mutation frequencies were concentration-dependent. The authors concluded that trichloroethylene induced base-pair as well as frameshift type mutations (Shahin & Von Borstel, 1977). Positive results have been reported in the same species for the induction of gene mutations and mitotic gene conversion (strain D7) in the presence of mammalian microsomes and for the host(mouse)-mediated assay (strain D4) (Bronzetti *et al.*, 1978).

Mice given single i.p. injections of half-LD_{50} doses of trichloro-ethylene in dimethylsulphoxide, or five repeated injections of one-sixth the LD_{50} at one-day intervals, showed no increase in the frequency of chromosome aberrations in their bone-marrow cells (Černá & Kypěnová, 1977).

In spot tests for somatic mutations, i.p. treatment of pregnant mice with 1 mM trichloroethylene induced coat colour mutations in exposed embryos (Fahrig, 1977).

[To what extent the positive mutagenic results reported with tri-chloroethylene are due to impurities in the test samples could not be determined by the Working Group].

(b) Humans

Numerous fatalities resulting from anaesthesia with trichloroethylene and from industrial intoxications have been compiled. Sudden death, probably due to ventricular fibrillation, has been reported on exertion shortly after intense exposure (Defalque, 1961).

Chronic inhalation of trichloroethylene affects the central nervous system (Grandjean *et al.*, 1955). Accidental ingestions produced inebriety, vomiting, diarrhoea, collapse and coma, followed either by death (pulmonary oedema and liver and kidney necrosis at autopsy) or recovery with transient neurological sequelae (amnesia, headache, numb-ness, weakness of extremities, psychosis or hemiparesis) (Defalque, 1961). Toxic effects on the liver (Schüttmann, 1970) and cutaneous reactions (Bauer & Rabens, 1974; Schirren, 1971; Stewart *et al.*, 1974) have been reported.

Psychophysiological function was depressed in volunteers exposed to 592 mg/m^3 (110 ppm) trichloroethylene for two 4-hr periods (Salvini *et al.*, 1971). Experimental exposure of 10 volunteers to 1070 mg/m^3 (200 ppm) trichloroethylene vapour for periods of 7 hrs over 5 days

produced fatigue and sleepiness (Stewart *et al.*, 1970).   Impairment of
neurological and psychological functions after acute and longer exposure was also reported by Gamberale *et al.* (1976) and Triebig *et al.*
(1977).   It has been suggested that the toxic action in humans was
due mainly to contaminants (Browning, 1965; Defalque, 1961).

There is an indication that the hepatotoxic effect of trichloroethylene is enhanced by concomitant exposure to ethanol or isopropyl
alcohol (Traiger & Plaa, 1974).

About 60% of inspired trichloroethylene is taken up by the body;
the arterial blood concentration increased linearly with the concentration in the alveolar air (Åstrand & Övrum, 1976).

Humans exposed to trichloroethylene excrete trichloracetic acid and
trichloroethanol in the urine (Kimmerle & Eben, 1973b; Nomiyama &
Nomiyama, 1971; Powell, 1945), and the concentration of trichloracetic
acid in the urine is an indication of trichloroethylene exposure
(Axelson *et al.*, 1978; Smith, 1978).   Kinetic studies of the formation
and excretion of trichloroacetic acid and trichloroethanol have been
reported (Fernandez *et al.*, 1977; Monster *et al.*, 1976; Müller *et al.*
1974).   Chloral hydrate was also identified as a trichloroethylene
metabolite in the blood (Cole *et al.*, 1975a; Scansetti *et al.*, 1959).

3.3 Case reports and epidemiological studies[1]

An epidemiological study of cancer mortality among 518 males exposed
occupationally to relatively low levels of trichloroethylene has been
reported.   Levels of exposure were estimated by concentrations of trichloroacetic acid in the urine: exposure categories with averages below
and above 100 mg/l trichloroacetic acid in the urine were used; 100 mg/
l corresponds roughly to an 8-hr time-weighted average exposure of 160 mg/
m^3 (30 ppm) trichloroethylene in air.   When compared with the national
population rates, 49 deaths from all causes were observed *versus* 62
expected.   With no consideration given to latency or intensity of
exposure, 11 deaths due to cancer at all sites were observed *versus*
14.5 expected.   When analyses were restricted to those with 10 or more
years since onset of exposure, no significant excess of cancer was
demonstrated, either for those exposed to high or lower levels of trichloroethylene.   It was concluded, however, that this study could not
rule out a cancer risk to humans, particularly for rare types of malig-
nancies such as liver cancer (Axelson *et al.*, 1978) [The small size of
the study group and the relatively short latent period (mainly less than
20 years) underline this conclusion].

---

[1]The Working Group was aware of 2 studies in progress: a cancer
mortality study of workers occupationally exposed to trichloroethylene
and a follow-up study of workers exposed to organochloride and alkyl-
chloride compounds, vinyl chloride, trichloroethylene and unsaturated
compounds (IARC, 1978b).

4. Summary of Data Reported and Evaluation

4.1 Experimental data

Trichloroethylene was tested in one experiment in mice and in one in rats by oral administration. In mice, it produced hepatocellular carcinomas and lung tumours in both males and females. The experiment in rats was considered to be inadequate. Preliminary results of a study in progress by oral administration to rats could not be evaluated.

Trichloroethylene is mutagenic in bacteria and yeast and in spot tests for somatic mutations in mice.

4.2 Human data[1]

No case reports were available to the Working Group. The only epidemiological study available reported no statistically significant excess of cancer associated with exposure to trichloroethylene. However, because of the small size of the group and the relatively short time since onset of exposure, no assessment of carcinogenicity could be made.

The extensive production of trichloroethylene for over 50 years, together with its use as an industrial solvent and metal cleaning agent, as an inhalational anaesthetic and as an additive in drugs, food and consumer products, indicate that widespread human exposure occurs. This is confirmed by many reports of its occurrence in air, water and foods and in human tissues and expired air.

4.3 Evaluation

There is *limited evidence* that trichloroethylene is carcinogenic in mice.

---

[1]Subsequent to the meeting of the Working Group, the Secretariat became aware of a study of 330 deceased laundry and dry-cleaning workers who had been exposed to carbon tetrachloride, trichloroethylene and tetrachloroethylene. An excess of lung, cervical and skin cancers and a slight excess of leukaemias and liver cancers were observed (Blair *et al.*, 1979).

5. References

Adams, E.M., Spencer, H.C., Rowe, V.K., McCollister, D.D. & Irish, D.D. (1951) Vapor toxicity of trichloroethylene determined by experiments on laboratory animals. AMA Arch. ind. Hyg. occup. Med., 4, 469-481

Allemand, H., Pessayre, D., Descatoire, V., Degott, C., Feldmann, G. & Benhamou, J.-P. (1978) Metabolic activation of trichloroethylene into a chemically reactive metabolite toxic to the liver. J. Pharmacol. exp. Ther., 204, 714-723

Anon. (1978) Trichloroethylene. Pestic. Tox. Chem. News, 10 May, p.2

Åstrand, I. & Övrum, P. (1976) Exposure to trichloroethylene. I. Uptake and distribution in man. Scand. J. Work Environ. Health, 4, 199-211

Austern, B.M., Dobbs, R.A. & Cohen, J.M. (1975) Gas chromatographic determination of selected organic compounds added to wastewater. Environ. Sci. Technol., 9, 588-590

Aviado, D.M., Zakhari, S., Simaan, J. & Ulsamer, A.G. (1976) Methyl Chloroform and Trichloroethylene in the Environment, Cleveland, OH, Chemical Rubber Co., pp. 47-89

Axelson, O., Andersson, K., Hogstedt, C., Holmberg, B., Molina, G. & de Verdier, A., (1978) A cohort study on trichloroethylene exposure and cancer mortality. J. occup. Med., 20, 194-196

Babenko, K.V. (1974) Sanitary hygienic assessment of the working conditions for operators involved in the chemical cleaning of clothes (Russ.). Gig. Sanit., 11, 77-79

Banerjee, S. & Van Duuren, B.L. (1978) Covalent binding of the carcinogen trichloroethylene to hepatic microsomal proteins and to exogenous DNA in vitro. Cancer Res., 38, 776-780

Barrett, H.M. & Johnson, J.H. (1939) The fate of trichloroethylene in the organism. J. biol. Chem., 127, 765-770

Barsoum, G.S. & Saad, K. (1934) Relative toxicity of certain chloride derivatives of the aliphatic series. Q. J. Pharm. Pharmacol., 7, 205-214

Battelle Columbus Laboratories (1977) Multimedia Levels. Trichloroethylene EPA 560/6-77-029, Washington DC, US Environmental Protection Agency. Available from Springfield, VA, National Technical Information Service, Report No. PB-276535

Bauer, M. & Rabens, S.F. (1974) Cutaneous manifestations of trichloro-
    ethylene toxicity. Arch. Dermatol., 110, 886-890

Bellar, T.A., Litchenberg, J.J. & Kroner, R.C. (1974) The occurrence of
    organohalides in chlorinated drinking waters. J. Am. Water Works
    Assoc., 66, 703-706

Blair, A., Decoufle, P. & Grauman, D. (1979) Causes of death among
    laundry and dry cleaning workers. Am. J. publ. Health, 69, 508-511

Bolt, H.M., Buchter, A., Wolowski, L., Gil, D.L. & Bolt, W. (1977)
    Incubation of ^{14}C-trichloroethylene vapor with rat liver microsomes:
    uptake of radioactivity and covalent protein binding of metabolites.
    Int. Arch. occup. environ. Health, 39, 103-111

Bonse, G. & Henschler, D. (1976) Chemical reactivity, biotransformation,
    and toxicity of polychlorinated aliphatic compounds. CRC Crit. Rev.
    Toxicol., 4, 395-409

Bonse, G., Urban, T., Reichert, D. & Henschler, D. (1975) Chemical
    reactivity, metabolic oxirane formation and biological reactivity of
    chlorinated ethylenes in the isolated perfused rat liver preparation.
    Biochem. Pharmacol., 24, 1829-1834

Bronzetti, G., Zeiger, E. & Frezza, D. (1978) Genetic activity of tricholor-
    oethylene in yeast. J. environ. Pathol. Toxicol., 1, 411-418

Browning, E. (1965) Toxicity and Metabolism of Industrial Solvents,
    Amsterdam, Elsevier, pp. 189-212

Bureau International Technique des Solvants Chlorés (1976) Standardization
    of methods for the determination of traces of some volatile chlorinated
    aliphatic hydrocarbons in air and water by gas chromatography. Anal.
    chim. acta, 82, 1-17

Butler, T.C. (1949) Metabolic transformations of trichloroethylene.
    J. Pharmacol. exp. Ther., 97, 84-92

Byington, K.H. & Leibman, K.C. (1965) Metabolism of trichloroethylene by
    liver microsomes. II. Identification of the reaction product as
    chloral hydrate. Mol. Pharmacol., 1, 247-254

Camisa, A.G. (1975) Analysis and characteristics of trichloroethylene
    wastes. J. Water Pollut. Control Fed., 47, 1021-1031

Carlson, G.P. (1974) Enhancement of the hepatotoxicity of trichloroethylene
    by inducers of drug metabolism. Res. Comm. Chem. Pathol. Pharmacol.,
    7, 637-640

Cerná, M. & Kypěnová, H. (1977) Mutagenic activity of chloroethylenes analysed by screening system tests (Abstract no. 36). Mutat. Res., 46, 214-215

Cole, W.J., Mitchell, R.G. & Salamonsen, R.F. (1975a) Isolation, characterization and quantitation of chloral hydrate as a transient metabolite of trichloroethylene in man using electron capture gas chromatography and mass fragmentography. J. Pharm. Pharmacol., 27, 167-171

Cole, W.J., Salamonsen, R.F. & Fish, K.J. (1975b) A method for the gas chromatographic analysis of inhalation anaesthetics in whole-blood by direct injection into a simple precolumn device. Br. J. Anaesth., 47, 1043-1047

Coleman, W.E., Lingg, R.D., Melton, R.G. & Kopfler, F.C. (1976) The occurrence of volatile organics in five drinking water supplies using gas chromatography/mass spectrometry. In: Keith, L.H., ed., Identification and Analysis of Organic Pollutants of Water, Ann Arbor, MI, Ann Arbor Science, pp. 305-327

Conkle, J.P., Camp, B.J. & Welch, B.E. (1975) Trace composition of human respiratory gas. Arch. environ. Health, 30, 290-295

Copelin, H.B. (1957) Stabilization of chlorinated hydrocarbons. US Patent 2,797,250, June 25 to E.I. Du Pont de Nemours & Co.

Corbett, T.H. (1973) Retention of anesthetic agents following occupational exposure. Anesth. Analg. Curr. Res., 52, 614-618

Cox, R.A., Derwent, R.G., Eggleton, A.E.J. & Lovelock, J.E. (1976) Photochemical oxidation of halocarbons in the troposphere. Atmos. Environ., 10, 305-308

Daniel, J.W. (1963) The metabolism of ^{36}Cl-labeled trichloroethylene and tetrachloroethylene in the rat. Biochem. Pharmacol., 12, 795-802

Defalque, R.J. (1961) Pharmacology and toxicology of trichloroethylene. A critical review of the world literature. Clin. Pharmacol. Ther., 2, 665-688

Dickson, A.G. & Riley, J.P. (1976) The distribution of short-chain halogenated aliphatic hydrocarbons in some marine organisms. Marine Biol. Pollut., 7, 167-169

Dowty, B.J., Carlisle, D.R. & Laseter, J.L. (1975) New Orleans drinking water sources tested by gas chromatography-mass spectrometry. Occurrence and origin of aromatics and halogenated aliphatic hydrocarbons. Environ. Sci. Technol., 9, 762-765

Drexler, H.-J. & Osterkamp, G. (1977) Head-space analysis for the
    quantitative determination of trichloroethylene and tetrachloro-
    ethylene in oils and liquid paraffin. J. Clin. Chem. Clin. Biochem.,
    15, 431-432

Ellison, W.K. & Wallbank, T.E. (1974) Solvents in sewage and industrial
    waste waters: identification and determination. Water Pollut. Control,
    73, 656-672

Eurocop-Cost (1976) A Comprehensive List of Polluting Substances Which
    Have Been Identified in Various Fresh Waters, Effluent Discharges,
    Aquatic Animals and Plants, and Bottom Sediments, 2nd ed., EUCO/MDU/
    73/76, XII/476/76, Luxembourg, Commission of the European Communities,
    p. 57

Ewing, B.B., Chian, E.S.K., Cook, J.C., Evans, C.A., Hopke, P.K. & Perkins,
    E.G. (1977) Monitoring to Detect Previously Unrecognized Pollutants
    in Surface Waters, EPA-560/6-77-015, Washington DC, US Environmental
    Protection Agency. Available from Springfield, VA, National Technical
    Information Service, pp. 63-64, 74

Fahrig, R. (1977) The sensitivity of the mammalian spot test to mutagens
    of different types of action (Abstract no. 17). Mutat. Res., 46, 202

Fernández, J.G., Droz, P.O., Humbert, B.E. & Caperos, J.R. (1977) Trichloro-
    ethylene exposure. Simulation of uptake, excretion, and metabolism
    using a mathematical model. Br. J. ind. Med., 34, 43-55

Fujii, T. (1977) Direct aqueous injection gas chromatography-mass spectro-
    metry for analysis of organohalides in water at concentrations below
    the parts per billion level. J. Chromatogr., 139, 297-302

Fuller, B.B. (1976) Air Pollution Assessment of Trichloroethylene, MTR-
    7142, Research Triangle Park, NC, US Environmental Protection Agency,
    Contract No. 68-02-1495. Available from Springfield, VA, National
    Technical Information Service, No. PB-256 730

Gamberale, F., Annwall, G. & Olson, B.A. (1976) Exposure to trichloro-
    ethylene. III. Psychological functions. Scand. J. Work Environ.
    Health, 4, 220-224

Gracián, J. & Martel, J. (1972) Determination of solvent residues in
    refined edible oils. I. (Sp.). Grasas CRC Aceites (Sevilla), 23,
    1-6

Grandjean, E., Münchinger, R., Turrain, V., Haas, P.A., Knoepfel, H.-K.
    & Rosenmund, H. (1955) Investigations into the effects of exposure
    to trichlorethylene in mechanical engineering. Br. J. ind. Med.,
    12, 131-142

Grasselli, J.G. & Ritchey, W.M., eds (1975)   CRC Atlas of Spectral Data and Physical Constants for Organic Compounds, 2nd ed., Vol. III, Cleveland, OH, Chemical Rubber Co., p. 283

Greim, H., Bonse, G., Radwan, Z., Reichert, D. & Henschler, D. (1975) Mutagenicity *in vitro* and potential carcinogenicity of chlorinated ethylenes as a function of metabolic oxirane formation. Biochem. Pharmacol., 24, 2013-2017

Grimsrud, E.P. & Rasmussen, R.A. (1975)   Survey and analysis of halocarbons in the atmosphere by gas chromatography-mass spectrometry. Atmos. Environ., 9, 1014-1017

Grob, K. & Grob, G. (1974)   Organic substances in potable water and in its precursor.   II. Applications in the area of Zürich.   J. Chromatogr. 90, 303-313

Hardie, D.W.F. (1964)   Chlorocarbons and chlorohydrocarbons.   Trichloro-ethylene.   In: Kirk, R.E. & Othmer, D.F., eds, Encyclopedia of Chemical Technology, 2nd ed., Vol. 5, New York, John Wiley & Sons, pp. 183-195

Hawley, G.G., ed. (1971)   Condensed Chemical Dictionary, 8th ed., New York, Van Nostrand-Reinhold, pp. 886-887

Henschler, D., Eder, E., Neudecker, T. & Metzler, M. (1977)   Carcino-genicity of trichloroethylene: fact or artifact?   Arch. Toxikol., 37, 233-236

Horwitz, W., ed. (1975)   Official Methods of Analysis of the Association of Official Analytical Chemists, 12th ed., Washington DC, Association of Official Analytical Chemists, pp. 383, 658-660

IARC (1976a)   IARC Monographs on the Evaluation of Carcinogenic Risk of Chemicals to Man, 11, Cadmium, Nickel, Some Epoxides, Miscellaneous Industrial Chemicals and General Consideration on Volatile Anaesthetics, Lyon, pp. 263-276

IARC (1976b)   IARC Monographs on the Evaluation of Carcinogenic Risk of Chemicals to Man, 11, Cadmium, Nickel, Some Epoxides, Miscellaneous Industrial Chemicals and General Considerations on Volatile Anaesthetics Lyon, pp. 131-139

IARC (1978a)   Information Bulletin on the Survey of Chemicals Being Tested for Carcinogenicity, No. 7, Lyon, p. 277

IARC (1978b)   Directory of On-Going Research in Cancer Epidemiology, 1978 (IARC Scientific Publications No. 26), Lyon, pp. 58 (Abstract No. 144), 148 (Abstract No. 377)

Irish, D.D. (1963) Aliphatic halogenated hydrocarbons. Trichloroethylene. In: Patty, F.A., ed., Industrial Hygiene and Toxicology, 2nd ed., Vol. II, New York, Interscience, pp. 1309-1313

Kimmerle, G. & Eben, A. (1973a) Metabolism, excretion and toxicology of trichloroethylene after inhalation. I. Experimental exposure in rats. Arch. Toxikol., 30, 115-126

Kimmerle, G. & Eben, A. (1973b) Metabolism, excretion and toxicology of trichloroethylene after inhalation. 2. Experimental human exposure. Arch. Toxikol., 30, 127-138

Klaassen, C.D. & Plaa, G.L. (1966) Relative effects of various chlorinated hydrocarbons on liver and kidney function in mice. Toxicol. appl. Pharmacol., 9, 139-151

Klaassen, C.D. & Plaa, G.L. (1967) Relative effects of various chlorinated hydrocarbons on liver and kidney function in dogs. Toxicol. appl. Pharmacol., 10, 119-131

Kleinfeld, M. & Tabershaw, I.R. (1954) Trichloroethylene toxicity. Report on five fatal cases. AMA Arch. ind. Hyg., 10, 134-141

Kotzias, D., Klein, W. & Korte, F. (1975) Ecological chemistry. CVI. Occurrence of xenobiotics in ground water of waste deposits (Germ.). Chemosphere, 5, 301-306

Kouer, F.D. (1975) Preliminary Study of Selected Potential Environmental Contaminants - Optical Brighteners, Methyl Chloroform, Trichloroethylene, Tetrachloroethylene and Ion Exchange Resins, EPA-560/2-75-002, Washington DC, US Environmental Protection Agency, pp. 81-86, 123-130. Available from Springfield, VA, National Technical Information Service, PB 243910

Kreuzer, L.B., Kenyon, N.D. & Patel, C.K.N. (1972) Air pollution: sensitive detection of ten pollutant gases by carbon monoxide and carbon dioxide lasers. Science, 177, 347-349

Krynska, A., Grabowski, Z. & Posniak, M. (1976) Determination of trichloroethylene, tetrachloroethylene, and tetrachloroethane in air by gas chromatography (Pol.). Pr. Cent. Inst. Ochr. Pr., 26, 293-306 [Chem. Abstr., 87, 140307b]

Kuchinskii, A.L. (1977) Gas-liquid chromatographic determination of perchloroethylene and trichloroethylene in air (Russ.). Gig. Sanit., 4, 57-58

Leibman, K.C. (1965) Metabolism of trichloroethylene in liver microsomes. I. Characteristics of the reaction. Mol. Pharmacol., 1, 239-246

Lillian, D., Singh, H.B., Appleby, A., Lobban, L., Arnts, R., Gumpert, R., Hague, R., Toomey, J., Kazazis, J., Antell, M., Hansen, D. & Scott, B. (1975) Atmospheric fates of halogenated compounds. Environ. Sci. Technol., 9, 1042-1048

Lloyd, J.W., Moore, R.M., Jr & Breslin, P. (1975) Background information on trichloroethylene. J. occup. Med., 17, 603-605

Lovelock, J.E. (1974) Atmospheric halocarbons and stratospheric ozone. Nature (Lond.), 252, 292-294

Lyman, W.J. (1978) Report on trichloroethylene. In: Berkowitz, J.B., Literature Review - Problem Definition Studies on Selected Chemicals, Cambridge, MA, Arthur D. Little, Inc., pp. 19-69

Maltoni, C. & Maioli, P. (1977) Long-term bioassay of carcinogenicity of trichloroethylene. Preliminary results (Ital.). Osp. Vita, 4, 108-110

McConnell, G., Ferguson, D.M. & Pearson, C.R. (1975) Chlorinated hydrocarbons and the environment. Endeavor, 34, 13-18

Mercier, M. (1977) Criteria (Exposure/Effect Relationships) for Organo-Solvents, V/F/177-4, Luxembourg, Commission of the European Communities, pp. 123-190

Monster, A.C., Boersma, G. & Duba, W.C. (1976) Pharmacokinetics of trichloroethylene in volunteers, influence of workload and exposure concentration. Int. Arch. occup. environ. Health, 38, 87-102

Mosinger, M. & Fiorentini, H. (1955) Hepatic, renal, ganglionic and splenic reactions in experimental intoxication with trichloroethylene in the cat (Fr.). C.R. Soc. Biol. (Paris), 149, 150-152

Moslen, M.T., Reynolds, E.S. & Szabo, S. (1977a) Enhancement of the metabolism and hepatotoxicity of trichloroethylene and perchloroethylene. Biochem. Pharmacol., 26, 369-375

Moslen, M.T., Reynolds, E.S., Boor, P.J., Bailey, K. & Szabo, S. (1977b) Trichloroethylene-induced deactivation of cytochrome P-450 and loss of liver glutathione in vivo. Res. Comm. chem. Pathol. Pharmacol., 16, 109-120

Müller, G., Spassovski, M. & Henschler, D. (1974) Metabolism of trichloroethylene in man. II. Pharmacokinetics of metabolites. Arch. Toxikol., 32, 283-295

Murray, A.J. & Riley, J.P. (1973) Occurrence of some chlorinated aliphatic hydrocarbons in the environment. Nature (Lond.), 242, 37-38

National Cancer Institute (1976) Carcinogenesis Bioassay of Trichloro-
     ethylene (Technical Report Series No. 2), DHEW Publication No. (NIH)
     76-802, Washington DC, US Department of Health, Education, & Welfare

National Institute for Occupational Safety & Health (1973) Criteria
     for a Recommended Standard - Occupational Exposure to Trichloro-
     ethylene, HSM-73-11025, Washington DC, US Department of Health,
     Education & Welfare, pp. 15-19

National Institute for Occupation Safety & Health (1977a) National
     Occupational Hazard Survey, Vol. III, Survey Analyses and Supple-
     mental Tables, DHEW (NIOSH) Publication 76, Draft, Cincinnati, OH,
     Table 50, pp. 11590-11600

National Institute for Occupational Safety & Health (1977b) Recommenda-
     tions for workplace exposure to waste anesthetic gases and vapors.
     Occup. Saf. Health Rep., 19 May, p. 1577

National Institute for Occupational Safety & Health (1977c) NIOSH
     Manual of Analytical Methods, 2nd ed., Part II, Standards Completion
     Program Validated Methods, Vol. 3, Method No. S336, Cincinnati, OH,
     US Department of Health, Education, & Welfare, pp. S336-1 - S336-9

Nicholson, A.A., Meresz, O. & Lemyk, B. (1977) Determination of free and
     total potential haloforms in drinking water. Anal. Chem., 49,
     814-819

Nomiyama, K. & Nomiyama, H. (1971) Metabolism of trichloroethylene in
     human. Sex difference in urinary excretion of trichloroacetic acid
     and trichloroethanol. Int. Arch. Arbeitsmed., 28, 37-48

Ohta, T., Morita, M. & Mizoguchi, I. (1976) Local distribution of
     chlorinated hydrocarbons in the ambient air in Tokyo. Atmos.
     Environ., 10, 557-560

Page, N.P. & Arthur, J.L. (1978) Special Occupational Hazard Review
     of Trichloroethylene, DHEW (NIOSH) Publication No. 78-130, Rockville,
     MD, US Department of Health, Education, & Welfare

Panel on Fumigant Residues in Grain (1974) Determination of residues of
     volatile fumigants in grain. Analyst (Lond.), 99, 570-578

Pearson, C.R. & McConnell, G. (1975) Chlorinated C_1 and C_2 hydrocarbons
     in the marine environment. Proc. R. Soc. Lond. B., 189, 305-332

Piotrowski, J.K. (1977) Exposure Tests for Organic Compounds in Industrial
     Toxicology, DHEW (NIOSH) Publication No. 77-144, Cincinnati, OH, US
     Department of Health, Education, & Welfare, National Institute for
     Occupational Safety & Health, pp. 86-97

Powell, J.F. (1945) Trichloroethylene: absorption, elimination and
    metabolism. Br. J. ind. Med., 2, 142-145

Prendergast, J.A., Jones, R.A., Jenkins, L.J., Jr & Siegel, J. (1967)
    Effects on experimental animals of long-term inhalation of trichloro-
    ethylene, carbon tetrachloride, 1,1,1-trichloroethane, dichlorodi-
    fluoromethane, and 1, 1-dichloroethylene. Toxicol. appl. Pharmacol.,
    10, 270-289

Rook, J.J., Meijers, A.P., Gras, A.A. & Noordsij, A. (1975) Headspace
    analysis of volatile trace compounds in the Rhine (Germ.). Vom
    Wasser, 44, 23-30

Russell, J.W & Shadoff, L.A. (1977) The sampling and determination of
    halocarbons in ambient air using concentration on porous polymer.
    J. Chromatogr., 134, 375-384

Salvini, M., Binaschi, S. & Riva, M. (1971) Evaluation of the psycho-
    physiological functions in humans exposed to trichloroethylene. Br.
    J. ind. Med., 28, 293-295

Scansetti, G., Rubino, G.F. & Trompeo, G. (1959) Studies on chronic
    trichloroethylene poisoning. III. Metabolism of trichloroethylene
    (Ital.). Med. Lav., 50, 743-754

Schehl, T.A. (1973) Trace Organic Impurities in Gaseous Helium, NASA
    Technical Note, D-6520, Washington DC, National Aeronautics & Space
    Administration

Schirren, J.M. (1971) Skin lesions caused by trichloroethylene in a metal
    working plant (Germ.). Berufs-Derm., 19, 240-254

Schnell, W. & Fischer, G. (1975) Carbon dioxide laser absorption co-
    efficients of various air pollutants. Appl. Optics, 14, 2058-2059

Schumacher, H. & Grandjean, E. (1960) Comparative studies on the narcotic
    effect and acute toxicity of nine solvents (Germ.). Arch. Gewer-
    bepathol. Gewerbehyg., 18, 109-119

Schüttmann, W. (1970) Liver damage after occupational exposure to
    trichloroethylene (Germ.). Dtsch. Z. Verd. Stoffwechseltr., 30,
    43-45

Schwetz, B.A., Leong, B.K.J. & Gehring, P.J. (1975) The effect of
    maternally inhaled trichloroethylene, perchloroethylene, methyl
    chloroform, and methylene chloride on embryonal and fetal development
    in mice and rats. Toxicol. appl. Pharmacol., 32, 84-96

Shackelford, W.M. & Keith, L.H. (1976) Frequency of Organic Compounds
    Identified in Water, EPA-600/4-76-062, Athens, GA, US Environmental
    Protection Agency, p. 133

Shahin, M.M. & Von Borstel, R.C. (1977) Mutagenic and lethal effects of
α-benzene hexachloride, dibutyl phthalate and trichloroethylene in
Saccharomyces cerevisiae. Mutat. Res., 48, 173-180

Simmon, V.F., Kauhanen, K. & Tardiff, R.G. (1977) Mutagenic activity
of chemicals identified in drinking water. In: Scott, D.,
Bridges, B.A. & Sobels, F.H., eds, Progress in Genetic Toxicology,
Amsterdam, Elsevier/ North Holland, pp. 249-258

Singh, H.B. (1976) Phosgene in the ambient air. Nature (Lond.), 264,
428-429

Smith, G.F. (1966) Trichlorethylene: a review. Br. J. ind. Med., 23,
249-262

Smith, G.F. (1978) Trichloroethylene - relationship of metabolite levels
to atmospheric concentrations: preliminary communication. J. R. Soc.
Med., 71, 591-595

Smyth, H.F., Jr, Carpenter, C.P., Weil, C.S., Pozzani, U.C., Striegel, J.A.
& Nycum, J.S. (1969) Range-finding toxicity data: List VII. Am. ind.
Hyg. Assoc. J., 30, 470-476

Starks, F.W. (1956) Stabilization of chlorinated hydrocarbons. US Patent
2,818,446, 25 October, to E.I. Du Pont de Nemours & Co.

Stewart, R.D., Dodd, H.C., Gay, H.H. & Erley, D.S. (1970) Experimental
human exposure to trichloroethylene. Arch. environ. Health, 20,
64-71

Stewart, R.D., Hake, C.L. & Peterson, J.E. (1974) 'Degreaser's flush'.
Dermal response to trichloroethylene and ethanol. Arch. environ.
Health, 29, 1-5

Takamatsu, M. (1962) Health hazards in workers exposed to trichloroethylene
vapor. II. Exposure to trichloroethylene during degreasing operation
in a communicating machine factory. Kumamoto med. J., 15, 43-54

Toxicology Information Program (1976) Study of the effects from repeated
inhalation of trichloroethylene vapor in rats and mice. Tox. Tips,
1 (5), 3

Tringer, G.J. & Plaa, G.L. (1974) Chlorinated hydrocarbon toxicity.
Potentiation by isopropyl alcohol and acetone. Arch. environ. Health,
28, 276-278

Triebig, G., Schaller, K.H., Erzigkeit, H. & Valentin, H. (1977) Biochemical investigations and psychological studies of persons
chronically exposed to trichloroethylene with regard to non-exposure
intervals (Germ.). Int. Arch. occup. environ. Health, 38, 149-162

Uehleke, H. & Poplawski-Tabarelli, S. (1977) Irreversible binding of
    ^{14}C-labelled trichloroethylene to mice liver constituents *in vivo*
    and *in vitro*. Arch. Toxikol., 37, 289-294

Uehleke, H., Tabarelli-Poplawski, S., Bonse, G. & Henschler, D. (1977)
    Spectral evidence for 2,2,3-trichloro-oxirane formation during
    microsomal trichloroethylene oxidation. Arch. Toxikol., 37, 95-105

US Department of Commerce (1977a) US Exports, Schedule B Commodity
    Groupings, Schedule B Commodity by Country, FT 410/December,
    Washington DC, US Government Printing Office, p. 2-85

US Department of Commerce (1977b) US General Imports, Schedule A
    Commodity by Country, FT 135/December 1976, Washington DC, US
    Government Printing Office, p. 2-91

US Food & Drug Administration (1977) Trichloroethylene. Removal from
    food additive use. Fed. Regist., 42, 49465-49471

US International Trade Commission (1977) Synthetic Organic Chemicals,
    US Production and Sales, 1976, USITC Publication 833, Washington DC,
    US Government Printing Office, pp. 303, 332

US Occupational Safety & Health Administration (1975) Occupational
    exposure to trichloroethylene. Fed. Regist., 40, 49032-49045

US Tariff Commission (1972) Synthetic Organic Chemicals, US Production
    and Sales, 1970, TC Publication 479, Washington DC, US Government
    Printing Office, pp. 215, 241

Van Duuren, B.L. & Banerjee, S. (1976) Covalent interaction of metabolites
    of the carcinogen trichloroethylene in rat hepatic microsomes. Cancer
    Res., 36, 2419-2422

Von Oettingen, W.F. (1964) The Halogenated Hydrocarbons of Industrial
    and Toxicological Importance, Amsterdam, Elsevier, pp. 240-271

Walter, P., Craigmill, A., Villaume, J., Sweeney, S. & Miller, G.L. (1976)
    Chlorinated Hydrocarbon Toxicity (1,1,1-Trichloroethane, Trichloro-
    ethylene, and Tetrachloroethylene): A Monograph, Report No. CPSC-
    BBSC-76-M1, Contract No. CPSC-C-75-0100, Bethesda, MD, Consumer
    Product Safety Commission, pp. 21-25, 138-172

Weast, R.C., ed. (1976) CRC Handbook of Chemistry and Physics, 57th ed.,
    Cleveland, OH, Chemical Rubber Co., p. C-298

Winell, M. (1975) An international comparison of hygienic standards for
    chemicals in the work environment. Ambio, 4, 34-36

FLAME RETARDANT

TRIS(2,3-DIBROMOPROPYL) PHOSPHATE

1. Chemical and Physical Data

1.1 Synonyms and trade names

Chem. Abstr. Services Reg. No.: 126-72-7

Chem. Abstr. Name: 2,3-Dibromo-1-propanol phosphate (3:1)

Synonyms: 2,3-Dibromo-1-propanol phosphate; (2,3-dibromopropyl) phosphate; tris(2,3-dibromopropyl) phosphoric acid ester; Tris

Trade names: Anfram 3PB; Apex 462-5; Bromkal P 67-6HP; ES 685; Firemaster LV-T 23P; Firemaster T 23P; Flacavon R; Flamex T 23P; Flammex AP; Flammex T 23P; T 23P; Zetofex ZN

1.2 Structural and molecular formulae and molecular weight

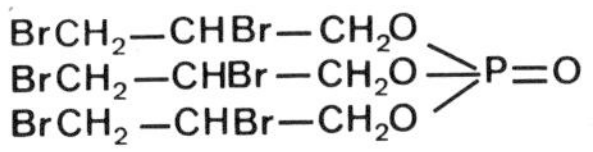

$$\begin{array}{l} BrCH_2-CHBr-CH_2O \\ BrCH_2-CHBr-CH_2O \\ BrCH_2-CHBr-CH_2O \end{array}\!\!>\!\!P=O$$

$C_9H_{15}Br_6O_4P$ Mol. wt: 697.7

1.3 Chemical and physical properties of the pure substance

From Lande *et al.* (1976), unless otherwise specified

(a) Description: Viscous, pale-yellow liquid (Hawley, 1977)

(b) Freezing-point: 5.5°C

(c) Density: d^{25} 2.27

(d) Spectroscopy data: Infra-red and nuclear magnetic resonance spectral data have been tabulated (Grasselli & Ritchey, 1975).

(e) Refractive index: n_D^{20} 1.5772 (Hawley, 1977)

(f) Solubility: Insoluble in water; miscible with carbon tetrachloride, chloroform and methylene chloride (Stauffer Chemical Co., 1972)

(g) Volatility: Vapour pressure is 0.00019 mm at 25°C.

(h) Stability: Stable to 200-250°C; major decomposition begins at 308°C; stable in sunlight

(i) Reactivity: Hydrolysed by acids and bases

1.4 Technical products and impurities

Tris(2,3-dibromopropyl) phosphate is available in the US in at least two grades. The high-purity grade has the following typical properties: a clear, pale-yellow viscous liquid; density at 25°C, 2.20-2.26; refractive index at 25°C, 1.576-1.577; viscosity at 25°C, 3900-4200 centistokes; acid number (mg KOH/g), 0.05 max; volatiles, 1.5%; max; bromine content, 68.7%; and phosphorus content, 4.4%. Typical properties for a lower grade are as follows: density at 25°C, 2.2-2.3; viscosity at 25°C, 1400-1700 centistokes; acid number (mg KOH/g), 0.05 max; and volatiles, 10% max.

Impurities in tris(2,3-dibromopropyl) phosphate include 2,3-dibromopropanol, 1,2,3-tribromopropane and 1,2-dibromo-3-chloropropane (see monograph, p. 83) (Blum & Ames, 1977).

2. Production, Use, Occurrence and Analysis

A review on haloalkyl phosphates has been published (US Environmental Protection Agency, 1976a).

2.1 Production and use

(a) Production

The first described preparation of tris(2,3-dibromopropyl) phosphate is believed to have been in 1950, when it was made by the addition of bromine to a solution of triallyl phosphate in benzene. It is prepared commercially in the US by a two-step process in which bromine is added to allyl alcohol and the resultant 2,3-dibromopropanol is reacted with phosphorous oxychloride (Overbeek & Namety, 1962) (possibly in the presence of an aluminium chloride catalyst).

Commercial production of tris(2,3-dibromopropyl) phosphate in the US was first reported in 1959 (US Tariff Commission, 1960). In 1976,

2 US companies reported production of an undisclosed amount (see preamble, p. 16) (US International Trade Commission, 1977).   US production in 1975 has been estimated to have been 4.1-5.4 million kg (US Environmental Protection Agency, 1976a).

No data on its production in Europe were available.

Japanese production of tris(2,3-dibromopropyl) phosphate is estimated to have been 100 thousand kg in 1976, the last year in which the single manufacturer made it; it is not imported.

(b) Use

Tris(2,3-dibromopropyl) phosphate is used primarily as a flame retardant additive for synthetic textiles and plastics (US Environmental Protection Agency, 1976a).   It has also been recommended for use in phenolic resins, paints, paper coatings and rubber (Agranoff, 1976).

Tris(2,3-dibromopropyl) phosphate is used mainly in polyester and cellulosic acetate fabrics, but it has also been used in acrylic fabrics; twice as much is used in polyester fabrics as in cellulosic acetate fabrics.   About 65% of the tris(2,3-dibromopropyl) phosphate used in the US in 1975 was applied to fabrics for children's clothing (US Environmental Protection Agency, 1976b).   It may be added to textiles by the producer, although addition by dyers and finishers is believed to be more usual, at a level of 6-10% by weight.

Its addition to polyurethane foams (see IARC, 1979a) is the major use in plastics;   relatively small amounts are believed to be used as an additive to polystyrene foam (see IARC, 1979b).   It is added to rigid foams and to a lesser extent to flexible polyurethane foams.   It has been estimated that fire-retarded polyurethane requires approximately 0.5% phosphorus and 4-7% bromine;   this is equivalent to about 10% tris-(2,3-dibromopropyl) phosphate (by weight) in the product (US Environmental Protection Agency, 1976a).

Flexible polyurethane foams are used primarily for cushioning. Cushioning treated with haloalkyl phosphates is found in automotive and aircraft interiors, institutional bedding, cushions and upholstered furniture.   Rigid foams containing tris(2,3-dibromopropyl) phosphate are used in insulation, furniture, automobile interior parts and water flotation devices.   Less expensive fire retardants are used for rigid foams used in building insulation (US Environmental Protection Agency, 1976a).

As a result of actions taken on 8 April and 1 June 1977, the US Consumer Product Safety Commission banned children's clothing treated with tris(2,3-dibromopropyl) phosphate, the chemical itself when used or intended to be used in children's clothing and fabric, yarn or fibre

containing it when intended for use in such clothing (US Consumer
Product Safety Commission, 1977a,b).   However, children's clothing
containing tris(2,3-dibromopropyl) phosphate is still available because
the ban has not yet been fully enforced (Anon., 1978; US Consumer
Product Safety Commission, 1978a,b).

In March 1978, the Consumer Product Safety Commission listed 22
products that contain tris(2,3-dibromopropyl) phosphate and are available to US consumers.   These included children's clothing, industrial
uniforms, draperies, tent fabric, automobile headliners, epoxy resins
for the electronics industry, Christmas decorations and polyester
thread (Anon., 1978).

No data on its use in Europe were available.   Until 1977, it was
used in Japan primarily as a fire retardant in polyester fibres and polyurethane plastics.

2.2 Occurrence

Tris(2,3-dibromopropyl) phosphate is not known to occur as a
natural product.

Although environmental levels of tris(2,3-dibromopropyl) phosphate
have not been measured, it has been estimated that as much as 10% of US
production reaches the environment from textile finishing plants and
laundries and that most of the rest will reach the environment as solid
waste (US Environmental Protection Agency, 1976b).   Several experimental
studies conducted on polyester and cellulose acetate fabrics treated
with tris(2,3-dibromopropyl) phosphate have shown that it can leach
into wash and rinse water during laundering (Lande *et al.*, 1976).   When
sheets treated with tris(2,3-dibromopropyl) phosphate were washed, up to
6 mg/l were found in the combined wash- and rinse-water (Gutenmann &
Lisk, 1975).

Approximately 180 µg/day (9 µg/kg bw) tris(2,3-dibromopropyl)
phosphate is absorbed through the skin of children wearing polyester
pyjamas (Blum *et al.*, 1978).

A 1974 National Occupational Hazard Survey indicated that workers
primarily exposed to tris(2,3-dibromopropyl) phosphate are those in the
telephone communication industry (National Institute for Occupational
Safety & Health, 1977).

2.3 Analysis

Methods used for the analysis of tris(2,3-dibromopropyl) phosphate
are listed in Table 1.

TABLE 1. METHODS FOR THE ANALYSIS OF TRIS(2,3-DIBROMOPROPYL) PHOSPHATE

SAMPLE TYPE	ANALYTICAL METHOD		
	EXTRACTION/CLEAN-UP	DETECTION	REFERENCE
Textiles	Pyrolysis	GC/flame photometry	Cope (1973)
Polyester flannel	Heat in distilled water; evaporate to dryness; hydrolyse by refluxing with hydrobromic acid; complex with molybdenum blue	Spectrophotometry	Gutenmann & Lisk (1975)

Abbreviation: GC - gas chromatography

3. Biological Data Relevant to the Evaluation

of Carcinogenic Risk to Humans

3.1 Carcinogenicity studies in animals

(a) Oral administration

Mouse: Groups of 50 male and 50 female B6C3F1 hybrid mice, 6 weeks of
age, were fed various concentrations of technical-grade tris(2,3-dibromo-
propyl) phosphate (containing no detectable 1,2-dibromo-3-chloropropane)
in the diet for 103 weeks followed by a 1-week observation period. The
experimental design of the study is shown in Table 2. Of the males, 43/50
high-dose, 38/50 low-dose and 44/55 matched control mice survived until
the end of the study; of the females, 38/50 high-dose, 37/50 low-dose
and 44/55 control mice survived. The compound increased the incidence of
squamous-cell carcinomas and papillomas of the forestomach and of adenomas
and carcinomas of the lungs in both male and female treated animals as
compared with controls; there was also an increased incidence of renal
tubular-cell adenomas and adenocarcinomas in treated male mice and of liver-
cell adenomas and carcinomas in treated female mice. Neoplastic lesions
associated with the administration of tris(2,3-dibromopropyl) phosphate
are summarized in Table 2. Renal tubular dysplasia was observed in 30/49
high-dose males, 37/50 low-dose males, 12/46 high-dose females and 1/50
low-dose females but in none of the controls (National Cancer Institute,
1978).

Rat: Groups of 55 male and 55 female Fischer 344 rats, 6 weeks old,
were fed diets containing various concentrations of technical-grade
tris(2,3-dibromopropyl) phosphate for 103 weeks, followed by a 1- or 2-
week observation period. The experimental design of the study is shown
in Table 2. Of the males, 40/55 high-dose, 35/55 low-dose and 39/55
control rats survived until the end of the study; of the females, 36/55
high-dose, 44/55 low-dose and 36/55 control rats survived. The
compound increased the incidence of renal tubular-cell adenomas in rats
of both sexes and of tubular-cell adenocarcinomas in high-dose males.
Neoplastic lesions associated with the administration of tris(2,3-dibromo-
propyl) phosphate are summarized in Table 2. Renal tubular dysplasia
was observed in 6/54 high-dose males and in 35/54 high-dose females, but
not in the control or low-dose groups (National Cancer Institute, 1978).

(b) Skin application

Mouse: Female ICR/Ha Swiss mice, 6-8 weeks old, were treated thrice
weekly with tris(2,3-dibromopropyl) phosphate (97% pure) in 0.2 ml acetone
applied to the shaved dorsal skin for 474-496 days. Most of the animals
survived to the end of the study. The compound increased the incidence
of tumours of the skin, lung, forestomach and oral cavity in treated mice

TABLE 2. TUMOUR INCIDENCES IN MICE AND RATS FED TRIS(2,3-DIBROMOPROPYL) PHOSPHATE

SPECIES	SEX	NO. OF ANIMALS TREATED	CONCENTRATION (mg/kg OF DIET)	DURATION (WEEKS)	NUMBER OF TUMOUR-BEARING ANIMALS/NUMBER OF ANIMALS EXAMINED			
					FORESTOMACH (SQUAMOUS-CELL CARCINOMAS OR PAPILLOMAS)	LUNG (ADENOMAS OR CARCINOMAS)	KIDNEY (TUBULAR-CELL ADENOMAS OR ADENOCARCINOMAS)	LIVER (ADENOMAS OR CARCINOMAS)
Mouse	M	55	0	105	$0/51^a$	12/54	0/54	28/54
	M	50	500	103	$10/47^b$	$18/44^e$	4/50	31/49
	M	50	1000	103	$13/48^b$	$25/50^d$	$14/49^e$	23/49
	F	55	0	105	$2/53^b$	4/55	0/55	$11/54^f$
	F	50	500	103	$14/48^b$	9/50	2/50	$23/50^f$
	F	50	1000	103	22/44	$17/50^d$	2/46	$35/49^f$
Rat	M	55	0	107	–	0/54	$0/53^e$	0/54
	M	55	50	103	–	3/55	$26/54^e$	1/55
	M	55	100	103	–	0/55	$29/54^e$	4/54
	F	55	0	107	–	–	0/52	–
	F	55	50	103	–	–	$4/54^e$	–
	F	55	100	103	–	–	$10/54^e$	–

Fisher analysis of treated group versus control:

[a] Squamous-cell papillomas; $P < 0.01$

[b] Squamous-cell carcinomas & papillomas; $P < 0.01$

[c] Alveolar/bronchiolar adenomas & carcinomas; $P < 0.05$

[d] Alveolar/bronchiolar adenomas & carcinomas; $P < 0.01$

[e] Tubular-cell adenomas & adenocarcinomas; $P < 0.01$

[f] Hepatocellular adenomas & carcinomas; $P < 0.01$

as compared with controls.   The experimental design and the neoplastic
lesions associated with the dermal application of tris(2,3-dibromopropyl)
phosphate are summarized in Table 3 (Van Duuren *et al.*, 1978).

TABLE 3.   TUMOUR INCIDENCES IN FEMALE SWISS MICE AFTER DERMAL
APPLICATION OF TRIS(2,3-DIBROMOPROPYL) PHOSPHATE

NUMBER OF ANIMALS TREATED	DOSE (mg/ ANIMALS)	NUMBER OF MICE WITH TUMOURS/NUMBER NECROPSIED[a]			
		FORESTOMACH	LUNG	SKIN	ORAL CAVITY
29	0	1/29	7/29	0/29	0/29
30	10	10/29	26/29	2/29	2/29
30	30	20/30	28/30	5/30	4/30

[a]Increases in incidences of tumours of forestomach, lung, skin and
oral cavity in treated animals were statistically significant when
compared with those in controls (P < 0.05).

3.2   Other relevant biological data

(a)   Experimental data

Toxic effects

    Tris(2,3-dibromopropyl) phosphate containing less than 1% volatile
impurities has an oral LD_{50} of 5.24 g/kg bw in rats and a dermal LD_{50}
of > 8 g/kg bw in rabbits.

    In rabbits, administration of 0.22 g/animal to the eye or 1.1 g/
animal to the skin caused no irritation (Daniher, 1976;   Kerst, 1974).
No evidence of skin sensitization was seen in guinea-pigs (Morrow *et
al.*, 1976).

    Application of commercial, high-purity (99.76%) tris(2,3-dibromo-
propyl) phosphate weekly for 3 months at a dose of 2.27 g/kg bw to
intact and abraded skin of the backs of female and male rabbits produced
a 50% decrease in testicular weight in 7/8 males, with spermatogonia
in the seminiferous tubules and occasional progression to secondary
spermatocytes.   In addition, chronic interstitial nephritis was seen
in 6/8 males (Osterberg *et al.*, 1977).

    No data on the embryotoxicity or teratogenicity of tris(2,3-dibromo-
propyl) phosphate were available.

Absorption, distribution, excretion and metabolism

Tris(2,3-dibromopropyl) phosphate was absorbed from the digestive system of male weanling rats fed 100 and 1000 mg/kg of diet for 28 days. Dose-related bromine concentrations were detected by neutron activation analysis in muscle, liver and fat after 28 days' feeding; these concentrations were reduced to control levels 6 weeks after administration of the compound was discontinued (Kerst, 1974). The absorption of tris(2,3-dibromopropyl) phosphate was dose-dependent in rabbits that received daily skin applications of 500, 1000 and 2000 mg/kg of diet, as shown by increased blood bromide levels (Daniher, 1976).

After application of fabric treated with ^{14}C-tris(2,3-dibromopropyl) phosphate to the clipped skin of rabbits, up to 17% of the radiolabel in the cloth penetrated the skin over a 96-hr period of exposure. Most of the radiolabel appeared in the urine. Even higher absorption of radiolabel occurred when cloth moistened with human urine was applied to the skin (Ulsamer *et al.*, 1978).

When a dose of 100 mg/animal was applied to the shaven skin of a male Lewis rat, a metabolic hydrolysis product, 2,3-dibromopropanol, was detected in free and conjugated form in the urine for several days (St John *et al.*, 1976).

Mutagenicity and other related short-term tests

Tris(2,3-dibromopropyl) phosphate is mutagenic in *Salmonella typhimurium* TA100 and TA1535, but not in TA1537 and TA1538, indicating that the mutations induced are of the base-pair substitution type (Blum & Ames, 1977; Brusick *et al.*, 1977; Prival *et al.*, 1977). In the study of Prival *et al.* (1977), although tris(2,3-dibromopropyl) phosphate behaved as a direct-acting mutagen at higher concentrations (> 1 µl/ plate), much lower concentrations (0.01 µl/plate) had significant genetic activity only when microsomal preparations were present. On a quantitative basis, no significant difference in mutagenic activity was observed among 9 different commercial samples.

The urine of rats treated orally or dermally with tris(2,3-dibromo-propyl) phosphate in doses of 500 and 5000 mg/kg bw also showed mutagenic activity in *Salmonella typhimurium* TA1535 (Brusick *et al.*, 1977).

Tris(2,3-dibromopropyl) phosphate was mutagenic in *Drosophila melanogaster*, inducing sex-linked recessive lethals in male germ-cell stages; the spermatids were the most sensitive (Valencia, 1978).

Results of a forward mutation assay with the thymidine kinase system in mouse lymphoma cells (L5178Y) were inconclusive, although a 2-3-fold increase in mutation frequency was obtained consistently with concentrations of 5 µg/ml (Brusick *et al.*, 1977).

Exposure to concentrations of 2 μl tris(2,3-dibromopropyl) phosphate per ml of growth medium for 4½ hrs induced reparable lesions (single-strand breaks) in the DNA of human cells (KB) in culture, as evidenced by a lowering of the sedimentation rate in alkaline sucrose gradients (Gutter & Rosenkranz, 1977).

2,3-Dibromo-1-propanol, a metabolite and also an impurity present in tris(2,3-dibromopropyl) phosphate, was mutagenic in *Salmonella typhimurium* TA100 and TA1535 but not in TA1538 (Carr & Rosenkranz, 1978).

A significant, dose-dependent increase in sister chromatid exchanges was observed in Chinese hamster V79 cells treated with tris(2,3-dibromo-propyl) phosphate; chromosome aberrations were not significantly increased (Furukawa *et al.*, 1978).

(b) Humans

No skin irritation or sensitization was seen among 52 people who received 10 patch-test applications of the compound (Kerst, 1974). In another study with undiluted tris(2,3-dibromopropyl) phosphate, sensitization reactions occurred in 8/24 subjects; with a concentration of 20% in petroleum jelly, 2/25 subjects were sensitized. Seven of 8 treated fabrics elicited a response in the sensitized subjects (Morrow *et al.*, 1976).

Tris(2,3-dibromopropyl) phosphate is absorbed through the skin in humans (Blum & Ames, 1977). Approximately 180 μg/day (9 μg/kg bw) is absorbed through the skin of children wearing pyjamas treated with tris-(2,3-dibromopropyl) phosphate. Up to 29 ng/ml 2,3-dibromo-1-propanol, a mutagenic metabolite of tris(2,3-dibromopropyl) phosphate, has been found in the urine of children wearing such pyjamas (Blum *et al.*, 1978).

3.3 Case reports and epidemiological studies

No data were available to the Working Group.

4. Summary of Data Reported and Evaluation

4.1 Experimental data

Tris(2,3-dibromopropyl) phosphate was tested in one experiment in mice and in one in rats by oral administration and in one experiment in female mice by skin application. In mice, following oral administration, it produced tumours of the forestomach and lung in animals of both sexes, benign and malignant liver tumours in females and benign and malignant tumours of the kidney in males. In rats, it produced benign and malignant tumours of the kidney in males and benign kidney tumours in females.

After skin application to female mice, it produced tumours of the skin, lung, forestomach and oral cavity.

Tris(2,3-dibromopropyl) phosphate is mutagenic in *Salmonella typhimurium* and *Drosophila melanogaster*.

4.2 Human data

No case reports or epidemiological studies were available to the Working Group.

The extensive production and use of tris(2,3-dibromopropyl) phosphate over the past two decades, primarily as a flame retardant for textiles and plastics, indicate that widespread human exposure occurs. The Working Group knew of no published attempts to determine levels of this compound in the environment; however, estimates of the amounts released from industrial operations and textile leaching suggest that it is widely distributed. Its widespread use in childrens' sleepwear was noted.

4.3 Evaluation

There is *sufficient evidence* that tris(2,3-dibromopropyl) phosphate is carcinogenic in mice and rats. In the absence of adequate data in humans, it is reasonable, for practical purposes, to regard tris(2,3-dibromopropyl) phosphate as if it presented a carcinogenic risk to humans.

5. References

Agranoff, J., ed. (1976) _Modern Plastics Encyclopedia 1976-1977_, Vol. 53
No. 10A, New York, McGraw-Hill, p. 662

Anon. (1978) CPSC lists products containing the suspect carcinogen tris.
Pestic. Tox. Chem. News, 6, 9

Blum, A. & Ames, B.N. (1977) Flame-retardant additives as possible cancer
hazards. _Science_, 195, 17-23

Blum, A., Gold, M.D., Ames, B.N., Kenyon, C., Jones, F.R., Hett, E.A.,
Dougherty, R.C., Horning, E.C., Dzidic, I., Carroll, D.I., Stillwell,
R.N. & Thenol, J.-P. (1978) Children absorb Tris-BP flame retardant
from sleepwear: urine contains the mutagenic metabolite, 2,3-dibromo-
propanol. _Science_, 201, 1020-1023

Brusick, D., Matheson, D. & Bakshi, K. (1977) _Evaluation of tris(2,3-
dibromopropyl)phosphate for mutagenic and transforming activity in a
battery of test systems_. In: _Proceedings of the Second International
Conference on Environmental Mutagens, Edinburgh, 1977_ (Abstracts),
p. 165

Carr, H.S. & Rosenkranz, H.S. (1978) Mutagenicity of derivatives of the
flame retardant tris(2,3-dibromopropyl)phosphate: halogenated
propanols. _Mutat. Res._, 57, 381-384

Cope, J.F. (1973) Identification of flame retardant textile finishes by
pyrolysis-gas chromatography. _Anal. Chem._, 45, 562-564

Daniher, F.A. (1976) The toxicology of tris-(2,3-dibromopropyl)phosphate.
Proceedings of a Symposium on Textile Flammability, Vol. 4, pp. 126-14:

Furukawa, M., Sirianni, S.R., Tan, J.C. & Huang, C.C. (1978) Sister
chromatid exchanges and growth inhibition induced by the flame
retardant tris(2,3-dibromopropyl)phosphate in Chinese hamster cells:
brief communication. _J. natl Cancer Inst._, 60, 1179-1181

Grasselli, J.G. & Ritchey, W.M., eds (1975) _CRC Atlas of Spectral Data and
Physical Constants for Organic Compounds_, 2nd ed., Vol. IV, Cleveland,
OH, Chemical Rubber Co., p. 134

Gutenmann, W.H. & Lisk, D.J. (1975) Flame retardant release from fabrics
during laundering and their toxicity to fish. _Bull. environ. Contam.
Toxicol._, 14, 61-64

Gutter, B. & Rosenkranz, H.S. (1977) The flame retardant tris(2,3-dibromo-
propyl)phosphate: alteration of human cellular DNA. _Mutat. Res._, 56,
89-90

Hawley, G.G., ed. (1977) The Condensed Chemical Dictionary, 9th ed., New
    York, Van Nostrand-Reinhold, p. 893

IARC (1979a) IARC Monographs on the Evaluation of the Carcinogenic Risk of
    Chemicals to Humans, 19, Some Monomers, Plastics and Synthetic
    Elastomers, and Acrolein, Lyon, pp. 303-340

IARC (1979b) IARC Monographs on the Evaluation of the Carcinogenic Risk of
    Chemicals to Humans, 19, Some Monomers, Plastics and Synthetic
    Elastomers, and Acrolein, Lyon, pp. 231-274

Kerst, A.F. (1974) Toxicology of tris(2,3-dibromopropyl)phosphate.
    J. Fire Flammability/Fire Retardant Chem., 1, 205-217

Lande, S.S., Santodonato, J., Howard, P.H., Greninger, D., Christopher,
    D.H. & Saxena, J. (1976) Investigation of Selected Potential Environ-
    mental Contaminants: Haloalkyl Phosphates, EPA-560/2-76-007,
    Washington DC, US Environmental Protection Agency. Available from
    Springfield, VA, National Technical Information Service, No. PB 257
    9100, pp. 4, 9, 20, 63-65, 73, 83-86, 89-91, 175, 182

Morrow, R.W., Hornberger, C.S., Kligman, A.M. & Maibach, H.I. (1976)
    Tris(2,3-dibromopropyl)phosphate: human contact sensitization. Am.
    ind. Hyg. Assoc. J., 37, 192-197

National Cancer Institute (1978) Bioassay of Tris (2,3-Dibromopropyl)
    Phosphate for Possible Carcinogenicity (Technical Report Series No.
    76), Publication No. (NIH) 78-1326, Washington DC, US Government
    Printing Office

National Institute for Occupational Safety & Health (1977) National
    Occupational Hazard Survey, Vol. III, Survey Analyses and Supplemental
    Tables, DHEW (NIOSH) Publication 76-Draft, Cincinnati, OH, p. 11,772

Osterberg, R.E., Bierbower, G.W. & Hehir, R.M. (1977) Renal and testicular
    damage following dermal application of the flame retardant tris(2,3-
    dibromopropyl)phosphate. J. Toxicol. environ. Health, 3, 979-987

Overbeek, D.E. & Nametz, R.C. (1962) Method for the preparation of tris-
    (2,3-dibromopropyl)phosphate. US Patent 3,046,297, 25 July, to
    Michigan Chemical Corporation

Prival, M.J., McCoy, E.C., Gutter, B. & Rosenkranz, H.S. (1977) Tris(2,3-
    dibromopropyl)phosphate: mutagenicity of a widely used flame retard-
    ant. Science, 195, 76-78

Stauffer Chemical Company (1972) Fyrol® HB-32, Product Data Sheet, Westport,
    CT, Specialty Chemical Division

St John, L.E., Jr, Eldefrawi, M.E. & Lisk, D.J. (1976) Studies of possible absorption of a flame retardant from treated fabrics worn by rats and humans. Bull. environ. Contam. Toxicol., 15, 192-197

Ulsamer, A.G., Porter, W.K. & Osterberg, R.E. (1978) Percutaneous absorption of radiolabeled tris from flame-retarded fabric. J. environ. Pathol. Toxicol., 1, 543-549

US Consumer Product Safety Commission (1977a) Children's wearing apparel containing tris; interpretation as banned hazardous substance. Fed. Regist., 42, 18850-18854

US Consumer Product Safety Commission (1977b) Children's wearing apparel containing tris; tris and fabric, yarn or fiber containing tris; withdrawal of interpretations as banned hazardous substances. Fed. Regist., 42, 61593-61594, 61621-61622

US Consumer Product Safety Commission (1978a) Standard for the flammability of children's sleepwear: sizes 7 through 14 (FF5-74). Fed. Regist., 43, 4849-4855

US Consumer Product Safety Commission (1978b) Flammability standards for children's sleepwear. Withdrawal of proposed amendment. Fed. Regist., 43, 31348-31349

US Environmental Protection Agency (1976a) Investigation of Selected Potential Environmental Contaminants. Haloalkyl Phosphates, PB-257 910, Springfield, VA, National Technical Information Service, pp. 32-35, 38, 46, 48, 54, 55

US Environmental Protection Agency (1976b) Summary Characterizations of Selected Chemicals of Near-Term Interest, EPA 560/4-76-004, Washington DC, Office of Toxic Substances, p. 53

US International Trade Commission (1977) Synthetic Organic Chemicals, US Production and Sales, 1976, USITC Publication 833, Washington DC, US Government Printing Office, p. 327

US Tariff Commission (1960) Synthetic Organic Chemicals, US Production and Sales, 1959, Report No. 206, Second Series, Washington DC, US Government Printing Office, p. 162

Valencia, R. (1978) Drosophila mutagenicity tests of saccharin, tris, PtCl₄ and other compounds (Abstract Cb-11). In: IX Annual Meeting of the American Environmental Mutation Society, San Francisco, 1978

Van Duuren, B.L., Loewengart, G., Seidman, I., Smith, A.C. & Melchionne, S. (1978) Mouse skin carcinogenicity tests of the flame retardants tris-(2,3-dibromopropyl)phosphate, tetrakis(hydroxymethyl)phosphonium chloride, and polyvinyl bromide. Cancer Res., 38, 3236-3240

Corrigenda covering Volumes 1-6 appeared in Volume 7, others appeared in Volumes, 8, 10, 11, 12, 13, 15, 16, 17, 18 and 19.

Volume 4

p. 253   1.3(*b*)   *add* 'at 1.4 mm' *after* '112°C'

Volume 18

p. 3   line 15   *replace* '29' *by* '37'

CUMULATIVE INDEX TO IARC MONOGRAPHS ON THE EVALUATION

OF THE CARCINOGENIC RISK OF CHEMICALS TO HUMANS

Numbers underlined indicate volume, and numbers in italics indicate page. References to corrigenda are given in parentheses. Compounds marked with an asterisk (*) were considered by the Working Groups, but monographs were not prepared because no adequate data on their carcinogenicity were available.

Cantharidin   <u>10</u>,*79*

Caprolactam   <u>19</u>,*115*

Carbaryl   <u>12</u>,*37*

Carbon tetrachloride   <u>1</u>,*53*
                                                                   <u>20</u>,*371*

Carmoisine   <u>8</u>,*83*

Catechol   <u>15</u>,*155*

Chlorambucil   <u>9</u>,*125*

Chloramphenicol   <u>10</u>,*85*

Chlordane   <u>20</u>,*45*

Chlordecone   <u>20</u>,*67*

Chlorinated dibenzodioxins   <u>15</u>,*41*

Chlormadinone acetate   <u>6</u>,*149*

Chlorobenzilate   <u>5</u>,*75*

Chloroform   <u>1</u>,*61*
                                                                   <u>20</u>,*401*

Chloromethyl methyl ether   <u>4</u>,*239*

Chloroprene   <u>19</u>,*131*

Chloropropham   <u>12</u>,*55*

Chloroquine   <u>13</u>,*47*

para-Chloro-*ortho*-toluidine and its hydrochloride   <u>16</u>,*277*

5-Chloro-*ortho*-toluidine*

Chlorpromazine*

Cholesterol   <u>10</u>,*99*

Chromium and inorganic chromium compounds   <u>2</u>,*100*
    Barium chromate
    Calcium chromate
    Chromic chromate
    Chromic oxide
    Chromium acetate
    Chromium carbonate
    Chromium dioxide
    Chromium phosphate
    Chromium trioxide
    Lead chromate
    Potassium chromate
    Potassium dichromate
    Sodium chromate
    Sodium dichromate

N-Nitrosofolic acid	17,217
N-Nitrosohydroxyproline	17,303
N-Nitrosomethylethylamine	17,221
N-Nitroso-N-methylurea	1,125
	17,227
N-Nitroso-N-methylurethane	4,211
N-Nitrosomethylvinylamine	17,257
N-Nitrosomorpholine	17,263
N'-Nitrosonornicotine	17,281
N-Nitrosopiperidine	17,287
N-Nitrosoproline	17,303
N-Nitrosopyrrolidine	17,313
N-Nitrososarcosine	17,327
Nitroxoline*	
Nivalenol*	
Norethisterone and its acetate	6,179
Norethynodrel	6,191
Norgestrel	6,201
Nylon 6	19,120
Nylon 6/6*	

O

Ochratoxin A	10,191
Oestradiol-17β	6,99
Oestradiol mustard	9,217
Oestriol	6,117
Oestrone	6,123
Oil Orange SS	8,165
Orange I	8,173
Orange G	8,181
Oxazepam	13,58
Oxymetholone	13,131
Oxyphenbutazone	13,185

Polyvinyl acetate	19,*346*
Polyvinyl alcohol	19,*351*
Polyvinyl chloride	7,*306*
	19,*402*
Polyvinylidene fluoride*	
Polyvinyl pyrrolidone	19,*463*
Ponceau MX	8,*189*
Ponceau 3R	8,*199*
Ponceau SX	8,*207*
Potassium bis(2-hydroxyethyl)dithiocarbamate	12,*183*
Prednisone*	
Progesterone	6,*135*
Pronetalol hydrochloride	13,*227* (corr. 16,*387*)
1,3-Propane sultone	4,*253* (corr. 13,*243*)
	(corr. 20,*591*)
Propham	12,*189*
β-Propiolactone	4,*259* (corr. 15,*341*)
n-Propyl carbamate	12,*201*
Propylene	19,*213*
Propylene oxide	11,*191*
Propylthiouracil	7,*67*
Pyrazinamide*	
Pyrimethamine	13,*233*

Q

para-Quinone	15,*255*
Quintozene (Pentachloronitrobenzene)	5,*211*

R

Reserpine	10,*217*
Resorcinol	15,*155*
Retrorsine	10,*303*
Rhodamine B	16,*221*